ANNALS OF THE NEW YORK ACADEMY OF SCIENCES

Volume 793

EDITORIAL STAFF

Executive Editor
BILL BOLAND

Managing Editor
JUSTINE CULLINAN

Associate Editor
COOK KIMBALL

The New York Academy of Sciences
2 East 63rd Street
New York, New York 10021

MYOCARDIAL PRESERVATION, PRECONDITIONING, AND ADAPTATION

ANNALS OF THE NEW YORK ACADEMY OF SCIENCES
Volume 793

MYOCARDIAL PRESERVATION, PRECONDITIONING, AND ADAPTATION

Edited by Dipak K. Das, Richard Engelman, and K. M. Cherian

The New York Academy of Sciences
New York, New York
1996

Library of Congress Cataloging-in-Publication Data

Myocardial preservation, preconditioning, and adaptation/edited by Dipak K. Das, Richard M. Engelman, and K. M. Cherian.
    p.   cm. —(Annals of the New York Academy of Sciences, ISSN 0077-8923; v. 793).
    Proceedings of a conference held Dec. 14–16, 1995 in Madras, India.
    Includes bibliographical references and indexes.
    ISBN 1-57331-024-7 (cloth: alk. paper). —ISBN 1-57331-025-5 (paper: alk. paper).
    1. Myocardium—Pathophysiology—Congresses. 2. Myocardium—Adaptation—Congresses. 3. Myocardial ischemia—Prevention—Congresses. I. Das, Dipak Kumar, 1946– . II. Engelman, Richard M. III. Cherian, K. M., M.D. IV. Series.
    [DNLM: 1. Myocardial Ischemia—physiopathology—congresses. 2. Myocardial Ischemia—prevention & control—congresses. 3. Myocardium—metabolism—congresses. 4. Heart—drug effects—congresses. 5. Adaptation, Physiological—congresses.   W1 AN626YL v.793 1996/WG 300 M997668 1996]
Q11.N5 vol. 793
[RC685.M9]
616.1'23—dc20
DNLM/DLC
for Library of Congress   96-21067
                                                           CIP

Bi-Comp/PCP
Printed in the United States of America
ISBN 1-57331-024-7 (cloth)
ISBN 1-57331-025-5 (paper)
ISSN 0077-8923

ANNALS OF THE NEW YORK ACADEMY OF SCIENCES

Volume 793
September 30, 1996

MYOCARDIAL PRESERVATION, PRECONDITIONING, AND ADAPTATION[a]

Conference Chair
DIPAK K. DAS

Editors
DIPAK K. DAS, RICHARD M. ENGELMAN, AND K. M. CHERIAN

CONTENTS

[a] This volume contains the papers from a conference entitled *Myocardial Preservation and Cellular Adaptation*, which was held by the local organizers in Madras, India on December 14–16, 1995.

Part II. Myocardial Preconditioning: Role of Intracellular Mediators

Part III. Heat Shock/Oxidative Stress Proteins in Myocardial Adaptation

Part IV. Signal Transduction in Ischemic Preconditioning/Adaptation

Part VII. Application of Preconditioning/Adaptation in Myocardial Protection

Contributed Papers

Financial assistance was received from:

Major Funders
- RIBI IMMUNOCHEM RESEARCH, INC.
- NOBUAKIRA TAKEDA, M.D., Ph.D.

Contributors
- PFIZER INTERNATIONAL INC.
- ELI LILLY & CO.
- MEDTRONIC INC.
- QUEST MEDICAL INC.
- ST. JUDE MEDICAL
- BAXTER HEALTH CARE CORPORATION (CARDIOVASCULAR
  GROUP)

Preface

The last decade has witnessed the development of a novel concept for myocardial preservation that uses the cell's inherent propensity for self-preservation by way of adaptation. The myocardium possesses a remarkable ability to readily adapt to a stressful situation by upregulating its defense systems, which can defend it against subsequent insult. This phenomenon, known as *ischemic preconditioning and myocardial adaptation* so far has been tested for ischemic heart disease. Myocardial protection by ischemic preconditioning has opened a new horizon; this concept is now believed to be one of the most powerful techniques for myocardial protection.

Almost sixty years ago, Weichardt[1] observed that "the administration of certain nonspecific damaging substances leads to the production of metabolites which increase the resistance of the organism against various diseases." Therefore, the concept of preconditioning/adaptation is certainly not a novel one; but only recently has it gained popularity, and studies have begun objectively under controlled laboratory conditions.

Professor Hans Selye[2] once said, "Stress is life and life is stress." He realized about fifty years ago that "adaptation to our surroundings is one of the most important physiologic reactions in life." We now realize how correct he was; we indeed live in a world surrounded by stress. Many diseases such as duodenal and gastric ulcers, diabetes, cancer, stroke and some heart diseases are stress related. Nevertheless, compared to the stressful situations in life, human beings are afflicted with such stress-related diseases far more rarely than they should be. This is because all living organisms (including human beings) possess a highly developed ability to adapt themselves to stressful situations. In Hindu mythology, God once tested the knowledge of a saint by asking him the question, "What is the most surprising thing in the world?" and the answer was "the ability to survive." Indeed, the very survival of an organism depends on its ability to successfully adapt to the continuously changing environment. This is the *ultimate truth* behind the phenomenon of *preconditioning and adaptation*.

Myocardial ischemia and reperfusion remain an unsolved problem despite a great deal of research to understand the mechanism of ischemia reperfusion injury. For centuries, conventional techniques for myocardial protection have focused on noninvasive extracellular interventions or increasingly complex invasive procedures. Recently, there was a surge of interest in testing the novel concept of myocardial preservation that is based on the fact that the enhancement of the endogenous cellular defense system provides each cell with new protein synthesis and thereby the means to protect itself when it is more susceptible. Using the concept, a number of investigators showed that preconditioning of the heart by repeated stunning can delay the onset of further irreversible injury, or even reduce subsequent postischemic ventricular dysfunction and incidence of arrhythmias. Such myocardial preservation by repeated short-term reversible ischemia led to the development of the concept of stress adaptation. Consequently, a number of investigators developed new ideas of preconditioning, which include adenosine, potassium channel opening, hypoxia, α-adrenergic receptor, and oxidative stress.

There is no doubt that ischemic preconditioning is a real phenomenon, but the mechanisms remain highly speculative. Of many hypotheses, the most popular has been the adenosine A_1 receptor. The other hypotheses include α_1-receptor, potassium channel, and protein kinase C. While the mechanisms of preconditioning remain speculative, it is universally believed that preconditioning is a short-term phenomena which lasts for several hours. The "adaptation to ischemia" also known as the "second window of protection" is, on the other hand, a long-term process that may occur after several hours and may last for several days. It is also believed that preconditioning is triggered by an as yet unknown endogenous factor or factors that propagate a cascade of intracellular reactions through signal transduction, while myocardial adaptation is mediated by the transcription of genes and their successful translation into protective proteins. Evidence suggests that these stress proteins involve heat shock and antioxidants.

Evidence also suggests that preconditioning triggers adaptive responses leading to ischemic adaptation mediated by the reprogramming of gene expression. The goal is to apply the preconditioning/adaptation technique to render hearts permanently resistant to subsequent ischemia; and, for this, the cellular and molecular link between preconditioning and adaptation must be identified. Protein kinase C is a likely candidate to meet such criteria, because it is activated by intracellular signaling and can induce gene expression. More recent studies implicated a downstream regulator of protein kinase C, MAPKAP kinase 2, as a potential link between ischemic preconditioning and myocardial adaptation to ischemia.

The successful application of the preconditioning/adaptation technique in clinical arenas depends on the clear understanding of the mechanism of action. Clinicians and basic scientists joined together at a recent international symposium on "Myocardial Preservation and Cellular Adaptation" held in Madras, India. The present volume of the *Annals of the New York Academy of Sciences* is the outcome of this important symposium, the aim of which is to familiarize readers with the status and potential application of the current techniques of preconditioning/adaptation in myocardial protection. A comprehensive list of topics has been carefully selected, which encompasses the pathophysiology as well as the cellular and molecular aspects of preconditioning/adaptation.

Dipak K. Das

REFERENCES

1. WEICHARDT, W. 1936. Die Grundlagen der unspezifischen therapie. Ergeb. Hyg. Bakt. Immunitätsforsch. Exp. Ther. **16:** 1–5.
2. SELYE, H. 1946. The general adaptation syndrome and the diseases of adaptation. J. Clin. Endocrinol. **6:** 117–230.

Alteration in Cardiac Sarcolemmal ATP Receptors by Oxyradicals[a]

SORIN MUSAT AND NARANJAN S. DHALLA[b]

Division of Cardiovascular Sciences
St. Boniface General Hospital Research Centre
and
Department of Physiology
Faculty of Medicine
University of Manitoba
Winnipeg, Manitoba R2H 2A6, Canada

INTRODUCTION

It is now widely accepted that adenosine triphosphate (ATP) is released from both adrenergic and cholinergic nerve terminals,[1] from platelets during degranulation,[2] from vascular endothelium in response to hypoxia or alpha$_1$-adrenergic stimulation,[3] and from cardiomyocytes in response to ischemia.[4–8] Extracellular ATP is known to affect heart function by directly modulating ionic currents, Ca^{2+} homeostasis and excitation-contraction coupling in the atrial and ventricular cardiomyocytes from several species.[2,4,5,9,10] These mechanisms have been proposed to mediate the positive inotropic and arrhythmogenic effects of extracellular ATP in the heart.[2,5,10,11] Specific receptors of extracellular ATP (P2-purinoceptors) and ecto-nucleotidases, which control its concentration, have been demonstrated basically on every major tissue and/or cell type[12,13] including mammalian cardiac myocytes.[2,5] While electrophysiological and/or calcium imaging studies in the heart have suggested the presence of P2Y[14], P2X[13,14] and P2U[15] purinoceptors, photoaffinity labeling of rat heart sarcolemma with 8Az-[α^{32}P]-ATP has identified two separate proteins of close molecular weights, probably representing two functionally different cardiac ATP-receptors.[16] In addition, binding studies from our laboratory[17] and others[18] have identified both high affinity and low affinity binding sites in various tissues including heart. Unfortunately, the presence of different types of ATP-binding proteins and the lack of specific agonists and antagonists for P2-purinoceptors are still hampering protein purification, characterization and even a satisfactory classification of ATP-receptors.[12]

Regardless of the receptor subtypes involved, the potent actions of ATP in the cardiovascular system are suggestive of an important role for extracellular ATP and P2-purinoceptors in cardiac pathophysiology.[5,11] However, to date the functional regulation of the cardiac P2-purinoceptors in normal and/or diseased myocardium is virtually an unexplored territory. In this respect, it is pointed out

[a] The research reported in this article was supported by a grant from the Medical Research Council of Canada (MRC Group in Experimental Cardiology).

[b] To whom correspondence should be addressed: Division of Cardiovascular Sciences, St. Boniface General Hospital Research Centre, 351 Tache Avenue, Winnipeg, Manitoba R2H 2A6 Canada. Tel.: (204)-235-3417; Fax: (204)-233-6723; E-mail: cvso@sbrc.umanitoba.ca.

1

that reactive oxygen metabolites and/or impairment of the antioxidant defence mechanisms are considered to play a major role in numerous pathologies[19] including myocardial ischemia and reperfusion.[20-22] Furthermore, the oxidative stress is known to interfere directly or indirectly with the functions of a wide variety of receptors, ionic channels, contractile proteins and enzymes[23-26] including cardiac ecto-ATPase.[27] Therefore, we have undertaken this study to investigate whether the high affinity specific ATP-binding with cardiac sarcolemma is modified by *in vitro* oxidative stress. In addition, we have examined the effects of some putative antagonists of P2-purinoceptors on the high affinity ATP-binding to test if these sites represent the ATP-receptors in cardiac sarcolemma.

MATERIALS AND METHODS

Chemicals

ATP-Tris salt, sodium hypochlorite, Cibacron blue 3GA, theophylline, verapamil, ouabain, *dl*-propanolol (racemic mixture), glibenclamide, 4,4'-diisothiocyanatostilbene(DIDS), 2-2,5'-*p*-fluorosulfonylbenzoyladenosine (FSBA), probenecid and atenolol were purchased from Sigma Chemical Co. (St. Louis, MO). Suramin was from Calbiochem-Novabiochem Corp. (San Diego, CA); Prazosin from Chas-Pfizer & Co., Inc. (New York, NY); 4-aminopyridine from Aldrich Chemical Co., Inc. (Milwaukee, WI); N,N-dimethylformamide from Fisher Scientific Ltd. (Fair Lawn, NJ); hydrogen peroxide (Perhydrol suprapur®, 30% H_2O_2) from E. Merck AG (Darmstadt, Germany); CytoScint ES™ from ICN Biochemicals, Inc. (Costa Mesa, CA) and [^{35}S]-adenosine 5'-(γ-thio)triphosphate, triethylammonium salt ([^{35}S]ATPγS) (specific activity = 65 Ci/mmol, radiochemical purity 97%) from DuPont Canada Inc. (Mississauga, ON, Canada). All other chemicals were of analytical grade.

Isolation of Sarcolemmal Membranes

Male Sprague-Dawley rats weighing 200–250 g were sacrificed by decapitation and hearts were rapidly excised and trimmed of atria and large vessels, and the ventricular tissue was processed for the isolation of "heavy" sarcolemmal membranes by the hypotonic shock-LiBr treatment method.[28] The sarcolemmal membranes were suspended in 250 mM sucrose, 50 mM Tris-HCl, pH 7.4, at a concentration of 3–5 mg/ml, frozen in liquid nitrogen, stored at −80°C, and used within 2–3 weeks.

ATP-Binding Assay

The sarcolemmal membrane (30–50 μg protein) was prewarmed at 37°C for 5 min, subjected to various treatments and then incubated in a final volume of 0.5 ml medium containing 10 nM [^{35}S]ATPγS and 50 M Tris-HCl, pH 7.5 at 37°C for 30 min as described previously.[17] The reaction was terminated by vacuum filtration through wet Whatman filters (GF/B) by using a cell harvester (M-24R, Brandel, Gaithersburg, MD). The filters were washed three times with 6 ml of ice-cold water and the radioactivity was counted with a Beckman scintillation counter using 10 ml CytoScint cocktail. The binding was determined in the absence (total) and presence (nonspecific) of 4 mM ATP; the specific binding was calculated by subtracting the nonspecific binding from the total binding. For avoiding possible artifacts, the binding of the radioligand to the GF/B filters (*i.e.*, in the absence of membrane protein) was also checked for all the compounds used in this study. Various inhibitors of cardiac receptors, cation channels and cation pumps tested in this study were incubated with heart membranes for 10 min before the addition of the radioligand, and unless otherwise stated, were dissolved in the buffer.

H_2O_2-Induced Oxidative Stress

Sarcolemmal membranes were incubated for different periods with various concentrations (0.05–10 mM) of H_2O_2 in the presence or absence of 10 μg/ml catalase before the addition of radioligand. Catalase activity and hydrogen peroxide concentration were determined spectrophotometrically before each experiment by a method[29] that tracks the decomposition of H_2O_2 at 240 nm using an extinction coefficient of 43.6 $M^{-1} \cdot cm^{-1}$. Since catalase increased both the specific and the nonspecific ATP-binding, albeit modestly, the control values in this set of experiments were taken as those obtained when catalase was present in the assay tubes; all other values were expressed as a percentage of these controls.

HOCl-Induced Oxidative Stress

Cardiac membranes were incubated with various concentrations (0.1–1 mM) of HOCl for 10 min before addition of the radioligand in the presence or absence of 0.3 or 1 mM *l*-methionine. It should be pointed out that *l*-methionine is a relatively specific protectant against the oxidative insult produced by HOCl.[23] HOCl was prepared by vacuum distillation of sodium hypochlorite at pH 6.2 (adjusted with H_2SO_4) as reported previously.[23] The concentration of HOCl was measured spectrophotometrically before each experiment using a molar absorptivity coefficient of 100 at 235 nm.

Statistical Methods

Each value (mean ± SE) represents the specific binding of at least 6 separate membrane preparations (performed in triplicate for total binding and in duplicate for nonspecific binding). The results were analyzed statistically by using the Student *t* test. A value of $p < 0.05$ was considered statistically significant.

RESULTS

Effects of P2 Antagonists on Specific ATP-Binding

The measurement of ATP-binding in the presence of various compounds such as Cibacron blue, suramin and DIDS, which are known to antagonize the effects of ATP, showed that all the putative P2 antagonists inhibited the high affinity site binding of ATPγS in a concentration-dependent manner (FIG. 1). The strongest antagonism was observed in the presence of Cibacron blue, whereas the least effective in inhibiting ATP-binding was DIDS. FSBA, a nonspecific inhibitor of different enzymes including ecto-ATPase,[12] failed to modify ATP-binding even at millimolar concentrations (FIG. 1). Inhibitors of different cardiac receptors, cation channels, cation pumps and other compounds, including theophylline (a putative P1 antagonist), showed no effect on ATP-binding with sarcolemmal membranes (TABLE 1).

Effects of H₂O₂ on Specific ATP-Binding

FIGURE 2 shows that incubation of sarcolemmal membranes with 0.05 mM H_2O_2 produced a gradual increase in specific ATP-binding (30% over control value at 45 min), while higher concentrations elicited a time- and concentration-dependent biphasic change. At 0.5 mM H_2O_2, the stimulation in specific ATP-binding became bell-shaped whereas at higher concentrations, H_2O_2 (2.5 mM)

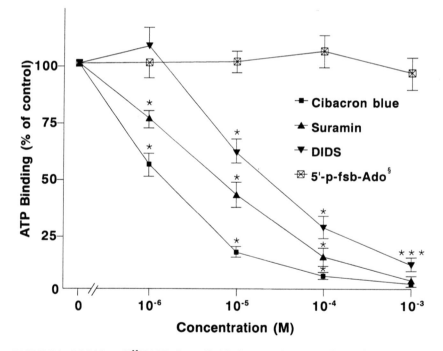

FIGURE 1. Inhibition of [³⁵S]ATPγS specific binding to rat heart sarcolemma in the presence of different concentrations of various P2-purinoceptor antagonists. Nonspecific binding in absence and presence of membrane protein was 0.22 ± 0.09 and 0.28 ± 0.11 pmol/mg protein, respectively. § - Specific binding in this case was expressed relative to controls in which *N,N*-dimethylformamide was added at a final concentration of 2.5% because this agent was used for the solubilization of FSBA. Each value is a mean ± SE of 6–8 experiments. *$p < 0.05$ when compared to control values.

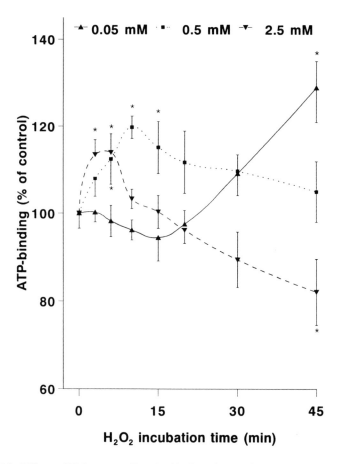

FIGURE 2. Effects of H_2O_2 on specific ATP-binding with cardiac sarcolemma as a function of time and concentration. All the values were normalized and expressed as a percentage of the control values for the corresponding time of incubation. Each value is a mean ± SE of 6–8 experiments. *p <0.05 when compared to control values.

produced not only a narrower peak, but when incubated for longer periods caused an inhibition in binding (20% after 45 min incubation). It should be pointed out that the specific ATP-binding with cardiac sarcolemma (control) decreased slightly, but significantly, as a function of the incubation time (data not shown); all values were normalized and expressed as a percentage of the control for a corresponding time of incubation.

In order to examine the concentration-response relationship of H_2O_2 on specific ATP-binding, cardiac sarcolemma was incubated for 10 min with various concentrations of H_2O_2 (0.05 to 10 mM). Lower concentrations of H_2O_2 stimulated while higher concentrations inhibited ATP-binding (FIG. 3). At concentrations of H_2O_2 lower than 1 mM, catalase pretreatment decreased the stimulatory response whereas the inhibition produced by higher concentrations of H_2O_2 was inhibited

TABLE 1. Effect of Various Inhibitors of Hormone Receptors, Cation Channels and Cation Pumps on [^{35}S]ATPγS Binding with Cardiac Sarcolemma[a]

	ATP-Binding (% of Control) at Different Inhibitor Concentrations			
	1 μM	10 μM	100 μM	1 mM
Verapamil	97.0 ± 5.4	109 ± 7.2	111 ± 11.3	118 ± 9.5
Propanolol	92.4 ± 2.8	99.2 ± 4.1	88.4 ± 4.3	101 ± 4.5
Atenolol	96.7 ± 3.9	105 ± 5.8	108 ± 9.1	101 ± 10.4
Prazosin[b]	92.6 ± 3.8	98.6 ± 6.3	90.2 ± 3.6	112 ± 9.6
Ouabain	97.0 ± 3.2	102 ± 2.4	93.7 ± 7.5	110 ± 10.8
Glibenclamide[c]	108 ± 4.9	92.2 ± 6.6	92.7 ± 7.3	—
4-Aminopyridine	102 ± 6.1	100 ± 4.0	104 ± 3.6	98.0 ± 2.5
Theophylline	89.5 ± 4.9	94.3 ± 4.0	99.0 ± 2.8	106 ± 3.2
Probenecid	100 ± 3.5	105 ± 2.6	107 ± 5.7	100 ± 3.8

[a] Values are mean ± SE of 6–8 experiments. The specific binding was calculated as a percentage relative to the control values.

[b] Prazosin was dissolved in ethanol; the final concentration in the samples was less than 0.25%; the values were compared with controls containing the same concentration of ethanol (unchanged from control).

[c] 5 mg of glybenclamide was dissolved in 0.2 ml 0.1 NaOH, sonnicated (40W) for 5 min and 4.8 ml distilled water was added while continuing sonnication. The final concentration of NaOH in these samples was negligible; higher concentration than 100 μM could not be tested due to poor solubility.

by catalase. As shown in FIGURE 3, catalase prevented the 85% inhibition produced by 10 mM H_2O_2 completely while at 5 mM H_2O_2 the 60% inhibition was reversed to an increase of 20% The highest stimulation of ATP-binding (30% of control values) was observed when cardiac sarcolemmal membranes were incubated in the presence of both catalase and 2.5 mM H_2O_2. Catalase also completely prevented the increase produced by H_2O_2 in nonspecific ATP-binding (data not shown).

Effects of HOCl on Specific ATP-Binding

As shown in FIGURE 4, HOCl inhibited the specific binding of ATPγS with cardiac sarcolemma in a concentration-dependent manner; inhibitions to the extent of 20, 40 and 60% of the control values were observed at 0.3, 0.5 and 1 mM HOCl, respectively. When l-methionine (a relatively specific "scavenger" of HOCl[23,30]) was present in the assay buffer, the inhibition in ATP-binding was significantly prevented; 0.3 mM l-methionine shifted the HOCl dose-response curve to the right while 1 mM l-methionine fully protected the cardiac sarcolemma against the decrease in specific ATP-binding produced by HOCl.

Other Interventions

The consequences of other reactive oxygen intermediates like the hydroxyl radical and superoxide radical (by employing a mixture of H_2O_2 plus Fe^{2+} and using the xanthine/xanthine oxidase generating system, respectively) on the specific ATP-binding could not be determined because of the interference due to Fe^{2+}

and xanthine oxidase. Fe^{2+} at concentrations higher than 10 μM produced the precipitation of more than 70% of the radioligand whereas xanthine oxidase, even when incubated without substrate, inhibited more than 60% of the specific ATP-binding. Likewise, we encountered another technical difficulty when addressing the possible involvement of thiol groups in the observed oxidant-induced alterations in specific ATP-binding because DTT, a well-known protectant against sulfhydryl group modification, inhibited ATP-binding almost completely.

DISCUSSION

It has become generally accepted that ATP provides intercellular routes of metabolic communication in an autocrine fashion in addition to its well-known role in cellular energy and intermediary metabolism, diverse phosphorylation reactions and cotransmitter function.[1] As is the case for other putative signaling agents, appreciable levels of extracellular ATP seem to occur only transiently in response to specific physiological and/or pathological stimuli.[4,31] Several compounds, which are known to interact with ATP-binding enzymes/proteins, have

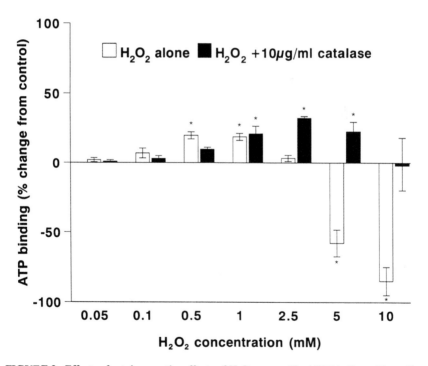

FIGURE 3. Effects of catalase on the effects of H_2O_2 on specific ATP-binding with cardiac sarcolemma. Sarcolemmal membranes were incubated for 10 min with various concentrations of H_2O_2 in the presence or absence of 10 $\mu g/ml$ catalase. The values are expressed as the percent change from the control. Each value is a mean $\pm$ SE of 6–8 experiments. *$p < 0.05$ when compared to control values.

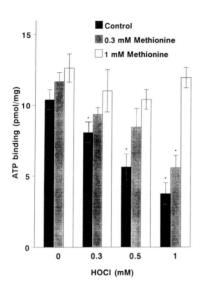

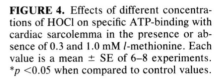

FIGURE 4. Effects of different concentrations of HOCl on specific ATP-binding with cardiac sarcolemma in the presence or absence of 0.3 and 1.0 mM *l*-methionine. Each value is a mean ± SE of 6–8 experiments. *$p < 0.05$ when compared to control values.

been used as functional antagonists and/or inhibitors of putative ATP-receptors (P2 purinoceptors).[2,12,13] However, all the compounds reported to exhibit antagonism/inhibition to P2-purinoceptors show nonselectivity, nonhomogeneity of the chemical composition, irreversibility of the antagonism, and significant inhibition of ecto-nucleotidase.[32] Among these, the most widely used are Cibacron blue 3GA, an anthraquinone-sulfonic acid derivative, suramin, a trypanocidal drug and DIDS, an impermeant anion-exchange blocker and a potent inhibitor of various hydrolytic and oxidative enzymes as well as of Na^+/K^+ ATPase.[13] In the present study we have shown that all these putative P2 antagonists inhibited [^{35}S]ATPγS binding in cardiac sarcolemma markedly. This effect on ATP-binding may be of some specific nature because the ATP-binding with cardiac sarcolemma was unaffected by several other agents that are well known to inhibit adrenergic receptors, cation channels, cation pumps and other enzymes present in the sarcolemmal membrane. These results along with previous observations regarding the potency of various nucleotides and nucleosides in inhibiting [^{35}S]ATPγS binding with the cardiac sarcolemma[17] suggest that the high affinity ATP-binding sites may represent the P2-purinoceptors in the heart cell membrane.

Incubation of cardiac sarcolemmal membranes with H_2O_2 resulted in a complex response, depending on the concentration employed and the time of incubation. The H_2O_2-induced effects (both the increase and the decrease) on the specific high affinity ATP-binding were significantly altered by catalase. The concentrations of H_2O_2 employed in this study are pathophysiologically relevant,[33,34] since millimolar concentrations of H_2O_2 are considered to be generated in the immediate vicinity of the target cells by stimulated neutrophils.[35] It should be pointed out that H_2O_2 is one of the most likely oxidants to penetrate cells and reach various cellular targets, including cell membranes and is considered responsible for post-ischemic myocardial derangements.[34] *In vitro* studies have suggested that cardiomyocyte necrosis during H_2O_2-induced oxidative stress progresses in an autocatalytic "chain reaction" manner,[34] since cardiomyocyte disruption required only a brief H_2O_2 "pulse." Although it has not been possible to identify a unifying mechanism that defines the initiation and progression of cell injury in response to H_2O_2, Ca^{2+}-overload has been postulated to be the mechanism of oxidant-induced cell damage.[36] Furthermore, a recent report has suggested that protein kinase C (PKC) may be a critical mediator of the H_2O_2-induced alterations in Ca^{2+} homeostasis.[37] It is noteworthy that an ATP-induced increase in Ca^{2+}-independent PKC isoform activity in cardiomyocytes has been confirmed.[5] Since both H_2O_2[21,36,38] and extracellular ATP[11] are known to promote the development of afterdepolarizations and triggered activity in the heart and are ascertained to be released in appreciable amounts in ischemia-reperfusion,[8,19,34,39] the present finding that H_2O_2 modulates the specific ATP-binding with the cardiac sarcolemma may be of some pathophysiological significance.

Another potent oxidant involved in various pathologies including myocardial ischemia is HOCl, which is produced by activated neutrophils and other phagocytic cells.[40] This agent has been shown to exert deleterious effects on a wide variety of biomolecules mainly through the oxidation of cysteine and methionine residues.[41,42] Recent studies have demonstrated that HOCl increases the myofibrillar Mg^{2+}-ATPase but decreases the Ca^{2+}-stimulated ATPase activities[23] in addition to depressing the sarcolemmal Na^+/Ca^{2+} exchange and Na^+/K^+-ATPase activities in the heart.[41] The notable inhibition produced by HOCl on the specific ATP-binding with cardiac sarcolemma in the present study was concentration-dependent and antagonized by a well-known antioxidant, methionine. Since DTT was found to inhibit the specific ATP-binding with cardiac sarcolemma significantly, it was not possible to clarify if the HOCl-induced alteration in ATP-receptors was mediated through the oxidation of critical SH groups. While our efforts to examine the effects of superoxide and hydroxyl radicals on ATP-receptors were not successful due to interference of the oxyradical generating system with the assay, the observed inhibition of ATP-binding due to DTT raises the possibility that the putative cardiomyocyte P2-purinoceptors may be modulated by the status of their sulfhydryl groups. This view is consistent with observations reported for the muscarinic, adrenergic, histaminergic, growth hormone and other receptors.[24] In addition, different cations such as Mg^{2+}, Ca^{2+}, Mn^{2+}, Cu^{2+} and Zn^{2+} have also been reported to modify the high affinity ATP-binding sites in cardiac sarcolemma.[43] Thus it appears that purinergic receptors in the cardiac sarcolemmal membrane are regulated by physiological, pharmacological and pathophysiological interventions.

SUMMARY

We previously demonstrated that cardiac sarcolemmal membranes bind [^{35}S]ATPγS at both low and high affinity binding sites. In this study we examined the effects of some P2-purinoceptor antagonists as well as of two oxidants (H_2O_2 and HOCl) on the high affinity ATP-binding sites under in vitro conditions. It was found that putative P2-purinoceptor antagonists such as Cibacron blue, suramin, and 4,4'-diisothiocyanatostilbene 2-2 acid markedly inhibited specific ATP-binding with sarcolemmal membrane. H_2O_2 produced a biphasic effect (first increase and then decrease) on the specific ATP-binding with cardiac sarcolemma in a time- and concentration-dependent manner; these effects were prevented by catalase. On the other hand, HOCl markedly inhibited ATP-binding; this inhibition was prevented by l-methionine. These results suggest that the high affinity ATP-binding sites in cardiac sarcolemma may represent the P2-purinoceptors, which are susceptible to modification by oxidative stress under pathophysiological conditions including myocardial ischemia-reperfusion injury.

REFERENCES

1. BURNSTOCK, G. 1972. Purinergic nerves. Pharmacol. Rev. **24:** 509–581.
2. DUBYAK, G. R. & C. EL-MOATASSIM. 1993. Signal transduction via P2-purinergic receptors for extracellular ATP and other nucleotides. Am. J. Physiol. **265:** C577–C606.
3. SHINOZUKA, K., M. HASHIMOTO, S. MASUMURA, R. A. BJUR, D. P. WESTFALL & K. HATTORI. 1994. *In vitro* studies of release of adenine nucleotides and adenosine from rat vascular endothelium in response to α_1-adrenoceptor stimulation. Br. J. Pharmacol. **113:** 1203–1208.
4. GORDON, J. L. 1986. Extracellular ATP: effects, sources and fate. Biochem. J. **233:** 807–815.
5. VASSORT, G., M. PUCÉAT & F. SCAMPS. 1994. Modulation of myocardial activity by extracellular ATP. Trends Cardiovasc. Med. **4:** 236–240.
6. VIAL, C., P. OWEN, L. H. OPIE & D. POSEL. 1987. Significance of release of adenosine triphosphate and adenosine induced by hypoxia or adrenaline in perfused rat heart. J. Mol. Cell. Cardiol. **19:** 187–197.
7. FORRESTER, T. & C. A. WILLIAMS. 1977. Release of adenosine triphosphate from isolated adult heart cells in response to hypoxia. J. Physiol. (London) **268:** 371–390.
8. POPESCU, L. M., S. MUSAT, O. C. TRIFAN, M. LEABU, C. M. TIGARET, M. POPESCU, A. POPESCU, M. E. HINESCU, I. I. MORARU & D. K. DAS. 1994. K^+-channel openers protect the myocardium against the ischemia-reperfusion injury. Ann. N. Y. Acad. Sci. **723:** 398–400.
9. FRIEL, D. D. & B. P. BEAN. 1988. Two ATP-activated conductances in bullfrog atrial cells. J. Gen. Physiol. **91:** 1–27.
10. PARKER, K. E. & A. SCARPA. 1995. An ATP-activated nonselective cation channel in guinea pig ventricular myocytes. Am. J. Physiol. **269:** H789–H797.
11. SONG, Y. & L. BELARDINELLI. 1994. ATP promotes development of afterdepolarizations and triggered activity in cardiac myocytes. Am. J. Physiol. **267:** H2005–H2011.
12. FREDHOLM, B. B., M. P. ABBRACCHIO, G. BURNSTOCK, J. W. DALY, T. K. HARDEN, K. A. JACOBSON, P. P. LEFF & M. WILLIAMS. 1994. Nomenclature and classification of purinoceptors. Pharmacol. Rev. **46:** 143–156.
13. DALZIEL, H. H. & D. P. WESTFALL. 1994. Receptors for adenine nucleotides and nucleosides: subclassification, distribution, and molecular characterization. Pharmacol. Rev. **46:** 449–466.
14. BJORNSSON, O. G., J. R. MONCK & J. R. WILLIAMSON. 1989. Identification of P2Y purinoceptors associated with voltage-activated cation channels in cardiac ventricular myocytes of the rat. Eur. J. Biochem. **186:** 395–404.
15. FROLDI, G., L. PANDOLFO, A. CHINELLATO, E. RAGAZZI, I. CAPARROTTA & G. FASSINA. 1994. Dual effect of ATP and UTP on rat atria: which types of receptors are involved? Naunyn Schmiedebergs Arch. Pharmacol. **349:** 381–386.
16. GIANNATTASIO, B., K. POWERS & A. SCARPA. 1992. Photoaffinity labeling and expression cloning of extracellular ATP receptors of cardiac myocytes. Ann. N. Y. Acad. Sci. **671:** 471–477.
17. ZHAO, D. & N. S. DHALLA. 1990. [^{35}S]ATPγS binding sites in the purified heart sarcolemma membrane. Am. J. Physiol. **258:** C185–C188.
18. MICHEL, A. D. & P. P. HUMPHREY. 1993. Distribution and characterization of [3H]alpha, beta-methylene ATP binding sites in the rat. Naunyn Schmiedebergs Arch. Pharmacol. **348:** 608–617.
19. COCHRANE, C. G. 1991. Cellular injury by oxidants. Am. J. Med. **91**(Suppl. 3C): 3C–23S.
20. KLONER, R. A., K. PRZYKLENK & P. WHITTAKER. 1989. Deleterious effects of oxygen radicals in ischemia/reperfusion. Circulation **80:** 1115–1127.
21. CURTIS, M. J., M. K. PUGSLEY & M. J. A. WALKER. 1993. Endogenous chemical

mediators of ventricular arrhythmias in ischemic heart disease. Cardiovasc. Res. **27:** 703–719.

22. ZWEIER, J. L., J. T. FALHERTY & M. L. WEISFELDT. 1987. Direct measurement of free radical generation following reperfusion of ischemic myocardium. Proc. Natl. Acad. Sci. USA **84:** 1404–1407.

23. SUZUKI, S., M. KANEKO, D. C. CHAPMAN & N. S. DHALLA. 1991. Alterations in cardiac contractile proteins due to oxygen free radicals. Biochim. Biophys. Acta **1074:** 95–100.

24. VAN DER VIELT, A. & A. BAST. 1992. Effect of oxidative stress on receptors and signal transmission. Chem. Biol. Interact. **85:** 95–116.

25. KANEKO, M., D. C. CHAPMAN, P. K. GANGULY, R. E. BEAMISH & N. S. DHALLA. 1991. Modification of cardiac adrenergic receptors by oxygen free radicals. Am. J. Physiol. **260:** H821–H826.

26. KANEKO, M., V. ELIMBAN & N. S. DHALLA. 1989. Mechanism for depression of heart sarcolemmal Ca^{2+}-pump activity by oxygen free radicals. Am. J. Physiol. **257:** H804–H811.

27. KANEKO, M., P. K. SINGAL & N. S. DHALLA. 1990. Alterations in heart sarcolemmal Ca^{2+}-ATPase and Ca^{2+} binding activities due to oxygen free radicals. Basic Res. Cardiol. **85:** 45–54.

28. DHALLA, N. S., M. B. ANAND & J. A. C. HARROW. 1976. Calcium binding and ATPase activities of heart sarcolemma. J. Biochem. **79:** 1345–1350.

29. CLAIRBORNE, A. 1985. Catalase activity. *In* Handbook of Methods for Oxygen Radical Research. R. A. Greenwald, Ed. 283–284. CRC. Boca Raton, FL.

30. KUKREJA, R. C., A. B. WEAVER & M. L. HESS. 1989. Stimulated human neutrophils damage cardiac sarcoplasmic reticulum function by generation of oxidants. Biochim. Biophys. Acta **990:** 198–205.

31. DUBYAK, G. R. & J. S. FEDAN. 1990. The biologic actions of extracellular adenosine triphosphate. Compr. Ther. **16:** 57–61.

32. CRACK, B. E., M. W. BEUKERS, K. C. MCKECHNIE, A. P. IJZERMAN & P. LEFF. 1994. Pharmacological analysis of ecto-ATPase inhibition: evidence for combined enzyme inhibition and receptor antagonism in P2x-purinoceptor ligands. Br. J. Pharmacol. **113:** 1432–1438.

33. JANERO, D. R., D. HRENIUK & H. H. SHARIF. 1991. Hydrogen peroxide-induced oxidative stress to the mammalian heart-muscle cell (cardiomyocyte): lethal peroxidative membrane injury. J. Cell. Physiol. **149:** 347–364.

34. HALLIVELL, B. 1991. Reactive oxygen species in living systems: sources, biochemistry, and role in human disease. Am. J. Med. **91**(Suppl. 3C): 3C–14S.

35. KRAEMER, R., B. SELIGMAN & K. M. MULLANE. 1990. Polymorphonuclear leukocytes reduce cardiac function *in vitro* by release of H_2O_2. Am. J. Physiol. **259:** H1330–H1336.

36. BERESEWICZ, A. & M. HORACKOVA. 1991. Alterations in electrical and contractile behaviour of isolated cardiomyocytes by hydrogen peroxide: possible ionic mechanisms. J. Mol. Cell. Cardiol. **23:** 899–918.

37. WARD, C. A. & M. P. MOFFAT. 1995. Role of protein kinase C in mediating effects of hydrogen peroxide in guinea-pig ventricular myocytes. J. Mol. Cell. Cardiol. **27:** 1089–1097.

38. DUAN, J. & M. P. MOFFAT. 1992. Potential cellular mechanisms of hydrogen peroxide-induced cardiac arrhythmias. J. Cardiovasc. Pharmacol. **19:** 593–601.

39. ZULUETA, J. J., F. YU, I. A. HERTIG, V. J. THANNICKAL & P. M. HASSOUN. 1995. Release of hydrogen peroxide on response to hypoxia-reoxygenation: role of an NAD(P)H oxidase-like enzyme in endothelial cell plasma membrane. Am. J. Respir. Cell Mol. Biol. **12:** 41–49.

40. LUCHESI, B. R., J. K. MICKELSON, J. W. HOMEISTER & C. V. JACKSON. 1987. Interaction of the formed elements of blood with the coronary vasculature *in vivo*. Fed. Proc. **46:** 63–72.

41. KAMINISHI, T., T. MATSUOKA, T. YANAGISHITA & J. KAKO. 1989. Increase vs. decrease of calcium uptake by isolated heart cells induced by H_2O_2 vs. HOCl. Am. J. Physiol. **256:** C598–C607.

42. ALBRICH, J. M., C. A. McCARTHY & J. K. HURST. 1981. Biological reactivity of hypochlorous acid. Implications for microbicidal mechanisms of leukocyte myeloperoxidase. Proc. Natl. Acad. Sci. USA **78:** 210–214.
43. MUSAT, S. & N. S. DHALLA. 1995. Modification of ATP-binding with cardiac sarcolemma by some cations. Exp. Clin. Cardiol. In press.

The Slowing of Ischemic Energy Demand in Preconditioned Myocardium[a]

KEITH A. REIMER[b]

Department of Pathology
Duke University Medical Center
Durham, North Carolina 27710

Facets of Ischemic Metabolism

A defining feature of myocardial ischemia is that high energy phosphate (HEP) requirements exceed the rate of ATP production, leading to progressive depletion of HEP. Myocardial HEP reserves of creatine phosphate (CP) and ATP are small; creatine phosphate is depleted almost completely within the first few seconds of ischemia and ATP content is rapidly depleted minutes thereafter. In severe regional ischemia in anesthetized dogs, ATP decreases to about 35% of control by 15 minutes and to less than 10% by 40 minutes.[1,2] The depletion of ATP is paralleled by degradation of the total adenine nucleotide pool.[2]

A second defining feature of ischemia is that the products of a variety of catabolic pathways progressively accumulate in the tissue. When aerobic respiration is inhibited, the principal source of ATP production is anaerobic glycolysis. Consequently, products of anaerobic glycolysis, in particular lactate, rapidly accumulate. Purine bases and inorganic phosphate also accumulate as a result of the breakdown of adenine nucleotides. Tissue acidosis develops due to several catabolic processes including glycolysis, lipolysis, and ATP hydrolysis.[3] Ammonia, produced by the deamination of adenosine, amino acids, etc., is detoxified by conversion of pyruvate to alanine. Both ammonia and alanine accumulate in totally ischemic myocardium.[4] The combined effect of this catabolite accumulation creates a substantial osmotic load within the ischemic myocyte.[5]

As these metabolic changes develop, they are associated with cellular injury, which initially is *reversible*, in that no necrosis develops if reperfusion is established, but which becomes *irreversible* with increasing duration, in that myocytes undergo necrosis despite reperfusion. The pathogenesis of the transition from reversible to irreversible (lethal) myocyte injury remains incompletely defined. However, in very general terms, the principal cause of irreversible myocyte injury must be either the depletion of ATP to critically low levels for a critical duration, or accumulation to toxic levels of one or more catabolites.[6]

Since high energy phosphate (HEP) is required to provide energy to support many of the complex functions of the myocyte, the hypothesis that depletion of HEP is directly or indirectly related to the development of the irreversible state

[a] Supported in part by NIH Grants HL 27416 and HL 23138.

[b] Address for correspondence: Dr. Keith A. Reimer, Department of Pathology, Box 3712, Duke University Medical Center, Durham, NC 27710. Tel.: (919) 684-3659, Ext. 221; Fax: (919) 684-3324 or 684-4352.

13

is attractive. This hypothesis is supported by observations that interventions which delay ATP depletion, such as hypothermia or treatment with calcium antagonists, delay cell death and vice versa. However, since energy depletion from myocytes within a region of ischemia in the intact heart is a heterogenous process, the precise relationship between energy state and the transition to irreversibility cannot be measured accurately.

The progressive accumulation of catabolites also could have lethal consequences. In particular, myocardial acidosis has a variety of potentially deleterious effects. For example, H^+ inhibits various metabolic pathways[7] including enzymes of the glycolytic pathway.

History and Definition of Ischemic Preconditioning

In the early 1980s, we hoped to determine which of these two general metabolic facets of ischemia, namely, 1) the continued use and progressive loss of high energy phosphates and 2) the progressive accumulation of a variety of potentially noxious catabolites is more important in the pathogenesis of *lethal* ischemic injury. To address this question, we designed a protocol in which myocardial infarct size was measured after a 40-minute test episode of ischemia. Control infarcts were compared with infarcts in which the 40-minute test episode was preceded by four 5-minute periods of ischemia, each separated by 5 minutes of reperfusion. We expected that, because repletion of adenine nucleotides is very slow in myocardium, the additional ischemia would accentuate high energy phosphate depletion. On the contrary, we expected the intermittent reperfusion to wash out catabolites, resulting in no cumulative increase and perhaps in reduced accumulation, if precursor substrate content became limiting.

We were amazed when we observed that infarct size in the experimental group was only 25% of the expected infarct size, despite the additional 20 minutes of ischemia to which the myocardium was subjected (FIG. 1).[8] Thus, it became evident that myocardium which has been subjected to one or several brief period(s) of ischemia, of insufficient duration to cause myocyte necrosis, rapidly (within minutes) develops markedly increased resistance to myocyte injury when subjected to a subsequent episode of ischemia. This rapid adaptation to ischemic stress was termed *ischemic preconditioning*.[8] We now know that similarly marked limitation of infarct size occurs with a single 5- to 15-minute preconditioning episode of ischemia and either a 40- or 60-minute test episode.[9–12] Ischemic preconditioning has been observed in several species in addition to dogs, including rats, rabbits, and pigs.[13–15] Clinical studies suggest that it most likely occurs in patients with ischemic heart disease.[16–18]

Moreover, subsequent reports have extended the use of the term "ischemic preconditioning" to include several endpoints in addition to the originally described phenomenon of infarct limitation in intact animals. Thus, it has been reported that preconditioning protects against dysrhythmias,[19–21] postischemic contractile dysfunction in isolated, perfused rat or rabbit hearts,[22–25] autonomic nerve dysfunction,[26] and microvascular dysfunction.[27] However, it should be noted that until the mechanism(s) underlying all facets of ischemic preconditioning is (are) known, it cannot be assumed that the mechanism of each facet is the same. Our discussion of ischemic preconditioning will emphasize results relating to its infarct-limiting facet.

The adaptive response to preconditioning occurs quickly (within minutes as demonstrated in the aforementioned protocols) but is relatively short lived. If the duration of reperfusion between preconditioning and the sustained 40- or 60-minute

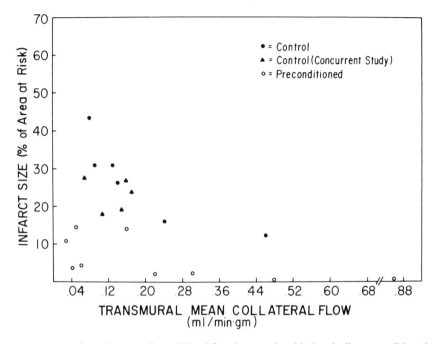

FIGURE 1. Infarct size vs collateral blood flow in control and ischemically preconditioned myocardium subjected to 40 minutes of circumflex coronary occlusion. Control dogs with the most severe ischemia (lowest collateral blood flow) had the largest infarcts, and vice versa. Ischemic preconditioning caused a marked limitation of infarct size irrespective of the collateral blood flow. (From Murry et al.[8] Reprinted by permission from *Circulation.*)

test period of ischemia is increased to two hours, the protective effect is largely lost.[9] Recent evidence suggests that there may be a slower adaptive response which also is initiated by preconditioning ischemia which results in a second window of protection ("SWOP") detectable in some experimental models at 24 hours.[28,29] The cardioprotection seen in the SWOP phenomenon is not as great and probably is explained by a molecular mechanism which is different from that of the early, classic preconditioning response.

Substantial progress has been made toward elucidation of the mechanism of the early preconditioning response by work in a large number of laboratories. These studies have focused on 1) the possible signaling pathway(s) through which rapid adaptation to ischemic stress occurs, and 2) identification of the resultant intracellular changes which make myocytes more resistant to ischemic injury. In regard to the second aspect, our studies have shown that the protective effect in dogs is associated with a marked slowing of the rate of energy metabolism.[30]

Effects of Ischemic Preconditioning on Ischemic Metabolism

We observed that dogs with repeated 10-minute episodes of ischemia had a much slower rate of decline of ATP and a much slower production of purine

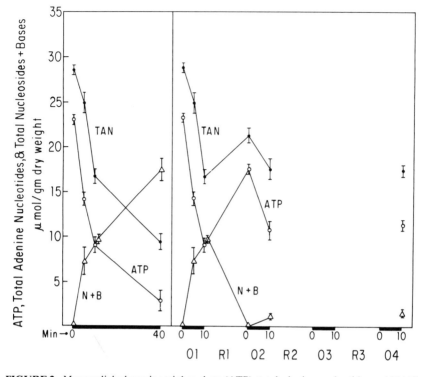

FIGURE 2. Myocardial adenosine triphosphate (ATP), total adenine nucleotide pool (TAN), and total pool of nucleosides and bases (N + B) during 40 minutes of continuous ischemia (*left*) and during 40 minutes of cumulative ischemia with intermittent reperfusion (*right*). Ten minutes of ischemia resulted in loss of 60% of the ATP and 40% of the adenine nucleotide pool. Reperfusion for 20 minutes then resulted in only partial repletion of ATP. Nevertheless, no cumulative loss of ATP occurred during three additional 10-minute episodes of ischemia. This is explained by a slower rate of ATP depletion in the later episodes. Note also that production of nucleosides and bases, the catabolites of adenine nucleotides, was substantial in the first ischemic episode but was markedly inhibited in later episodes. (From Reimer *et al.*[31] Reprinted by permission from the *American Journal of Physiology*.)

nucleosides and bases during later ischemic episodes vs the first episode (FIG. 2).[31] Moreover, we observed that both the rate of ATP depletion and the rate of accumulation of purine nucleosides and bases and catabolites of anaerobic glycolysis (FIG. 3) during a sustained 40-minute period of ischemia occurred much more slowly during ischemia following ischemic preconditioning.[30] That ATP depletion occurs more slowly, despite the fact that high energy phosphate (HEP) production via anaerobic glycolysis must also be slowed, indicates a marked reduction in high energy phosphate utilization during ischemia following ischemic preconditioning.

The metabolic slowing which we have observed in dogs also has been observed by others in a variety of animal species. In pigs, preconditioning slows both the rate of ATP utilization and the rate of development of intra- and extracellular acidosis.[32,33] In dogs, preconditioning results in less interstitial adenosine release during a subsequent episode of ischemia, as assessed by microdialysis sampling.[34]

In rat hearts studied either *in vivo* or *in vitro*, preconditioning has been reported by several groups to result in a reduction of tissue acidosis and in glycogen utilization during the prolonged ischemic test period.[23,24,35] Thus, preservation of ATP despite depressed glycogen utilization is a common feature of the preconditioned state, whether studied in hearts of large or small animal species, and whether studied during regional ischemia, *in vivo*, or total ischemia, *in vitro* in canine myocardium. Recently, it was reported that preconditioning attenuated the rate of ATP loss during ischemia of human myocardium, based on sequential biopsies obtained following repeated brief episodes of global ischemia (preceding coronary bypass surgery).[17]

The following explanations for the energy-sparing and infarct-limiting effects of ischemic preconditioning can be excluded:

1) Ischemic preconditioning does not cause a measurable increase in collateral blood flow and the marked limitation of infarct size in canine myocardium is observed at equivalent levels of collateral flow measured during the test episode.[8]

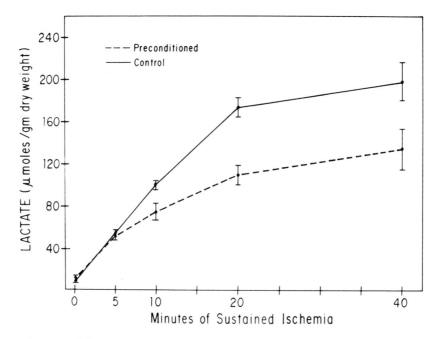

FIGURE 3. Subendocardial lactate content vs duration of ischemia in control and ischemically preconditioned myocardium. Anaerobic glycolysis is the principal pathway through which ATP can be formed in ischemic tissue, and lactate is its end product. Since much less lactate accumulates in preconditioned vs control myocardium during a 40-minute ischemic challenge, the slower depletion of ATP shown in FIGURE 2 cannot be explained by an accelerated rate of anaerobic glycolysis. The slower accumulation of lactate and other catabolites of glycolysis (data not shown), together with the slower degradation of adenine nucleotides shown in FIGURE 2, indicates a general reduction in the rate of ischemic metabolism in preconditioned myocardium. These data were obtained from groups with severe ischemia (subendocardial flow ≤ 0.07 ml/min · gm). (From Murry *et al.*[30] Reprinted by permission from *Circulation Research*.)

Moreover, preconditioning has been observed in species with minimal native collateral blood flow such as pigs, rabbits and rats.

2) Cellular stores of high energy phosphates are not enhanced in preconditioned myocardium at the onset of the test episode. Although it is known that a 10- or 15-minute episode of ischemia, followed by reperfusion, results in an "overshoot" in creatine phosphate content,[36] this increase in creatine phosphate is counterbalanced by the partial depletion of ATP and ADP.[2,30]

3) ATP production cannot be increased through an acceleration of anaerobic glycolysis, since reduced accumulation of the products of anaerobic glycolysis during ischemia is one of the hallmarks of preconditioned myocardium.[30]

Thus, the slower rate of high energy phosphate depletion during ischemia is likely explained by a slowing of one or more energy utilizing reactions.

Pathways of Energy Utilization in Ischemic Myocardium

Many cellular processes and reactions contribute to the progressive decline in ATP during ischemia. Those thought to be of particular importance include continued attempts at myofibrillar contraction, transport ATPases, adenylate cyclase, and the mitochondrial ATPase (reverse function of the mitochondrial ATP synthase).

Under aerobic conditions, the major use of HEP is in support of the contractile process. Under ischemic conditions, effective contraction ceases within a few seconds. Nevertheless, energy still is utilized by cross-bridge cycling in response to continuing electrical activation. In turn, these processes are accompanied by Na^+, K^+, and Ca^{2+} ion cycling, which drives the various ion transport ATPases.

Another important pathway of ATP consumption in ischemia is a reaction that does not occur in aerobic myocardium, namely, mitochondrial ATPase activity. The mitochondrial ATP synthase is the macromolecular complex of proteins comprising the F1-F0 particles of mitochondria. Under aerobic conditions this enzyme complex *synthesizes* ATP, but under nonenergizing conditions, such as those experienced under conditions of myocardial ischemia, the reaction occurs in the reverse direction and ATP is *hydrolyzed*. This reaction is a major cause of early ATP depletion in ischemic myocardium.[37,38] However, ATP depletion would occur *more* quickly than it does, were it not for the existence of an endogenous inhibitor of the ATPase. This inhibitor, the F1-ATPase inhibitory subunit (IF1), is present in slow-heart-rate species including dogs, and binds to the ATPase to effect partial inhibition of ATPase activity that otherwise would occur during ischemic conditions.[39]

Norepinephrine is released from sympathetic nerve endings during the first few minutes of ischemia. Stimulation of beta adrenergic receptors on ventricular myocytes activates *adenylate cyclase* and thereby accelerates a variety of energy-utilizing reactions. In addition, activation of alpha$_1$ receptors also may increase myocardial energy demand. Alpha$_1$ receptor stimulation activates phospholipase C (PLC) through a G protein-mediated mechanism. Enhanced function of PLC increases production of the second messengers inositol triphosphate (IP$_3$) and diacylglycerol (DAG), which, in turn, increase the release of Ca^{++} from intracellular stores and activate protein kinase C. The net effect of PLC activation under aerobic conditions is increased contractility and increased intracellular calcium cycling.[40] The net effect under ischemic conditions is unknown. Activation of PKC hypothetically could either increase or reduce the demand for high energy phosphate depending on the net effect of PKC-mediated phosphorylation, and consequent increase or decrease of the activities, of various ATP-utilizing enzymes and ion channels.

At present, the relative contribution of each of these various processes to overall ATP utilization in ischemic myocardium is not clear, nor is it known which of these, if any, might be slowed in preconditioned myocardium.

Hypothetical Explanations for the Energy-Sparing Effects of Ischemic Preconditioning

Concomitant Myocardial Stunning

The brief episodes of ischemia that induce the preconditioning effect also cause myocardial "stunning" (reduced postischemic systolic contractile function that develops even though no infarction is present). Thus, one explanation for the slowing of energy depletion characteristic of ischemically preconditioned myocardium is that the myocardium is concurrently stunned and therefore uses less ATP attempting to contract in the initial phases of a subsequent episode of ischemia.

In one study to test this hypothesis, we assessed energy metabolism during total ischemia, in vitro, after first preconditioning myocardium in vivo.[41] Hearts were arrested with KCl to abolish electrical and contractile activity. Control and preconditioned regions of these quiescent hearts were excised and subjected to total ischemia at 37°C. The initial rates of both ATP depletion and anaerobic glycolysis were much slower in preconditioned vs control myocardium from the same hearts, even though possible differences in contractile effort between regions had been abolished.

Both indirect and direct evidence from in vivo studies indicates that the metabolic and antiinfarct effects of ischemic preconditioning are not manifestations of concomitant myocardial stunning. For example, the cardioprotective effect of preconditioning is a relatively transient phenomenon that dissipates after one to two hours of reperfusion,[9] whereas stunning may persist for hours or days. In addition, four 5-minute episodes of coronary occlusion, which formed the first preconditioning protocol, causes relatively mild stunning in canine myocardium.[42] The discrepancy between the mild degree of stunning and the marked limitation of infarct size provides indirect evidence that preconditioning is not simply a consequence of stunning.

Direct evidence against a causal relation between stunning and preconditioning is provided by a study in which dobutamine was administered after preconditioning to overcome the postischemic contractile dysfunction.[42] Dobutamine infusion easily restored contractile function to baseline values, but the protective effect of ischemic preconditioning on infarct size was preserved. Although these results do *not* exclude the possibility that an underlying cellular defect that causes the contractile dysfunction of stunning could also cause the cardioprotective effect of preconditioning, they do indicate that the metabolic and cardioprotective effects of preconditioning are not simply a consequence of reduced contractile effort.

Inhibition of the Mitochondrial ATPase

Hypothetically, the reduction of demand for HEP induced by ischemic preconditioning might be explained by earlier or more complete inhibition of the mitochondrial ATPase. However, we have observed that, even in nonpreconditioned myocardium, mitochondrial ATPase activity becomes inhibited very quickly (within 90 seconds) following the onset of severe ischemia and that inhibition of the ATPase, induced by preconditioning episodes of ischemia, does not persist following 5 minutes of arterial reperfusion.[43] It also should be noted that rat myocardium can be preconditioned[15] even though it has markedly reduced mitochondrial ATPase inhibitor activity compared with the activity present in slow-heart-rate species such as dogs. In short, early inhibition of the mitochondrial ATPase in ischemia is an endogenous protective mechanism which occurs even in non-preconditioned myocardium, but it seems unlikely that inhibition of the mitochondrial ATPase can explain the energy-sparing effects of ischemic preconditioning.[44]

Antiadrenergic Effects

Norepinephrine is released from sympathetic nerve endings during the first few minutes of ischemia and stimulation of beta adrenergic receptors on ventricular myocytes activates adenylate cyclase and thereby accelerates a variety of energy-utilizing reactions.[40] Therefore, either a reduction in norepinephrine release from sympathetic nerve endings, or reduced alpha- or beta-receptor responsiveness to norepinephrine could have an energy-sparing effect during the early phase of myocardial ischemia.

One hypothetical scenario involves the release of adenosine which, through activation of an inhibitory G protein (G_i),[45] both inhibits exocytotic release of norepinephrine from cardiac nerve endings[46,47] and counteracts in cardiac myocytes the stimulatory effect of beta adrenergic receptor stimulation on adenylate cyclase[48,49] and hence on protein kinase A-dependent reactions.

If the energy-sparing and infarct-limiting effects of ischemic preconditioning are mediated through an antiadrenergic mechanism, elimination of myocardial catecholamines before ischemia should have the same effects as ischemic preconditioning. However, using an *in vivo* model of regional ischemia, we found that although infarct size was slightly smaller in reserpine-treated (catecholamine-depleted) than in control hearts, the protective effect was not nearly as great as observed with preconditioning. Moreover, the combination of reserpine and preconditioning was no better than reserpine alone and was less effective than preconditioning alone.[12]

These results are consistent with the following hypotheses: 1) A stimulation of one or more catecholamine-mediated pathways is necessary during the *preconditioning episodes* of ischemia to trigger the adaptive response, *and* 2) An inhibition of one or more catecholamine-mediated pathways during the *test episode* of ischemia could explain part, but not all of the energy-sparing and infarct-limiting effects of preconditioning.

Inhibition of K_{ATP}^+ Channels

Another hypothesis to explain both the cardioprotective and metabolic effects of ischemic preconditioning involves ATP-dependent K^+ (K_{ATP}^+) channels. It has been proposed that preconditioning may accelerate or enhance the opening of these channels.[11] Activation of (K_{ATP}^+) channels does occur during ischemia.[50] The decrease in ATP opens the channel and results in an efflux of potassium, which decreases the duration of the plateau phase of the cardiac action potential.[51-53]

Thus, the time during which inward flux of Ca^{++} occurs is shortened. This decreases contractile effort, and at the subcellular level reduces the amount of high energy phosphate required to support cellular Ca^{++} cycling.[54]

Evidence supporting the K_{ATP}^+ channel hypothesis of preconditioning has been reported from studies using dogs[11] and pigs (Heusch, G.; personal communication). Glibenclamide (an inhibitor of the K_{ATP}^+ channel), when administered either before or after a brief episode of ischemia, abolished the protective effect of ischemic preconditioning. However, conflicting results have been reported from studies using rabbits.[55]

Hypothetical Signaling Mechanisms in Ischemic Preconditioning

Possible signaling mechanisms through which ischemic preconditioning could be coupled to its metabolic and infarct-limiting effects have been extensively investigated in rodents. The preponderance of this evidence suggests that the mechanism of preconditioning may involve activation of the protein kinase C (PKC) regulatory pathway. Activation of phospholipase C or phospholipase D in the cell membrane leads to the formation of the second messenger, diacylglycerol (DAG). DAG activates protein kinase C (PKC) which phosphorylates a variety of other cellular proteins, with diverse functions.[56-58] A growing number of isoforms of PKC have been identified. At least four different isoforms are present in cardiac muscle, including α, δ, ε and zeta. The activation of PKC occurs through the translocation of the enzyme from the cytosol to the cell membrane via microtubules.[58,59] Several surface receptors are known to induce activation of cardiac PKC, including α_1-adrenergic, muscarinic, endothelin, angiotensin II, and adenosine A_1 receptors.[58,60-62] Many proteins are phosphorylated by PKC and such phosphorylation modulates the activities of several enzyme systems including adenylate cyclase, L-type calcium channels, the Na^+/Ca^{++} exchanger, AMP deaminase and at least one K^+ channel.[63-67]

Several pathways modulated by the PLC-PKC system, such as sensitization of adenylate cyclase,[66] would likely increase, rather than decrease energy utilization. In addition, phospholipase C produces not only diacyl glycerol (DAG), but another second messenger, inositol triphosphate (IP_3), which is known to enhance calcium mobilization.[68] Thus, it is not known if, or how the consequences of activating the PLC-PKC pathway might result in reduced ischemic metabolism and consequent cardioprotection. Whether and how PKC also modulates the activity of the K_{ATP}^+ channel is less clear. It is known that these channels are coupled via a G_i protein to the adenosine A_1 receptor[67] and to myocardial muscarinic receptors.[69]

Nevertheless, it has been reported that preconditioning episodes of ischemia are sufficient to induce the translocation and activation of PKC in rat or rabbit hearts.[60,66,70] We have shown that it is translocated during acute ischemia in the dog heart (Strasser, R. H., Reimer, K. A. & Jennings, R. B.; unreported data). Direct activators of PKC such as phorbol myristate acetate (PMA) or the diacyl glycerol analog, oleoylacetate glycerol (OAG), have been reported to limit myocardial infarct size in rabbits, and the infarct-limiting effects of both preconditioning and direct PKC activators are reportedly blocked by inhibitors of PKC.[60,71-73] In addition, the PKC inhibitor calphostin C blocked preconditioning induced by substrate deficiency in isolated cardiac myocytes.[74] In contrast, several preliminary reports regarding the possible role of PKC activation in the mechanism of ischemic preconditioning in large animal models have had negative results.[75–78]

Potential Clinical Implications

The results of many clinical studies support the now generally accepted view that morbidity and mortality from myocardial infarction are related directly to the size of a myocardial infarct.[79,80] Thus, elucidation of mechanisms of ischemic injury has important clinical ramifications in that such knowledge should permit the development of methods to delay the onset of irreversibility that could be applied as adjunctive therapy pending reperfusion. Such therapy could be used to enhance cardioplegia for myocardial protection during surgery, or to delay myocardial injury in patients with acute myocardial infarction, pending reperfusion. Although these clinical possibilities remain speculative, the fact that ischemic preconditioning does result in slower injury during a subsequent period of ischemia is proof that the process of ischemic injury can be delayed. It also must be emphasized that in experimental models, ischemic preconditioning has been consistently reproducible and that this endogenous cardioprotective mechanism has more potent infarct-limiting efficacy than any of a myriad of pharmacologic interventions tested to date as possible adjuncts to early reperfusion.[81]

It also is likely that patients who suffer a sustained coronary occlusion after one or more brief episodes of ischemia (*e.g.*, as might occur in unstable, preinfarction angina), may undergo infarction in a setting of spontaneous preconditioning. In such patients, infarction should develop more slowly than occurs following an abrupt occlusion.

For these reasons, studies of ischemic preconditioning remain an exciting and potentially fruitful area of research.

SUMMARY

One or several brief episodes of myocardial ischemia (ischemic preconditioning; IP) rapidly induces tolerance to a later ischemic challenge. This endogenous cardioprotective effect is characterized by a slower onset of cell death. A key feature and probable proximate mechanism of IP is reduced ischemic energy demand which is evident by slower use of ATP and slower accumulation of ischemic catabolites. Several mechanisms for IP and the associated metabolic slowing have been studied: The mitochondrial ATPase is a major cause of ATP hydrolysis in ischemic myocardium but slower ATP depletion in preconditioned myocardium is *not* due to persistent inhibition of this ATPase. Brief episodes of ischemia in dogs induce stunning as well as IP. Stunning, however, is neither necessary nor sufficient to establish the protective effects of IP. Release of norepinephrine from adrenergic cardiac nerves causes beta adrenergic receptor-mediated stimulation of adenylate cyclase, which stimulates energy-dependent processes. However, IP in dogs that were depleted of catecholamines by pretreatment with reserpine was less effective than IP in control hearts. Thus, an antiadrenergic mechanism does not fully account for the preconditioned state. Another proposed mechanism involves earlier or more complete opening of ATP-sensitive potassium (K_{ATP}^+) channels. Which of these (or other) pathways mediate the energy sparing effects of ischemic preconditioning remains unknown.

REFERENCES

1. JENNINGS, R. B., H. K. HAWKINS, J. E. LOWE, M. L. HILL, S. KLOTMAN & K. A. REIMER. 1978. Relation between high energy phosphate and lethal injury in myocardial ischemia in the dog. Am. J. Pathol. **92:** 187–214.
2. REIMER, K. A., M. L. HILL & R. B. JENNINGS. 1981. Prolonged depletion of ATP and of the adenine nucleotide pool due to delayed resynthesis of adenine nucleotides following reversible myocardial ischemic injury in dogs. J. Mol. Cell. Cardiol. **13:** 229–239.
3. GEVERS, W. 1977. Generation of protons by metabolic processes in heart cells. Editorial. J. Mol. Cell. Cardiol. **9:** 867–874.
4. TAEGTMEYER, H., A. G. FERGUSON & M. LESCH. 1977. Protein degradation and amino acid metabolism in autolyzing rabbit myocardium. Exp. Mol. Pathol. **26:** 52–62.
5. JENNINGS, R. B., K. A. REIMER & C. STEENBERGEN. 1986. Myocardial ischemia revisited. The osmolar load, membrane damage, and reperfusion. Editorial comment. J. Mol. Cell. Cardiol. **18:** 769–780.
6. JENNINGS, R. B., C. E. MURRY, C. STEENBERGEN, JR. & K. A. REIMER. 1990. Development of cell injury in sustained acute ischemia. Circulation **82**(Suppl. 2): II-2–II-12.
7. WILLIAMSON, J. R., S. W. SCHAFFER, C. FORD & B. SAFER. 1976. Contribution of tissue acidosis to ischemic injury in the perfused rat heart. Circulation **53:** I3–I14.
8. MURRY, C. E., R. B. JENNINGS & K. A. REIMER. 1986. Preconditioning with ischemia: a delay of lethal cell injury in ischemic myocardium. Circulation **74:** 1124–1136.
9. MURRY, C. E., V. J. RICHARD, R. B. JENNINGS & K. A. REIMER. 1991. Myocardial protection is lost before contractile function recovers from ischemic preconditioning. Am. J. Physiol. (Heart Circ. Physiol.) **260:** H796–H804.
10. LI, G. C., J. A. VASQUEZ, K. P. GALLAGHER & B. R. LUCCHESI. 1990. Myocardial protection with preconditioning. Circulation **82:** 609–619.
11. GROSS, G. J. & J. A. AUCHAMPACH. 1992. Blockade of ATP-sensitive potassium channels prevents myocardial preconditioning in dogs. Circulation **70:** 223–233.
12. VANDER HEIDE, R. S., L. M. SCHWARTZ, R. B. JENNINGS & K. A. REIMER. 1995. Effect of catecholamine depletion on infarct size in dogs: role of catecholamines in ischemic preconditioning. Cardiovasc. Res. **30:** 656–667.
13. SCHOTT, R. J., S. ROHMANN, E. R. BRAUN & W. SCHAPER. 1990. Ischemic preconditioning reduces infarct size in swine myocardium. Cir. Res. **66:** 1133–1142.
14. THORNTON, J. D., S. STRIPLIN, G. S. LIU, A. SWAFFORD, A. W. H. STANLEY, D. M. VAN WINKLE & J. M. DOWNEY. 1990. Inhibition of protein synthesis does not block myocardial protection afforded by preconditioning Am. J. Physiol. (Heart Circ. Physiol.) **259:** H1822–H1825.
15. YELLON, D. M., A. M. ALKHULAIFI, E. E. BROWNE & W. B. PUGSLEY. 1992. Ischaemic preconditioning limits infarct size in the rat heart. Cardiovasc. Res. **26:** 983–987.
16. DEUTSCH, E., M. BERGER, W. G. KUSSMAUL, J. W. HIRSHFELD, JR., H. C. HERMANN & W. K. LASKEY. 1990. Adaptation to ischemia during PTCA: clinical, hemodynamic and metabolic features. Circulation **82:** 2044–2051.
17. YELLON, D. M., A. M. ALKHULAIFI & W. B. PUGSLEY. 1993. Preconditioning the human myocardium. Lancet **342:** 276–277.
18. KLONER, R. A., T. SHOOK, K. PRZYKLENK, V. G. DAVIS, L. JUNIO, R. V. MATTHEWS, S. BURSTEIN, M. GIBSON, W. K. POOLE, C. P. CANNON, C. H. MCCABE, E. BRAUNWALD & TIMI 4 Investigators. 1995. Previous angina alters in-hospital outcome in TIMI 4: a clinical correlate to preconditioning. Circulation **91:** 37–47.
19. SHIKI, K. & D. J. HEARSE. 1987. Preconditioning of ischemic myocardium: reperfusion-induced arrhythmias. Am. J. Physiol. **253:** H1470–H1476.
20. HAGAR, J. M., S. L. HALE & R. A. KLONER. 1991. Effect of preconditioning ischemia on reperfusion arrhythmias after coronary artery occlusion and repefusion in the rat. Circ. Res. **68:** 61–68.
21. VEGH, A., S. KOMORI, L. SZEKERES & J. R. PARRATT. 1992. Antiarrhythmic effects of preconditioning in anaesthetised dogs and rats. Cardiovasc. Res. **26:** 487–495.

22. CAVE, A. C. & D. J. HEARSE. 1992. Ischaemic preconditioning and contractile function: studies with normothermic and hypothermic global ischaemia. J. Mol. Cell. Cardiol. **24:** 1113–1123.

23. ASIMAKIS, G. K., K. INNERS-MCBRIDE, G. MEDELLIN & V. R. CONTI. 1992. Ischemic preconditioning attenuates acidosis and postischemic dysfunction in isolated rat heart. Am. J. Physiol. **263:** H887–H894.

24. STEENBERGEN, C., M. E. PERLMAN, R. E. LONDON & E. MURPHY. 1992. Mechanism of preconditioning. Ionic alterations. Circ. Res. **71:** 112–125.

25. BANERJEE, A., C. LOCKE-WINTER, K. B. ROGERS, M. B. MITCHELL, E. C. BREW, C. B. CLAIRNS, D. D. BENSARD & A. H. HARKEN. 1993. Preconditioning against myocardial dysfunction after ischemia and reperfusion by an α_1-adrenergic mechanism. Circ. Res. **73:** 656–670.

26. MIYAZAKI, T. & D. P. ZIPES. 1989. Protection against autonomic denervation following acute myocardial infarction by preconditioning ischemia. Circ. Res. **64:** 437–448.

27. BAUER, B., B. Z. SIMKHOVICH, R. A. KLONER & K. PRZYKLENK. 1993. Does preconditioning protect the coronary vasculature from subsequent ischemia/reperfusion injury? Circulation **88:** 659–672.

28. MARBER, M. S., D. S. LATCHMAN, J. M. WALKER & D. M. YELLON. 1994. Cardiac stress protein elevation 24 hours after brief ischemia or heat stress is associated with resistance to myocardial infarction. Circulation **1264:** 1272.

29. KUZUYA, T., S. HOSHIDA, N. YAMASHITA, H. FUJI, H. OE, M. HORI, T. KAMADA & M. TADA. 1993. Delayed effects of sublethal ischemia on the acquisition of tolerance to ischemia. Circ. Res. **72:** 1293–1299.

30. MURRY, C. E., V. J. RICHARD, K. A. REIMER & R. B. JENNINGS. 1990. Ischemic preconditioning slows energy metabolism and delays ultrastructural damage during a sustained ischemic episode. Circ. Res. **66:** 913–931.

31. REIMER, K. A., C. E. MURRY, I. YAMASAWA, M. L. HILL & R. B. JENNINGS. 1986. Four brief periods of myocardial ischemia cause no cumulative ATP loss or necrosis. Am. J. Physiol. **251:** H1306–H1315.

32. KIDA, M., H. FUJIWARA, M. ISHIDA, C. KAWAI, M. OHURA, I. MIURA & Y. YABUUCHI. 1991. Ischemic preconditioning preserves creatine phosphate and intracellular pH. Circulation **84:** 2495–2503.

33. FLEET, W. F., T. A. JOHNSON, C A. GRAEBNER & L. S. GETTES. 1985. Effect of serial brief ischemic episodes on extracellular K +, pH, and activation in the pig. Circulation **72:** 922–932.

34. DORHEIM, T. A., R. M. MENTZER, JR. & D. G. L. VAN WYLEN. 1991. Preconditioning reduces interstitial fluid purine metabolites during prolonged myocardial ischemia (abstract). Circulation **84**(Suppl. 2): II-191.

35. WOLFE, C. L., R. E. SIEVERS, F. L. VISSEREN & T. J. DONNELLY. 1993. Loss of myocardial protection after preconditioning correlates with the time course of glycogen recovery within the preconditioned segment. Circulation **87:** 881–892.

36. SWAIN, J. L., R. L. SABINA, P. A. MCHALE, J. C. GREENFIELD, JR. & E. W. HOLMES. 1982. Prolonged myocardial adenine nucleotide depletion after brief ischemia in the open-chest dog. Am. J. Physiol. **242:** H818–H826.

37. JENNINGS, R. B., K. A. REIMER & C. STEENBERGEN, JR. 1991. Effect of inhibition of the mitochondrial ATPase on net myocardial ATP in total ischemia. J. Mol. Cell. Cardiol. **23:** 1383–1395.

38. ROUSLIN, W., J. L. E. ERICKSON & R. J. SOLARO. 1986. Effects of oligomycin and acidosis on rates of ATP depletion in ischemic heart muscle. Am. J. Physiol. **250:** H503–H508.

39. ROUSLIN, W. 1991. Mini-review. Regulation of the mitochondrial ATPase *in situ* in cardiac muscle: role of the inhibitor subunit. J. Bioenerg. Biomembr. **23:** 873–887.

40. FLEMING, J. W., P. L. WISLER & A. M. WATANABE. 1992. Signal transduction by G proteins in cardiac tissues (review). Circulation **85:** 420–423.

41. JENNINGS, R. B., K. A. REIMER, C. STEENBERGEN, JR. & J. SCHAPER. 1989. Total ischemia III: effect of inhibition of anaerobic glycolysis. J. Mol. Cell. Cardiol. **21**(Suppl. I): 137–154.

42. MATSUDA, M., T. G. CATENA, R. S. VANDER HEIDE, R. B. JENNINGS & K. A. REIMER. 1993. Cardiac protection by ischemic preconditioning is not mediated by myocardial stunning. Cardiovasc. Res. 27: 585–592.

43. VANDER HEIDE, R. S., M. L. HILL, K. A. REIMER & R. B. JENNINGS. 1996. Effect of reversible ischemia on the activity of the mitochondrial ATPase: relationship to ischemic preconditioning. J. Mol. Cell. Cardiol. 28: 103–112.

44. VANDER HEIDE, R. S., M. L. HILL, C. STEENBERGEN, JR., K. A. REIMER & R. B. JENNINGS. 1991. Effect of reversible ischemia on mitochondrial ATPase activity in canine myocardium (abstract). Circulation 84(Suppl. 4): II-192.

45. NEER, E. J. & D. E. CLAPHAM. 1992. Signal transduction through G proteins in the cardiac myocyte. Trends Cardiovasc. Med. 2: 6–11.

46. WAKADE, A. R. & T. D. WAKADE. 1978. Inhibition of noradrenaline release by adenosine. J. Physiol. 282: 35–49.

47. FREDHOLM, B. B. & P. HEDQUIST. 1980. Modulation of neurotransmission by purine nucleotides and nucleosides. Biochem. Pharmacol. 29: 1635–1643.

48. ROMANO, F. D. & J. G. DOBSON, JR. 1990. Adenosine modulates B-adrenergic signal transduction in guinea pig heart ventricular membranes. J. Mol. Cell. Cardiol. 22: 1359–1370.

49. DOBSON, J. G., JR. & R. A. FENTON. 1987. Antiadrenergic effects of adenosine in the heart. In Regulatory Function of Adenosine. R. M. Berne, T. W. Rall & R. Rubio, Eds. 363–376. Martinus Nijhoff Publishers. The Hague/Boston/London.

50. HEARSE, D. J. 1995. Activation of ATP-sensitive potassium channels: a novel pharmacological approach to myocardial protection? (review). Cardiovasc. Res. 30: 1–17.

51. NOMA, A. 1983. ATP-regulated K+ channels in cardiac muscle. Nature 305: 147–148.

52. RICHER, C., J. PRATZ, P. MULDERM, S. MONDOT, J. F. GIUDICELLI & I. CAVERO. 1990. Cardiovascular and biological effects of K+ channel openers, a class of drugs with vasorelaxant and cardioprotective properties. Life Sci. 47: 1693–1705.

53. COLE, W. C., C. D. MCPHERSON & D. SONTAG. 1991. ATP-regulated K+ channels protect the myocardium against ischemia/reperfusion damage. Circ. Res. 69: 571–581.

54. ASHCROFT, S. J. H. & F. M. ASHCROFT. 1990. Properties and functions of ATP-sensitive K-channels. Mini review. Cell. Signalling 2: 197–214.

55. THORNTON, J. D., C. S. THORNTON, D. L. STERLING & J. M. DOWNEY. 1993. Blockade of ATP-sensitive potassium channels increases infarct size but does not prevent preconditioning in rabbit heart. Circ. Res. 72: 44–49.

56. NISHIZUKA, Y. 1986. Studies and perspectives of protein kinase C. Science 233: 308–312.

57. NISHIZUKA, Y. 1992. Intracellular signaling by hydrolysis of phospholipids and activation of protein kinase C. Science 258: 607–614.

58. STABLE, S. & P. J. PARKER. 1991. Protein kinase C. Pharmacol. Ther. 51: 71–95.

59. YUAN, S., F. A. SUNAHARA & A. K. SEN. 1987. Tumor-promoting phorbol esters inhibit cardiac functions and induce redistribution of protein kinase C in perfused beating rat heart. Circ. Res. 61: 372–378.

60. YTREHUS, K., Y. LIU & J. M. DOWNEY. 1994. Preconditioning protects ischemic rabbit heart by protein kinase C activation. Am. J. Physiol. 266: H1145–H1152.

61. BOGOYEVITCH, M. A., P. J. PARKER & P. H. SUGDEN. 1993. Characterization of protein kinase C isotype expression in adult rat heart. Protein kinase C-epsilon is a major isotype present, and it is activated by phorbol esters, epinephrine and endothelin. Circ. Res. 72: 757–767.

62. PRASAD, M. R. & R. M. JONES. 1992. Enhanced membrane protein kinase C activity in myocardial ischemia. Basic Res. Cardiol. 87: 19–26.

63. DÖSEMECI, A., R. S. DHALLAN, N. M. COHEN, W. J. LEDERER & T. B. ROGERS. 1988. Phorbol ester increases calcium current and stimulates the effects of angiotensin II on cultured neonatal rat heart myocytes. Circ. Res. 62: 347–357.

64. ZHENG, J-S., A. CHRISTIE, M. N. LEVY & A. SCARPA. 1992. Ca^{2+} mobilization by extracellular ATP in rat cardiac myocytes: regulation by protein kinase C and A. Am. J. Physiol. 263: C933–C940.

65. THAKKAR, J. K., D. R. JANERO, C. YARWOOD & H. M. SHARIF. 1993. Modulation of mammalian cardiac AMP deaminase by protein kinase C-mediated phosphorylation. Biochem. J. **291:** 523–527.
66. STRASSER, R. H., R. BRAUN-DULLAEUS, H. WALENDZIK & R. MARQUETANT. 1992. α_1-Receptor-independent activation of protein kinase C in acute myocardial ischemia: mechanisms for sensitization of the adenylyl cyclase system. Circ. Res. **70:** 1304–1312.
67. KIRSCH, G. E., J. CODINA, L. BIRNBAUMER & A. M. BROWN. 1990. Coupling of ATP-sensitive K^+ channels to A_1 receptors by G proteins in rat ventricular myocytes. Am. J. Physiol. **259:** H820–H826.
68. MOUTON, R., B. HUISAMEN & A. LOCHNER. 1991. The effect of ischaemia and reperfusion on sarcolemmal inositol phospholipid and cytosolic inositol phosphate metabolism in the isolated perfused rat heart. Mol. Cell. Biochem. **105:** 127–135.
69. YAO, Z. & G. J. GROSS. 1994. The ATP-dependent potassium channel: an endogenous cardioprotective mechanism. J. Cardiovasc. Pharmacol. **24:** S28–S34.
70. MITCHELL, M. B., X. MENG, L. AO, J. M. BROWN, A. H. HARKEN & A. BANERJEE. 1995. Preconditioning of isolated rat heart is mediated by protein kinase C. Circ. Res. **76:** 73–81.
71. LIU, Y., K. YTREHUS & J. M. DOWNEY. 1994. Evidence that translocation of protein kinase C is a key event during ischemic preconditioning of rabbit myocardium. J. Mol. Cell. Cardiol. **26:** 661–668.
72. TSUCHIDA, A., Y. LIU, G. S. LIU, M. V. COHEN & J. M. DOWNEY. 1994. α_1-Adrenergic agonists precondition rabbit ischemic myocardium independent of adenosine by direct activation of protein kinase C. Circ. Res. **75:** 576–585.
73. SPEECHLY-DICK, M. E., M. M. MOCANU & D. M. YELLON. 1994. Protein kinase C: its role in ischemic preconditioning in the rat. Circ. Res. **75:** 586–590.
74. ARMSTRONG, S., J. M. DOWNEY & C. E. GANOTE. 1994. Preconditioning of isolated rabbit cardiomyocytes: induction by metabolic stress and blockade by the adenosine antagonist SPT and calphostin C, a protein kinase inhibitor. Cardiovasc. Res. **28:** 72–77.
75. SIMKHOVICH, B. Z., R. A. KLONER & K. PRZYKLENK. 1994. Brief preconditioning ischemia does not trigger translocation of protein kinase C in canine myocardium (abstract). Circulation **90:** I-208.
76. VOGT, A., M. BARANCIK, D. WEIHRAUCH, M. ARRAS, T. PODZUWEIT & W. SCHAPER. 1994. Activation of protein kinase C fails to protect ischemic porcine myocardium from infarction *in vivo* (abstract). J. Mol. Cell. Cardiol. **26:** 118.
77. VOGT, A., M. BARANCIK, D. WEIHRAUCH, M. ARRAS, T. PODZUWEIT & W. SCHAPER. 1994. Protein kinase C inhibitors reduce infarct size in pig hearts *in vivo* (abstract). Circulation **90:** I-647.
78. PRZYKLENK, K., M. A. SUSSMAN, B. Z. SIMKHOVICH & R. A. KLONER. 1995. Does ischemic preconditioning trigger translocation of protein kinase C in the canine model? Circulation **92:** 1546–1557.
79. CERQUEIRA, M. D., C. MAYNARD, J. L. RITCHIE, K. B. DAVIS & J. W. KENNEDY. 1992. Long-term survival in 618 patients from Western Washington Streptokinase in Myocardial Infarction Trials. J. Am. Coll. Cardiol. **20:** 1452–1459.
80. BERNING, J. & F. STEENSGAARD-HANSEN. 1990. Early estimation of risk by echocardiographic determination of wall motion index in an unselected population with acute myocardial infarction. Am. J. Cardiol. **65:** 567–576.
81. MARBER, M., D. WALKER & D. YELLON. 1994. Editorial. Ischaemic preconditioning. Br. Med. J. **308:** 1–2.

Cardioprotection by Ischemic and Nonischemic Myocardial Stress and Ischemia in Remote Organs

Implications for the Concept of Ischemic Preconditioning[a]

PIETER D. VERDOUW,[b] BEN C. G. GHO,
MONIQUE M. G. KONING, REGIEN G. SCHOEMAKER,[c]
AND DIRK J. DUNCKER

Experimental Cardiology, Thoraxcenter
and
[c]Department of Pharmacology
Cardiovascular Research Institute (COEUR)
Erasmus University Rotterdam
Rotterdam, The Netherlands

INTRODUCTION

Traditionally, ischemic preconditioning studies have employed one or more brief abrupt total coronary artery occlusion and reperfusion sequences to reduce myocardial infarct size produced by a subsequent prolonged coronary artery occlusion. Evidence is now emerging that stimuli other than total coronary artery occlusions can induce a protected state of the myocardium. We will present the results of studies from our own laboratory that support the hypothesis that a number of distinctly different stimuli can protect the myocardium against irreversible injury. Based on those findings we propose that ischemic preconditioning is only one feature of a more general form of protection, that can be triggered by ischemic as well as nonischemic stresses.

Preconditioning by a Partial Coronary Artery Occlusion without Intervening Reperfusion

Ischemic preconditioning studies usually employ one or multiple brief total coronary artery occlusion(s) to precondition myocardium before infarction is produced by a prolonged coronary artery occlusion.[1-3] If partial coronary artery occlusions could also be shown to precondition myocardium this would greatly

[a] The research of Dr. Dirk J. Duncker has been made possible by a fellowship of the Royal Netherlands Academy of Arts and Sciences. Supported by Grant 92.144 from the Netherlands Heart Foundation and by Grant CIPA-CT-92-4009 of the European Economic Community.

[b] Correspondence to: P. D. Verdouw, PhD, Experimental Cardiology, Thoraxcenter, Erasmus University Rotterdam, P.O. Box 1738, 3000 DR Rotterdam, The Netherlands. Tel.: +31-10-4088029; Fax: +31-10-4365607; E-mail: Verdouw@tch.fgg.eur.nl.

increase the clinical relevance of ischemic preconditioning, especially if protection could be demonstrated without the need of a period of complete reperfusion between the partial and prolonged total occlusion. Harris showed some 40 years ago that a brief partial coronary occlusion preceding a prolonged total coronary occlusion without a period of intervening reperfusion (*i.e.*, a two-stage coronary artery occlusion) was an effective method to suppress the incidence of ventricular fibrillation during the complete occlusion.[4] Arrhythmias occur mostly between 4–9 min and 15–20 min following occlusion, and it was believed that reducing the level of ischemia during the first 30 min would increase the number of animals surviving this life-threatening period. Once those 30 min had passed, the artery could be totally occluded with a minimal threat of ventricular tachycardia and fibrillation. In view of what is known about the effect of ischemic preconditioning on ventricular arrhythmias[5,6] we can now hypothesize that during the partial occlusion the myocardium became preconditioned, which resulted in the lower incidence of ventricular fibrillation during the subsequent total occlusion. Moreover, data have been presented that a partial coronary artery occlusion can precondition myocardium against irreversible damage.[7] However, in this study a period of complete reperfusion separating the partial from the total prolonged coronary artery occlusion was mandatory for protection to occur. Because only one level of partial occlusion was examined it appears premature to generalize this conclusion to all levels of partial occlusion. We therefore investigated the necessity of an intervening reperfusion period by studying coronary flow reductions of different severity and duration preceding a 60 min coronary artery occlusion without a period of intervening reperfusion. The experiments were performed in anesthetized instrumented pigs, which were allocated to 8 different groups (FIG. 1).[8,9] Inflation of a fluid-filled balloon positioned around the proximal left anterior descending coronary artery was used to reduce coronary blood flow, as measured with a Doppler flow meter, to either 30% or 70% of baseline. At the end of the experiments the area at risk was identified by an intraatrial injection of fluorescein sodium and the infarcted area determined by staining the viable tissue with para-nitrobluetetrazolium after the heart was removed and divided into 5 rings of equal thickness. To determine the transmural distribution of infarct size the myocardium was divided into two layers of equal thickness.

When the hearts were preconditioned by a 10 min total coronary artery occlusion and 15 min of reperfusion, infarct size produced by the 60 min total coronary artery occlusion (60 min TCO) was reduced similarly in the subendocardium and the subepicardium.[9] This is not a surprising finding as pigs do not have a significant coronary collateral circulation and a total occlusion therefore reduces perfusion to less than 3% of baseline in both the subendocardium and the subepicardium. Consequently the degree of ischemia was likely to be similar in the two layers. FIGURE 2 shows that when the 60 min TCO was preceded by a 70% flow reduction (70% FR) without intervening reperfusion, infarct size was reduced independent of whether the duration of the 70% FR lasted 30 min or 90 min. The beneficial effect of the 90 min 70% FR on the infarct size produced by the 60 min TCO is of particular interest as irreversible damage already started to develop during this long period of low-flow ischemia (FIG. 2). The same figure also reveals that the 30 min 70% FR reduced infarct size in both the subendocardial and subepicardial halves. With the 90 min 70% FR the protection was larger in the subepicardial than in the subendocardial half. An explanation may be that the irreversible damage produced by the 90 min 70% FR was more pronounced ($p < 0.01$) in the subendocardium than in the subepicardium. The additional necrosis produced by the 60 min TCO was not only similar for both myocardial halves ($p > 0.20$), but also so little

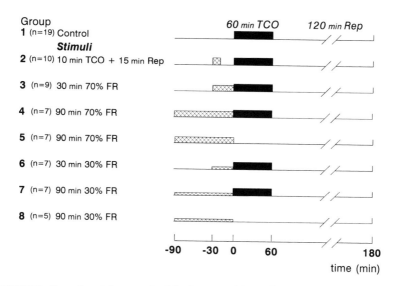

FIGURE 1. Experimental protocols of the 8 groups of domestic pigs in which the distribution of infarction size was determined after ischemic preconditioning by a partial coronary artery occlusion without intermittent reperfusion. TCO, total coronary artery occlusion (*filled bars*); Rep, reperfusion; FR, flow reduction (*hatched bars*). The number of animals which completed the experimental protocols is presented in parentheses. (From Koning *et al.*[9] Reprinted by permission from *Cardiovascular Research*.)

that infarct size at the end of the 60 min TCO was still less than in the control group. The larger protection in the subepicardium in this group of animals was thus a consequence of the less severe necrosis in the subepicardium during the 90 min 70% FR period rather than more irreversible damage during the additional 60 min TCO.

When the flow was reduced by only 30% of its baseline value for 30 min (30 min 30% FR) prior to the 60 min TCO, infarct size did not differ from that of the control animals. Extending the duration of the 30% FR period to 90 min still did not provide an adequate stimulus for cardioprotection in either the subendocardium or the subepicardium during the subsequent 60 min TCO (FIG. 3).

The results of these studies indicate that partial coronary artery occlusions can precondition the myocardium without the requirement of intervening reperfusion provided that the reduction in blood flow is sufficiently severe.[8] When the flow reduction is not severe enough to precondition the myocardium, prolonging the duration of that flow reduction appears not to be sufficient to obtain an effective stimulus.[9]

Thus the data of these experiments suggest that in this two-stage coronary occlusion model the severity of ischemia during the first stage rather than its duration is critical for the partial occlusion to be cardioprotective. It is beyond any doubt that the 30% FR resulted in myocardial ischemia as this amount of flow reduction resulted in a decreased oxygen consumption, increase in the arterio-coronary venous difference in pH (a reliable marker for lactate production by anaerobic metabolism in this model[10]), a decrease in segment shortening and the

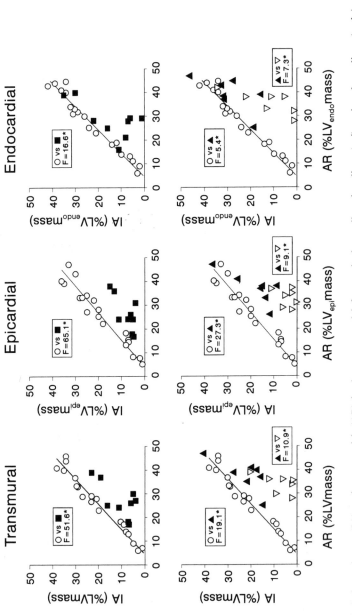

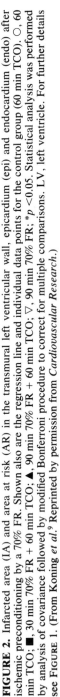

FIGURE 2. Infarcted area (IA) and area at risk (AR) in the transmural left ventricular wall, epicardium (epi) and endocardium (endo) after ischemic preconditioning by a 70% FR. Shown also are the regression line and individual data points for the control group (60 min TCO). ○, 60 min TCO; ■, 30 min 70% FR + 60 min TCO; ▲, 90 min 70% FR + 60 min TCO; ▽, 90 min 70% FR; *p <0.05. Statistical analysis was performed by analysis of covariance followed by modified Bonferroni procedure to correct for multiple comparisons. LV, left ventricle. For further details see FIGURE 1.[9] Reprinted by permission from *Cardiovascular Research*.)

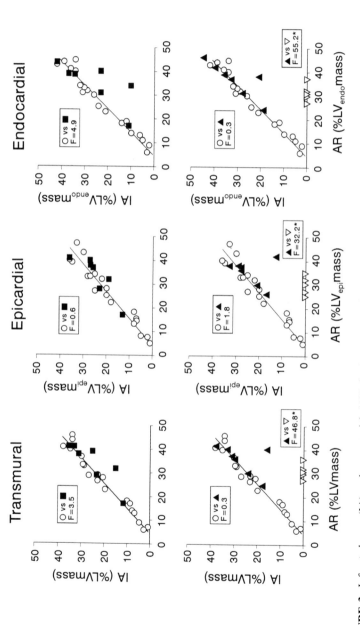

FIGURE 3. Infarcted area (IA) and area at risk (AR) in the transmural left ventricular wall, epicardium (epi) and endocardium (endo) after ischemic preconditioning by a 30% FR. ○, 60 min FR. ○ vs ■, 30 min 30% FR + 60 min TCO; ■, 90 min 30% FR + 60 min TCO; ▲, 90 min 30% FR + 60 min TCO; ▽, 90 min 30% FR; *p <0.05. For further details see FIGURE 2. (From Koning *et al.*[9] Reprinted by permission from *Cardiovascular Research*.)

appearance of post-systolic segment shortening, although the changes were less pronounced than with the 70% FR (FIG. 4).

Because partial coronary artery occlusions affect perfusion of the subendocardial layers more profoundly than of the subepicardial layers and consequently cause more severe ischemia in the subendocardial than in the subepicardial layers, we hypothesized that the protection by partial coronary artery occlusions might not be homogeneously distributed over the transmyocardial layers. For

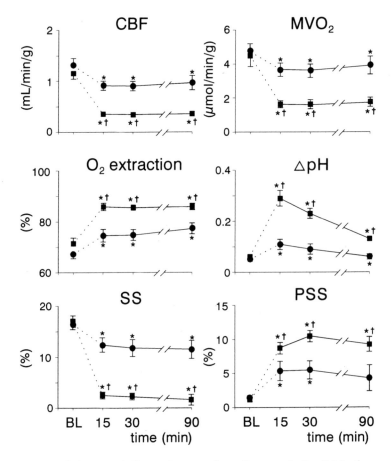

FIGURE 4. Perfusion, metabolism and contractile performance in the distribution area of the left anterior descending coronary artery during 30% (*circles*) and 70% (*squares*) coronary blood flow reductions (FR). Data are from all animals which underwent either 30% FR (n = 19) or 70% FR (n = 14). CBF, left anterior or descending coronary artery blood flow; MVO_2, myocardial oxygen consumption; O_2, myocardial oxygen extraction (the arterio-coronary venous oxygen content difference divided by the arterial oxygen content); $\triangle pH$, difference in pH of the arterial and local coronary venous blood; SS, systolic shortening; PSS, post-systolic segment shortening. *$p < 0.05$ vs baseline; †$p < 0.05$ for 70% FR vs 30% FR. (From Koning et al.[9] Reprinted with permission from *Cardiovascular Research*.)

instance, mild flow reductions could produce an insufficient degree of ischemia to precondition the subepicardium but a sufficient degree of ischemia to precondition the subendocardium. If true, this hypothesis would predict that, at least in a species with a lack of coronary collaterals, partial flow reductions preceding a total coronary artery occlusion could protect the subendocardial layers, while providing an ineffective stimulus for the subepicardial layers. On the other hand, Przyklenk *et al.*[11] showed that a brief coronary artery occlusion can also precondition the myocardium outside its own perfusion territory ("protection of virgin myocardium"), and it may therefore be argued that in the present study this "protection of virgin myocardium" negated a preferential protection for the subendocardium.

Remote Organ Protection

The observation by Przyklenk *et al.*[11] that myocardium can become protected by brief coronary artery occlusions in adjacent myocardium prompted us to investigate whether not only brief periods of ischemia in neighboring myocardium but also ischemia in other organs can precondition the myocardium. This question is even more opportune if one considers that brief periods of ischemia in organs such as kidney,[12] brain,[13] skeletal muscle,[14] and liver[15] will alleviate signs of ischemia in these organs during subsequent periods of hypoperfusion. The possibility of interorgan protection was first addressed by McClanahan *et al.*,[16] who showed that in rabbits a brief renal artery occlusion followed by reperfusion preceding a 45 min coronary artery occlusion reduced myocardial infarct size. In a number of pilot experiments we could confirm the beneficial effect of a 15 min left renal artery occlusion on infarct size produced by a 60 min coronary artery occlusion in anesthetized rats,[17] but the results of our experiments may have been affected by the body temperature of the animals as this was not rigorously controlled throughout the experiments. The effect of body temperature on both infarct size and the effectiveness of a pharmacological intervention which aims to limit infarct size has received considerable attention lately.[18-20] We therefore designed a new series of experiments in which the body temperature of the rats was rigorously controlled. In addition we not only investigated whether a brief renal artery occlusion but also whether a brief mesenteric artery occlusion could lead to cardioprotection, *i.e.*, a reduction in infarct size produced by a 60 min coronary artery occlusion.[21] The effect of brief remote organ ischemia on myocardial infarct size was investigated in the 9 groups of pentobarbital-anesthetized rats depicted in FIGURE 5. Eight groups underwent a 60 min occlusion of the left anterior descending coronary artery followed by 180 min of reperfusion during either normothermia (body core temperature 36–37°C) (groups 1–4) or hypothermia (body core temperature 30–31°C) (groups 6–9). Groups 1 and 6 served as control and underwent a 25 min sham period prior to the 60 min coronary occlusion. The other six groups underwent a 15 min occlusion of either the left anterior descending coronary artery (15 min CAO, groups 2 and 7), the mesenteric artery (15 min MAO, groups 3 and 8), or the left renal artery (15 min RAO, groups 4 and 9) followed by 10 min reperfusion before the left anterior descending coronary artery was occluded for 60 min. The normothermic rats of group 5 underwent a 15 min CAO followed by 250 min of reperfusion to determine if this brief coronary occlusion already caused irreversible myocardial damage.

The animals were instrumented for measurement of heart rate and mean arterial blood pressure, while temperature was controlled in the designated range by using

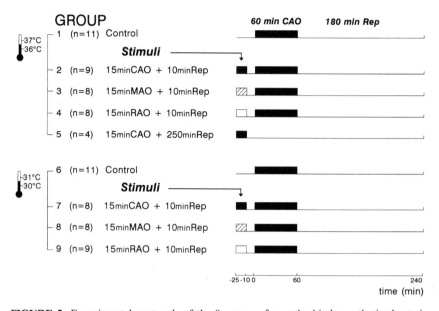

FIGURE 5. Experimental protocols of the 9 groups of pentobarbital anesthetized rats in which remote organ protection was studied. CAO, left anterior descending coronary artery occlusion (*closed bars*); MAO, mesenteric artery occlusion (*hatched bars*); RAO, left renal artery occlusion (*open bars*); Rep, reperfusion. Groups 1–5 were studied during normothermia (36–37°C) and groups 6–9 during hypothermia (30–31°C).

either heating pads or ice-filled packages. Animals that encountered ventricular fibrillation were allowed to complete the study protocol when conversion to normal sinus rhythm occurred spontaneously within 1 minute or resuscitation via gentle thumping of the thorax was successful within 2 min after the onset of ventricular fibrillation. Because of these criteria 8 out of the 84 rats had to be excluded. The excluded animals were equally distributed over all groups. At the end of the experiment, the area at risk (AR) and infarcted area (IA) were determined with standard techniques.[22,23]

There was a strong linear relationship between IA and AR of control rats which underwent only the 60 min coronary occlusion during normothermia (IA = 0.76 AR − 1.93; r^2 = 0.98, p <0.0001) (FIG. 6). Infarct size produced by the 60 min coronary occlusion in control rats was 68 ± 2% of the area at risk. A 15 min CAO, which itself resulted in negligible necrosis (IA/AR = 3 ± 1%), decreased infarct size of the subsequent 60 min coronary occlusion to 50 ± 3% (mean ± SEM, p <0.001 vs control group). A 15 min MAO produced a similar degree of protection (IA/AR = 52 ± 4%, p <0.001), but a 15 min RAO failed to protect the myocardium (IA/AR = 72 ± 5%).

In the hypothermic control group the relation between IA and AR was again highly linear, and (almost) identical to that of the normothermic control group (IA = 0.74 AR − 1.80; r^2 = 0.90, p <0.0001). The protection by 15 min CAO during hypothermia was greater (IA/AR = 22 ± 3%, p <0.001) than during normo-

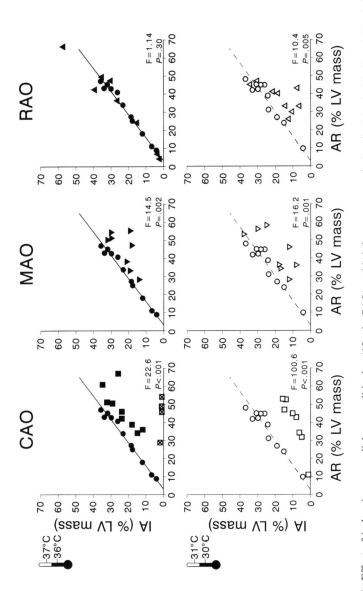

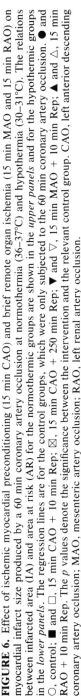

FIGURE 6. Effect of ischemic myocardial preconditioning (15 min CAO) and brief remote organ ischemia (15 min MAO and 15 min RAO) on myocardial infarct size produced by a 60 min coronary artery occlusion at normothermia (36–37°C) and hypothermia (30–31°C). The relations between infarcted area (IA) and area at risk (AR) for the normothermic groups are shown in the *upper panels* and for the hypothermic groups in the *lower panels*. The regression lines are for the control groups, which were only subjected to the 60 min coronary artery occlusion. ● and ○, control; ■ and □, 15 min CAO + 10 min Rep; ⊠, 15 min CAO + 250 min Rep; ▼ and ▽, 15 min MAO + 10 min Rep; ▲ and △, 15 min RAO + 10 min Rep. The *p* values denote the significance between the intervention and the relevant control group. CAO, left anterior descending coronary artery occlusion; MAO, mesenteric artery occlusion; RAO, left renal artery occlusion.

thermia (p <0.01). During hypothermia, 15 min MAO decreased IA/AR from 67 ± 3% to 44 ± 6% (p <0.005), which was not different from the protection by 15 min MAO during normothermia. The 15 min RAO, which was ineffective during normothermia, decreased IA/AR to 46 ± 6% (p <0.01) during hypothermia (FIG. 6).

During normothermia baseline values of heart rate (354 ± 5 bpm), mean aortic blood pressure (88 ± 3 mmHg), and the product of heart rate and systolic arterial pressure (35400 ± 1400 bpm · mmHg) did not differ between groups 1–4. Hypothermia had no significant effect on mean aortic pressure (83 ± 3 mmHg) but lowered heart rate (289 ± 8 bpm, p <0.01) and consequently the heart rate-pressure product (28400 ± 160 bpm · mmHg, p <0.01). There were also no differences between the baseline values of heart rate and blood pressure of groups 6–9.

Multivariate regression analysis revealed that the area at risk explained 99% and 96% of the variability in the infarcted area, in the normothermic and hypothermic control and 15 min MAO groups, respectively, and that the contributions of temperature or rate-pressure product *at the onset* of the 60 min coronary occlusion were therefore negligible. In both the 15 min CAO and 15 min RAO groups the area at risk alone explained 87% and 85% of the variability in the infarcted area, respectively. When also the temperature was taken into account in both groups 94% of the variability of the infarcted area could be explained, implying that the contribution of the rate-pressure product was again negligible. Thus, temperature but not different hemodynamic conditions explain the enhanced protection observed in the hypothermic 15 min RAO and 15 min CAO groups compared to the corresponding normothermic groups.

Many questions arise from this study. In the first place we have not yet addressed the mechanism by which the 15 min MAO and the 15 min RAO (during hypothermia) exert their protection, and it is therefore unknown whether their mechanism of protection differs from that of the classical ischemic preconditioning stimulus 15 min CAO. Furthermore, it is unknown whether partial or permanent occlusions of the left renal or mesenteric artery are able to protect the myocardium. If the latter would be true one could hypothesize that the cardioprotection might not be secondary to a circulating substance, released at the onset of renal or mesenteric reperfusion. The reason for the ineffectiveness of the 15 min renal artery occlusion at normothermia compared to the protection by the 15 min mesenteric artery occlusion is not clear. It must be kept in mind that although the flow through both arteries is similar, the renal artery occlusion produces less likely severe ischemia, because only approximately 10% of the renal flow serves as nutritional flow as kidney weight is approximately one eighth of the weight of the perfusion area of the mesenteric artery.

The differences in the degree of protection during normothermia and hypothermia also deserves further attention. Several earlier studies showed a dependency of body temperature on infarct size in rabbits[18] and pigs,[19] but in these animals the temperature range was varied between 35°C and 42°C (against 30°C to 36°C in our studies), while the durations of the prolonged occlusion were 30 min[18] and 45 min[19], respectively. Infarct size of the normothermic control animals was not different from that of the hypothermic control animals. On the other hand, during hypothermia the protection by 15 min CAO was considerably larger than during normothermia, while the 15 min RAO was effective only at the lower temperature. These data suggest that not the lower temperature during the 60 min TCO, but the hypothermia during the 15 min CAO and 15 min RAO was decisive. One possibility is that hypothermia inactivated enzymes involved in the processes leading to irreversible cell damage.

Ventricular Pacing

Thus it has now become evident that myocardium can become protected not only by undergoing a brief period of ischemia itself, but also by ischemia in adjacent myocardium[11] or other organs.[21] Since local ischemia is not a prerequisite for myocardial protection the question arises whether stimuli that do not produce ischemia can also protect myocardium during a subsequent prolonged coronary artery occlusion. The question was first addressed by Ovize *et al.*,[24] who showed that in anesthetized dogs increased left ventricular wall stress produced by volume overload reduced infarct size during a subsequent coronary artery occlusion. We have extended these studies by investigating the effect of ventricular pacing at a rate of 200 bpm on infarct size produced by a subsequent 60 min occlusion of the left anterior descending coronary artery in anesthetized pigs.[25] Studies were performed in anesthetized pigs, which were allocated to the experimental groups depicted in FIGURE 7. FIGURE 8 shows that when a 60 min coronary artery occlusion (60 min TCO) was preceded by a 10 min RVP + 15 min of normal sinus rhythm (NSR), myocardial infarct size was $79 \pm 3\%$, which was not different from that of the control group which underwent only the 60 min TCO ($84 \pm 2\%$). When the duration of the pacing period was increased to 30 min there was a small reduction in infarct size ($71 \pm 2\%$, $p < 0.05$ vs control), but the cardioprotective effect was most pronounced when the 60 min TCO followed the 30 min RVP without an intervening period of normal sinus rhythm ($63 \pm 4\%$, $p < 0.05$). The protection by ventricular pacing was significant but considerably less than after ischemic preconditioning by a 10 min TCO + 15 min Rep.[8,9] Similarly, the duration of the

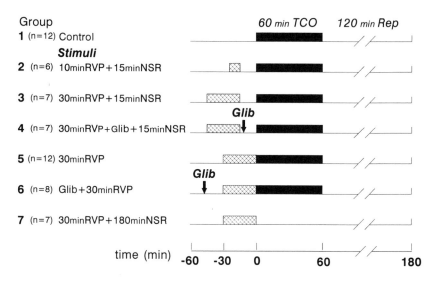

FIGURE 7. Experimental protocols of the 7 groups of domestic swine in which the effect of rapid ventricular pacing at 200 bpm on infarct size produced by a subsequent 60 min total coronary artery occlusion was studied. *Filled bars,* 60 min total coronary artery occlusion (60 min TCO); *hatched bars,* rapid ventricular pacing (RVP). NSR, normal sinus rhythm; Rep, reperfusion; Glib, glibenclamide (1 mg/kg, iv). (From Koning *et al.*[25] Reprinted by permission from *Circulation.*)

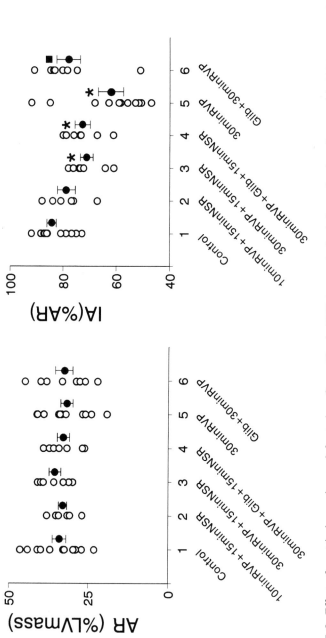

FIGURE 8. Effect of ventricular pacing on infarct size after a 60 min TCO in anesthetized domestic pigs. Area at risk (AR) expressed as percentage of left ventrical mass and the infarct area (IA) expressed as percentage of the area at risk are presented for each group. Individual data are indicated by *open circles*; mean data (± SEM) of each group are indicated by the *solid circles*. *p <0.05 vs control, ■p <0.05 vs 30 min RVP. (From Verdouw *et al.*[21] Reprinted by permission from *Basic Research in Cardiology*.)

protection by ventricular pacing was also considerably shorter than after ischemic preconditioning with 10 min TCO + 15 min Rep. With the latter the protective effect was not attenuated when the duration of the intermittent reperfusion period was increased to 60 min.[26] To investigate whether, in analogy to ischemic preconditioning,[27-29] activation of K^+_{ATP} channels was involved in the protection by ventricular pacing, the effect of 30 min RVP on infarct size produced by a 60 min TCO was also studied after pretreatment with 1 mg/kg glibenclamide, a dose sufficient to abolish the protection by ischemic myocardial preconditioning in pigs.[29] In FIGURE 8 it is shown that pretreatment with glibenclamide abolished the protection by 30 min RVP. However, continued activation of K^+_{ATP} channels proved not to be mandatory, as administration of glibenclamide after the 30 min RVP during the 15 min of normal sinus rhythm did not attenuate the protection in this group of animals (73 ± 3% vs 71 ± 2%, ns). These data are at variance with the results obtained with ischemic preconditioning by a brief coronary artery occlusion, as glibenclamide abolished the protective effect of the brief coronary artery occlusion irrespective of whether treatment occurred before or after the brief coronary occlusion.[29]

In earlier studies it was shown that 2 min of ventricular pacing protected the myocardium against the occurrence of ventricular arrhythmias and fibrillation during a subsequent coronary occlusion.[30] In that study dog hearts were paced at 300 bpm, which increased left ventricular end-diastolic pressure and produced ST segment changes indicative of myocardial ischemia. The authors concluded that ventricular pacing produced ischemia and therefore protected the myocardium by ischemic preconditioning. In the present study the left ventricle was paced at a lower rate (200 bpm), which may explain why left ventricular end-diastolic pressure did not increase.[25] Furthermore, a number of functional and metabolic parameters failed to indicate the presence of ischemia during ventricular pacing. Thus, (i) transmural myocardial blood flow remained normally distributed across the left ventricular wall, (ii) the decrease in systolic shortening was entirely due to a decrease in end-diastolic length, (iii) post-systolic shortening did not develop and (iv) there were no changes in myocardial levels of ATP and phosphocreatine, energy charge and arterial or coronary venous pH and PCO_2. Further evidence that ischemia did not occur during ventricular pacing was the absence of (v) no reactive hyperemia and (vi) the immediate recovery of systolic segment shortening, *i.e.*, no development of myocardial stunning after pacing was stopped. Even if myocardial ischemia went undetected by these parameters, it is unlikely that in view of the inability of the 30% flow reduction, which showed all the signs of ischemia (FIG. 4), to precondition the myocardium, the severity of ischemia would have been sufficient to precondition the myocardium. Therefore, we wish to conclude that ventricular pacing protected the myocardium during the subsequent 60 min TCO by activation of K^+_{ATP} channels via a mechanism not involving myocardial ischemia.

CONCLUSIONS

The major conclusions from these studies are that under proper conditions myocardium can be protected against irreversible damage by partial coronary occlusions without intermittent reperfusion and stimuli that produce ischemia in organs remote from the heart as well as stimuli which do not lead to ischemia at all. These findings broaden the concept of cardioprotection and suggest that ischemic myocardial preconditioning may be just one of many triggers capable of reducing infarct size produced by a prolonged coronary occlusion. Many points remain unresolved, as we have not investigated whether all these stimuli operate via a common end point, possibly activated by different triggers. Interestingly, it was recently shown that stretch-induced cardioprotection was abolished when animals were pretreated with the K^+_{ATP} channel blocker glibenclamide, suggesting that K^+_{ATP} channels could be such an intermediate.[31]

The present observations definitely complicate the interpretation of clinical studies that try to find proof of the occurrence of ischemic preconditioning in man,[32-34] as not only angina prior to infarction, but also transient ischemia in other organs and forms of stress which do not produce ischemia can determine infarct size.

SUMMARY

Ischemic preconditioning studies employ one or more brief total coronary artery occlusions separated by complete reperfusion to limit infarct size during a subsequent prolonged coronary artery occlusion. We now present evidence that in anesthetized pigs a partial coronary artery occlusion without intervening reperfusion between the partial and prolonged total occlusions can also precondition the myocardium provided that the reduction in coronary blood flow is sufficiently severe. Thus infarct size was reduced after a 60 min total coronary artery occlusion when the total occlusion was preceded by a partial coronary occlusion that reduced coronary blood flow by 70% but not when the flow reduction was only 30%. In this two-stage coronary occlusion model the degree of protection appears greater in the epicardial than in the endocardial half.

In view of evidence that brief occlusions of a coronary artery also protect myocardium outside its perfusion territory, we subsequently investigated whether ischemia in remote organs can protect myocardium. Because of reports that development of infarct size may be temperature dependent, we also investigated whether the cardioprotection by remote organ ischemia was temperature dependent. In anesthetized rats a 15 min coronary artery occlusion was more effective in reducing infarct size produced by a subsequent 60 min total coronary artery occlusion when the experiments were performed at a body core temperature of 30–31°C than at 36–37°C, while infarct size of animals which were subjected to only the 60 min total coronary artery occlusion was the same for the two body core temperatures. In rats with a body core temperature of 36–37°C a 15 min mesenteric artery occlusion, but not a 15 min renal artery occlusion, reduced infarct size produced by a subsequent 60 min coronary artery occlusion. When the experiments were performed at 30–31°C both the mesenteric and renal artery occlusions were protective. These observations indicate the local myocardial ischemia is not required to protect the myocardium during a prolonged coronary occlusion.

We further investigated whether myocardium could also be protected by a cardiac stimulus which does not produce ischemia at all. For this purpose we electrically paced the left ventricle of anesthetized pigs to produce heart rates of 200 bpm (which did not lead to ischemia as assessed by a number of functional and biochemical variables) and found that 30 min of ventricular pacing reduced myocardial infarct size produced by a subsequent 60 min coronary artery occlusion. The protection by ventricular pacing involved activation of K^+_{ATP} channels as pretreatment with glibenclamide abolished the protection by ventricular pacing.

We conclude that a number of distinctly different stimuli can protect the myocardium suggesting that ischemic myocardial preconditioning could be just one feature of a more general protection phenomenon.

REFERENCES

1. MURRY, C. E., R. B. JENNINGS & K. A. REIMER. 1986. Preconditioning with ischemia: a delay of lethal cell injury in ischemic myocardium. Circulation **74:** 1124–1136.
2. LAWSON, C. S. & J. M. DOWNEY. 1993. Preconditioning: state of art myocardial protection. Cardiovasc. Res. **27:** 542–550.
3. SCHOTT, R. J., S. ROHMANN, E. R. BRAUN & W. SCHAPER. 1990. Ischemic preconditioning reduces infarct size in swine myocardium. Circ. Res. **66:** 1133–1142.
4. HARRIS, A. S. 1950. Delayed development of ventricular ectopic rhythms following experimental coronary occlusion. Circulation **1:** 1318–1328.
5. HAGAR, J. M., S. L. HALE & R. A. KONER. 1991. Effect of preconditioning ischemia on reperfusion arrhythmias after coronary artery occlusion and reperfusion in the rat. Circ. Res. **68:** 61–68.
6. VEGH, A., S. KOMORO, L. SZEKERES & J. R. PARRATT. 1992. Antiarrhythmic effects of preconditioning in anaesthetised dogs and rats. Cardiovasc. Res. **26:** 487–495.
7. OVIZE, M., K. PRZYKLENK & R. A. KONER. 1992. Partial coronary stenosis is sufficient and complete reperfusion is mandatory for preconditioning the canine heart. Circ. Res. **71:** 1165–1173.
8. KONING, M. M. G., L. A. J. SIMONIS, S. DE ZEEUW, S. NIEUKOOP, S. POST & P. D. VERDOUW. 1994. Ischaemic preconditioning by partial occlusion without intermittent reperfusion. Cardiovasc. Res. **28:** 1146–1151.
9. KONING, M. M. G., B. C. G. GHO, E. VAN KLAARWATER, D. J. DUNCKER & P. D. VERDOUW. 1995. Endocardial and epicardial infarct size after preconditioning by a partial coronary artery occlusion without intervening reperfusion. Cardiovasc. Res. **30:** 1017–1027.
10. SCHAMHARDT, H. C., P. D. VERDOUW & P. R. SAXENA. 1981. Effects of oxyfedrine on global haemodynamics and myocardial lactate balance in acute ischaemia of the porcine hearts preparation. Arzneim. Forsch./Drug Res. **31:** 1091–1095.
11. PRZYKLENK, K., B. BAUER, M. OVIZE, R. A. KONER & P. WHITTAKER. 1993. Regional ischemic "preconditioning" protects remote virgin myocardium from subsequent sustained coronary occlusion. Circulation **87:** 893–899.
12. ZAGER, R. A., L. A. BALTES, H. M. SHARMA & M. S. JURKOWITHZ. 1984. Responses of the ischemic acute renal failure kidney to additional ischemic events. Kidney Int. **26:** 689–700.
13. KITAGAWA, K., M. MATSUMOTO, M. TAGAYA, R. HTA, H. UEDA, M. NIINOBE, N. HANDA, R. FUKUNAGA, K. KIMURA, K. MIKOSHIBA & T. KAMADA. 1990. 'Ischemic tolerance' phenomenon found in the brain. Brain Res. **528:** 21–24.
14. MOUNSEY, R. A., C. Y. PANG & C. FORREST. 1992. Preconditioning: a new technique for improved muscle flap survival. Otolaryngol. Head Neck Surg. **107:** 549–552.
15. LLORIS-CARSI, J. M., D. CEJALVO, L. H. TOLEDO-PEREYRA, M. A. CALVO & S. SUZUKI. 1993. Preconditioning: effect upon lesion modulation in warm liver ischemia. Transplant. Proc. **25:** 3303–3304.
16. MCCLANAHAN, T. B., B. S. NAO, L. J. WOLKE, B. J. MARTIN, T. E. METZ & K. P. GALLAGHER. 1993. Brief renal occlusion and reperfusion reduces myocardial infarct size in rabbits. FASEB J. **7:** A118,682 (abstract).
17. GHO, B. C. G., R. G. SCHOEMAKER, C. VAN DER LEE, H. S. SHARMA & P. D. VERDOUW. 1994. Cardioprotection by transient renal ischemia, an *in vivo* study in rats. Circulation **90:** 1476 (abstract).
18. CHIEN, G. L., R. A. WOLFF, R. F. DAVIS & D. M. VAN WINKLE. 1994. "Normothermic range" temperature affects myocardial infarct size. Cardiovasc. Res. **28:** 1014–1017.
19. DUNCKER, D. J., C. L. KLASSEN, Y. ISHIBASHI, S. H. HERRLINGER, T. J. PAVEK &

R. J. BACHE. 1995. Effect of temperature on myocardial infarction in swine. Am. J. Physiol. In press.

20. McCLANAHAN, T. B., T. E. MERTZ, B. J. MARTIN & K. P. GALLAGHER. 1994. Pentostatin reduces infarct size in pigs only when combined with mild hypothermia. Circulation **90:** 1478 (abstract).

21. VERDOUW, P. D., B. C. G. GHO & D. J. DUNCKER. 1996. Cardioprotection by organs in stress or distress. Basic Res. Cardiol. **91:** 44–46.

22. FISHBEIN, M. C., D. MacLEAN & P. R. MAROKO. 1978. Experimental myocardial infarction in the rat. Am. J. Pathol. **90:** 57–70.

23. SCHOEMAKER, R. G., J. URQUHART, J. J. M. DEBETS, H. A. J. STRUYKER-BOUDIER & J. F. M. SMITS. 1990. Acute hemodynamic effects of coronary artery ligation in conscious rats. Basic Res. Cardiol. **85:** 9–20.

24. OVIZE, M., R. A. KLONER & K. PRZYKLENK. 1994. Stretch preconditions canine myocardium. Am. J. Physiol. **266:** H137–H146.

25. KONING, M. M. G., B. C. G. GHO, E. VAN KLAARWATER, R. L. J. OPSTAL, D. J. DUNCKER & P. D. VERDOUW. 1996. Rapid ventricular pacing produces myocardial protection by non-ischemic activation of K^+_{ATP} channels. Circulation. **93:** 178–186.

26. KONING, M. M. G., S. DE ZEEUW, S. NIEUKOOP, J. W. DE JONG & P. D. VERDOUW. 1994. Is myocardial infarct size limitation by ischemic preconditioning an "all or nothing" phenomenon? In Cellular, Biochemical and Molecular Aspects of Reperfusion Injury. D. K. Das, Ed. Ann. N. Y. Acad. Sci. **723:** 333–336.

27. GROSS, G. J. & J. A. AUCHAMPACH. 1992. Blockade of ATP-sensitive potassium channels prevents myocardial preconditioning. Circ. Res. **70:** 223–233.

28. ROHMANN, S., H. WEYGANDT, P. SCHELLING, L. K. SOEI, K. H. BECKER, P. D. VERDOUW, I. LUES & G. HAUSLER. 1994. Effect of Bimakalim (EMD 52692), an opener of ATP-sensitive potassium channels, on infarct size, coronary blood flow, regional wall function, and oxygen consumption in swine. Cardiovasc. Res. **28:** 858–863.

29. ROHMANN, S., H. WEYGANDT, P. SCHELLING, L. K. SOEI, P. D. VERDOUW & L. LUES. 1994. Involvement of ATP-sensitive potassium channels in ischemic preconditioning protection. Basic Res. Cardiol. **89:** 563–576.

30. VEGH, A., L. SZEKERES & J. R. PARRATT. 1991. Transient ischaemia induced by rapid cardiac pacing results in myocardial preconditioning. Cardiovasc. Res. **25:** 1051–1053.

31. MARGONARI, H., M. OVIZE, G. RIOUFOL, A. GYSEMBERGH, C. POP, X. ANDRE-FOUET & Y. MINAIRE. 1995. Blockade of K^+_{ATP} channels prevents stretch-induced preconditioning. Circulation **92**(Suppl): I251 (abstract).

32. KLONER, R. A. & D. YELLON. 1994. Does ischemic preconditioning occur in patients? J. Am. Coll. Cardiol. **24:** 1133–1142.

33. LAWSON, C. S. Does ischemic preconditioning occur in the human heart? Cardiovasc. Res. **28:** 1133–1142.

34. VERDOUW, P. D., B. C. G. GHO & D. J. DUNCKER. 1995. Ischemic preconditioning: is it clinically relevant? Eur. Heart J. **16:** 1169–1176.

Contribution to the Factors Involved in the Protective Effect of Ischemic Preconditioning

The Role of Catecholamines and Protein Kinase C[a]

TANYA RAVINGEROVÁ,[b] MIROSLAV BARANČÍK,
DEZIDER PANCZA, JÁN STYK, ATTILA ZIEGELHÖFFER,
WOLFGANG SCHAPER,[c] AND JÁN SLEZÁK

Institute for Heart Research
Slovak Academy of Sciences
Bratislava, Slovakia
and
[c]Max Planck Institute
Department of Experimental Cardiology
Bad Nauheim, Germany

INTRODUCTION

A novel approach to myocardial protection against ischemia by way of adaptation of the heart to ischemia during preceding brief episodes of the same ischemic stress triggering endogenous protective mechanisms has been recently developed and termed ischemic preconditioning (IP).[1,2] Short-term adaptation induced by IP includes attenuation of myocardial dysfunction and reduction of cell necrosis and of life-threatening arrhythmias.[3–5] Protection is believed to be mediated by the mechanisms of cell signaling, suggesting that different parts of the signal transduction cascade might represent the targets for the pharmacological induction of IP. A number of substances, both protective and deleterious, are known to be released in the myocardium during early ischemia and to modulate the severity of ischemic injury.[6,7] As a matter of fact, a general approach to the pharmacological induction of preconditioning was either to potentiate the effects of protective substances or to antagonize the deleterious effects of the toxic substances. Some of these potentially protective substances (*e.g.*, adenosine) have been implicated as mediators of IP, and stimulation of the A1 receptors by selective adenosine analogues has been shown to induce the IP-like effect and to reduce infarct size.[4,8] However, this does not seem to be a universal mechanism of protection, since in the rat heart IP has not been found to be mediated by adenosine.[3] Furthermore, it does not account for the antiarrhythmic effect of IP in the canine model.[9]

An alternative approach to trigger the IP-like protection pharmacologically is to utilize potentially deleterious substances, such as catecholamines, as a tool to

[a] This study was supported, in part, by the EC COST Grant "Endogenous Cardioprotection" (CIPA CT 92 4009) and by Slovak Grant Agency for Science Grants Nos. 2/1257/95 and 2/1258/95.

[b] Address for correspondence: Dr. T. Ravingerová, Institute for Heart Research, Slovak Academy of Sciences, Dubravska cesta 9, 842 33 Bratislava, Slovakia. Fax: 427 376 637.

43

induce a short-term stress, but without harmful consequences of the ischemic stress. In other words, preconditioning can be simulated by either endogenously released catecholamines or by exogenous catecholamines applied shortly before the induction of long-lasting ischemia. Recent reports have shown that preconditioning with catecholamines can protect the heart against postischemic myocardial stunning in rats[10,11] and reduce infarct size in rabbits,[12] and that the effect is mediated mainly via stimulation of α1-adrenergic receptors. Although several lines of evidence indicate that under certain conditions catecholamines might exert a protective effect in the myocardium, their role in the mechanisms of protection is not fully understood.

Both, α1-adrenergic and A1 receptor stimulation can activate parallel pathways in the myocardium leading to a common effector. Protein kinase C (PKC) is believed to play the key role in signal transduction mechanisms underlying IP since it serves as a link between different pathways. There is some experimental evidence that IP cascade involves α1-adrenergic (or A1) stimulation and G protein-mediated activation of PKC and its translocation (at least of some of its isoforms) from the cytosol to the cellular membrane leading to phosphorylation of some (yet unknown) proteins.[13–15] Moreover, pharmacological activation of PKC has been shown to cause protection against infarction in rabbits[16] and rats.[17] However, this protection has not been found in pigs.[18] Neither did exogenous activation of PKC protect the rat heart against arrhythmias,[17] indicating that different effects might be mediated by different signaling pathways.

The present study was designed to evaluate some possibilities of pharmacological induction of preconditioning. We have chosen different end points of preconditioning and different mechanisms of preconditioning cascade. Most of the studies of the IP-like effect of catecholamines have used the recovery of contractile function or infarct size limitation, as the end points, and only a few have investigated the effect of catecholamine-induced preconditioning on ischemic arrhythmias. In the rat model we have chosen arrhythmias as an end point. Since indirect evidence indicates that catecholamines can stimulate the Na/K pump and prevent the loss of K^+ from the cells during ischemia,[19,20] we hypothesized that any intervention capable of improving the transport of ions through the cell membrane might contribute to the antiarrhythmic effect. Preconditioning with adenosine has been found to protect the pig heart against infarction.[8] However, the role of PKC in pharmacologically induced preconditioning (e.g., by adenosine analogues, or by catecholamines) has not been elucidated so far. Accordingly, our aims were to investigate: i) whether stimulation of adrenergic receptors with exogenous norepinephrine can afford protection against arrhythmias in rats, and whether it is accompanied by changes in the activity of Na/K ATPase in the cell membrane; and ii) whether stimulation of A1 receptors in porcine heart by adenosine analogue resulting in the infarct size limitation involves activation of PKC.

METHODS

Isolated Heart Preparation

Perfusion Technique

All studies were performed in accordance with the Guide for the Care and Use of Laboratory Animals published by the US National Institutes of Health (NIH publication No 85-23, revised 1985). Male Wistar rats (250–300 g) were heparinized (500 IU, i.p.) and anesthetized (sodium pentobarbitone, 40 mg/kg, i.p.). Ten minutes later the hearts were excised and perfused (Langendorff mode) at a constant flow of 10 ml/min. Krebs-Henseleit solution contained (in mM): NaCl 118.0; KCl 3.2; $MgSO_4$ 1.2; $NaHCO_3$ 25.0; NaH_2PO_4 1.18; $CaCl_2$ 2.5; glucose 11.1; Na pyruvate 2.0; it was gassed (95% O_2 + 5% CO_2) and maintained at 37°C; pH 7.4. Epicardial ECG was recorded by means of two stainless steel electrodes attached to the apex of the heart and the aortic cannula. Heart rate was calculated from the ECG and continuously monitored on Mingograph ELEMA (Sweden).

Perfusion Protocol

After stabilization of the hearts for 20 min, regional ischemia lasting 30 min was induced by occlusion of the LAD coronary artery (n = 15). Efficacy of occlusion was confirmed by a 45% increase in perfusion pressure. Arrhythmias were analyzed in accordance with Lambeth Conventions[21] by counting the total number of ventricular premature beats (VPB), by determining the incidences of ventricular tachycardia (VT) and fibrillation (VF) and their duration. VF lasting more than 2 min was considered as sustained, and in such hearts normal sinus rhythm has never been restored. In addition, severity of arrhythmias was evaluated by means of an arrhythmia score ranging from 1 (for VPBs) to 5 (for sustained VF).

To simulate ischemic preconditioning, exogenous norepinephrine (Arterenol, SIGMA, NE) was introduced before the onset of ischemia in the following way: a short 5-min infusion (1 μM) followed by a 10-min washout (n = 18). After 30 min of ischemia the hearts were freeze-clamped and stored at -70°C for the estimation of Na/K ATPase activity. The same procedure was also performed in the time-matched treated and untreated controls (n = 9 for each group).

Na/K ATPase Activity

The fraction of cardiac sarcolemma was prepared by the method of hypotonic shock combined with the treatment with NaJ.[22] The protein content was assayed according to Lowry *et al.*[23] using bovine serum albumin as a standard. The activity of Na/K ATPase was measured at 37°C in the presence of ATP (0.08–6.0 mM) by incubating 30–50 μg of membrane proteins in a total volume of 0.5 ml of medium containing 50 mM imidazole (pH 7.4) and metallic cofactors (in mM): $MgCl_2$ 4, NaCl 100, KCl 10. Following 10 min of preincubation in substrate free medium, the reaction was started by addition of ATP, and after a reaction period of 20 min it was terminated by 1 ml of 12% ice cold trichloroacetic acid. The inorganic phosphate (Pi) liberated by ATP splitting was determined by the method of Tausski and Shorr.[24] Enzyme activity was determined as the difference between the amount of Pi liberated in the presence of all three cofactors and of Mg only.

Preconditioning in Pigs

The model of IP in pigs inducing a significant reduction of infarct size has already been described.[18] The same degree of protection has been demonstrated with A1-receptor agonist N^6-cyclohexyladenosine (CHA).[8] In brief, to mimic preconditioning, CHA (1.5 mM) was microinfused for 10 minutes to the left ventricle of the pigs. The samples for investigation of PKC activity were obtained from the treated and untreated myocardium by drill biopsy immediately after the end of infusion and frozen in liquid N_2.

Assay of Protein Kinase C (PKC) Activity

The biopsy samples from the control and CHA-treated myocardial tissue were homogenized in buffer A containing 20 mM Tris-HCl, 0.25 M sucrose, 1.0 mM EDTA, 1.0 mM EGTA, 1.0 mM DTT, 0.5 mM PMSF (pH 7.4) and the homogenate was centrifuged at 1000 × g for 10 min at 4°C. The supernatant after this low-speed centrifugation was centrifuged again for 60 min at 150,000 × g (4°C). The resulting supernatant represented the cytosolic fraction, the pellet was designed as a particulate (membrane) fraction. After solubilization of particulate proteins with 1% Triton X-100, proteins from both cytosolic and membrane fractions were subjected to DEAE-Sephacel minicolumns equilibrated with buffer B (20 mM Tris-HCl, 0.5 mM EGTA, 0.5 mM DTT and 0.5 mM PMSF (pH 7.4)). The bound proteins were eluted with buffer B containing 400 mM NaCl, and the eluate was used for determination of PKC activity. PKC activity was assayed by measuring the incorporation of ^{32}P into lysine-rich histone III-S. The standard assay mixture contained 20 mM Tris-HCl (pH 7.4), 10 mM magnesium chloride, 400 μg/ml histone III-S, 35 μl of DEAE-Sephacel fraction with or without phosphatidylserine (80 μg/ml), diacylglycerol (16 μg/ml) and calcium (2 mM). The incubation was started by addition of 50 μM [χ-^{32}P] ATP (400–1000 cpm/pmol) and terminated after 15 min by spotting of aliquots of the reaction mixtures to phosphocellulose P81 filters. The filters were extensively washed with phosphoric acid and the amount of ^{32}P-labeled histone III-S on the P81 filter was quantitated by liquid scintillation counting. PKC activity was calculated as a difference between basal activity (without calcium and lipids) and the stimulated PKC activity per miligram proteins. Protein concentrations were determined according to the method of Bradford[25] using bovine serum albumin as a standard.

Statistical evaluation was performed using a one-way analysis of variance (ANOVA) followed by the unpaired Student's t test for Gaussian distributed data, as well as a χ^2 test for binomially distributed variables. $p < 0.05$ was considered as significant.

RESULTS

Isolated Heart Preparation

In the control group, severe ventricular arrhythmias including VT and VF occurred between 10 and 20 min of ischemia in 87% and 73% of hearts, respectively (Fig. 1, top). A total number of VPBs was 542 ± 84 (Fig. 1, bottom). In contrast, in the NE-treated group, only 44% of hearts exhibited VT, VF occurred in 11% of hearts ($p < 0.05$), and a total number of VPBs was significantly reduced to 25 ± 11 ($p < 0.01$).

In addition, duration of both VT and VF was significantly decreased after NE treatment (TABLE 1): VT lasted 4.5 ± 2 s (vs 82 ± 30 s in controls), duration of VF was 96 ± 24 s (vs 216 ± 24 s in the control group). Accordingly, the severity of arrhythmias was significantly lower after administration of NE (TABLE 1). Arrhythmia score in this group was reduced to 1.8 ± 0.4 from 3.9 ± 0.8 in the control group ($p < 0.01$).

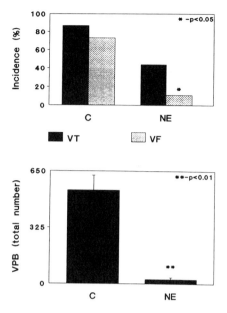

FIGURE 1. Ischemia-induced ventricular arrhythmias in the isolated rat heart. VT—ventricular tachycardia, VF—ventricular fibrillation, VPB—ventricular premature beat, C—untreated controls, NE—norepinephrine-treated hearts. Data are means ± SEM of 15–18 experiments. *p <0.05, **p <0.01 vs untreated controls.

Hemodynamic Effects of Norepinephrine

Infusion of NE in the isolated hearts caused a transient increase in heart rate and in perfusion pressure by approximately 15–20%. These effects, however, were short-lasting and completely disappeared by the end of a 10-min washout period.

Na/K ATPase Activity

Infusion of NE did not change the enzyme activity in the heart sarcolemmal fraction before the induction of ischemia (FIG. 2). Ischemia led to a considerable depression in the activity of Na/K ATPase in the untreated group. In contrast, in the NE-treated group, no decrease in the activity of the enzyme was observed after 30 min of ischemia. It was maintained on the initial preischemic level (with a tendency to a slight increase), as compared to both untreated and treated controls before ischemia.

TABLE 1. Effect of Acute Pretreatment with Norepinephrine on Duration and Severity of Ischemic Arrhythmias[a]

	Control Hearts	NE-Treated Hearts
Duration (sec):		
VT	82 ± 30	4.5 ± 2*
VF	216 ± 24	96 ± 24*
Severity (AS)	3.9 ± 0.8	1.8 ± 0.4*

[a]Abbreviations as in FIGURE 1. Data are means ± SEM of 15–18 experiments. *p <0.01.

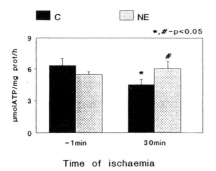

Time of ischaemia

FIGURE 2. The effect of norepinephrine on the activity of the sarcolemmal Na/K ATPase in the rat heart subjected to ischemia. C—untreated groups; NE—norepinephrine-treated groups. Data are means ± SEM of 9–12 experiments expressed in μmol ATP/mg prot./h. *$p < 0.05$ vs nonischemic untreated group; #$p < 0.05$ vs ischemic untreated group.

Protein Kinase C Activity

Protein kinase C activity was assessed in cytosolic (C) and membrane (M) preparations isolated from control and CHA-treated myocardium and expressed as the ratio of membrane-bound to total specific PKC activity (M/[M + C]). As demonstrated in FIGURE 3, treatment of porcine myocardium with A1-receptor agonist N6-cyclohexyladenosine (CHA) did not change significantly the myocardial PKC activity.

DISCUSSION

The main objective of this study was to evaluate some possibilities to induce a short-term adaptation to ischemic stress by utilizing mechanisms of cell signaling operating in ischemic preconditioning. We chose different approaches towards pharmacological induction of protection by applying either potentially protective (adenosine) or potentially deleterious (noradrenaline) substance in two different models and by following two different end-points of preconditioning—reduction in the size of infarction and in the incidence of severe arrhythmias. These pharmacological interventions activate different pathways of signal transduction by stimulating either A1 or adrenergic receptors. However, in spite of these differences, they may share common postreceptor transduction leading through central mediators (G proteins, coupled to both A1 and α1 receptors) to common effector protein kinase C. Our further objective was, therefore, to investigate whether PKC is involved in protection against infarction induced by A1 agonist (CHA) in porcine myocardium. In the rat model of preconditioning, PKC has not been implicated

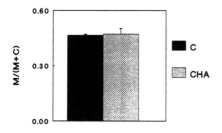

FIGURE 3. Protein kinase C (PKC) activity in the porcine myocardium. PKC activity was determined in the membraneous (M) and cytosolic (C) preparations isolated from the left ventricular drill biopsies taken from the control (n = 5) tissue and after N6-cyclohexyladenosine (CHA; n = 5) microinfusion. PKC activity was expressed as the ratio of membrane-bound to total specific PKC activity [M/(M + C)]. Data are means ± SEM.

as a main mechanism of protection against arrhythmias,[17] probably due to its proarrhythmic properties. Therefore, in this model, our interest was turned to other factors modulating arrhythmogenesis during ischemia. A disturbed homeostasis of ions is considered as a main source of electrical instability of the heart. We recently demonstrated that stimulation of the Na/K pump by pretreatment with 7-oxo prostacyclin can lead to a significant suppression of arrhythmias.[26] From this point of view, the role of Na/K ATPase as a possible target for catecholamine action in the cell membrane is extremely important.

Endogenous catecholamines have been shown to be released early in the course of myocardial ischemia.[27] Accordingly, the protective effect of a brief ischemia-induced stress has been suggested to be mediated via endogenously released catecholamines, and, therefore, to be mimicked by exogenously applied catecholamines.[12] In general, it is believed that under conditions of myocardial ischemia, excess catecholamines exacerbate arrhythmias by facilitating calcium influx into the cells and enhancing automaticity and triggered activity.[28,29] Moreover, high concentrations of catecholamines can damage the myocardium and cause leucocyte infiltration, myofibrillar degeneration, and cell necrosis.[30] However, electrophysiological response of the heart to catecholamines may be different, depending on the species differences, location in the myocardium, and whether myocardium is normal or injured. Stimulation of β-adrenergic receptors induces proarrhythmic effects in the normal myocardium, such as refractory period shortening. On the other hand, α1-adrenergic stimulation (which is more important under pathological conditions) prolongs refractoriness, increases action potential duration and conduction velocity, and decreases automaticity, the effects which in general are considered to be antiarrhythmic.[31] In partially depolarized myocardium arrhythmogenic effects of catecholamines might be attenuated.[32] In addition, a large number of controversial reports have shown that antiadrenergic/sympathetic interventions sometimes have little or no effect on arrhythmias.[33]

The results of this study demonstrate that ischemia-induced severe ventricular arrhythmias can be suppressed by a pharmacological induction of preconditioning. Administration of noradrenaline served as a tool to simulate a brief ischemia-induced stress, but without the harmful consequences of ischemia. An antiarrhythmic effect has been demonstrated in acute experiments mimicking "classical" IP, in which both the incidence and the duration of sustained ischemia-induced VF and VT were significantly attenuated (FIG. 1, TABLE 1).

These results are consistent with the finding of Parratt *et al.*[34] that infusion of exogenous catecholamines can protect the rat heart against ischemia-induced arrhythmias *in vivo*. Other evidence that catecholamines can mimic the effect of preconditioning on ischemia-induced ventricular arrhythmias has been provided in the study by Vegh *et al.*[35] in anesthetized dogs. Furthermore, as we showed recently,[36] pretreatment of rats with norepinephrine *in vivo* can afford a delayed protection against arrhythmias 24 h after administration and consequently improve the survival of the animals. Delayed protection afforded by administration of norepinephrine seems to resemble the "second window of protection," which also appears several hours after preconditioning,[37,38] when the acute effect is already lost.

The antiarrhythmic effect of preconditioning with NE was accompanied by the preservation of the activity of Na/K ATPase after ischemia on the preischemic level, while in the control hearts ischemia resulted in a significant decrease of the enzyme activity (FIG. 2). This finding is consistent with the results of Clausen[39] showing that catecholamines can activate electrogenic transport of Na^+ and K^+ through the cell membrane leading to its hyperpolarization. Since the loss of

K^+ from the cells is considered an important factor of arrhythmogenesis during ischemia,[40] preservation of the ionic homeostasis due to an improved function of the Na/K pump could contribute to the maintenance of electrical stability of the cell membranes. This is in agreement with a recent finding of Tosaki *et al.*[41] that α-adrenergic stimulation of the rat heart not only preconditions it against reperfusion-induced arrhythmias, but also reduces ischemia- and reperfusion-induced Na^+ and Ca^{2+} gains and prevents K^+ and Mg^{2+} loss.

On the other hand, we cannot exclude a direct adrenergic effect of catecholamines on the myocardium triggering adaptive processes mediated via the signal transduction system. It was recently demonstrated by Richard *et al.*[42] that adrenergic stimulation of isolated rat heart by exogenous noradrenaline stimulates adenosine formation in the heart, similarly to ischemia-induced nonexocytotic noradrenaline release. The effect of noradrenaline on the release of adenosine has been shown to be mediated via β-adrenoceptor stimulation. It can be inferred thus that activation of adenosine receptors may occur before the onset of ischemia and trigger a further cascade of events. On the other hand, Winter *et al.*[43] have demonstrated that in rats, α-adrenoceptor-mediated preconditioning does not involve adenosine receptors. Thus, the role of adenosine (or A1 agonists) in myocardial preconditioning in rats has to be discounted, and it has been also confirmed by Asimakis *et al.*[3]

On the contrary, in the species like rabbits, dogs and pigs the role of adenosine in mediating protection has been well documented.[4,8,44] Stimulation of A1 receptors with adenosine analogues has been found to protect the heart against infarction and postischemic myocardial dysfunction. It was recently suggested[16] that both noradrenaline and adenosine endogenous ligands can initiate a pathway leading to the translocation and activation of PKC and subsequently to PKC-dependent phosphorylation of some effector proteins inducing protection. However, in our study of A1 agonist-induced protection against infarction in pigs, pretreatment of the porcine myocardium with CHA, despite its infarct size-reducing effect, did not cause any change in the activity of PKC. In the present study we measured total activity of all isoforms of PKC in the myocardium that can use histone III as a substrate. However, as was shown previously,[45] CHA-treatment did not exert an effect on the redistribution of $PKC\alpha$ and $PKC\varepsilon$ isoforms between the cytosol and membrane and their subsequent activation as well. Thus, these findings indicate that A1 agonist-induced protection in the porcine model seems to be mediated by a PKC-independent mechanism. Moreover, it has been found that pharmacological activation of PKC with phorbol myristate acetate (PMA) failed to protect porcine myocardium against infarction, while PKC inhibition reduced the extent of ischemic damage and did not abolish the protective effect of IP.[46,47] Similar results have been demonstrated by Lasley *et al.*[48] in a rabbit model of infarction and stunning showing that inhibition of PKC improved postischemic functional recovery and reduced the size of infarction. Different results can be attributed to the presence of several PKC isoforms in the myocardium with a different time-course of activation during ischemia. In addition, PKC improved postischemic functional recovery and reduced the size of infarction. Different results can be attributed to the presence of several PKC isoforms in the myocardium with a different time-course of activation during ischemia. In addition, some isoforms can be translocated into the nucleus, where they can activate many oncogenes and transcription factors with a consequent synthesis of some protective proteins believed to be responsible for the late phase of protection (reviewed by Yellon and Baxter[38]).

Moreover, controversial reports may result from differences in experimental settings, variabilities in the preconditioning protocols utilized and in the end-points, and to a great extent these discrepancies can be explained by the multifactorial nature of ischemic stress and complexity of the protective mechanisms operating in each case.

In summary, this study demonstrated that stimulation of adrenergic and adenosine receptors could afford a short-term adaptation to ischemic stress in different experimental models. However, the exact mechanisms of this protection require further exploration. This may offer new approaches to pharmacological induction of preconditioning and contribute to the development of new therapeutic strategies.

REFERENCES

1. DAS, D. K. 1993. Ischaemic preconditioning and myocardial adaptation to ischaemia. Cardiovasc. Res. **27:** 2077–2079.
2. MURRY, C. E., R. B. JENNINGS & K. A. REIMER. 1986. Preconditioning with ischemia: a delay of lethal cell injury in ischemic myocardium. Circulation **74:** 1124–1136.
3. ASIMAKIS, G. K., K. INNERS-MCBRIDE & V. R. CONTI. 1993. Attenuation of postischaemic dysfunction by ischaemic preconditioning is not mediated by adenosine in the isolated rat heart. Cardiovasc. Res. **27:** 1522–1530.
4. LIU, G. S., J. THORNTON, D. M. VAN WINKLE, A. W. H. STANLEY, R. A. OLSSON & J. M. DOWNEY. 1991. Protection against infarction afforded by preconditioning is mediated by A_1 adenosine receptors in rabbit heart. Circulation **84:** 350–356.
5. VEGH, A., S. KOMORI, L. SZEKERES & J. R. PARRATT. 1992. Antiarrhythmic effects of preconditioning in anaesthetised dogs and rats. Cardiovasc. Res. **26:** 487–495.
6. PARRATT, J. R. 1993. Endogenous myocardial protective (antiarrhythmic) substances. Cardiovasc. Res. **27:** 693–702.
7. CURTIS, M. J., M. K. PUGSLEY & M. J. A. WALKER. 1993. Endogenous chemical mediators of arrhythmogenesis in ischaemic heart disease. Cardiovasc. Res. **27:** 703–719.
8. VOGT, A., M. BARANCIK, D. WEIHRAUCH, M. ARRAS, T. PODZUWEIT & W. SCHAPER. 1994. Protection of ischemic porcine myocardium from infarction by an A1-receptor agonist is not mediated by protein kinase C. Circulation **90:** I-371.
9. VEGH, A., J. GY. PAPP & J. R. PARRATT. 1995. Pronounced antiarrhythmic effects of preconditioning in anaesthetised dogs: Is adenosine involved? J. Mol. Cell. Cardiol. **27:** 349–356.
10. BANERJEE, A., C. LOCKE-WINTER, K. B. ROGERS *et al.* 1993. Preconditioning against myocardial dysfunction after ischemia and reperfusion by an α1-adrenergic mechanism. Circ. Res. **73:** 656–670.
11. ASIMAKIS, G. K., K. INNERS-MCBRIDE, V. R. CONTI *et al.* 1994. Transient β adrenergic stimulation can precondition the rat heart against postischaemic contractile dysfunction. Cardiovasc. Res. **28:** 1726–1734.
12. BANKWALA, Z., S. L. HALE & R. A. KLONER. 1994. α-Adrenoceptor stimulation with exogenous norepinephrine or release of endogenous catecholamines mimics ischemic preconditioning. Circulation **90:** 1023–1028.
13. HU, K. & S. NATTEL. 1994. Signal transduction systems underlying ischemic preconditioning in rat hearts. Circulation **90:** I-108.
14. BOGOYEVITCH, M. A., P. J. PARKER & P. H. SUGDEN. 1993. Characterization of protein kinase C isotype expression in adult rat heart. Circ. Res. **72:** 757–767.
15. TSUCHIDA, A., Y. LIU, G. S. LIU *et al.* 1994. Alpha 1-adrenergic agonists precondition rabbit ischemic myocardium independent of adenosine by direct activation of protein kinase C. Circ. Res. **75:** 76–85.
16. YTREHUS, K., Y. LIU & J. M. DOWNEY. 1994. Preconditioning protects ischemic rabbit heart by protein kinase C activation. Am. J. Physiol. **266** (Heart Circ. Physiol. **35**): H1145–H1152.

17. SPEECHLY-DICK, M. E., M. M. MOCANU & D. M. YELLON. 1994. Protein kinase C. Its role in ischemic preconditioning in the rat. Circ. Res. **75:** 586–590.

18. SCHOTT, R. J., S. ROHMAN, E. R. BROWN & W. SCHAPER. 1990. Ischemic preconditioning reduces infarct size in swine myocardium. Circ. Res. **66:** 1133–1142.

19. WILDE, A. A. M., R. J. G. PETERS & M. J. JANSE. 1988. Catecholamine release and potassium accumulation in the isolated globally ischemic rabbit heart. J. Mol. Cell. Cardiol. **20:** 887–896.

20. HAAG, M., W. GEVERS & R. G. BÖHMER. 1985. The interaction between calcium and the activation of Na^+,K^+-ATPase by noradrenaline. Mol. Cell. Biochem. **66:** 111–116.

21. WALKER, M. J. A., M. J. CURTIS, D. J. HEARSE et al. 1988. The Lambeth conventions: guidelines for the study of arrhythmias in ischemia, infarction, and reperfusion. Cardiovasc. Res. **22:** 447–455.

22. VRBJAR, N., J. SOOS & A. ZIEGELHOFFER. 1984. Secondary structure of heart sarcolemmal proteins during interaction with metallic cofactors of (Na,K) ATPase. Gen. Physiol. Biophys. **3:** 317–325.

23. LOWRY, O. H., N. J. ROSEBROUGH, A. L. FARR & R. J. RANDALL. 1953. Protein measurement with the folin phenol reagent. J. Biol. Chem. **193:** 265–275.

24. TAUSSKI, H. H. & E. E. SHORR. 1953. A microcolorimetric method for determination of inorganic phosphorus. J. Biol. Chem. **202:** 575–585.

25. BRADFORD, M. 1976. A rapid and sensitive method for the quantitation of microgram quantities of protein utilizing the principle of protein-dye-binding. Anal. Biochem. **72:** 248–254.

26. RAVINGEROVA, T., N. TRIBULOVA, A. ZIEGELHOEFFER, J. STYK & L. SZEKERES. 1993. Suppression of reperfusion induced arrhythmias in the isolated rat heart: pretreatment with 7-oxo prostacyclin in vivo. Cardiovasc. Res. **27:** 1051–1055.

27. SCHÖMIG, A., S. FISCHER, T. KURZ et al. 1987. Nonexocytotic release of endogenous noradrenaline in the ischemic and anoxic rat heart: mechanism and metabolic requirements. Circ. Res. **60:** 194–205.

28. JANSE, M. J. 1992. The premature beat. Cardiovasc. Res. **26:** 89–100.

29. PENNY, W. J. 1984. The deleterious effects of myocardial catecholamines on cellular electrophysiology and arrhythmias during ischaemia and reperfusion. Eur. Heart J. **5:** 960–973.

30. JIANG, J. P. & S. E. DOWNING. 1990. Catecholamine cardiomyopathy: review and analysis of pathogenetic mechanisms. Yale J. Biol. Med. **63:** 581–591.

31. WENDT, D. J. & J. B. MARTINS. 1990. Autonomic neural regulation of intact Purkinje system of dogs. Am. J. Physiol. 258 (Heart Circ. Physiol. **27**): H1420–H1426.

32. LI, H. G., D. L. JONES, R. YEE et al. 1993. Arrhythmogenic effects of catecholamines are decreased in heart failure induced by rapid pacing in dogs. Am. J. Physiol. 265 (Heart Circ. Physiol. **34**): H1654–H1662.

33. CURTIS, M. J., J. H. BOTTING, D. J. HEARSE et al. 1989. The sympathetic nervous system, catecholamines and ischemia-induced arrhythmias: dependence upon serum potassium concentration. In Adrenergic System and Ventricular Arrhythmias in Myocardial Infarction. J. Brachman & A. Schömig, Eds. 205–219. Springer-Verlag, Berlin.

34. PARRATT, J. R., C. CAMPBELL & O. FAGBEMI. 1981. Catecholamines and early post-infarction arrhythmias: the effects of α- and β-adrenoceptor blockade. In Catecholamines and the Heart. W. Delius, E. Gerlach, H. Grobecker & W. Kübler, Eds. 269–284. Springer-Verlag. Berlin.

35. VEGH, A., J. GY. PAPP & J. R. PARRATT. 1994. Intracoronary noradrenaline suppresses ischaemia-induced ventricular arrhythmias in anaesthetized dogs. J. Mol. Cell. Cardiol. **26:** LXXXVII.

36. RAVINGEROVA, T., W. SONG, A. ZIEGELHOEFFER & J. PARRATT. 1995. Delayed antiarrhythmic effect of pretreatment with norepinephrine in rats: the role of Na/K ATPase. J. Mol. Cell. Cardiol. **27**(6): A162.

37. SZEKERES, L., J. PATARICZA, Z. SZILVASSY, E. UDVARY & A. VEGH. 1992. Cardioprotection: endogenous protective mechanisms promoted by prostacyclin. Basic Res. Cardiol. **87:** 215–221.

38. YELLON, D. M. & G. F. BAXTER. 1995. "Second window of protection" or delayed preconditioning phenomenon: future horizons for myocardial protection? J. Mol. Cell. Cardiol. **27:** 1023–1034.
39. CLAUSEN, T. 1983. Adrenergic control of Na^+-K^+-homeostasis. Acta Med. Scand. Suppl. **672:** 111–115.
40. CURTIS, M. J. & D. J. HEARSE. 1989. Ischemia-induced and reperfusion-induced arrhythmias differ in their sensitivity to potassium: implications for mechanisms of initiation and maintenance of ventricular fibrillation. J. Mol. Cell. Cardiol. **21:** 21–40.
41. TOSAKI, A., N. S. BEHJET, D. T. ENGELMAN, R. M. ENGELMAN & D. K. DAS. 1995. Alpha-1 adrenergic receptor agonist-induced preconditioning in isolated working rat hearts. J. Pharmacol. Exp. Ther. **273:** 689–694.
42. RICHARD, G., R. BLESSING & A. SCHÖMIG. 1994. Cardiac noradrenaline release accelerates adenosine formation in the ischemic rat heart: role of neuronal noradrenaline carrier and adrenergic receptors. J. Mol. Cell. Cardiol. **26:** 1321–1328.
43. WINTER, C. B., M. B. MITCHELL, C. R. LOCKE-WINTER *et al.* 1992. Adenosine induced preconditioning is dependent upon $\alpha1$ adrenoreceptor activation. Circulation **86**(Suppl. I): I-25.
44. KITAKAZE, M., M. HORI & T. KAMADA. 1993. Role of adenosine and its interaction with α adrenoceptor activity in ischaemic and reperfusion injury of the myocardium. Cardiovasc. Res. **27:** 18–27.
45. BARANCIK, M., A. VOGT & W. SCHAPER. Differential activation of protein kinase C isoforms and mitogen-activated protein kinases during ischemia. Protein kinase C activation is not involved in adenosine A1-receptor agonist-mediated protection of porcine myocardium against ischemia. Circ. Res. In press.
46. VOGT, A., M. BARANCIK, D. WEIHRAUCH, M. ARRASS, T. PODZUWEIT & W. SCHAPER. 1994. Activation of protein kinase C fails to protect ischemic porcine myocardium from infarction *in vivo*. J. Mol. Cell. Cardiol. **26**(6): CXVIII.
47. VOGT, A., M. BARANCIK, D. WEIHRAUCH, M. ARRASS, T. PODZUWEIT & W. SCHAPER. 1994. Protein kinase C inhibitors reduce infarct size in pig hearts *in vivo*. Circulation **90**(2): I-647.
48. LASLEY, R. D., M. A. NOBLE, P. J. KONYN & R. M. MENTZER. 1995. The protein kinase C inhibitor bisindolylmaleimide reduces myocardial interstitial purine accumulation and infarct size in the rabbit. Circulation **92**(8): I-136.

Molecular Motor Mechanics in the Contracting Heart

V_1 versus V_3 Myosin Heavy Chain[a]

JON N. PETERSON AND NORMAN R. ALPERT

Department of Molecular Physiology and Biophysics
University of Vermont College of Medicine
Burlington, Vermont 05405

INTRODUCTION

In small mammals, ventricular myosin heavy chain (MHC) type is a major determinant of myocardial muscle mechanics. There are two distinct ventricular MHC's, α and β. V_1 myosin is a homodimer made up of two α MHC's, while V_3 contains two β MHC's.[1-4] Hormonal, hemodynamic and developmental states, as well as species, are important in determining the myocardial composition of myosin isoenzymes. Functionally, V_1 has substantially higher myosin[5] and myofibrillar[5-7] ATPase activity compared to V_3, as well as an increased maximum velocity of muscle shortening.[5,8-10] Other indications of kinetic difference include increased frequency of minimum stiffness[11,12] and tension dependent heat per unit tension[13-15] under isometric conditions for V_1 compared to V_3.

It seems clear, based on the above work, that the cross-bridge cycle is different between muscles containing V_1 and V_3. Our goal in this report is to determine what aspects of the cycle have changed. This study is based on intact papillary muscles, rather than skinned or *in vitro* preparations, to maintain the filament superstructure seen by the individual cross-bridges. Using myothermal techniques, we have already demonstrated that isometric cross-bridge tension-time integral (TTI) per ATP hydrolyzed[16] is greater for muscles containing V_3. In the work presented below, we have supplemented the myothermal protocol with measurements of maximum Ca^{2+} activated force (MCAF) and the time course of twitch relaxation. This additional information allows a more detailed analysis of the cross-bridge cycle in intact muscle, allowing us to estimate mechanical and kinetic parameters for muscles containing V_1 and V_3 MHC. With this more detailed view, we can also correlate our intact muscle data with that obtained in *in vitro* motility assays.

METHODS

Experimental Preparation

Experiments were conducted on right ventricular papillary muscles from male New Zealand white rabbits. The thyroid state of these animals was altered

[a] Supported in part by USPHS Grants R29HL50603 and P01HL28001.

by adding propylthiouracil (0.8 mg/ml) (PTU) to the drinking water over a period of three weeks, or daily injection of L-thyroxine (T_4) for a period of 2 weeks. Treatment with these drugs causes opposite shifts in the predominant myosin heavy chain isoform, towards 100% V_3 for PTU[17] or 100% V_1 for T_4.[18]

The basic experimental apparatus for myothermal measurements has been described in detail elsewhere.[19] Here we use a similar myothermal apparatus, where the muscle is mounted horizontally rather than vertically. The animals were anesthetized with CO_2, then the heart was removed and exsanguinated with repeated changes in superfusate. The bathing solution was a modified Krebs-Ringer, consisting of (in mM): 152 Na^+, 3.6 K^+, 135 Cl^-, 25 HCO_3^-, 0.6 Mg^{2+}, 1.3 H_2PO_4, 0.6 SO_4^{2-}, 2.5 Ca^{2+}, 5.0 glucose, continuously bubbled with 95% O_2–5% CO_2. The heart was transferred to a dissection chamber at room temperature, where the right ventricle was opened and a suitably thin papillary muscle was selected. After ligature electrodes were attached with loops of 4.0 noncapillary braided silk, the muscle was excised and horizontally mounted in the thermopile chamber which contained the same solution as above.

Protocols

All protocols were under computer control (IBM PC), with force, length and temperature signals digitized every 2 ms. The muscle was paced at a rate of 0.2 Hz with a 3-ms, 10% supra maximal rectangular stimulus pulse, applied end-to-end through the ligature electrodes. Over a period of two hours, the muscle was incrementally stretched to L_0, the length at which developed force was maximum. Student unpaired t test ($p < 0.05$) was used to test for statistical significance of all parameters between the PTU and T_4 groups. All experiments were performed at 21°C.

Muscle temperature was measured with an 8-junction, Hill-type thermopile fabricated by vacuum deposition of bismuth and antimony junctions on a mica substrate.[20] The thermopile used for this series of experiments had a sensitivity of 0.6 mV/°C. During heat measurements, the chamber was drained to minimize extraneous heat transfer paths. The muscle was kept moist by bubbling moisturized, temperature equilibrated 95% O_2–5% CO_2 gas through a 2-mm layer of Krebs-Ringer solution at the bottom of the chamber. Stimulus amplitude could be markedly reduced, since the conducting pathway through the bathing solution was eliminated in the drained chamber.

Initial heat, consisting of tension dependent (TDH: cross-bridge) and tension independent (TIH: mainly Ca^{2+} transport) components, is derived from the thermopile temperature signal as described previously.[21] Briefly, TIH is extracted from initial heat by selectively inhibiting cross-bridge cycling with 2 and 4 mM butanedione monoxime (BDM);[19] TDH is then obtained by subtracting this tension independent heat signal from the initial heat.

After heat measurements were complete, we measured maximum Ca^{2+} activated force (MCAF) by applying a 10-Hz stimulus pulse train after a 20-minute incubation in Krebs solution containing 10 mM Ca^{2+}, 50 μM cyclopiazonic acid, and 1 μM ryanodine.[22] This resulted in a fused tetanus of maximum amplitude; several muscles were also subjected to 12–15 mM Ca^{2+}, which did not increase tetanic force.

Analysis

The above data are used to estimate average cross-bridge kinetic and mechanical parameters. In this brief treatment, we assume a 2-state cross-bridge cycle consisting of an attached, force generating state and a detached state.

Maximum activation implies that all available cross-bridges are contributing to muscle force, so we estimated average cross-bridge force (F_{avg}) as the ratio of MCAF to the number of cross-bridges in a half sarcomere (N_{XBr}):

$$N_{XBr} = (160 \ \mu M) \cdot \text{weight} \cdot N_A/L_0$$

$$F_{avg} = MCAF/N_{XBr} \tag{1}$$

where N_A is Avagadro's number. Here, myosin concentration is taken as $160 \ \mu M$.[23]

The number of cross-bridge cycles during a given time period can be computed from the cross-bridge enthalpy change (tension dependent heat) by assuming the enthalpy of creatine phosphate hydrolysis to be 34 kJ/mole.[24] The number of cycles during a contraction, in the muscle (NC_m) and in the half sarcomere (NC_{hs}), are:

$$NC_m = \Delta TDH/34 \text{ kJ/mole}$$

$$NC_{hs} = NC_m/(L_0 \cdot 1000) \tag{2}$$

where L_0 is in mm and a half sarcomere is taken as $1 \ \mu m$; the quantity ($L_0 \cdot 1000$) defines the number of half sarcomeres in the muscle.

Cross-bridge force-time integral (FTI_{XBr}) is computed as integrated muscle twitch force (muscle tension-time integral) normalized to the number of cross-bridge cycles occurring in a half sarcomere (NC_{hs}).[16] In a 2-state model, FTI_{XBr} is the product of unitary cross-bridge force (F_{uni}) and attachment time (T_{att}). Thus,

$$FTI_{XBr} = TTI_{muscle}/NC_{hs} = F_{uni} \cdot T_{att} \tag{3}$$

Average force (F_{avg}) depends on F_{uni}, and the duty cycle (DC, or fraction of time attached during the cycle):

$$F_{avg} = F_{uni} \cdot DC = F_{uni} \cdot T_{att}/T_{cycle} = F_{uni} \cdot T_{att} \cdot CR \tag{4}$$

Note that cycle time (T_{cycle}) is simply the inverse of cycling rate (CR). Rearranging (4), and substituting (3) into (4), we can solve for cycling rate:

$$CR = F_{avg}/(F_{uni} \cdot T_{att}) = F_{avg}/FTI_{XBr} \tag{5}$$

We now have F_{avg}, FTI_{XBr}, and CR, but cannot separate FTI_{XBr} into F_{uni} and T_{att}. In the 2-state model, attachment time is simply the inverse of detachment rate g ($T_{att} = 1/g$). We have chosen to estimate g by considering the time course of late force relaxation in the twitch. Since little or no Ca^{2+} is bound to the thin filaments this late in the twitch,[25] we assume that late relaxation is controlled by cross-bridge detachment. Cross-bridge detachment rate g is then equal to $1/\tau_{relax}$, where τ_{relax} is the time constant of a single exponential curve fit to late force decline

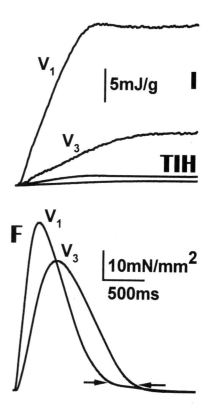

FIGURE 1. Time course of twitch force, initial heat (I) and tension independent heat (TIH) in V_1 and V_3 papillary muscles. I is derived from the raw temperature tracings, as discussed in the text. TIH is computed as explained in the text, and shown in FIGURE 2. Note that I and TIH evolve more rapidly in the V_1 muscle, as does force. *Arrows* indicate when force has fallen to 5% of its peak value; the force time course subsequent to this point is fit with a single exponential τ_{relax} to estimate cross-bridge detachment rate.

(force time course corresponding to <5% of peak force; see FIG. 1; also see the Discussion for caveats regarding this approach). T_{att} is equal to τ_{relax} ($T_{att} = 1/g = \tau_{relax}$); knowing T_{att}, we can solve for duty cycle (DC) and unitary cross-bridge force (F_{uni}):

$$DC = T_{att} \cdot CR \qquad (6)$$

$$F_{uni} = FTI_{XBr}/T_{att} \qquad (7)$$

RESULTS

FIGURE 1 shows the time course of initial heat (I) and force (F) for representative V_1 and V_3 muscles. As expected, both heat and force evolve more slowly in the V_3 preparation. Calculated tension independent heat (TIH) is also shown. A sample dataset for calculating TIH is shown in FIGURE 2, where the initial heat evolved at the end of the twitch is plotted as a function of twitch tension-time integral (TTI). As discussed in Methods, TTI was varied using 2 and 4 mM BDM. Tension dependent heat (TDH), which is used to calcualte all cross-bridge parameters presented below, is simply the difference between I and TIH. TIH is actually a

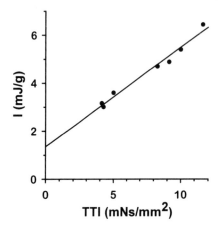

FIGURE 2. Determination of TIH. Integrated tension (TTI) for several twitches are plotted against the value of I obtained at the end of each twitch. TTI is reduced using 2 and 4 mM BDM, as explained in the text. Extrapolation of a linear fit to these data through 0 TTI yields a tension independent heat (TIH) value of 1.36 mJ/g for this muscle.

fairly small component of I, with TDH making up $85 \pm 4\%$ of I in the V_1 muscle, and $91 \pm 1\%$ in the V_3 muscle (p = n.s.).

A comparison of muscle dimensions, as well as myothermal and mechanical twitch parameters, is shown in TABLE 1. Peak twitch tension is not different between the two groups, but timing parameters (time to peak tension (TPT) and twitch time (TT)) are significantly slower for the V_3 muscle. Neither TTI nor TDH are significantly different between groups, though FIGURE 3 demonstrates that cross-bridge force-time integral (which is proportional to the ratio of TTI to TDH) is quite different.

FIGURE 3 shows a comparison of the derived cross-bridge parameters for each group. As shown previously,[16] cross-bridge force-time integral is twice as large in the V_3 muscle. Cycling rate is almost 3 times faster in the V_1 muscle, which is consistent with other indices of cycling kinetics (see the Discussion). Given the changes in FTI and CR, though, we were somewhat surprised to find that average force is not different between the two groups.

TABLE 1. Comparison of Mechanical and Myothermal Parameters[a]

	PTU (n = 5)	T_4 (n = 4)
L_0 (mm)	5.3 ± 0.4	5.8 ± 0.6
P_0 (mN/mm^2)	42.5 ± 5.6	54.5 ± 11.3
CSA (mm^2)	0.64 ± 0.09	$0.36 \pm 0.11^*$
TPT (ms)	589 ± 20	$318 \pm 19^*$
TT (ms)	1780 ± 130	$1230 \pm 160^*$
TTI (mN $\cdot$ s/mm^2)	40.0 ± 6.7	33.5 ± 8.8
I (mJ/g)	8.6 ± 1.2	15.2 ± 4.1
TIH (mJ/g)	0.45 ± 0.2	$2.0 \pm 0.6^*$
TDH	7.8 ± 1.1	13.8 ± 4.0

[a] Muscle dimensions (mean $\pm$ SEM) and twitch parameters for the PTU (V_3) and T_4 (V_1) groups. CSA, muscle cross-sectional area. *Asterisks* indicate statistical significance ($p <0.05$).

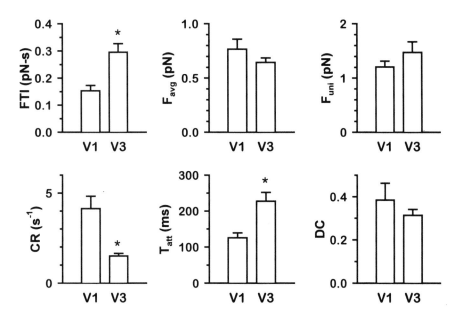

FIGURE 3. Comparison of isometric cross-bridge parameters. While cross-bridge force-time integral is significantly higher for V_3, both average force and unitary force are unchanged. This increased FTI is explained primarily by a significantly increased attachment time. Cycling rate decreases with increased T_{att}, leading to a constant duty cycle.

It should be noted here that the derived duty cycle for two of the T_4 muscles was greater than 1.0. For this analysis, these experiments were excluded from calculations of T_{att}, DC and F_{uni}. Note that, even with n = 2, attachment time was significantly less in the T_4 group, while unitary force and duty cycle were unaffected by the MHC population.

DISCUSSION

This paper presents a determination of cross-bridge properties for the two major cardiac myosin isoenzymes, at the level of the papillary muscle. Our approach complements *in vitro* systems, with the advantage of maintaining an intact myofibrillar superstructure. These estimated cross-bridge parameters represent population averages, rather than individual cross-bridge events or small populations as seen in the *in vitro* assays.

Our findings are shown schematically in FIGURE 4. We have demonstrated that isometric cross-bridge cycling rate is 2.5 times faster in the T_4 group, which is consistent with a factor of 2 increase in the frequency of minimum stiffness magnitude during constant isometric activation.[11,12] This result is also consistent with nonisometric kinetic indices, such as increased ATPase[5-7] and maximum shortening velocity[5,8-10] for the V_1 versus V_3 MHC.

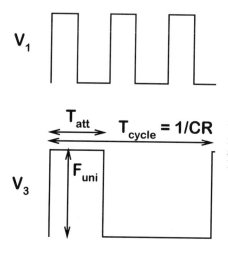

FIGURE 4. Schematic V_1 and V_3 cross-bridge cycles. The data of FIGURE 3 are summarized in this representation, where cross-bridge attachment is shown as a step increase in force. While unitary force is similar, both attachment time and cycle time are much longer for V_3.

Average cross-bridge force is not different in the two groups. This finding is supported by *in vitro* measurements using a centrifuge microscope,[26] but is contradicted by *in vitro* myosin mixture experiments looking at velocity[27] and *in vitro* microneedle experiments measuring force.[28] This contradiction has yet to be explained, but it may result from differences in the animal model used to obtain V_3 myosin. Specifically, Sugiura *et al.*[26] employed PTU as we did to push the MHC population towards 100% V_3, whereas Harris *et al.*[27] and VanBuren *et al.*[28] utilized pressure overload hypertrophy.

Our assessment of cross-bridge attachment time derives from the time course of final twitch force decline. Force decline could be affected by the inherent properties of the contractile proteins (cross-bridge attachment/detachment), regulatory processes (Ca^{2+} removal), or passive mechanical processes (viscoelastic elements). Previous work[25] suggests that Ca^{2+} is not significantly bound to troponin C during the final half of relaxation in rabbit papillary muscle, but force decline during the final 5% of force could still be affected by passive components. If this were the case, we would expect increased cross-bridge kinetics to have no effect on τ_{relax}. The fact that we did observe a decrease in τ_{relax} for V_1 with respect to V_3 indicates that the V_3 force decline is minimally contaminated with passive processes. This may not be the case in the V_1 preparation, since estimated T_{att} was actually longer than the cycle time (1/CR) in two experiments, leading to duty cycles greater than unity. We have chosen to interpret this as contamination from passive processes, and have therefore discarded these two data points for the calculation of T_{att}, F_{uni} and DC. These values, then, should be viewed with some caution for the T_4 group. With this caveat, we still show a significant decrease in T_{att} for the V_1 muscle.

It is well known that myosin heavy chain isoform is a major determinant of cardiac muscle kinetics in small mammals. We previously showed that myothermal economy is well correlated with % V_3 across several animal species,[16] but have been unable to determine whether changes in economy (*i.e.*, cross-bridge force-time integral) are due to changes in cross-bridge unitary force, attachment time, or both. Based on the present work, we now propose that cross-bridge unitary force is unaffected by MHC type. The only effect of MHC isoform shifts appears to be kinetic, with V_1 preparations having proportionately decreased attachment time and cycle time, such that duty cycle remains constant. As a result of this constant duty cycle and unitary force, average cross-bridge force also remains constant.

One way to gain insight into the molecular differences between V_1 and V_3 is to directly compare the deduced primary amino acid sequences, obtained from cloned cDNA's.[29] Despite profound differences in the kinetic behavior of the two myosins as discussed above, only 131 (or 6.76%) of their 1,938 amino acids are nonidentical. This implies that the few differing amino acids must be situated at crucial functional sites. In fact, two-thirds of the differing amino acids fall into clusters that are situated at presumed strategic sites throughout the molecule. Three of these clusters of difference occur at sites that have been implicated in nucleotide binding, strong attachment of the cross-bridge to actin, and a putative conformational change associated with force generation (*i.e.*, the proposed "hinge" region; for a review of myosin domain mapping see Warrick & Spudich[30]). Thus, variation at each of these domains could play a key role in determining the distinct kinetic and energetic functions of their parent isoforms.

ACKNOWLEDGMENTS

We wish to thank Rich Lachapelle and Lisa Akins for technical support.

REFERENCES

1. Hoh, J., G. Yeoh, M. Thomas & L. Higginbottom. 1979. Structural differences in the heavy chains of rat ventricular myosin isoenzymes. FEBS Lett. **97**: 330–334.
2. Sinha, A., P. Umeda, C. Kavinsky, C. Rajamanickham, H. Hsu, S. Jakovcic & M. Rabinowitz. 1982. Molecular cloning of mRNA sequences for cardiac alpha- and beta-form myosin heavy chains. Expression in normal, hypothyroid and thyrotoxic rabbits. Proc. Natl. Acad. Sci. USA **79**: 5847–5851.
3. Everett, A., R. Chizzonite, W. Clark & R. Zak. 1982. Cardiac isomyosins: influence of thyroid hormone on their distribution and rate of synthesis. *In* Muscle Development: Molecular and Cellular Control. M. Pearson & H. Epstein, Eds. 35–41. Cold Spring Harbor Laboratory. Cold Spring Harbor, NY.
4. Everett, A., A. Sinha, P. Umeda, S. Jakovcic, M. Rabinowitz & R. Zak. 1984. Regulation of myosin synthesis by thyroid hormone: relative change in the alpha- and beta-myosin heavy chain mRNA levels in rabbit heart. Biochemistry **23**: 1596–1599.
5. Capelli, V., R. Botinelli, C. Pogessi, R. Moggio & C. Regiani. 1989. Shortening velocity and myosin and myofibrillar ATPase activity related to myosin isoenzyme composition during postnatal development in rat myocardium. Circ. Res. **65**: 446–457.
6. Litten, R. Z., B. J. Martin, E. R. Howe, N. R. Alpert & R. J. Solaro. 1981. Phosphorylation and adenosine triphosphatase activity of myofibrils from thyrotoxic rabbit hearts. Circ. Res. **48**: 498–501.
7. Pope, B., J. Hoh & W. Weeds. 1980. The ATPase activity of rat cardiac myosin isoenzymes. FEBS Lett. **118**: 205–208.
8. Pagani, E. D. & F. J. Julian. 1984. Rabbit papillary muscle myosin isozymes and the velocity of muscle shortening. Circ. Res. **54**: 586–594.
9. Schwartz, K., Y. Lecarpentier, J. Martin, A. Lompre, J. Mercadier &

      B. SWYNGHEDAUW. 1981. Myosin isoenzyme distribution correlates with speed of
      myocardial contraction. J. Mol. Cell. Cardiol. **13:** 1071–1075.
10. KORECKY, B. & M. BEZNAK. 1971. Effect of thyroxine on growth and function of
      cardiac muscle. *In* Cardiac Hypertrophy. N. Alpert, Ed. 55–64. Academic Press.
      New York.
11. ROSSMANITH, G. H., J. F. Y. HOH, A. KIRMAN & L. J. KWAN. 1986. Influence of V_1
      and V_3 isomyosins on the mechanical behavior of rat papillary muscle as studied by
      pseudo-random binary noise modulated length perturbations. J. Muscle Res. Cell
      Motil. **7:** 307–319.
12. SHIBATA, T., W. C. HUNTER & K. SAGAWA. 1987. Dynamic stiffness of barium-
      contractured cardiac muscles with different speeds of contraction. Circ. Res. **60:**
      770–779.
13. ALPERT, N. R., L. A. MULIERI & R. Z. LITTEN. 1979. Functional significance of
      altered myosin adenosine triphosphatase activity in enlarged hearts. Am. J. Cardiol.
      44: 947–953.
14. LOISELLE, D. S., I. R. WENDT & J. F. Y. HOH. 1982. Energetic consequences of
      thyroid modulated shifts in ventricular isomyosin distribution in the rat. J. Muscle
      Res. Cell Motil. **3:** 5–23.
15. HOLUBARSCH, C., R. P. GOULETTE, R. Z. LITTEN, B. J. MARTIN, L. A. MULIERI &
      N. R. ALPERT. 1985. The economy of isometric force development, myosin isoen-
      zyme pattern and myofibrillar ATPase activity in normal and hypothyroid rat myocar-
      dium. Circ. Res. **56:** 78–86.
16. HASENFUSS, G., L. A. MULIERI, E. M. BLANCHARD, C. HOLUBARSCH, B. J. LEAVITT,
      F. ITTLEMAN & N. R. ALPERT. 1991. Energetics of isometric force development in
      control and volume-overload human myocardium. Comparison with animal species.
      Circ. Res. **68:** 836–846.
17. LING, E., P. J. O'BRIEN, T. SALEMO & C. D. IANUZZO. 1988. Effects of different
      thyroid treatments on the biochemical characteristics of rabbit myocardium. Can.
      J. Cardiol. **4:** 301–306.
18. LITTEN, R. Z., B. J. MARTIN, R. B. LOW & N. R. ALPERT. 1982. Altered myosin
      isozyme patterns from pressure-overloaded and thyrotoxic hypertrophied rabbit
      hearts. Circ. Res. **50:** 856–864.
19. ALPERT, N. R., E. M. BLANCHARD & L. A. MULIERI. 1989. Tension-independent heat
      in rabbit papillary muscle. J. Physiol. (London) **414:** 433–453.
20. MULIERI, L. A., G. LUHR, J. TREFRY & N. R. ALPERT. 1977. Metal-film thermopiles for
      use with rabbit right ventricular papillary muscles. Am. J. Physiol. **233:** C146–C156.
21. PETERSON, J. N & N. R. ALPERT. 1991. Time course of mechanical efficiency during
      afterloaded contractions in isolated cardiac muscle. Am. J. Physiol. **261:** 27–29.
22. DOBRUNZ, L. E., P. H. BACKX & D. T. YUE. 1995. Steady-state $[Ca^{2+}]_i$-force relation-
      ship in intact twitching cardiac muscle: direct evidence for modulation by isoprotere-
      nol and EMD 53998. Biophys. J. **69:** 189–201.
23. BARSOTTI, R. & M. FERENCZI. 1988. Kinetics of ATP hydrolysis and tension production
      in skinned cardiac muscle of the guinea pig. J. Biol. Chem. **263:** 16750–16756.
24. WOLEDGE, R. C. & P. J. REILLY. 1988. Molar enthalpy change for hydrolysis of
      phosphorylcreatine under conditions in muscle cells. Biophys. J. **54:** 97–104.
25. PETERSON, J. N., W. C. HUNTER & M. R. BERMAN. 1991. Estimated time course of
      Ca^{2+} bound to troponin C during relaxation in isolated cardiac muscle. Am. J. Physiol.
      260: H1013–H1024.
26. SUGIURA, S., H. YAMASHITA, M. SATA, S. MOMOMURA, T. SERIZAWA, K. OIWA,
      S. CHAEN, T. SHIMMEN & H. SUGI. 1995. Force-velocity relations of rat cardiac
      myosin isozymes sliding on algal cell actin cables *in vitro*. Biochim. Biophys. Acta
      1231: 69–75.
27. HARRIS, D. E., S. S. WORK, R. K. WRIGHT, N. R. ALPERT & D. W. WARSHAW. 1994.
      Smooth, cardiac and skeletal muscle myosin force and motion generation assessed
      by cross-bridge mechanical interaction *in vitro*. J. Muscle Res. Cell Motil. **15:** 11–19.
28. VANBUREN, P., D. HARRIS, N. ALPERT & D. WARSHAW. 1995. Cardiac V_1 and V_3
      myosins differ in their hydrolytic and mechanical activities *in vitro*. Circ. Res. **77:**
      439–444.

29.   McNally, E. M., R. Kraft, M. Bravo-Zehnder, D. A. Taylor & L. A. Leinwand. 1989. Full length rat alpha and beta cardiac myosin heavy chain sequences: comparisons suggest a molecular basis for functional differences. J. Mol. Biol. **210:** 665–671.
30.   Warrick, H. M. & J. A. Spudich. 1995. Myosin structure and function in cell motility. Ann. Rev. Cell Biol. **3:** 379–421.

The Contractile Response of the Ventricular Myocardium to Adenosine A_1 and A_2 Receptor Stimulation[a]

JAMES G. DOBSON, JR.,[b] RICHARD A. FENTON, AND
DARRELL R. SAWMILLER

Department of Physiology
University of Massachusetts Medical School
and
Graduate School of Biomedical Sciences
Worcester, Massachusetts

INTRODUCTION

Adenosine has been implicated as having both negative and positive inotropic responses in the ventricular myocardium. These actions of the naturally occurring nucleoside are in addition to its other known actions in the heart, which include coronary vasodilation,[1,2] antiarrhythmogenesis,[3] angiogenesis[4,5] and cardioprotection.[6] The latter actions of adenosine have been reviewed elsewhere.[3,7]

Both adenosine A_1 and A_2 receptors appear to be present on the ventricular myocyte.[8] However, the functional significance of adenosinergic activation of these receptors is far from fully understood. The negative inotropic action of adenosine, at physiological concentrations, is mediated by adenosine A_1 receptors and results in the well-known antiadrenergic effect of the nucleoside.[9–11] The antiadrenergic action of adenosine involves reductions in β-adrenoceptor-mediated increases in adenylyl cyclase activity,[8,12] cyclic AMP formation,[13,14] intracellular Ca^{2+} transient magnitude,[15] protein kinase A activation,[10] myocardial protein phosphorylation,[16,17] glycogen phosphorylase activation[10,11,14] and ventricular contractility.[10,13,18,19] Evidence indicates that as the interstitial level of adenosine[20–23] is increased, the antiadrenergic effect of adenosine is also increased.[24,25] Thus, adenosine functions as a negative-feedback modulator of β-adrenoceptor-mediated contractile and glycogenolytic responses in the myocardium.[9,14] The importance of adenosine in its role as an antiadrenergic agent in the heart is garnered from reports suggesting that adenosine protects the heart from β-adrenergic overstimulation whether the heart is normoxic,[24] hypoxic[26] or ischemic.[27] Recently, adenosine via A_2 receptors was found to increase cardiac adenylyl cyclase activity[8] and the formation of cyclic AMP.[28,29] However, there is not universal agreement on whether adenosine A_2 receptor stimulation manifests an increase in ventricular contractility.[29–32]

This paper focuses on some of our recent studies indicating that endogenous adenosine has both negative and positive inotropic actions in the contracting

[a] This work was supported by PHS Grants HL-22828 and AG-11491.

[b] Please mail all correspondence to: James G. Dobson, Jr., Department of Physiology, University of Massachusetts Medical School, 55 Lake Avenue North, Worcester, MA 01655-0127.

ventricular myocardium by interacting with adenosine A_1 and A_2 receptors, respectively. The results indicate that endogenous adenosine attenuates the β-adrenoceptor-mediated positive inotropic responses in the contracting oxygenated heart through adenosine A_1 receptors. Furthermore, endogenous adenosine, also via adenosine A_1 receptors, fosters an enhanced recovery of mechanical function upon reperfusion of the underperfused β-adrenergic-stimulated heart. In addition endogenous adenosine, via adenosine A_2 receptors, appears to potentiate the β-adrenoceptor-mediated positive inotropic response in the heart.

RESULTS

Adenosine A_1 Receptor Stimulation in Normoxic Heart Curtails the β-Adrenergic-Elicited Positive Inotropic Response

The isolated constant flow perfused rat heart was employed to assess the effect of endogenous adenosine on β-adrenergic catecholamine-elicited inotropic responses. The hearts were perfused with physiological saline solution (PSS) at 16 ml/min, and the contractile state of the hearts was assessed by recording left ventricular pressure (LVP) and the maximal rates of left ventricular pressure development ($+dP/dt_{max}$) and relaxation ($-dP/dt_{max}$). The adenosine A_1 receptor antagonist, 1,3-dipropyl-8-cyclopentylxanthine (DPCPX), potentiated the isoproterenol-elicited increase in both LVP and $\pm dP/dt_{max}$ as illustrated in FIGURE 1. Administration of isoproterenol, a β-adrenergic receptor agonist, at a final concen-

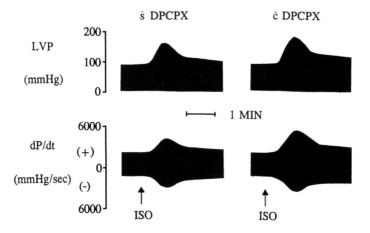

FIGURE 1. Typical recordings illustrating the potentiation of the isoproterenol (ISO)-elicited positive inotropic response caused by the adenosine A_1 receptor antagonist DPCPX in the isolated rat heart. Hearts were perfused at 16 ml/min with PSS, paced at 300 contractions/min and LVP and $\pm dP/dt_{max}$ recorded as indicated. The PSS contained (in mM) 118.4 NaCl, 4.69 KCl, 2.52 $CaCl_2$, 25.0 $NaHCO_3$, 1.18 $MgSO_4$, 1.2 KH_2PO_4, and 10 glucose and maintained at a pH of 7.4 by gassing with 95% O_2–5% CO_2. The heart was exposed to 10^{-8} M isoproterenol for 10 sec in either the absence ($\bar{s}$ DPCPX) or presence ($\bar{c}$ DPCPX) of 10^{-7} M DPCPX.

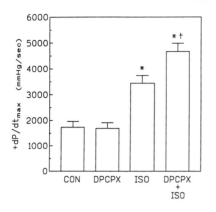

FIGURE 2. The effect of DPCPX on the isoproterenol-elicited positive inotropic response in isolated perfused rat hearts. See the legend of FIGURE 1 for details. Hearts were perfused either in the absence (CON) or presence (DPCPX) of 10^{-7} M DPCPX in the PSS. Isoproterenol (ISO) was administered at a final concentration of 10^{-8} M for 10 sec. Each value represents the mean ± SE for 6 hearts. *Asterisks* denote a statistically significant difference from the appropriate CON or DPCPX value. The *dagger* denotes a statistically significant difference from the ISO value.

tration of 10^{-8} M for 10 sec produced a peak increase in $+dP/dt_{max}$ of 99% (FIG. 2). While DPCPX alone did not influence basal $+dP/dt_{max}$, the adenosine A_1 receptor antagonist potentiated the isoproterenol elicited increase in $+dP/dt_{max}$ by 36%. These results suggest that endogenous myocardial adenosine does not permit full expression of β-adrenoceptor-mediated positive inotropic responses in the normoxic heart. Thus, the antiadrenergic action of endogenous adenosine appears to cause a negative inotropic effect in the oxygenated heart exposed to β-adrenergic stimulation.

Rather than antagonizing the action of adenosine on A_1 receptors, an alternative approach was to administer adenosine deaminase with the intent of reducing the endogenous myocardial level of adenosine. The use of adenosine deaminase to lower tissue adenosine was successful in the past using *in vitro* cardiac atrial[26] and ventricular[24] preparations. Adenosine deaminase potentiated the isoproterenol-induced positive inotropic response in oxygenated perfused rat hearts (FIG. 3). Adenosine deaminase was administered to the perfusion solution of isolated hearts at a level of 1.5 U/ml of PSS. Isoproterenol at 10^{-8} M

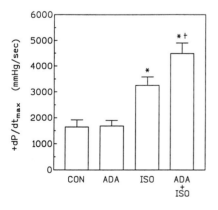

FIGURE 3. Effect of adenosine deaminase on the isoproterenol-elicited positive inotropic response in isolated perfused rat hearts. See the legend of FIGURE 1 for details. Hearts were perfused either in the absence (CON) or presence (ADA) of 1.5 U adenosine deaminase/ml PSS. Isoproterenol (ISO) was administered at a final concentration of 10^{-8} M for 10 sec. Each value represents the mean ± SE for 6 hearts. *Asterisks* denote a statistically significant difference from the appropriate CON or ADA value. The *dagger* denotes a statistically significant difference from the ISO value.

produced a 98% increase in $+dP/dt_{max}$ in the absence of adenosine deaminase and a 169% increase in $+dP/dt_{max}$ in the presence of the deaminase. Adenosine deaminase in the absence of isoproterenol had no effect on the basal level of contractility, but potentiated the isoproterenol-elicited response by 38%. These results suggest that adenosine deaminase lowered the endogenous myocardial level of adenosine and thereby potentiated the positive inotropic effect of isoproterenol. These findings confirm the results obtained with adenosine A_1 receptor antagonist DPCPX, indicating that endogenous adenosine probably serves an important antiadrenergic function in the normoxic heart subjected to β-adrenergic stimulation.

Adenosine A_1 Receptor Stimulation Enhances Mechanical Recovery of the Ischemic Heart Exposed to β-Adrenergic Catecholamines

Endogenous levels of adenosine are sufficient to protect the myocardium from the deleterious effects of elevated β-adrenergic stimulation. This conclusion was reached after investigating the effect of administering 10^{-6} M isoproterenol during low-flow ischemia on contractile recovery during subsequent isoproterenol-free reperfusion. Isolated rat hearts were perfused with oxygenated PSS and then subjected to ischemic conditions for 45 min (FIG. 4). The ischemic conditions were initiated by perfusing the hearts at 0.5 ml/min, whereupon hearts were exposed to 10^{-6} M isoproterenol. Throughout most of the ischemic period,

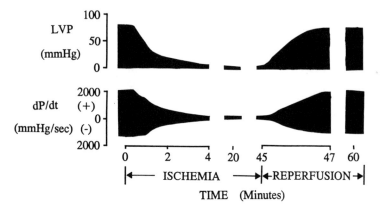

FIGURE 4. A typical recording illustrating the contractile function of an isolated rat heart subjected to low-flow ischemia followed by reperfusion. Hearts were perfused at 14 ml/min with PSS, paced at 300 contractions/min and both LVP and $\pm dP/dt_{max}$ recorded as indicated. After 30 min the hearts were subjected to low-flow ischemia by perfusing the hearts at 0.5 ml/min (ISCHEMIA) in either the absence or presence of 10^{-6} M isoproterenol for 45 min. The recording presented is from a heart not exposed to isoproterenol. Reperfusion at 14 ml/min was initiated at the end of the low-flow ischemic period devoid of isoproterenol and the level to which mechanical function returned was assessed at 60 min (15 min of reperfusion).

$\pm dP/dt_{max}$ was reduced to approximately 5% of the preischemic value. With reperfusion isoproterenol administration was discontinued and the return of mechanical function was continuously monitored.

Hearts in the absence of exogenously administered adenosine antagonists or agonists displayed a full recovery upon 15 min of reperfusion (FIG. 5), as evidenced by the return of $+dP/dt_{max}$ to the preischemic value whether or not isoproterenol was present during the low-flow ischemic period. Hearts stimulated with isoproterenol in the presence of the adenosine A_1 agonist phenylisopropyladenosine (PIA) also displayed full recovery upon reperfusion. However, when the adenosine A_1 receptor antagonist DPCPX was present throughout the ischemic and reperfusion periods there was incomplete recovery of mechanical function in that $+dP/dt_{max}$ was significantly depressed by approximately 43%. DPCPX partially depressed recovery even with PIA present. These results indicate that the presence of endogenous adenosine which is known to accumulate with ischemia[21] facilitates the mechanical recovery upon reperfusion of the low-flow ischemic myocardium subjected to β-adrenergic stimulation. Even the addition of PIA did not improve upon the facilitation. This is presumably a cardioprotective role of endogenous adenosine involving A_1 receptors. It is possible that the antiadrenergic action of adenosine is operational in the ischemic myocardium.

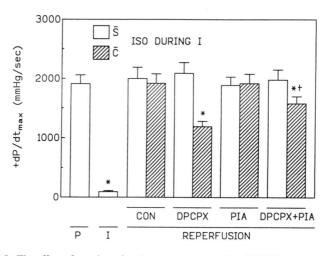

FIGURE 5. The effect of an adenosine A_1 receptor antagonist, DPCPX, and agonist, phenylisopropyladenosine (PIA), on the restoration of contractile function during reperfusion following 45 min of low-flow ischemia in either the absence ($\bar{s}$) or presence ($\bar{c}$) of 10^{-6} M isoproterenol (ISO). ISO was never present during the reperfusion period and only present during the low-flow ischemia period. The values of $+dP/dt_{max}$ at the end of the 30 min preischemic period (P) and after 45 min of low-flow ischemia (I) are given. The $+dP/dt_{max}$ values are also given at the 15 min time point of reperfusion (REPERFUSION) with either no additions (CON), 10^{-7} M DPCPX, 10^{-6} M PIA, or DPCPX + PIA present throughout the entire experiment. The values represent the mean $\pm$ SE for 5 hearts. *Asterisks* denote a statistically significant difference from the preischemic value (P) and the appropriate corresponding value in the absence of ISO. The *dagger* denotes a statistically significant difference from the DPCPX value in the presence of ISO.

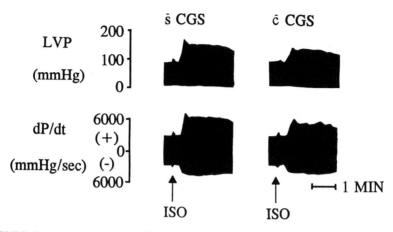

FIGURE 6. A typical recording illustrating the attenuation of the isoproterenol-elicited positive inotropic response caused by the adenosine A_2 receptor antagonist CGS-15943 in isolated rat hearts. Hearts were perfused with physiological saline solution at a constant pressure of 70 mm Hg which resulted in a coronary flow of 16 ml/min. The hearts were paced at 280 contractions/min and both LVP and $\pm dP/dt_{max}$ recorded as indicated. The hearts were exposed to 10^{-8} M isoproterenol (ISO) for 1 to 2 min in either the absence (s̄ CGS) or presence (c̄ CGS) of 10^{-6} M CGS-15943.

Adenosine A_2 Receptor Stimulation Potentiates β-Adrenoceptor-Mediated Increase in Heart Contractility

The adenosine normally present in the heart may also potentiate the inotropic state by interacting with adenosine A_2 receptors. The isolated constant flow perfused rat heart was used to assess the effect of endogenous adenosine on the β-adrenergic-elicited inotropic response in the presence of an adenosine A_2 receptor antagonist, 9-chloro-2-(2-furyl)[1,2,4]triazolo[1,5-c]quinazolin-5-amine (CGS-15943). The adenosine A_2 receptor antagonist attenuated the isoproterenol-induced increase in LVP and $\pm dP/dt_{max}$ as illustrated in FIGURE 6. Administration of isoproterenol at a final concentration of 10^{-8} M for 1 to 2 min produced a peak increase in $+dP/dt_{max}$ of 82% (FIG. 7). While CGS-15943 alone did not influence basal $+dP/dt_{max}$, the isoproterenol administration elicited only a 62% increase in $+dP/dt_{max}$ in the presence of the adenosine A_2 receptor antagonist. Thus, if CGS-15943 is preventing adenosine A_2 receptor activation, it could be concluded that endogenous adenosine is contributing approximately 8% to isoproterenol-elicited positive inotropy in these hearts. While there is concern that CGS-15943 may also block adenosine A_1 receptors, the antagonist has been reported[33] to be adenosine A_2 selective in the heart. Moreover, replacement of CGS-15943 with 0.5–1 × 10^{-6} M 1,3,7-trimethyl-8-(3-chlorostyryl)xanthine (CSC), a selective adenosine A_2 receptor antagonist,[34] produced comparable results. These results suggest that endogenous myocardial adenosine may also be shown to exert a positive inotropic effect in the heart under appropriate experimental conditions.

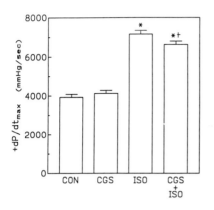

FIGURE 7. The effect of CGS-15943 on the isoproterenol-elicited positive inotropic response in isolated perfused rat hearts. See legend of FIGURE 6 for details. Hearts were perfused in either the absence (CON) or presence (CGS) of 10^{-6} M CGS-15943. Isoproterenol (ISO) was administered at a final concentration of 10^{-8} M for 1 to 2 min. Each value represents the mean ± SE for 7 hearts. *Asterisks* denote a statistically significant difference from the appropriate CON or CGS value. The *dagger* denotes a statistically significant difference from the ISO value.

DISCUSSION

The recent findings presented here suggest that endogenous adenosine exerts multiple actions in the contracting myocardium (FIG. 8). The antiadrenergic action of adenosine is well known.[9-11] The notion that endogenous adenosine is antiadrenergic was reported previously.[24] However, the results presented herein indicate that even the well oxygenated heart has a sufficient amount of endogenous adenosine present to exert an antiadrenergic effect. Since the adenosine A_1 receptor

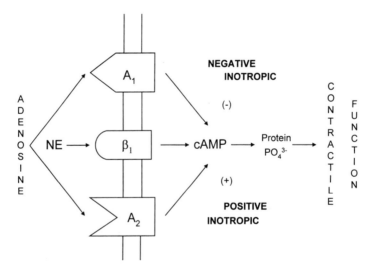

FIGURE 8. A scheme illustrating both the negative and positive inotropic responses of adenosine in the heart. The negative inotropic effect results from adenosine interacting with adenosine A_1 receptors. In this manner the antiadrenergic action of adenosine may play a cardioprotective role. The positive inotropic effect results from adenosine interacting with adenosine A_2 receptors possibly independently of β-adrenergic stimulation.

antagonist DPCPX was used to divulge this phenomenon, the participation of adenosine A_1 receptors is suggested. Thus, the antiadrenergic effect of endogenous adenosine would then appear to be a negative inotropic response when the heart is stimulated with β-adrenergic catecholamines.

The antiadrenergic action of endogenous adenosine appears to be important in the recovery of contractile function upon reperfusion of the ischemic heart subjected to β-adrenergic stimulation. Myocardial levels of norepinephrine may reach 10^{-6} M with ischemia.[35] This level is potentially cardiotoxic if permitted to stimulate the myocardium.[36] Isoproterenol administered to the heart during low-flow ischemia elicited no lasting depression of contractile function during the subsequent isoproterenol-free reperfusion until adenosine A_1 receptor activity was inhibited by DPCPX. When modulation of β-adrenoceptor activity by endogenous adenosine was absent, isoproterenol stimulation during ischemia resulted in a depressed recovery of contractile function after 15 min of reperfusion. These findings indicate that the endogenous adenosine which presumably accumulated during the ischemic period was protecting the myocardium from the detrimental effects of continuous β-adrenergic stimulation. This was reflected in a full recovery of contractile function upon reperfusion. Therefore, endogenously released adenosine, acting via adenosine A_1 receptors, possibly exerts an antiadrenergic action which results in cardioprotection during severe ischemic episodes when interstitial levels of catecholamine would be expected to be elevated.[37]

The results suggesting that endogenous adenosine potentiates the β-adrenergic-elicited positive inotropic response in the heart are of interest, because adenosine A_2 receptor stimulation appears to be involved. The administration of the adenosine A_2 receptor antagonists, either CGS-15943 or CSC, attenuated the positive inotropic contractile response caused by isoproterenol stimulation in well oxygenated perfused hearts. These results suggest that adenosine A_2 receptor stimulation causes a positive inotropic effect or may facilitate the β-adrenergic-induced inotropy in the heart. The notion that adenosine A_2 receptor stimulation is capable of eliciting a positive inotropic effect is supported by reports of studies in which isolated mammalian[32] and avian[31,38] ventricular myocytes have been used.

CONCLUSION

Endogenous myocardial adenosine appears to play several important roles in the contracting heart. First, by interacting with adenosine A_1 receptors in the oxygenated myocardium, endogenous adenosine is antiadrenergic in that it attenuates β-adrenergic-elicited positive inotropy. Second, interacting with the same receptors, endogenous adenosine may be cardioprotective by fostering recovery of contractile function upon reperfusion of the catecholamine-stimulated ischemic heart. Third, interacting with adenosine A_2 receptors in the oxygenated heart, endogenous myocardial adenosine may be a positive inotrope that potentiates β-adrenoceptor-mediated increases in contractility. The relative importance of each of these roles for endogenous adenosine remains to be determined.

REFERENCES

1. BERNE, R. M. 1980. The role of adenosine in the regulation of coronary blood flow. Circ. Res. **47**: 807–813.
2. FEIGL, E. O. 1983. Coronary physiology. Physiol. Rev. **63**: 1–205.

3. BELARDINELLI, L., J. LINDEN & R. M. BERNE. 1989. The cardiac effects of adenosine. Prog. Cardiovasc. Dis. **32:** 73–97.
4. MEININGER, C. J., M. E. SCHELLING & H. J. GRANGER. 1988. Adenosine and hypoxia stimulate proliferation and migration of endothelial cells. Am. J. Physiol. **255:** H554–H562.
5. ETHIER, M. F., V. CHANDER & J. G. DOBSON, JR. 1993. Adenosine stimulates proliferation of human endothelial cells in culture. Am. J. Physiol. **265:** H131–H138.
6. MULLANE, K. & D. BULLOUGH. 1995. Harnessing an endogenous cardioprotective mechanism: cellular sources and sites of action of adenosine. J. Mol. Cell. Cardiol. **27:** 1041–1054.
7. PARRATT, J. R. 1995. Possibilities for the pharmacological exploitation of ischaemic preconditioning. J. Mol. Cell. Cardiol. **27:** 991–1000.
8. ROMANO, F. D., S. G. MACDONALD & J. G. DOBSON, JR. 1989. Adenosine receptor coupling to adenylate cyclase of rat ventricular myocyte membranes. Am. J. Physiol. **257:** H1088–H1095.
9. DOBSON, J. G., JR. & R. A. FENTON. 1983. Antiadrenergic effects of adenosine in the heart. *In* Regulatory Function of Adenosine. R. M. Berne, T. W. Rall & R. Rubio, Eds. 363–376. Nijhoff. Boston.
10. DOBSON, J. G., JR. 1983. Mechanism of adenosine inhibition of catecholamine-induced elicited responses in heart. Circ. Res. **52:** 151–160.
11. DOBSON, J. G., JR., R. A. FENTON & F. D. ROMANO. 1987. The antiadrenergic actions of adenosine in the heart. *In* Topics and Perspectives in Adenosine Research. E. Gerlach & B. F. Becker, Eds. 356–368. Springer-Verlag. Berlin.
12. LAMONICA, D. A., N. FROHLOFF & J. G. DOBSON, JR. 1985. Adenosine inhibition of catecholamine-stimulated cardiac membrane adenylate cyclase. Am. J. Physiol. **248:** H737–H744.
13. SCHRADER, J., G. BAUMANN & E. GERLACK. 1977. Adenosine as inhibitor of myocardial effects of catecholamines. Pflugers Arch. **372:** 29–35.
14. DOBSON, J. G., JR. 1978. Reduction by adenosine of the isoproterenol-induced increase in cyclic adenosine 3′,5′-monophosphate formation and glycogen phosphorylase activity in rat heart muscle. Circ. Res. **43:** 785–792.
15. FENTON, R. A., E. D. W. MOORE, F. S. FAY & J. G. DOBSON, JR. 1991. Adenosine reduces the Ca^{2+} transients of isoproterenol-stimulated rat ventricular myocytes. Am. J. Physiol. **261:** C1107–C1114.
16. FENTON, R. A. & J. G. DOBSON, JR. 1984. Adenosine and calcium alter adrenergic-induced intact heart protein phosphorylation. Am. J. Physiol. **246:** H559–H565.
17. GEORGE, E. E., F. D. ROMANO & J. G. DOBSON, JR. 1991. Adenosine and acetylcholine reduce isoproterenol-induced protein phosphorylation of rat myocytes. J. Mol. Cell. Cardiol. **23:** 749–764.
18. ENDOH, M. & S. YAMASHITA. 1980. Adenosine antagonizes the positive inotropic action mediated via β-, but not α-adrenoceptors in the rabbit papillary muscle. Eur. J. Pharmacol. **65:** 445–448.
19. BOHM, M., R. BRUCKNER, W. MEYER, M. NOSE, W. SCHMITZ, H. SCHOLZ & J. STARBATTY. 1985. Evidence for adenosine receptor-mediated isoprenaline antagonistic effects of the adenosine analogs PIA and NECA on force of contraction in guinea-pig atrial and ventricular cardiac preparations. Naunyn-Schmiedebergs Arch. Pharmacol. **331:** 131–139.
20. DOBSON, J. G., JR. & J. SCHRADER. 1984. Role of extracellular and intracellular adenosine in the attenuation of catecholamine evoked responses in guinea pig heart. J. Mol. Cell. Cardiol. **16:** 813–822.
21. FENTON, R. A. & J. G. DOBSON, JR. 1987. Measurement by fluorescence of interstitial adenosine levels in normoxic, hypoxic and ischemic perfused rat hearts. Circ. Res. **60:** 177–184.
22. FENTON, R. A. & J. G. DOBSON, JR. 1990. Influence of β-adrenergic stimulation and contraction frequency on heart interstitial adenosine. Circ. Res. **66:** 457–468.
23. FENTON, R. A. & J. G. DOBSON, JR. 1992. Fluorometric quantitation of adenosine concentration in small samples of extracellular fluid. Anal. Biochem. **207:** 134–141.

24. DOBSON, J. G., JR., R. W. ORDWAY & R. A. FENTON. 1986. Endogenous adenosine inhibits catecholamine contractile responses in normoxic hearts. Am. J. Physiol. **251:** H455–H462.

25. DOBSON, J. G., JR., R. A. FENTON & F. D. ROMANO. 1990. Increased myocardial adenosine production and reduction of β-adrenergic contractile response in aged hearts. Circ. Res. **66:** 1381–1390.

26. DOBSON, J. G., JR. 1983. Adenosine reduces catecholamine contractile responses in oxygenated and hypoxic atria. Am. J. Physiol. **245:** H468–H474.

27. FENTON, R. A., K. J. GALECKAS & J. G. DOBSON, JR. 1995. Endogenous adenosine reduces depression of cardiac function induced by β-adrenergic stimulation during low flow perfusion. J. Mol. Cell. Cardiol. **27:** 2373–2383.

28. STEIN, B., U. MENDE, J. NEUMANN, W. SCHMITZ & H. SCHOLZ. 1993. Pertussis toxin unmasks stimulatory myocardial A₂-adenosine receptors on ventricular cardiomyocytes. J. Mol. Cell. Cardiol. **25:** 655–659.

29. STEIN, B., W. SCHMITZ, H. SCHOLZ & C. SEELAND. 1994. Pharmacological characterization of A₂-adenosine receptors in guinea pig ventricular myocytes. J. Mol. Cell. Cardiol. **26:** 403–414.

30. SHRYOCK, J., Y. SONG, D. WANG, S. P. BAKER, R. A. OLSSON & L. BELARDINELLI. 1993. Selective A₂-adenosine receptor agonists do not alter action potential duration, twitch shortening, or cyclic AMP accumulation in guinea pig, rat, or rabbit isolated ventricular myocytes. Circ. Res. **72:** 194–205.

31. LIANG, B. T. & B. HALTIWANGER. 1995. Adenosine A₂ₐ and A₂ᵦ receptors in cultured fetal chick heart cells. High- and low-affinity coupling to stimulation of myocyte contractility and cAMP accumulation. Circ. Res. **76:** 242–251.

32. DOBSON, J. G., JR. & R. A. FENTON. 1994. Adenosine A₂-receptor agonists elicit a positive inotropic response and increase adenylyl cyclase activity in rat ventricular myocytes. Drug Dev. Res. **31:** 265 (abstract).

33. GHAI, G., J. E. FRANCIS, M. WILLIAMS, R. A. DOTSON, M. F. HOPKINS, D. T. COTE, F. R. GOODMAN & M. B. ZIMMERMAN. 1987. Pharmacological characterization of CGS15943A: a novel nonxanthine adenosine antagonist. J. Pharmacol. Exp. Ther. **242:** 784–790.

34. JACOBSON, K. A., O. NIKODIJEVIC, W. L. PADGETT, C. GALLO-RODRIGUEZ, M. MAILLARD & J. W. DALY. 1993. 8-(3-Chlorostyryl) caffeine (CSC) is a selective A₂-adenosine antagonist *in vitro* and *in vivo*. Fed. Eur. Biochem. Soc. **323:** 141–144.

35. SCHOMIG, A., A. M. DART, R. DIETZ, E. MAYER & W. KUBLER. 1984. Release of endogenous catecholamines in the ischemic myocardium of the rat. Part A: Locally mediated release. Circ. Res. **55:** 689–701.

36. RONA, G. 1985. Catecholamine cardiotoxicity. J. Mol. Cell. Cardiol. **17:** 291–306.

37. SCHOMIG, A. 1990. Catecholamines in myocardial ischemia: systemic and cardiac release. Circulation **82**(Suppl. II): 13–22.

38. XU, D., H. KONG & B. T. LIANG. 1992. Expression and pharmacological characterization of a stimulatory subtype of adenosine receptor in fetal chick ventricular myocytes. Circ. Res. **70:** 56–65.

Depletion of Preischemic Glycogen Reduces the Increase of Low Molecular Weight Iron during Ischemia

JOHAN F. KOSTER,[a,c] ARTHUR VOOGD,[a]
TOM J. C. RUIGROK,[b] AND WIM SLUITER[a]

[a]Department of Biochemistry
Cardiovascular Research Institute
Erasmus University Rotterdam (COEUR)
Rotterdam, The Netherlands
and
[b]Department of Experimental Cardiology
University Hospital Utrecht
Interuniversity Cardiology Institute
Utrecht, The Netherlands

INTRODUCTION

The generation of reactive oxygen species upon reoxygenation of ischemic tissue contributes to the detrimental events that together constitute reperfusion injury.[1-5] The toxicity of superoxide and hydrogen peroxide is thought to be caused by the generation of the highly oxidizing hydroxyl radical mediated through transition metal dependent reactions.[6] The most abundant intracellular transition metal, iron, is safely deposited in ferritin or bound to haem proteins[7] and as such is not available for Haber-Weiss chemistry. Only a very small amount is present in what is known as the low molecular weight (LMW) pool,[8-11] in which form it can participate in the Haber-Weiss reactions.[12,13] In a recent study from our laboratory[14] we showed that iron is released into the LMW pool during ischemia, in the heart tissue. Prasad *et al.*[15] have reported that iron is released in the perfusate. However, this phenomenon was shown earlier by Nohl *et al.*[16] We showed[14] that this iron reallocation does not occur during anoxia. We have hypothesized that the ischemic reperfusion damage is closely related to the amount of iron in the LMW pool.

It is known that recovery after ischemia is inversely related to glycolytic activity, measured as the amount of lactate that accumulates during ischemia, but independent of tissue ATP just before reperfusion.[17] This was achieved by preschemic glycogen depletion through anoxic perfusion immediately before ischemia. By now, it is well established that short periods of ischemia protect against a longer ischemic insult, and the concept is known as ischemic preconditioning.[18,19] Among the explanations proposed for this phenomenon are reduced energy demand,[20] the induction of stress proteins and effects mediated through oxygen

[c] Correspondence to: Prof. Dr. J. F. Koster, Dept. of Biochemistry, Cardiovascular Research Institute Erasmus University Rotterdam (COEUR), P. O. Box 1738, 3000 DR Rotterdam, The Netherlands. Tel.: (31)104087327; Fax: (31)104360615.

radicals, adenosine receptor and arachidonic acid metabolites.[18,19] However, glycogen depletion is a common feature of all these experimental approaches and is known to attenuate acidification and metabolite accumulation during ischemia.[21,22]

Since ischemia induces an iron release into the LMW pool,[14] we investigated whether preconditioning would result in a reduction in the amount of iron that is released into the LMW pool. As stated, preconditioning resulted in a depletion of glycogen, and we investigated whether there is a correlation between the amount of glycogen present at the start of ischemia and the amount of iron released into the LMW pool during ischemia. We also applied conditions consisting of glycogen depletion by anoxia and glucagon administration before the actual ischemia insult.

MATERIALS AND METHODS

Animals and Langendorff Perfusion Protocol

Twelve- to fourteen-week-old male Wistar rats were used. After a brief anesthesia with diethyl ether the hearts were excised and placed in ice cold Tyrode buffer. The hearts were cannulated through the aorta and perfused retrogradely according to Langendorff[23] while beating spontaneously. Perfusions were carried out at 37°C with Tyrode buffer containing 128 mM NaCl, 4.7 mM KCl, 1.25 mM $CaCl_2$, 20.2 mM $NaHCO_3$, 0.4 mM NaH_2PO_4, 1 mM $MgCl_2$ and 11 mM glucose, pH 7.4. The buffer was saturated with 95% O_2 and 5% CO_2. Tyrode buffer was made anoxic by saturation with 95% N_2 and 5% CO_2 for at least one hour. Perfusion pressure was kept constant at 80 cm water pressure.

In order to investigate the effects of preischemic glycogen depletion hearts were subjected to three different protocols that are known to decrease cardiac glycogen content and subjected to fifteen minutes of no-flow ischemia. Preischemic glycogen depletion was achieved by preperfusion before ischemia with 1) anoxic buffer for fifteen minutes,[17] 2) three five-minute periods of no-flow ischemia interrupted by ten minutes reperfusion[21] and 3) perfusion with 250 μg/l glucagon for five minutes.[24] These groups were compared to control hearts, which were subjected to fifteen minutes of no-flow ischemia after perfusion with only normoxic Tyrode for one hour. Separate sets of experiments were performed in order to determine different parameters. Functional recovery, LDH and lactate release were determined in one set of four groups (n = 6 in each group) of hearts. Glycogen content was determined in one group (n = 5) after fifteen minutes of normoxic perfusion. A further eight groups of hearts (n = 5 in each group) were used to determine cardiac glycogen immediately before ischemia just after pretreatment and at the end of ischemia in all four experiments. LMW iron was determined in each group (n = 6 in each group) of hearts at the end of the ischemic period. Nuclear magnetic resonance (^{31}P NMR) measurements were performed using the final set of four groups (n = 3 in each group).

Glycogen, Lactate, LMW Iron and pH Determination

Hearts were frozen in freezing isopentane and homogenized in 5% perchloric acid. Glycogen was determined in the neutralized homogenate as described elsewhere.[25] Glycogen values are expressed as a percentage of normoxic control hearts which contained 2.21 ± 0.11 mg glycogen per g wet wt.

Lactate was determined in the coronary effluent as described elsewhere[26] and cumulative release is expressed as μmoles per gram wet weight (μmole/g wet wt).

Low molecular weight iron was determined as described in detail elsewhere[14] and expressed as picomoles per milligram protein (pmole/mg protein).

Intracellular pH values were calculated from the chemical shift of the intracellular inorganic phosphate peak in the ^{31}P NMR spectra as described in detail elsewhere.[27]

Functional Parameters

Lactate dehydrogenase (LDH) release, as a measure of tissue damage, and coronary flow were measured as described earlier.[28] Apex displacement was detected with a smooth muscle transducer. Contractility, as a measure of cardiac work, was calculated as the product of apex-amplitude and apex-frequency, which were recorded every thirty seconds. The mean value of the contractility of each heart during five minutes before ischemia was set at 100%.

Chemicals

Glucagon was obtained from NOVO Nordisk A/S, Copenhagen, Denmark, and dissolved in Tyrode at a concentration of 250 μg/l.

Statistics

Intergroup differences were evaluated with analysis of variance using the Bonferroni option for multiple comparisons (STATA release 2.0).

RESULTS

Glycogen Depletion and Functional Recovery

To establish the relationship between glycogen depletion and functional recovery after reperfusion separate groups of hearts were subjected to preperfusion with anoxic Tyrode and with Tyrode containing 250 μg/l glucagon and to a standard "preconditioning" protocol consisting of three five-minute periods of ischemia interrupted by ten minutes of reoxygenation. The glycogen content was determined directly before ischemia and after fifteen minutes of ischemia.

Control hearts perfused with normoxic Tyrode for fifteen minutes contained 2.11 ± 0.10 mg/g wet weight glycogen. After a further forty-five minutes of normoxic perfusion glycogen content was 2.21 ± 0.11 mg/g wet wt (n.s., n = 5, Fig. 1). After fifteen minutes of ischemia, glycogen content decreased to 38.7 ±

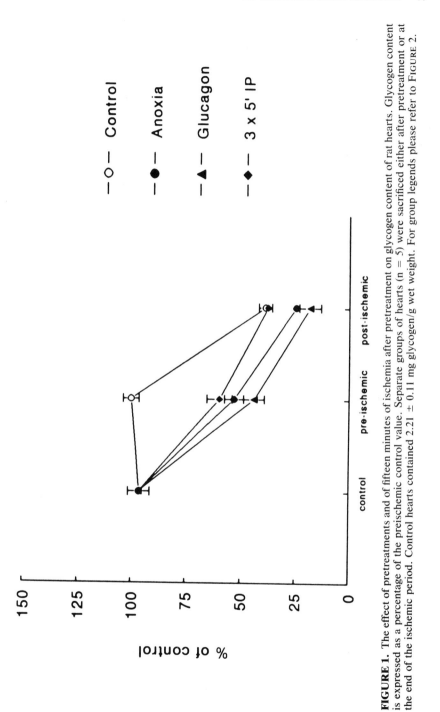

FIGURE 1. The effect of pretreatments and of fifteen minutes of ischemia after pretreatment on glycogen content of rat hearts. Glycogen content is expressed as a percentage of the preischemic control value. Separate groups of hearts (n = 5) were sacrificed either after pretreatment or at the end of the ischemic period. Control hearts contained 2.21 ± 0.11 mg glycogen/g wet weight. For group legends please refer to FIGURE 2.

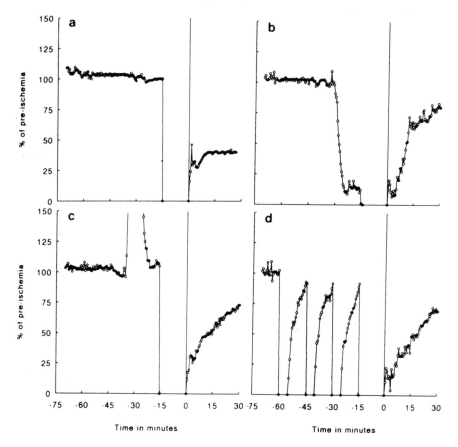

FIGURE 2. The effect of pretreatment on postischemic recovery. Data acquisition starts at time = −70. Contractility is expressed as percentage of the contractility between time = −65 and time = −60. All hearts were perfused with normoxic Tyrode buffer before treatment. Pretreatments: **(a)** none (control); **(b)** anoxia Tyrode for fifteen minutes starting at time = −30 (anoxia); **(c)** normoxic Tyrode containing 0.25 mg/l glucagon for five minutes starting at time = −35 followed by fifteen minutes without glucagon (glucagon); **(d)** three five-minute periods of ischemia and ten minutes of reperfusion (3 × 5′ IP).

2.1% of the original glycogen content (FIG. 1), and the function of the heart recovered to 44.0 ± 3.8% of preischemic contractility after thirty minutes of reoxygenation (FIG. 2a). Preperfusion with anoxic Tyrode for fifteen minutes depleted the cardiac glycogen stores to 52.9 ± 4.3% and this decreased further to 24.6 ± 2.1% (p <0.05, n = 5) after fifteen minutes of ischemia (FIG. 1), while the contractility recovered to 80 ± 5.2% after thirty minutes of reperfusion (FIG. 2b). Glucagon perfusion during five minutes depleted glycogen stores down to 43.8 ± 4.8% and this decreased further to 18.1 ± 5.2% (p <0.05, n = 5) during ischemia (FIG. 1). Perfusion with glucagon led to a transient increase in contractility up to 285% of control level due to the positive inotropic action of glucagon. After stabilization for fifteen minutes by changing to buffer without glucagon, the hearts were then made ischemic, which treatment led to a recovery of 81 ± 6.2% after thirty minutes of reperfusion (FIG. 2c). Treatment with three short periods of ischemia depleted glycogen stores to 59.7 ± 5.7% of the normoxic value which decreased further to 38.4 ± 1.7% after fifteen minutes of ischemia (p <0.05, n = 5; FIG. 1), and led to a recovery of 73 ± 5.6% of preischemic contractility (FIG. 2d).

Lactate Release

To assess lactic acid that is released by the ischemic heart upon reperfusion is a reflection of the glycolytic activity that has taken place during ischemia. Therefore the cumulative amount of lactic acid in the coronary effluent during thirty minutes of reperfusion was determined. All three of the pretreated groups released less lactate than the control group (FIG. 3, p <0.05 for the difference between the control group, n = 6 in each group).

Intracellular pH

To evaluate the influence of glycogen depletion on the development of ischemic acidosis, pH was measured by ^{31}P NMR in the four groups of hearts. In control hearts intracellular pH decreased from 7.04 ± 0.02 immediately before ischemia to 5.95 ± 0.05 after fifteen minutes of ischemia. In the three glycogen-depleted groups there was a significant attenuation of the acidosis (p <0.05 for the pH after fifteen minutes ischemia in control versus each group, n = 3). In these groups of hearts pH decreased during ischemia from 6.97 ± 0.02 to 6.24 ± 0.05 (anoxic

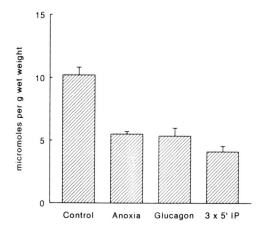

FIGURE 3. The effect of pretreatments on the total amount of lactate released in the coronary effluent during thirty minutes of reperfusion after ischemia. Cumulative lactate release was lower in pretreated hearts compared to control hearts (n = 6 hearts in each group, p <0.05 one-way analysis of variance using the Bonferroni correction for multiple comparisons). For group legends please refer to FIGURE 2.

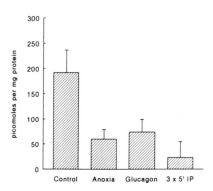

FIGURE 4. The effect of pretreatment on LMW iron in rat hearts at the end of fifteen minutes of ischemia. LMW iron was lower in pretreated groups than in control hearts (n = 6 hearts in each group, $p < 0.05$ one-way analysis of variance using the Bonferroni correction for multiple comparisons). For group legends please refer to FIGURE 2.

preperfusion), from 7.05 ± 0.01 to 6.12 ± 0.01 (glucagon) and from 7.07 ± 0.03 to 6.18 ± 0.05 (3 × 5 min ischemia).

LMW Iron

To investigate whether the amount of iron in the LMW pool upon reoxygenation, which is thought to be related to tissue damage and functional recovery, is affected by glycogen depletion, the effect of the pretreatment on the amount of LMW iron after fifteen minutes of ischemia was determined in separate groups of hearts. Control hearts contained 192 ± 45 pmoles of LMW iron per mg protein (FIG. 4). Pretreatment with anoxia, glucagon and three ischemic periods all led to a reduction in the amount of iron that was released into the LMW pool during ischemia (60 ± 19, 74 ± 25 and 23 ± 32 pmole/mg protein respectively, $p < 0.05$ for the difference between control and each group, n = 6).

LDH Release

To assess tissue damage induced by ischemia after glycogen depletion, cumulative LDH release was measured in the coronary effluent during thirty minutes of reperfusion. Control hearts released 5.23 ± 1.13 (means $\pm$ SD, n = 6) units LDH during thirty minutes of reperfusion (FIG. 5). Tissue damage was markedly

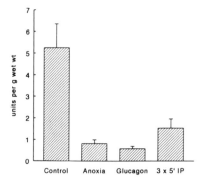

FIGURE 5. The effect of pretreatment on the total amount of LDH released in the coronary effluent during thirty minutes of reperfusion after fifteen minutes ischemia of rat hearts that were not pretreated (control) or pretreated with anoxic Tyrode for fifteen minutes (anoxia), normoxic Tyrode containing 0.25 mg/l glucagon for five minutes followed by fifteen minutes without glucagon (glucagon) and three five-minute periods of ischemia and ten minutes of reperfusion (3 × 5' IP).

attenuated by pretreatment with fifteen minutes of anoxic perfusion, five minutes preperfusion with glucagon and with three short periods of ischemia (0.81 ± 0.20, 0.57 ± 0.11 and 1.52 ± 0.36 U/g wet weight, respectively, $p < 0.01$ for the difference between each group and the control group, n = 6 in each group).

DISCUSSION

The important finding of the present study is that partial glycogen depletion before ischemia (which is known to improve postischemic cardiac function) led to a decrease in magnitude of the LMW iron pool. Presently, the mechanism of the iron release during ischemia is not known. Direct mobilization of ferritin iron by biological chelators is a slow process.[29-31] Reductive iron release is much faster,[32-34] and several of the metabolites accumulating during ischemia may be involved in this process. *In vitro* it has been shown[33,34] that flavins can act as reducing agents and their action is enhanced by a lower pH. In the present study glycogen depletion led to only a small attenuation of the acidosis which could hardly account for a decrease in iron release. However, lactate accumulation was markedly reduced, which also led to an attenuated NADH accumulation. In that respect it is worth noting that liver homogenate contains NADH-, NADPH- or xanthine-dependent ferrireductase activity, which have been shown to release iron from ferritin.[35] The NADH-dependent activity from rat liver has a K_m for NADH of 2.79 mM. In rat myocytes cytosolic NADH concentration has been estimated to be 0.89 mM,[36] which increases during ischemia. The presence of such an NADH-dependent ferrireductase activity in rat hearts then enhances iron release during ischemia, and glycogen depletion by reduction in lactate accumulation and subsequent NADH accumulation prevent iron release. Furthermore, during anoxic perfusion no cytosolic NADH accumulates, because lactate is removed. In this situation no increment of LMW iron is observed.[14]

Earlier studies showed that pretreatment with short periods of ischemia reduced the glycogen level,[21,22] which led to a better recovery of the contractility after an ischemic insult. We found here that this protocol, and also the reduction of the amount of glycogen through a previous glucagon administration and by applying a previous anoxia, all reduce the increment of LMW iron during the ischemic insult. Apparently, the magnitude of the LMW iron pool is directly related to the amount of glycogen present when ischemia starts. This might be highly relevant for the improvement in recovery of cardiac function after ischemia, because LMW iron catalyzes the generation of hydroxyl radicals that aggravate tissue damage.

SUMMARY

The amount of iron in the low molecular weight pool (LMW) increases during no-flow ischemia and is thought to be essential to oxygen radical-derived damage upon reperfusion. Applying three short ischemic periods (5 min) preconditioning before 15 min ischemia results in an improved contractility compared to a direct 15 min ischemic insult. This raises the question whether preconditioning leads to a decrease in the LMW iron pool. We therefore investigated the change in the LMW iron pool during ischemic insult after applying preconditioning. It is assumed that an increase in LMW iron is dependent on the accumulation of reduction equivalents derived from the anaerobic glycolysis. Therefore the glycogen content was also reduced by administration by anoxia and glucagon administration to study the effect on the LMW iron pool.

Methods and Results

Isolated rat hearts were depleted of glycogen by perfusion with (group 1) anoxic buffer, (group 2) buffer containing glucagon and (group 3) by three short periods of ischemia (15 min) before being subjected to various times of no-flow ischemia. All these treatments resulted in a decreased glycogen level respectively for group 1, $52.9 \pm 4.8\%$; group 2, $43.8 \pm 4.8\%$ and group 3, $59.7 \pm 5.7\%$. After 15 min of no-flow ischemia the LMW iron pool amounted to 192 ± 45 pmol/mg protein, while pretreated hearts contained 60 ± 19 (group 1), 74 ± 25 (group 2) and 23 ± 32 (group 3) pmol/mg protein ($p < 0.05$ control vs each group n = 6). All three pretreated groups show a better recovery in contractility than the control group.

Conclusion

Our results suggest that the amount of iron released in the LMW pool is determined by the amount of glycogen present at the beginning of ischemia. It is therefore tempting to conclude that the decreased amount of LMW iron pool after applying preconditioning is one of the mechanisms by which an improved recovery of the heart is obtained.

ACKNOWLEDGMENTS

The expert technical assistance of C. W. A. van der Kolk, M. G. J. Nederhoff, R. G. Kraak-Slee and L. E. A. van de Merbel-de Wit is gratefully acknowledged.

REFERENCES

1. BOLLI, R. 1991. Oxygen derived free radicals in myocardial reperfusion injury: an overview. Cardiovasc. Drugs Ther. 5(Suppl. 2): 249–269.
2. WERNS, S. W. & B. R. LUCCHESI. 1989. Free radicals and ischemic tissue injury. TIPS 11: 161–166.
3. MCCORD, J. 1988. Free radicals and myocardial ischemia; overview and outlook. Free Radical Biol. Med. 4: 9–14.
4. KLONER, R. A., K. PRZYKLENK & P. WHITTAKER. 1989. Deleterious effects of oxygen radicals in ischemia/reperfusion. Resolved and unresolved issues. Circulation 80: 1115–1127.
5. SIMPSON, P. J. & B. R. LUCCHESI. 1987. Free radicals and myocardial ischemia and reperfusion injury. J. Lab. Clin. Med. 110: 13–30.
6. HALLIWEL, B. & J. M. C. GUTTERIDGE. 1991. Role of free radicals and catalytic metal ions in human disease: an overview. Methods Enzymol. 186: 1–85.
7. CRICHTON, R. R. & M. CHARLOTEAUX-WAUTERS. 1987. Iron transport and storage. Eur. J. Biochem. 164: 485–506.
8. KOZLOV, A. V., D. Y. YEGOROV, Y. A. VLADIMIROV & O. A. AZIZOVA. 1992. Intracellular free iron in liver tissue and liver homogenate: studies with electron paramagnetic resonance on the formation of paramagnetic complexes with desferral and nitric oxide. Free Radical Biol. Med. 13: 9–16.

9. FONTECAVE, H. & J. L. PIERRE. 1991. Iron metabolism: the low molecular mass iron pool. Biol. Metals **4**: 133–135.
10. WEAVER, J. & S. POLLACK. 1986. Low Mr iron isolated from guinea pig reticulocytes as AMP-Fe and ATP-Fe complexes. Biochem. J. **261**: 787–792.
11. MULLIGAN, M., B. ALTHAUS & M. C. LINDER. 1986. Non-ferritin, non-heme iron pools in rat tissue. Int. J. Biochem. **18**: 791–798.
12. RUSH, J. D., Z. MASKOS & W. H. KOPPENOL. 1990. Reactions of iron (II) nucleotide complexes with hydrogenperoxide. FEBS Lett. **261**: 121–123.
13. FLOYD, R. A. & A. LEWIS. 1983. Hydroxyl radical formation from hydrogenperoxide by ferrous iron nucleotide complexes. Biochemistry **22**: 2645–2649.
14. VOOGD, A., W. SLUITER, H. G. VAN EIJK & J. F. KOSTER. 1992. Low molecular weight iron and the oxygen paradox in isolated rat hearts. J. Clin. Invest. **90**: 2050–2055.
15. PRASAD, M. R., X. LIU, J. A. ROUSOU, R. M. ENGELMAN, R. JONES, A. GEORGE & D. K. DAS. 1992. Reduced free radical generation during reperfusion of hypothermically arrested hearts. Mol. Cell. Biochem. **111**: 97–102.
16. NOHL, H., K. STOLZE, S. NAPETSCHNIG & T. ISHIKAWA. 1991. Is oxidative stress primarily involved in reperfusion injury of the ischemic heart? Free Radical Biol. Med. **11**: 581–588.
17. NEELY, J. R. & L. W. GROTYOHAN. 1992. Role of glycolytic products in damage to the ischemic myocardium. Circ. Res. **55**: 816–824.
18. DOWNEY, J. M. 1992. Ischemic preconditioning: nature's own protective mechanism. Trends Cardiovasc. Med. **2**: 170–176.
19. WALKER, D. M. & D. M. YELLON. 1992. Ischemic preconditioning: from mechanism to exploitation. Cardiovasc. Res. **26**: 734–739.
20. MURRY, C. E., V. J. RICHARD, K. A. REIMER & R. B. JENNINGS. 1990. Ischemic preconditioning slows energy metabolism and delays ultrastructural damage during a sustained ischemic episode. Circ. Res. **66**: 913–931.
21. VOLOVSEK, A., R. SUBRAMANIAN & D. REBOUSSIN. 1992. Effects of duration of ischaemia during preconditioning on mechanical function, enzyme release and energy production in the isolated working rat heart. J. Mol. Cell. Cardiol. **24**: 1011–1019.
22. KUPRIYANOV, V. V., V. L. LAKOMKIN, A. YA. STEINSCHNEIDER, M. YA. SEVERINA, V. I. KAPELKO, E. K. RUUGE & V. A. SAKS. 1988. Relationship between preischemic ATP and glycogen content and postischemic recovery of rat heart. J. Mol. Cell. Cardiol. **20**: 1151–1162.
23. LANGENDORFF, O., 1895. Untersuchungen am überlebenden Säugetierherzen. Pflügers Arch. Physiol. **61**: 225–241.
24. CORNBLATH, M., J. P. RANDLE, A. PARMEGGIANI & H. E. MORGAN. 1963. Regulation of glycogenolysis in muscle: effects of glucagon and anoxia on lactate production, glycogen content and phosphorylase activity in the perfused isolated rat heart. J. Biol. Chem. **238**: 1592–1597.
25. HUIJING, F. 1970. A rapid enzymic method for glycogen estimation in very small tissue samples. Clin. Chim. Acta **30**: 567–572.
26. BERGMEYER, H. U. 1963. Methods in Enzymatic Analysis. Academic Press. New York.
27. SCHREUR, J. H. M., J. H. KIRKELS, C. J. A. VAN ECHTELD & T. J. C. RUIGROK. 1992. Postischaemic metabolic and functional recovery of rat heart after transient reperfusion with various low calcium concentrations. Cardiovasc. Res. **26**: 687–693.
28. VAN DER KRAAIJ, A. M. M., L. J. MOSTERT, H. G. VAN EIJK & J. F. KOSTER. 1988. Iron load increases the susceptibility of rat hearts toward reperfusion damage. Protection by the anti oxidant (+)-cyanidanol-3 and deferoxamine. Circulation **78**: 442–449.
29. MAZUR, A., S. BAEZ & E. SCHORRE. 1955. The mechanism of iron release from ferritin as related to its biological properties. J. Biol. Chem. **213**: 147–160.
30. PAPE, L., J. D. MULTANI, C. STITT & P. SALTMAN. 1968. The mobilization of iron from ferritin by chelating agents. Biochemistry **7**: 613–616.
31. DOGNIN, J. & R. R. CRICHTON. 1975. Mobilization of iron from ferritin fractions of defined iron content by biological reductants. FEBS Lett. **54**: 234–236.
32. FUNK, F., J. P. LENDERS, R. R. CRICHTON & W. SCHNEIDER. 1985. Reductive mobilisation of ferritin iron. Eur. J. Biochem. **152**: 167–172.

33. SIRIVECH, S., E. FRIEDEN & S. OSAKI. 1974. The release of iron from horse spleen ferritin by reduced flavins. Biochem. J. **143:** 311–315.
34. JONES, T., R. SPENCER & C. WALSH. 1978. Mechanism and kinetics of iron release from ferritin by dihydroflavins and dihydroflavin analogs. Biochemistry **17:** 4011–4017.
35. TOPHAM, R., M. GOGER, K. PEARCE & P. SCHULTZ. 1989. The mobilisation of ferritin iron by liver cytosol. A comparison of xanthine and NADH as reducing substrates. Biochem. J. **261:** 137–143.
36. ESUMI, K., M. NISHIDA, D. SHAW, T. W. SMITH & J. D. MARSH. 1991. NADH measurements in adult rat myocytes during simulated ischemia. Am. J. Physiol. **260:** H1743–H1752.
37. MURRY, C. E., V. J. RICHARD, K. A. REIMER & R. B. JENNINGS. 1990. Ischemic preconditioning slows energy metabolism and delays ultrastructural damage during a sustained ischemic episode. Circ. Res. **66:** 913–931.

Metabolic Effects of Ischemic Preconditioning and Adenosine Receptor Blockade in Dogs[a]

OLEG I. PISARENKO,[b] OLGA V. TSKITISHVILY,
IRINA M. STUDNEVA, LARISA I. SEREBRYAKOVA,
AND OLGA V. KORCHAZHKINA

Institute of Experimental Cardiology
Cardiology Research Center
121552 Moscow, Russia

INTRODUCTION

Mechanisms of cardioprotection afforded by ischemic preconditioning (IPC) remain obscure. It was proposed that adenosine released during brief periods of coronary occlusion interacting with extracellular receptors may provide protection against ischemia/reperfusion injury.[1-3] However, effects of IPC on metabolism of risk area during regional ischemia and reperfusion remain controversial, varying among animals species and experimental designs.[4-9] Despite an abundance of investigations with various adenosine receptor agonists and antagonists,[1-3,10,11] the metabolic effects of these compounds on the ischemic preconditioned myocardium have not been systematically analyzed. Our previous study showed that a single cycle of IPC in the dog, 5-min occlusion of the left ventricular anterior descending coronary artery followed by 10-min reperfusion, improved postischemic recovery of regional contractile function. This effect was accompanied by a transient increase in interstitial adenosine during preconditioning followed by less release of adenine nucleotide breakdown products into the interstitium during subsequent sustained ischemia.[12] We undertook the present study to assess changes in myocardial contents of high-energy phosphates, creatine (Cr) and lactate (Lact) and inorganic phosphate (P_i) in the same dog model using conventional biopsy technique and cardiac microdialysis. The other aim of this work was to examine metabolic responses of pretreatment of the preconditioned myocardium with theophylline (Theo), the adenosine A_1/A_2 receptor antagonist, potentially capable of attenuating adenosine influence on glycolytic flux.[13]

METHODS

Animal Preparation

Animal care and experimental conduct conformed to the guidelines of the National Institutes of Health.[14] Adult mongrel dogs of either sex weighing 15–20 kg

[a] This work was supported by Grant No. 95004-12913a from the Russian Foundation for Basic Research.

[b] Address for correspondence: Dr. Oleg I. Pisarenko, Cardiology Research Center, 3rd Cherepkovskaya Str. 15A, 121552 Moscow, Russia. Tel.: (095)414-67-37.

were lightly sedated with dpoperidol (1 mg/kg s.c.), anesthetized with intravenous sodium thiopental (30 mg/kg i.v.), intubated and artificially ventilated with room air enriched with oxygen at 3–4 litre/min. Right internal jugular vein was cannulated for administration of heparin (5000 IU) to prevent thrombosis formation and to give small doses of sodium thiopental as necessary. A catheter was introduced through the right carotid artery into the left ventricular cavity for measurement of the left ventricular pressure, its first derivatives ($\pm$ dP/dt) and heart rate. All indices were recorded on a Siemens Elema 8-channel recorder (Mingograph 804). Left thoracotomy was performed at the 5th intercostal space, pericardium was incised and the heart was suspended in pericardial cradle. The proximal left anterior descending coronary artery or one of its diagonal branches (LAD) was isolated, and loose ligature was placed around it. Arterial blood pH and pCO_2 were maintained within physiological range by adjusting tidal volume, and O_2 supplementation and injection of sodium bicarbonate were carried out using an acid-base analyzer ABL-30 (Radiometer).

Cardiac Microdialysis

Two microdialysis probes were implanted in the area perfused by LAD to be occluded and one was inserted into intact LV wall, using techniques described previously.[15] After implantation, the inflow silica tubes of each probe were connected to a glass syringe of a CMA/100 microinjection pump (Carnegye Medicine). The syringe was filled with Ringer's solution (in mmol: NaCl 147; KCl 4.0; $CaCl_2$ 2.3) and each probe was perfused at a constant flow rate of 3 μl/min. After the equilibration period of forty minutes, the effluent referred to as the dialysate, was collected every 10 min from the outflow tube in Eppendorff tubes and frozen until metabolite analysis. *In vitro* experiments showed that this perfusion rate provides the average dialysis recovery for Lact, Cr and P_i equal to 28.6 $\pm$ 2.4, 46.5 $\pm$ 3.1, and 33.6 $\pm$ 2.8%, respectively.

Experimental Protocol

The dogs were randomly divided into three groups: control, preconditioned (PC) and treated with Theo prior to IPC (Theo-PC). After isolation of LAD branch and implantation of microdialysis probes, all groups underwent 40-min baseline period for stabilization of hemodynamic variables and collection of the initial dialysate samples (FIG. 1). In the control group there was an additional period of 15-min control perfusion before ischemia-reperfusion instead of IPC. In the PC and Theo-PC groups IPC was achieved using a single 5-min LAD occlusion followed by 10-min reperfusion. Animals in all groups were then subjected to 40 min of LAD occlusion and 60 min of reperfusion. During short-time and sustained occlusion, the ligature around the coronary artery was tightened to produce a zone of regional left ventricular ischemia, which was confirmed by regional cyanosis and diskinetic movement. In the Theo-PC group, 5 mg/kg of Theo were given intravenously over 30 sec 20 min before IPC. Theo solution was prepared according to Jeremy[16] and was passed through a Millipore filter (pore size = 0.22 μm) before the intravenous injection. At the end of each experimental period biopsies from risk area were taken. After the final reperfusion period, myocardial biopsies were also taken from the control area. All tissue specimens were immediately frozen in liquid

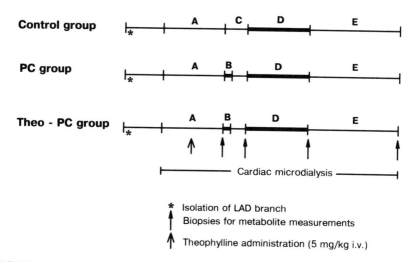

FIGURE 1. Schematic illustration of the experimental design. LAD, left anterior coronary artery. A, 40-min baseline period; B, 5-min occlusion of LAD branch followed by 10-min reperfusion; C, 15-min control perfusion; D, 40-min period of LAD ischemia; E, 60-min reperfusion of LAD region. *Arrows* indicate collections of biopsies from ischemic area for metabolite analysis and Theo administration. At the end of the reperfusion period biopsy was also taken from the nonischemic area of the left ventricle. Cardiac dialysate was collected throughout the experiment beginning from baseline period.

nitrogen until biochemical analysis. Hemodynamic variables were monitored throughout the experiment.

Tissue Sampling and Metabolite Analysis

The frozen tissue was quickly homogenized in a cooled 6% perchloric acid (10 ml/g tissue), and proteins were centrifuged at 3,000 g for 10 min at 4°C. Supernatants were neutralized with 5 M K_2CO_3 to pH 7.4. Tissue dry weights were determined by weighing the portion of pellets after extraction with $HClO_4$ and drying overnight at 110°C. Concentrations of ATP, phosphocreatine (PCr), creatine (Cr), glycogen (Gly), glucose and Lact in neutralized tissue extracts were measured enzymatically.[17] Modified spectrophotometric micromethods were used to assay dialysate samples for Lact, Cr and P_i.[17-19] All solutions were prepared using deionized water (Mili Ro4-Mili-Q).

Statistical Analysis

Data are reported as mean ± SEM. Multiple comparisons of the experimental groups were performed by one-way analysis of variance (ANOVA) with a Student-Newman-Keuls test. The differences between group variables for different time periods of measurements were tested by repeated measures ANOVA. A value of $p < 0.05$ was considered to be significant.

RESULTS

Cardiac Hemodynamics and Metabolic State of the Nonischemic Area

No significant differences in the left ventricular systolic pressure (LVSP), heart rate (HR), an index of cardiac contractile function evaluated by LVSP-HR product, and the maximum rate of rise or fall of left ventricular pressure development (+ dP/dt or − dP/dt, respectively) were found between the groups during the entire experiment (data not shown).

Tissue levels of high-energy phosphates, Cr, Gly and Lact in a normally perfused circumflex bed after the final reperfusion did not differ from the initial ones for ischemic area (TABLES 1, 2). Dialysate Cr, Lact and P_i concentrations did not change throughout the experiment, remaining very close to the baseline levels (FIGS. 2–4). These data mean that the animals remained hemodynamically stable, and adequate aerobic metabolism was persisted in nonischemic myocardium throughout the protocols in all groups.

Effects of PC on the Metabolism of the Risk Area

The single cycle of IPC reduced myocardial content of ATP and PCr to 72 and 74% of the initial values, respectively (TABLE 1). However, during sustained

TABLE 1. Effects of Ischemic Preconditioning and Theophylline Pretreatment on Myocardial Contents of ATP, PCr and Cr in Risk Area[1]

Time Period	Control	PC	Theo-PC
ATP			
Initial	25.86 ± 0.86	26.12 ± 0.94	24.74 ± 1.38
Preischemic	24.47 ± 1.18	18.84 ± 0.97[a]	17.42 ± 0.88[a]
Postischemic	10.04 ± 1.36	11.78 ± 1.12	8.06 ± 1.02
Reperfusion	11.18 ± 1.12[b,c,d]	15.64 ± 1.17[a,c,d]	7.34 ± 0.98[a,b,c]
Phosphocreatine			
Initial	30.39 ± 1.48	32.15 ± 1.64	29.34 ± 1.82
Preischemic	31.57 ± 1.69	23.78 ± 2.18[a]	19.54 ± 1.54[a]
Postischemic	5.73 ± 0.85	8.82 ± 1.02[a]	3.55 ± 0.68[a,b]
Reperfusion	14.00 ± 1.88[c,d]	17.58 ± 1.11[c,d]	8.94 ± 0.94[a,b,c]
Creatine			
Initial	64.90 ± 3.03	65.32 ± 2.14	65.02 ± 2.46
Preischemic	63.66 ± 2.31	60.94 ± 3.08	58.06 ± 2.59
Postischemic	89.32 ± 4.25	74.08 ± 4.37[a]	85.64 ± 4.46[b]
Reperfusion	56.08 ± 3.65[b,d]	64.63 ± 4.02	51.57 ± 3.64[b,c]
Total creatine			
Initial	95.51 ± 4.12	97.18 ± 5.09	94.30 ± 3.96
Preischemic	94.96 ± 3.21	84.78 ± 3.12[a]	77.82 ± 2.63[a]
Postischemic	95.05 ± 4.63	97.30 ± 3.86	89.19 ± 3.65
Reperfusion	70.17 ± 2.99[b,c]	83.04 ± 3.54[a,d]	61.25 ± 3.21[b,c]

[1] Values are the means ± SEM for 12–14 experiments and expressed in μmol/g dry weight. Transmural biopsies were taken after baseline period (initial); after control perfusion or the cycle of IPC (preischemic); after 40-min period of LAD occlusion (postischemic); and at the end of the final reperfusion (reperfusion) as indicated in FIGURE 1. PC and Theo-PC: groups receiving 5-min LAD occlusion followed by 10-min reperfusion without and with Theo pretreatment (5 mg/kg i.v.) before IPC. Total creatine = phosphocreatine + creatine. Significant difference from: [a]control, [b]PC, [c]baseline and [d]Theo-PC value ($p < 0.05$).

TABLE 2. Effects of Ischemic Preconditioning and Theophylline Pretreatment on Myocardial Contents of Glycogen and Glycolytic Metabolites in Risk Area[1]

Time Period	Control	PC	Theo-PC
Glycogen, μmol glucosyl units/g dry wt			
Initial	190.6 ± 15.2	191.8 ± 14.7	188.8 ± 12.6
Preischemic	188.7 ± 15.0	160.7 ± 13.6^c	164.5 ± 15.4
Postischemic	120.9 ± 13.2^c	121.8 ± 11.9^c	134.7 ± 13.0^c
Reperfusion	$147.2 \pm 11.8^{b,c}$	$175.2 \pm 17.2^{a,c}$	144.5 ± 13.8^c
Glucose, μmol/g dry wt			
Initial	1.63 ± 0.18	1.76 ± 0.19	1.93 ± 0.18
Preischemic	1.85 ± 0.21	$9.06 \pm 1.05^{a,c}$	$4.36 \pm 0.38^{a,b,c}$
Postischemic	$8.26 \pm 0.81^{b,c,d}$	$4.38 \pm 0.50^{a,c}$	$3.78 \pm 0.31^{a,c}$
Reperfusion	2.02 ± 0.23^c	1.90 ± 0.21	2.58 ± 0.26^c
Lactate, μmol/g dry wt			
Initial	12.28 ± 0.92	12.56 ± 1.03	13.02 ± 1.20
Preischemic	13.07 ± 1.04	15.38 ± 1.28	12.13 ± 0.97
Reperfusion	$120.83 \pm 8.45^{b,c,d}$	$82.41 \pm 6.54^{a,c}$	$73.80 \pm 5.13^{a,c}$
60-min reperfusion	$16.88 \pm 1.17^{b,c,d}$	13.16 ± 1.24^a	10.28 ± 1.13^a

[1] Values are the means $\pm$ SEM for 12–14 experiments. Other abbreviations are as in TABLE 1. Significant difference from: [a]control, [b]PC, [c]baseline and [d]Theo-PC value ($p < 0.05$).

ischemia the average rates of ATP and PCr depletion were 2-fold lower than in the control. After subsequent reperfusion recovery of ATP and PCr was greater in the preconditioned region.

A partial PCr breakdown induced by IPC was accompanied by a rise in Cr concentration in dialysate (FIG. 2). A lesser PCr depletion after IPC corresponded to a significant reduction in dialysate Cr concentration following sustained ischemia (FIG. 2) and reduced Cr accumulation in ischemic tissue by the end of occlusion period (TABLE 2). In both groups dialysate Cr concentrations decreased during reperfusion, but to lower values in the preconditioned tissue during the initial reperfusion (FIG. 2). At the end of reperfusion, the total creatine pool (TCr) was greater in the preconditioned region than that in control and contained a greater portion of PCr. Besides improved energy supply, this reflects a lesser loss of Cr from myocytes, thus suggesting a reduction of cell membrane damage.[20]

Dialysate P_i profiles in control and PC group agreed with changes in ATP and PCr. In nonpreconditioned myocardium, dialysate P_i increased transiently during ischemia and then gradually decreased remaining higher than the preischemic value at the end of reperfusion (FIG. 4). In PC group, P_i concentration in dialysate was significantly increased after a brief period of LAD occlusion. However, during sustained ischemia, the second transient increase in P_i was markedly reduced. After 20 min of reperfusion dialysate P_i concentration returned to the initial level.

IPC led to a rise of preischemic dialysate Lact, but substantially reduced Lact release into the interstitial fluid during sustained ischemia (FIG. 3). Accordingly, by the end of ischemia, the preconditioned bed contained almost 1.5-fold less of myocardial Lact compared to the control one (TABLE 2). Reperfusion decreased dialysate Lact concentration in both groups. However, in the preconditioned region, dialysate and myocardial Lact returned to baseline levels with reperfusion, while in nonpreconditioned myocardium these indices remained significantly higher than the initial values (TABLE 2, FIG. 3).

At the onset of sustained ischemia, myocardial content of glucose in the preconditioned tissue was nearly 5-fold higher than the baseline value, while in the control

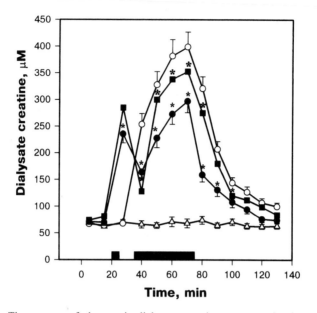

FIGURE 2. Time course of changes in dialysate creatine concentration in the region of LAD occlusion and nonischemic area. Values are the means ± SEM of 12–14 experiments (in some cases SEM is so small that it is hidden within the symbol). *Black bands* indicate periods of preconditioned and sustained ischemia. Nonischemic area, *open triangles*; risk area: control group, *open circles*; PC group, *closed circles*; Theo-PC group, *closed squares*. $p < 0.05$: *Theo-PC vs PC; *PC vs control.

tissue it did not differ from the initial level (TABLE 2). By the end of 40-min LAD occlusion, the glucose level decreased 2-fold in the preconditioned tissue and increased 4.5-fold in the control tissue. Reperfusion decreased glucose content to the baseline value in both groups.

IPC led to the Gly depletion (TABLE 2) expected with a rise in dialysate Lact (FIG. 3) and the tendency to a rise of its tissue level prior to sustained ischemia. During the period of sustained ischemia, Gly breakdown in the preconditioned tissue was reduced by 1.75-fold compared to that in the control. At the end of reperfusion Gly content in the PC group did not differ from the preischemic value, whereas it was significantly lower than the baseline level in the control.

Effects of Theo on the Metabolism of Preconditioned Tissue

Theo administration markedly reduced Lact concentrations in dialysate collected for the cycle of IPC (FIG. 3). At the onset of sustained ischemia, the Theo-PC group exhibited a 2-fold decrease in glucose consumption compared to that in the PC group (TABLE 2). During sustained ischemia, less Lact release into the interstitium and the attenuation of Gly breakdown were found in this group compared to those in the PC group. At the end of the ischemic period, glucose content in Theo-treated hearts did not differ from the preischemic value and Lact accumulation was less than in the preconditioned myocardium. After reperfusion, Theo-treated hearts showed a tendency to lower Lact and higher glucose contents compared to preconditioned ones, while Gly remained close to the value found after sustained ischemia and did not show an upward trend as in the PC group (TABLE 2).

Pretreatment with Theo increased concentrations of Cr and P_i in dialysate collected for the cycle of IPC (FIGS. 2, 4) and reduced myocardial PCr and TCr before 40-min LAD occlusion compared to these indices in the PC group (TABLE 1). During sustained ischemia, Theo-treated hearts demonstrated enhanced Cr and P_i release into the interstitial fluid which did not differ from the values found in the control (FIGS. 2, 4). This was accompanied by a more pronounced PCr and ATP breakdown and enchanced Cr accumulation in myocardial tissue by the end of ischemia (TABLE 1). During the initial phase of reperfusion, the Theo-PC group showed significantly greater Cr and P_i release in dialysate than the PC one (FIGS. 2, 4). By the end of the reperfusion, the contents of ATP, PCr and TCr in this group were substantially lower than in control and the PC group (TABLE 1).

DISCUSSION

The present study demonstrates a complex of metabolic effects of IPC which may account for enhanced regional myocardial contractile function following reperfusion observed previously in the same protocol.[12] They include retardation of energy wastage and Gly consumption during sustained ischemia

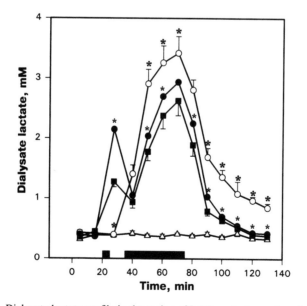

FIGURE 3. Dialysate lactate profile in the region of LAD occlusion and nonischemic area. Values are the means ± SEM of 12–14 experiments. Other symbols are as in FIGURE 2, $p<0.05$: *control vs Theo-PC; *PC vs control.

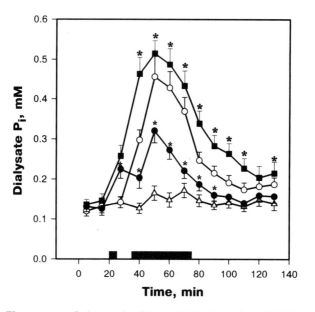

FIGURE 4. Time course of changes in dialysate P_i in the region of LAD occlusion and nonischemic area. Values are the means $\pm$ SEM of 12–14 experiments. Other symbols are as in FIGURE 2. $p < 0.05$: *Theo-PC vs PC; *PC vs control.

accompanied by diminished Lact, P_i and Cr accumulation in caridomyocytes. During reperfusion, the preconditioned tissue recovers energy stores (ATP, PCr and Gly) more rapidly and shows a greater integrity of cell membranes judging by less TCr loss. Abolishment of these metabolic effects by the nonselective adenosine receptor antagonist Theo indicates that improvement of the energy state of the preconditioned myocardium is mediated in part by adenosine receptor activation. The data from the present study, combined with those of previous ones, suggest an importance of coupling of reduced energy utilization with the rate of glycolysis/glycogenolysis for acquisition of tolerance to ischemia/reperfusion injury.

Mechanisms of Energy Sparing Effect

The reduction of ATP and PCr depletion in the PC group during prolonged LAD occlusion (TABLE 1, FIG. 3) principally agrees with previous reports showing a relatively better preservation of adenine nucleotides and PCr in preconditioned hearts of different species *in situ* after sustained ischemia.[5,7,9,21] Though a reduction of energy demand is transient,[6,22] it potentially increases ATP and PCr availability for myocyte functions, thus limiting ischemic injury. Reasons of the "downregulation" of energy metabolism in the preconditioned myocardium are not well known. Using hyperkalemic arrest of canine heart, Jennings *et al.*[22] demonstrated that this effect is not related to a difference in contractile effort between control and preconditioned myocardium. Activation of K_{ATP} channels by adenosine A_1

receptor stimulation may result in an energy sparing effect due to shortening of the action potential duration.[2,10] The latter decreases inward Ca^{2+} current through voltage-dependent Ca^{2+} channels and thus diminishes ATP demand for myosin ATPase. The other sources of reduced energy utilization may be decreased activities of sarcolemmal Na-K-ATPase, Ca-ATPase of the sarcoplasmic reticulum, and certain metabolic pathways consuming ATP. However, the quantitative contribution of these mechanisms in the total energy demand of ischemic heart has not been evaluated.

There is a growing body of evidence that regulation of mitochondrial F_1F_0-ATPase activity is of critical importance for ATP preservation in preconditioned heart. This is supported by the fact that activity of mitochondrial ATPase (a reversible H^+-ATPase) can be easily modulated by changes in electrochemical H^+ gradient across the mitochondrial membrane.[23] Moreover, an inhibition of this enzyme with oligomycin slows ATP depletion in ischemic canine heart,[24,25] and the affinity of the specific endogenous inhibitor to this ATPase was found to increase with tissue acidosis.[22] Recent direct measurements of mitochondrial ATPase activity in isolated rat heart showed that IPC causes enzyme inhibition to persist during the sustained ischemia.[24] It is known that mitochondrial adenine nucleotides are rapidly depleted during ischemia or hypoxia.[26,27] Although the intramitochondrial pool of ATP does not exceed 10% of the total adenine nucleotides in mitochondria, its relative decrease is the most dramatic among other nucleotides.[34] Therefore, it is possible that preliminary reduction of ATP in mitochondria induced by IPC may additionally decrease ATP accessibility to F_1F_0-ATPase during sustained ischemia. It is noteworthy that different types of PC (hypoperfusion, total ischemia, hypoxia or pacing) resulting in "deenergization" of mitochondria would lead to mitochondrial ATPase inhibition.[23] This may not only favor ATP and PCr preservation in ischemia, but contribute to a better postischemic energy state of the heart as confirmed by the present work and that of others.[5,9]

Reduced Glycogenolysis and Tissue Acidosis

Our study demonstrates that IPC attenuates Gly depletion and reduces Lact and glucose concentrations in dialysate and tissue during sustained ischemia (TABLE 2, FIG. 3). These findings are in accordance with previous works[21,22,29] showing less accumulation of glucose-6-phosphate, glucose-1-phosphate and α-glycerol phosphate in ischemic myocardium after IPC. Lower levels of phosphorylated intermediates of glycolysis along with reduced Gly utilization suggest inhibition of glycogenolysis. This may be related to either reduced availability of Gly and/or decreased glycogen phosphorylase activity. Probably, reduced Gly availability was not the main reason for the decreased rate of glycogenolysis in our study. After IPC, Gly stores were reduced only by 15% (TABLE 2) and remained high enough in control and the PC group by the end of sustained ischemia (about 63% of the initial value). In contrast, glycogen phosphorylase activity may be dramatically inhibited even by a brief (5-min) period of ischemia.[30] Furthermore, the conversion of the enzyme from inactive form (phosphorylase *a*) to the active form (phosphorylase *b*) is regulated by phosphorylase kinase via activation of protein kinase by adenosine 3',5'-cyclic monophosphate (cAMP).[29] Since IPC involves stimulation of adenosine A_1 receptors inhibiting adenylate cyclase,[1-3,24] retardation of glycogenolysis could result from reduced phosphorylase kinase activity due to reduction of cAMP.

Limitation of intracellular acidosis has been observed in several studies of IPC carried out on different experimental species including dogs.[6,29,31,32] Preservation of cytosolic pH can be the obvious consequence of reduced H^+ production and/or improved proton buffering capacity during ischemia. The last possibility was suggested by Kida *et al.*,[31] who speculated that "overshoot" of PCr, a proton buffer, can attenuate the extent of acidosis during subsequent ischemia. However, measures of intracellular pH by ^{31}P and ^{13}C NMR spectroscopy under different acid-loading conditions revealed no significant difference in the myocardial proton buffering capacity between ischemic preconditioned and control hearts.[33] PCr store does not always exhibit an "overshoot" with IPC[5,7-9] (TABLE 1) and is depleted within minutes after the onset of ischemia. Therefore, PCr "overshoot" is unable to maintain H^+ balance during prolonged ischemic episode.

Generation of acidosis in ischemic myocardium is usually attributed to anaerobic glycolysis/glycogenolysis and ATP hydrolysis. Theoretically, neither anaerobic lactate-producing glycolysis nor glycogenolysis should be proton sourcers.[34] Thus, the most likely H^+ producer is a degradation of ATP. Since the rate of ATP turnover is coupled with the rate of glycogenolysis in cardiac muscle,[35] reduced ATP demand may be closely related to reduced glycogenolysis. Therefore, the resulting proton accumulation in the preconditioned myocardium may depend on the balance between ATP production in glycolysis/glycogenolysis and ATP utilization. To date, there is no experimental evidence indicating that limitation of acidosis is the causal factor in IPC. However, normalization of pH attenuates some mechanisms of ischemic injury, such as Ca^{2+} overload and contracture development, which are probably capable of facilitating the metabolic and functional recovery of the preconditioned heart.

Alterations in Metabolism Induced by Adenosine Receptor Blockade

Pretreatment with the nonselective adenosine receptor antagonist Theo increased energy wastage during ischemia and impaired postischemic recovery of high-energy phosphates (TABLES 1, 2; FIGS. 2, 3). These results are consistent with observations indicating that blockade of adenosine A_1/A_2 receptors eliminates the cardioprotective effects of IPC in some species including dog (see Ref. 36 for references). In accordance with this, Vander Heide *et al.*[37] found that in canine myocardium IPC can be mimicked by intracoronary adenosine infusion slowing ATP and Gly depletion during ischemia. Subsequent works demonstrated a tight relationship between occupation of adenosine A_1 (and possibly A_3) receptors during IPC at the onset of sustained ischemia and the realized protection.[38,39] Additionally, our data indicate the importance of adenosine receptor activation for metabolic protection of preconditioned myocardium.

Blockade of adenosine receptors with Theo prior to IPC twice decreased the myocardial content of glucose and only slightly affected Gly depletion before sustained ischemia. By the end of ischemia, the Theo-PC group showed reduced Lact production, unchanged high content of glucose and practically the same Gly content as in the PC group (TABLE 2, FIG. 3). These findings suggest a reduction of both myocardial uptake of glucose and its utilization under the effect of Theo and the lack of influence of adenosine receptor blockade on Gly depletion. They are in close agreement with the results of Wyatt *et al.*,[13] who demonstrated that 8-(sulfophenyl)-theophylline decreased glycolytic flux in isolated rat heart perfused under anoxic conditions. In this study glycolytic flux was measured by incorporation of the tritium label from D-[3-^{3}H]glucose into ^3H_2O under constant coronary flow that provided simultaneous assessment of myocardial glucose uptake and metabolism. The involvement of A_1 receptor was testified by the fact that R-phenylisopropyladenosine (PIA), an adenosine A_1 receptor agonist, increased glycolytic flux in this preparation, while 5'-N-ethylcarboxamidoadenosine (NECA), an adenosine A_2 receptor agonist, was ineffective. Reasons for the regulatory influence of Theo and its derivatives over the glycolytic pathway are not apparent. These polar compounds can hardly penetrate cells or exhibit effects on the cAMP system, probably interacting with membrane glucose transporters.[13] Irrespective of potential mechanisms of Theo action, analysis of these results allows one to assume that IPC reducing Gly digestion favors glucose utilization for maintaining sufficient glycolytic flux during ischemia. Adenosine A_1 receptor blockade with Theo results in uncoupling of the rate of glycolysis/glycogenolysis to the rate of high-energy phosphate utilization. The most prominent consequence of this effect is enhanced APT and PCr depletion in the Theo-PC group during sustained ischemia and poor recovery of aerobic metabolism on reperfusion (TABLE 1). These metabolic events may be critical for myocyte viability and functional recovery of the heart.

CONCLUDING COMMENTS

IPC reduces energy utilization and the rate of glycogenolysis during regional ischemia in canine myocardium. This leads to sparing of high-energy phosphates, less catabolite accumulation, and very likely contributes to improved recovery of oxidative metabolism. Elimination of these beneficial effects by Theo supports the concept that cardioprotection by IPC in the dog involves adenosine receptor activation. However, the subtype of receptor responsible for decreased metabolic demand remains unknown because of the nonselectivity of the antagonist. This problem deserves further investigation for elaborating pharmacological correction of metabolic disturbances following prolonged coronary artery occlusion and subsequent reperfusion.

REFERENCES

1. MIURA, T. & O. IIMURA. 1993. Infarct size limitation by preconditioning: its phenomenological features and the key role of adenosine. Cardiovasc. Res. **27:** 36–42.
2. WALKER, D. M. & D. M. YELLON. 1993. Ischaemic preconditioning: from mechanisms to exploitation. Cardiovasc. Res. **26:** 734–739.
3. LAWSON, C. S. & J. A. DOWNEY. 1993. Preconditioning: state of the art myocardial protection. Cardiovasc. Res. **27:** 542–550.
4. COHEN, M. V., G. S. LIU & J. M. DOWNEY. 1991. Preconditioning caused improved wall motion as well as smaller infarcts after transient coronary occlusion in rabbits. Circulation **84:** 341–349.
5. SCHOTT, R. J., S. ROUHMANN, E. R. BRAUN & W. SCHAPPER. 1990. Ischemic preconditioning reduces infarct size in swine myocardium. Circ. Res. **66:** 1133–1142.
6. MURRY, C. E., V. J. RICHARD, K. A. REIMER & R. B. JENNINGS. 1990. Ischemic preconditioning slows energy metabolism and delays ultrastructural damage during a sustained ischemic episode. Circ. Res. **66:** 913–931.
7. SWAIN, J. L., R. L. SABINA, P. A. MCHALE, J. C. GREENFIELD & E. W. HOLMES. 1982. Prolonged myocardial nucleotide depletion after brief ischemia in open-chest dog. Am. J. Physiol. **242:** H818–H826.
8. HAGAR, J. M., S. L. HALE & R. A. KLONER. 1991. Effect of preconditioning ischemia

on reperfusion arrhythmias after coronary artery occlusion and reperfusion in the rat. Circ. Res. **68:** 61–68.

9. FLACK, J. E., Y. KIMURA, R. M. ENGELMAN, J. A. ROUSOU, J. IYENGAR, R. JONES & D. K. DAS. 1991. Preconditioning of the heart by repeated stunning improves myocardial salvage. Circulation **84**(Suppl. III): III-369–374.

10. LIU, G. S., J. THORNTON, D. VAN WINKLE, A. W. H. STANLEY, R. A. OLSSON & J. M. DOWNEY. 1991. Protection against infarction afforded by preconditioning is mediated by adenosine A_1 receptors in rabbit heart. Circulation **84:** 350–356.

11. BAXTER, G. F., M. S. MARBER, V. C. PATEL & D. M. YELLON. 1994. Adenosine receptor involvement in a delayed phase of myocardial protection 24 hours after ischemic preconditioning. Circulation **90:** 2993–3000.

12. KUZMIN, A. I., D. D. MATSIEVSKY, E. A. TOLMACHEVA, O. V. TSKITISHVILI, L. I. SEREBRYAKOVA & V. I. KAPELKO. 1996. Protective effects of preconditioning against myocardial stunning and no-reflow in the dog heart. Cardiovasc. Res. Submitted.

13. WYATT, D. A., M. C. EDMUNDS, R. RUBIO, R. M. BERNE, R. D. LASLEY & J. R. MENTZER. 1989. Adenosine stimulates glycolytic flux in isolated perfused rat heart by A_1-adenosine receptors. Am. J. Physiol. **257:** H1952–H1957.

14. National Institutes of Health. 1985. Guide for the Care and Use of Laboratory Animals. NIH publication No. 85-23, revised.

15. KUZMIN, A. I., O. V. TSKITISHVILI, L. I. SEREBRYAKOVA, T. V. SAPRYGINA, V. I. KAPELKO & O. S. MEDVEDEV. 1992. Cardiac microdialysis measurement of extracellular adenine nucleotide breakdown products during regional ischemia and reperfusion in canine heart: Protective effect of propranolol against reperfusion injury. J. Cardiovasc. Pharmacol. **20:** 961–968.

16. JEREMY, R. W., L. STAHL, M. GILLINOV, M. LITT, T. R. AVERSANO & L. C. BECKER. 1989. Preservation of coronary flow reserve in stunned myocardium. Am. J. Physiol. **256:** H1303–H1310.

17. BERGMEYER, H. U, Ed. 1974. Methods of Enzymatic Analysis. 4th edit. Vol. 3: 1510–1514, Vol. 4: 1772–1776, 1777–1781, 2101–2110. Academic Press. New York, NY.

18. MOMOZE, T., Y. OHKURA, K. KOHASHI, Y. YANO, K. OHASHI, R. NAGATA & K. OHTA. 1964. Improved methods of microdetermination of creatinine and creatine in serum. Yakugaku Zasshi **84:** 525–530.

19. ARMIGER, L. C., T. B. ELLIOT, S. FITZGERALD, S. M. HUMPHREY, P. MORRISON & R. SEELYE. 1983. Effects of proton release from adenine nucleotide degradation during ischemic necrosis of myocardium *in vitro*. Biochem. Med. **29:** 265–277.

20. REIMER, K. A., M. L. HILL & R. B. JENNINGS. 1981. Prolonged depletion of ATP and of the adenine nucleotide pool due to delayed resynthesis of adenine nucleotides following reversible myocardial ischemic injury in dogs. J. Mol. Cell. Cardiol. **13:** 229–239.

21. REIMER, K. A., C. E. MURRY, I. YAMASAWA, M. L. HILL & R. B. JENNINGS. 1986. Four brief periods of myocardial ischemia cause no cumulative ATP loss or necrosis. Am. J. Physiol. **251:** H1306–H1315.

22. JENNINGS, R. B., C. E. MURRY & K. A. REIMER. 1991. Energy metabolism in preconditioned and control myocardium: effect of total ischemia. J. Mol. Cell. Cardiol. **23:** 1449–1458.

23. DAS, A. M. & D. A. HARRIS. 1989. Reversible modulation of the mitochondrial ATP synthase with energy demand in cultured rat cardiomyocytes. FEBS Lett. **256:** 91–100.

24. VUORINEN, K., K. YLITALO, K. PEUHKURINEN, P. RAATIKAINEN, A. ALA-RAMI & I. E. HASSINEN. 1995. Mechanisms of ischemic preconditioning in rat myocardium. Role of adenosine, cellular energy state, and mitochondrial F_1F_0-ATPase. Circulation **91:** 2810–2818.

25. JENNINGS, R. B., K. A. REIMER & S. STEENBERGEN. 1991. Effect of inhibition of the mitochondrial ATPase on net myocardial ATP in total ischemia. J. Mol. Cell. Cardiol. **23:** 1383–1395.

26. ASIMAKIS, G. K. & V. R. CONTI. 1984. Myocardial ischemia: correlation of mitochondrial adenine nucleotide and respiratory function. J. Mol. Cell. Cardiol. **16:** 439–448.

27. PISARENKO, O. I., E. S. SOLOMATINA, I. M. STUDNEVA & V. I. KAPELKO. 1987. The relationship between the cardiac contractile function, adenine nucleotides and amino acids of cardiac tissue and mitochondria at acute respiratory hypoxia. Eur. J. Physiol. **409:** 169–174.
28. PISARENKO, O. I., I. M. STUDNEVA, E. S. SOLOMATINA & V. I. KAPELKO. 1986. Adenine nucleotides, glutamate and respiratory function of heart mitochondria during acute hypoxia. Biochem. Int. **13:** 51–58.
29. SCHAEFER, S., L. J. CARR, E. PRUSSEL & R. RAMASAMY. 1995. Effects of glycogen depletion on ischemic injury in isolated rat hearts: insights into preconditioning. Am. J. Physiol. **268:** H935–H944.
30. MEINKE, M. H. & R. D. EDSTROM. 1991. Muscle glycogenolysis: regulation of the interconversion of phosphorylase *a* and phosphorylase *b*. J. Biol. Chem. **26:** 2259–2266.
31. KIDA, M., H. FUJIWARA & M. ISHIDA. 1991. Ischemic preconditioning preserves creatine phosphate and intracellular pH. Circulation **84:** 2495–2503.
32. DE ALBUQUERQUE, C. P., G. GERSTENBLITH & R. G. WEISS. 1994. Importance of metabolic inhibition and cellular pH in mediating preconditioning contractile and metabolic effects in rat hearts. Circ. Res. **74:** 139–150.
33. DE ALBUQUERQUE, C. P., G. GERSTENBLITH & R. G. WEISS. 1995. Myocardial buffering capacity in ischemia preconditioned rat hearts. J. Mol. Cell. Cardiol. **27:** 777–781.
34. GEVERS, W. 1977 Generation of protons by metabolic processes in heart cells. J. Mol. Cell. Cardiol. **9:** 867–873.
35. REN, J. M. & E. HULTMAN. 1990. Regulation of phosphorylase *a* activity in human skeletal muscle. J. Appl. Physiol. **69:** 919–923.
36. CAVE, A. C., C. S. COLLIS, J. M. DOWNEY & D. J. HEARSE. 1993. Improved functional recovery by ischaemic preconditioning is not mediated by adenosine in the globally ischaemic isolated rat heart. Cardiovasc. Res. **27:** 663–668.
37. VANDER HEIDE, R. S., K. A. REIMER & R. B. JENNINGS. 1993. Adenosine slows ischaemic metabolism in canine myocardium *in vitro*: relationship to ischaemic preconditioning. Cardiovasc. Res. **27:** 669–673.
38. DOWNEY, J. M., M. V. COHEN, K. YTREHUS & Y. LIU. 1994. Cellular mechanisms in ischemic preconditioning: the role of adenosine and protein kinase C. Ann. N. Y. Acad. Sci. **723:** 82–98.
39. JEROME, S. N., T. AKIMITSU, D. C. GUTE & R. J. KORTHUIS. 1995. Ischemic preconditioning attenuates capillary no-reflow induced by prolonged ischemia and reperfusion. Am. J. Physiol. **268:** H2063–H2067.

Protection by Preconditioning and Cardiac Pacing against Ventricular Arrhythmias Resulting from Ischemia and Reperfusion[a]

JAMES R. PARRATT,[b,c] AGNES VEGH,
KAROLY KASZALA, AND JULIUS GY. PAPP

Department of Pharmacology
Albert Szent-Gyorgyi Medical University
Szeged, Hungary
and
[c]Department of Physiology and Pharmacology
University of Strathclyde
Glasgow, United Kingdom

Ischemic preconditioning is a form of myocardial adaptation through which the heart is protected, by short periods of ischemic stress, against the serious consequences of a subsequent prolonged period of ischemia.[1-4] This increased tolerance of the heart following subjection to brief periods of ischemic stress is manifested by a reduced area of myocardial necrosis,[1] by enhanced recovery of contractile function during reperfusion[5] and by a reduced severity of the life-threatening ventricular arrhythmias that arise during a period of ischemia and reperfusion.[6-8] There are good reasons for believing that the antiarrhythmic effect of ischemic preconditioning is an even more important manifestation of this protection than is the reduction in myocardial ischemic damage.[8] This review summarizes the evidence that preconditioning reduces the severity of these ventricular arrhythmias, that this protection is both acute and delayed and that the mechanisms involve the release of mediators from endothelial cells.

There was, even before the onset of the preconditioning era, evidence that brief periods of ischemia can suppress the arrhythmias that result from a subsequent period of ischemia. These include the findings that the reduction in the ventricular fibrillation threshold, which occurs during ischemia, becomes less pronounced with successive coronary artery occlusions,[9] that increased ventricular pacemaker activity resulting from intramyocardial infusions of noradrenaline are abolished when the artery supplying that region is occluded,[10] that dogs are more likely to survive a coronary artery occlusion if this is performed in two stages,[11] and that brief repeated periods (5 min) of ischemia result in fewer ventricular premature beats during ischemia[12] and reperfusion[13] during a second, and subsequent, brief occlusions of the same artery. Particularly important were the

[a] Supported by the British Council (in association with the Hungarian Committee for Technical Development), the European Commission (Network Grant ERB CT 924009) and the Hungarian State Government (OTKA).

[b] Please address all correspondence to: Professor J. R. Parratt, Department of Physiology and Pharmacology, University of Strathclyde, Glasgow Gl 1XW, Scotland, UK.

98

subsequent findings that brief periods of ischemia could protect against those arrhythmias arising during a subsequent, more prolonged period of ischemia that would normally result in myocardial necrosis.[7,8]

The Antiarrhythmic Effects of Classical Preconditioning

This was first shown in an anesthetized rat model.[7,14] When the main left coronary artery is occluded in anesthetized rats there is a resultant marked ventricular ectopic activity and a high incidence of, usually reversible, ventricular fibrillation.[15] If such a 30-min occlusion of the left coronary artery is preceded by a much shorter period of occlusion (*e.g.*, 3 min although not 1 min) then the severity of arrhythmias during this prolonged occlusion is markedly reduced.[7,14] However, this protection is rather short lived. If the time interval between the initial short (preconditioning) occlusion and the prolonged coronary artery occlusion is increased then the protection disappears.[7] This means that protection against these life-threatening arrhythmias is powerful but transient.

As one might expect, a similar protection is observed in other species.[6,8] We have been particularly concerned with the antiarrhythmic effects of ischemic preconditioning in mongrel dogs anesthetized with a mixture of chloralose and urethane, which avoids the marked detrimental effects of barbiturate anesthetics on myocardial function. We have used such a canine model because of the possibility of exploring the mechanisms of this protection in a more appropriate way. FIGURE 1 shows the effects of a 25-min period of coronary artery occlusion on

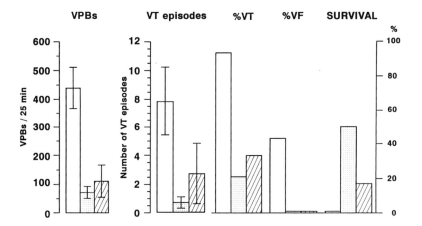

FIGURE 1. Ventricular arrhythmias (number of ventricular premature beats, number of episodes of ventricular tachycardia, the incidences of ventricular tachycardia (VT) and ventricular fibrillation (VF)) during a 25-min period of coronary artery occlusion in anesthetized open-chest dogs when this occlusion is preceded by either 1 (*hatched columns*) or 2 (*stippled columns*) brief (5-min) occlusions of the same anterior descending branch of the left coronary artery 20 min previously (control: *open columns*). Also shown is the survival from the combined 25-min period of ischemia followed by rapid reperfusion. One or two preconditioning coronary artery occlusions markedly reduce the severity of arrhythmias which occurred during a subsequent prolonged period of ischemia and reperfusion.

the severity of ventricular arrhythmias in this anesthetized canine model and how this severity is markedly reduced if the prolonged occlusion is preceded by either one or two short (5-min) preconditioning occlusions. It is quite clear that there is a marked suppression of arrhythmia activity with a lower incidence of ventricular tachycardia and ventricular fibrillation, fewer episodes of ventricular tachycardia and a significantly lower number of ventricular premature beats during the occlusion period. The most significant effect is the complete absence of ventricular fibrillation in such preconditioned dogs (FIG. 1). When two preconditioning occlusions are used there is also an increased survival from the combined ischemia-reperfusion insult; none of the control dogs survives this insult but around 50% of preconditioned dogs do so.[6,7]

This protection is not only powerful but real. This was demonstrated by prolonging the occlusion period from 25 min to 1 h in order to determine whether the arrhythmias were simply shifted to a later time. The total number of ventricular premature beats was considerably less over the entire 1-h period in preconditioned dogs than over a 25-min period in control dogs and again, there was no ventricular fibrillation.[7]

Although, as in the rat model, this protection against ischemia-induced arrhythmias is extremely powerful it is also short-lasting. Thus if the time interval between the preconditioning occlusion(s) and the prolonged occlusion is increased from 20 min (as in FIG. 1) to 1 h then the protection is largely lost.[7] This clearly limits the potential usefulness of the phenomenon.

This protection against arrhythmias does not depend upon the presence of blood, nor on an intact autonomic innervation since preconditioning against arrhythmias is easily demonstrated in isolated perfused hearts.[16,17] Under such conditions, as *in vivo*, the antiarrhythmic effect of short periods of ischemia (either global or local) leads to a marked, real but transient protection against arrhythmias during both ischemia and subsequent reperfusion. More recently, we have been concerned with determining whether this endogenous protective mechanism is present at birth and, if not, when during cardiac development it becomes apparent. It seems, using recovery of contractile function from a period of ischemia as an index of the preconditioning phenomenon, that preconditioning is not present at birth, is certainly present at day 7 and, in some hearts, is present at day 4 of postnatal development.[18] Such studies may throw light on the possible mechanisms involved in this protection.

Because of the marked influence of the endothelium on the function of cardiac myocytes we have also been interested in the role the endothelium plays in this phenomenon.[19] Removal of the endothelium in rat isolated hearts markedly increases the severity of arrhythmias during a subsequent 30-min coronary artery occlusion, indicating 'cross-talk' between protective mediators derived from the endothelium and cardiac myocytes.[20]

Protection against ventricular arrhythmias can also be achieved by means other than short periods of coronary artery occlusion. Using a pacing catheter in the right ventricle, dogs were subjected to rapid cardiac pacing either at 300 beats per min for two 2-min periods[21] or at a pacing rate of 220 beats per min for four 5-min periods.[22] The coronary artery was then occluded at different times following the cessation of cardiac pacing. The results are illustrated in FIGURE 2. When the coronary artery is occluded immediately after the cessation of pacing there is, as with classical preconditioning, a marked suppression of ischemia-induced ventricular arrhythmias (*e.g.*, lower incidences of ventricular fibrillation (0% v 47%), ventricular tachycardia (30% v 80%) and a reduction in the number of ventricular premature beats (*e.g.*, from 528 ± 40 to 136 ± 45; $p < 0.05$). This

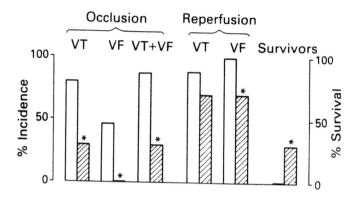

FIGURE 2. Severity of arrhythmias during a 25-min occlusion of the left anterior descending coronary artery in anesthetized dogs (*open columns*, n = 15) is reduced if the occlusion is preceded by rapid ventricular pacing (*hatched columns*, n = 10). There is also an increased survival from the combined ischemia-reperfusion insult. *$p < 0.05$. (Adapted from Vegh et al.[6])

protection is apparent using pacing rates of either 300 or 220 beats min^{-1} and is also illustrated, for the incidence of ventricular fibrillation during occlusion, in FIGURE 3. When the artery is occluded immediately, or 5 min, after the end of the pacing stimulus, there is no ventricular fibrillation. This protection, as with classical preconditioning, is transient and there is no protection by pacing if the coronary artery is occluded 15 min after the end of the stimulus.[23]

Possible Mechanisms of the Antiarrhythmic Effect of Ischemic Preconditioning and Cardiac Pacing

Little is known at present concerning the mechanisms of the antiarrhythmic effect of ischemic preconditioning. The evidence, such as it is, suggests that the endothelium (or at least endothelium-derived protective substances) play a particularly important part in this protection. The hypothesis is illustrated in FIGURE 4. It is that during brief periods of ischemia, and possibly also under conditions of cardiac pacing, bradykinin is generated in the coronary circulation, acts on specific (B2) receptors on the surface of endothelial cells and triggers the generation of nitric oxide through the L-arginine nitric oxide pathway and constitutive nitric oxide synthase. This nitric oxide diffuses to the cardiac myocytes, stimulates soluble guanylyl cyclase and elevates cyclic GMP. Elevated levels of cGMP within cardiac myocytes might influence arrhythmogenesis in a number of ways, *e.g.*, by stimulating the cyclic GMP dependent cyclic AMP phosphodiesterase (thereby lowering cAMP levels), by inhibiting the entry of calcium through L-type channels or by depressing myocardial contractility (nitric oxide is one of the reasons for depressed myocardial function under conditions of sepsis). The evidence for the above hypothesis is circumstantial and depends primarily on the use of drugs that inhibit various steps in the above process. These include the marked attenuation of the antiarrhythmic effects of ischemic preconditioning in the canine model (a) by the bradykinin B2 receptor blocking drug icatibant,[24] (b) by inhibitors of the L-arginine nitric oxide pathway,[25] and (c) by the local intracoronary administration of methylene blue[26] which inhibits both soluble guanylyl cyclase and the L-arginine nitric oxide pathway in endothelial cells. Nitric oxide is clearly a key mediator of this protection and there is now considerable evidence, in a variety of experimental models, that nitric oxide generation is beneficial under conditions of ischemia and reperfusion.[27] Adenosine, which is a major contributory factor in the protective effects of ischemic preconditioning against myocardial ischemic damage[2-4] is not involved in the antiarrhythmic effects of this phenomenon, since protection against arrhythmias is unaffected by drugs that block relevant adenosine receptors.[28]

Delayed Antiarrhythmic Effects of Ischemic Preconditioning

One of the disappointments of classical ischemic preconditioning discussed above is the transient nature of the protection. This depends on the nature of the experimental model, but in most experimental situations the protection is lost if the time interval between the preconditioning stimulus and the prolonged ischemic insult is increased to 1 or 2 h. The transient nature of the protection afforded by cardiac pacing is well illustrated in FIGURE 3. If the time interval between the end of the pacing stimulus and the first coronary artery occlusion is increased from 5

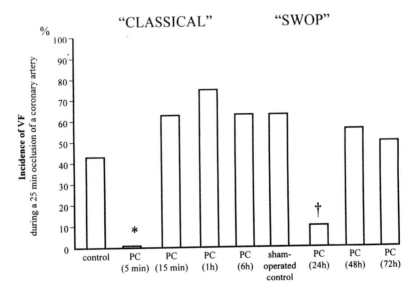

FIGURE 3. The incidence of ventricular fibrillation during a 25-min occlusion of the left anterior descending coronary artery in control dogs and in dogs subjected to rapid cardiac pacing (4 × 5 min at 220 beats min^{-1}) at different times prior to the coronary occlusion. The incidence of ventricular fibrillation during occlusion is reduced 5 min after cessation of pacing (classical preconditioning) and also 24 h after cessation of pacing (delayed protection) but not at intermediate or later times. *$p < 0.05$ vs control; †$p < 0.05$ vs sham-operated control.

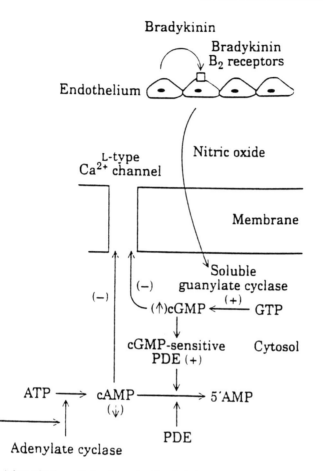

FIGURE 4. A hypothesis outlining the role of endothelium-derived protective substances under conditions of ischemic preconditioning and cardiac pacing. There is an early release of bradykinin, probably from endothelial cells which, by way of stimulation of bradykinin (B2 receptors) on the surface of adjacent endothelial cells stimulates the production of nitric oxide from L-arginine by activating constitutive nitric oxide synthase. This nitric oxide then 'talks' to cardiac myocytes, stimulates soluble guanylyl cyclase and increases cyclic GMP. The result is a reduction in cAMP levels within cardiac myocytes and inhibition of calcium entry. (Adapted from Parratt & Vegh.[19])

to 15 min then protection against ventricular fibrillation is completely lost. It was a very important step forward therefore when it was discovered[29,30] that this protection returned several hours later, a phenomenon well described by Yellon and his co-workers as 'a second window of protection.'[31] They, and others, showed that brief periods of coronary artery occlusion resulted in both early (and transient) protection against myocardial necrosis and a delayed protection with a time course of many hours.[29-31] We have shown[22,23] a similar delayed protection against ischemia-induced arrhythmias as a result of cardiac pacing, and this is also well illustrated in FIGURE 3. The marked reduction in ventricular fibrillation that occurs when the coronary artery is occluded 5 min after the cessation of pacing returns 24 h later. Although protection against ventricular fibrillation is not maintained if the coronary artery is occluded 48 or 72 h after the end of the pacing stimulus there is evidence, even at these times, for a reduction in other indices of arrhythmia severity during ischemia such as the number of ventricular premature beats and the number of episodes of ventricular tachycardia.[23]

We know little about the optimum conditions required for this delayed protection and it could well be that, as with classical preconditioning these depend upon the number of preconditioning occlusions (or pacing periods) as well as on the severity of ischemia during the preconditioning stimulus itself. Although there is some evidence[23] that right ventricular cardiac pacing results in subendocardial ischemia in the left ventricle, this induced ischemia is not marked and is certainly transient. This raises the question as to whether ischemia alone is the main stimulus for protection afforded by preconditioning, or whether it results from the endothelial release of mediators, not necessarily triggered by ischemia, or by the stretch of cardiac myocytes, as suggested by Kloner and his colleagues.[32]

These studies have resurrected the interest in delayed myocardial protection afforded by stimuli other than ischemic preconditioning. There is a long and interesting history on this which has recently been reviewed.[33] Thus, delayed cardiac protection also results from catecholamine administration; indeed, this might be another explanation for the protection afforded by cardiac pacing and by brief periods of ischemia referred to above. Historically, this probably represents the earliest example of delayed cardioprotection. Thus, following the early studies of Rona, Poupa, Selye and Balazs (reviewed in Ref. 33) that the myocardium can be protected against the toxic effects of large doses of isoprenaline by the prior administration of smaller doses of isoprenaline, Beckmann and his colleagues[34] showed that dogs that developed long-term tolerance to adrenaline were also resistant to coronary embolization with microspheres, with a particularly marked reduction in the incidence of ventricular fibrillation during myocardial ischemia.

Other examples of delayed myocardial protection include those following the administration of prostacyclin and its stable derivatives, such as 7-oxo-prostacyclin, and of bacterial endotoxin, or the nontoxic lipid-A derivative monophosphoryl lipid-A (MLA) (reviewed in Ref. 33). For example, if endotoxin is given to rats and then, after sacrifice several hours later, the hearts are removed, perfused according to the Langendorff mode and the left coronary artery occluded, then the ventricular arrhythmias that normally result in such preparations are much less severe.[35] This is a time-dependent phenomenon. Unlike ischemic preconditioning, there is no immediate protection by endotoxin; this first appears between 4 and 8 h after endotoxin administration with optimum protection between 8 and 12 h following administration. This is illustrated in FIGURE 5. This protection is sensitive to dexamethasone, which virtually abolishes the protection if given prior to endotoxin administration.[35] We now know that one nontoxic lipid A derivative also suppresses ischemia-induced arrhythmias, as it does infarct size, in a canine model of ischemia and reperfusion.[36]

We know even less about the mechanisms of delayed cardioprotection than we do about those involved in classical ischemic preconditioning. However, there is some evidence that endothelium-derived mediators are involved in this delayed protection. Thus, the protection against arrhythmias afforded by cardiac pacing is not seen in the presence of either icatibant,[37] implying that bradykinin release is involved, or after dexamethasone administration[38] perhaps suggesting the

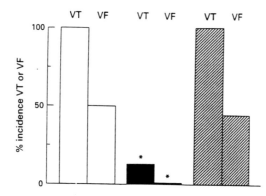

FIGURE 5. The incidence of ventricular tachycardia (VT) and of ventricular fibrillation (VF) in hearts removed from rats administered either saline (*open columns*), endotoxin (*solid columns*), or a combination of endotoxin and dexamethasone (*hatched columns*) 8 h previously, and then subjected to coronary artery occlusion. There is a marked reduction in the incidence of these arrhythmias in hearts removed from rats given endotoxin, a protection abolished by the prior administration of dexamethasone. $*p < 0.01$. (Modified from Wu et al.[35])

involvement of induced nitric oxide synthase or cyclooxygenase II. Other potential explanations for delayed cardiac protection include changes in $Na^+ K^+$ ATPase,[33] the induction of phsophodiesterase enzymes,[33] increased antioxidant status[39] and the formation of heat/stress proteins.[40]

Although such delayed protection lasts longer than that achieved by classical ischemic preconditioning it is still *relatively* transient (hours rather than days). However, if we understood the mechanisms involved and, since it is possible to reintroduce protection for a longer period of time during the 'waning' period of delayed protection,[41] then it might be possible to maintain the myocardium in a tolerant state for a considerable period of time. This might be particularly possible if the mechanisms involved in, say, cardiac pacing and in preconditioning resulting from coronary artery occlusion were dissimilar, as those involved in the myocardial protection resulting from chronic hypoxia and acute hypoxia (ischemia) appear to be.[42]

REFERENCES

1. MURRY, C. E., R. B. JENNINGS & K. A. REIMER. 1986. Preconditioning with ischemia: a delay in lethal injury in ischemic myocardium. Circulation **74:** 1124–1136.
2. BAXTER, G. F. & D. M. YELLON. 1994. Ischaemic preconditioning of myocardium: a new paradigm for clinical cardioprotection? Br. J. Clin. Pharmacol. **38:** 381–387.
3. PARRATT, J. R. 1994. Protection of the heart by ischaemic preconditioning: mechanisms and possibilities for pharmacological exploitation. Trends Pharmacol. Sci. **15:** 19–25.
4. WAINWRIGHT, C. L. & J. R. PARRATT. Eds. 1996. Myocardial Preconditioning. Springer. Berlin.
5. CAVE, A. C. & D. J. HEARSE. 1992. Ischaemic preconditioning and contractile function: studies with normothermic and hypothermic global ischaemia. J. Mol. Cell. Cardiol. **24:** 1113–1123.
6. VEGH, A., L. SZEKERES & J. R. PARRATT. 1990. Protective effects of preconditioning

of the ischaemic myocardium involves cyclooxygenase products. Cardiovasc. Res.
4: 1020–1023.

7. VEGH, A., S. KOMORI, L. SZEKERES & J. R. PARRATT. 1992. Antiarrhythmic effects of preconditioning in anaesthetised dogs and rats. Cardiovasc. Res. **26:** 487–495.
8. PARRATT, J. R. & A. VEGH. 1994. Pronounced antiarrhythmic effects of ischaemic preconditioning. Cardioscience **5:** 9–18.
9. GULKER, H., B. CRAMER, K. STEFHAN & W. MEESMANN. 1977. Changes in ventricular fibrillation threshold during repeated short-term coronary occlusion and release. Basic Res. Cardiol. **72:** 547–562.
10. PODZUWEIT, T., K. H. BINZ, P. NENNSTIEL & W. FLAIG. 1989. The anti-arrhythmic effects of myocardial ischaemia. Relation to reperfusion arrhythmias? Cardiovasc. Res. **23:** 81–90.
11. HARRIS, A. G. 1950. Delayed development of ventricular ectopic rhythms following experimental coronary occlusion. Circulation **1:** 1318–1326.
12. BARBER, M. J. 1983. Effect of time interval between repeated brief coronary artery occlusions on arrhythmias, electrical activity and myocardial blood flow. J. Am. Coll. Cardiol. **2:** 699–705.
13. SHIKI, K. & D. J. HEARSE. 1987. Preconditioning of ischemic myocardium: reperfusion-induced arrhythmias. Am. J. Physiol. **253:** H11470–H11476.
14. KOMORI, S., S. FUJIMAKI, H. IJILI & J. R. PARRATT. 1990. Inhibitory effect of ischemic preconditioning on ischemic arrhythmias using a rat coronary artery ligation model. Jpn. J. Electrocardiol. **10:** 774–782.
15. CLARK, C., M. I. FOREMAN, K. A. KANE, F. M. MCDONALD & J. R. PARRATT. 1980. Coronary artery ligation in anaesthetised rats as a method for the production of experimental dysrrhythmias and for the determination of infarct size. J. Pharmacol. Methods **3:** 357–368.
16. PIACENTINI, L., C. L. WAINWRIGHT & J. R. PARRATT. 1993. The antiarrhythmic effect of ischaemic preconditioning in isolated rat hearts involves a pertussis toxin sensitive mechanism. Cardiovasc. Res. **27:** 674–680.
17. LAWSON, C. S., D. J. COLTART & D. J. HEARSE. 1993. Dose-dependency and temporary characteristics of protection by ischaemic preconditioning against ischaemia-induced arrhythmias in rat hearts. J. Mol. Cell. Cardiol. **25:** 1391–1402.
18. OSTADALOVA, I., F. KOLAR, B. OSTADAL & J. R. PARRATT. 1996. Ischaemic preconditioning in neo-natal rat hearts. J. Physiol. **491:** 6P–7P.
19. PARRATT, J. R. & A. VEGH. 1996. Endothelial cells, nitric oxide and ischaemic preconditioning. Basic Res. Cardiol. **91:** 27–30.
20. FATEHI-HASSANABAD, Z., B. L. FURMAN & J. R. PARRATT. 1996. The effect of the endothelium on coronary artery occlusion-induced arrhythmias in rat isolated perfused hearts. J. Physiol. In press.
21. VEGH, A., L. SZEKERES, J. GY. PAPP & J. R. PARRATT. 1991. Transient ischaemia induced by rapid cardiac pacing results in myocardial preconditioning. Cardiovasc. Res. **25:** 1051–1053.
22. KASZALA, K., A. VEGH, J. R. PARRATT & J. GY. PAPP. 1995. Time course of pacing induced preconditioning in dogs. J. Mol. Cell. Cardiol. **27:** A145.
23. KASZALA, K., A. VEGH, J. GY. PAPP & J. R. PARRATT. 1996. Time course of the protection against ischaemia and reperfusion-induced ventricular arrhythmias resulting from brief periods of cardiac pacing. J. Mol. Cell. Cardiol. In press.
24. VEGH, A., J. GY. PAPP & J. R. PARRATT. 1994. Attenuation of the antiarrhythmic effects of ischaemic preconditioning by blockade of bradykinin B2 receptors. Br. J. Pharmacol. **113:** 1167–1172.
25. VEGH, A., L. SZEKERES & J. R. PARRATT. 1992. Preconditioning of the ischaemic myocardium; involvement of the L-arginine nitric oxide pathway. Br. J. Pharmacol. **107:** 648–652.
26. VEGH, A., J. GY. PAPP, L. SZEKERES & J. R. PARRATT. 1992. The local intracoronary administration of methylene blue prevents the pronounced antiarrhythmic effect of ischaemic preconditioning. Br. J. Pharmacol. **107:** 910–911.
27. MAULIK, N., D. T. ENGLEMAN, M. WATANABE, R. M. ENGLEMAN, G. MAULIK, G. A.

CORDIS & D. K. DAS. 1995. Nitric oxide signalling in ischaemic heart. Cardiovasc. Res. **30**: 593–601.

28. VEGH, A., J. GY. PAPP & J. R. PARRATT. 1995. Pronounced antiarrhythmic effects of preconditioning in anaesthetised dogs: is adenosine involved? J. Mol. Cell. Cardiol. **27**: 349–356.

29. KUZUYA, T., A. HOSHIDA & N. YAMASHITA. 1993. Delayed effects of sub-lethal ischemia on the acquisition of tolerance to ischemia. Circ. Res. **72**: 1293–1299.

30. MARBER, M. S., D. S. LATCHMAN, D. M. WALKER & D. M. YELLON. 1993. Cardiac stress protein elevation 24 hours following brief ischemia or heat stress is associated with resistance to myocardial infarction. Circulation **88**: 1264–1272.

31. YELLON, D. M. & G. F. BAXTER. 1995. A "second window of protection" or delayed preconditioning phenomenon; future horizons for myocardial protection? J. Mol. Cell. Cardiol. **27**: 1023–1034.

32. OVIZE, M., R. A. KLONER & K. PRZYKLENK. 1994. Stretch preconditions canine myocardium. Am. J. Physiol. **266**: H137–H146.

33. PARRATT, J. R. & L. SZEKERES. 1995. Delayed protection of the heart against ischaemia. Trends Pharmacol. Sci. **16**: 351–355.

34. BECKMAN, C. B., Z. NIAZI, R. H. DIETZMAN & R. C. LILLEHI. 1981. Protective effect of epinephrine tolerance in experimental cardiogenic shock. Circ. Shock **8**: 137–149.

35. WU, S., B. L. FURMAN & J. R. PARRATT. 1994. Attenuation by dexamethasone of endotoxin protection against ischaemic-induced ventricular arrhythmias. Br. J. Pharmacol. **113**: 1083–1084.

36. VEGH, A., J. GY. PAPP, G. T. ELLIOTT & J. R. PARRATT. 1996. Pretreatment with monophosphoryl lipid A (MPL-C) reduces ischaemia-reperfusion induced arrhythmias in dogs. J. Mol. Cell. Cardiol. **28**: A217.

37. VEGH, A., K. KASZALA, J. GY. PAPP & J. R. PARRATT. 1995. Delayed myocardial protection by pacing-induced preconditioning: a possible role for bradykinin. Br. J. Pharmacol. **116**: 288P.

38. VEGH, A., J. GY. PAPP & J. R. PARRATT. 1994. Prevention by dexamethasone of the marked antiarrhythmic effects of preconditioning induced 20 h after rapid cardiac pacing. Br. J. Pharmacol. **113**: 1081–1082.

39. STEARE, S. E. & D. M. YELLON. 1995. The potential for endogenous myocardial anti-oxidants to protect the myocardium against ischaemia-reperfusion injury: refreshing parts exogenous anti-oxidants cannot reach? J. Mol. Cell. Cardiol. **27**: 65–74.

40. YELLON, D. M. & D. S. LATCHMAN. 1992. Stress proteins and myocardial protection. J. Mol. Cell. Cardiol. **24**: 113–124.

41. KIS, A., A. VEGH, J. GY. PAPP & J. R. PARRATT. 1996. Repeated pacing widens the time window of delayed protection against ventricular arrhythmias in dogs. J. Mol. Cell. Cardiol. **28**: A229.

42. TAJIMA, M., D. KATAYOSE, M. BESSHO & S. ISOYAMA. 1994. Acute ischaemic preconditioning and chronic hypoxia independently increase myocardial tolerance to ischaemia. Cardiovasc. Res. **28**: 312–319.

Free Radicals and Heat Shock Protein in the Heart[a]

RAKESH C. KUKREJA,[b] MICHAEL C. KONTOS, AND
MICHAEL L. HESS

Eric Lipman Laboratories of Molecular and Cellular Cardiology
Division of Cardiology, Department of Medicine
Medical College of Virginia
Virginia Commonwealth University
Richmond, Virginia 23298

INTRODUCTION

The exposure of cells to harmful events or agents creating a noxious stress is met by several different cellular defense mechanisms including detoxifying enzymes like cytochrome P450[1] or catalase and SOD removing oxygen radicals.[2,3] A frequent consequence of noxious stresses, like hypoxia, is an accumulation of proteins that are not correctly folded.[4] Malfolded proteins do not remain soluble and become denatured proteins. Induction of stress or heat shock proteins (HSPs) protect the cells against harmful consequences of protein denaturation.[5,6] "Stress" or 'heat-stress' proteins were originally identified because of increased synthesis by many cell types after exposure to elevated temperatures. These proteins, formerly usually designated as heat shock proteins, are intracellular proteins well conserved during evolution, present in low or negligible amounts in unstressed cells. The major HSPs are divided according to their molecular weight into the small HSPs (26–28 kd), the HSP 60 family, which are located in the mitochondria, and the HSP 70, HSP 90 and HSP 100 gene families. It is now believed that heat-stress proteins may play an essential part in normal cells and in cells' responses to stress.[7] The HSP 70 family is the most abundant and best known among stress proteins. The HSP 70 gene family includes HSP 70c (70–71 kd), which are always present in cells. HSP 70c plays an important role by associating with nascently formed proteins that have not reached their permanent folding state and prevents their denaturation.[8] In addition, it serves as an unfoldase by associating with proteins being incorporated into mitochondria and placing them into a translocation competent configuration.[9] These effects of HSP 70 have been termed its chaperone function.[10] HSP 70 heat-stress protein was identified in neonatal and adult heart tissue from several species, including dog, rat and rabbit.[11] Studies in different species have shown that increased quantities of heat-stress proteins may protect the heart against subsequent damage. Similarly, a wide variety of other stressful stimuli have been shown to increase HSP 70 synthesis in cadiac tissue. These

[a] This work was supported in part by Grants HL 46763 and 51045 from the National Institutes of Health. MCK was supported by a fellowship from the American Heart Association Virginia Affiliate.

[b] Address for correspondence: Rakesh C. Kukreja, Ph.D., Associate Professor, Box 282, Cardiology Division, Medical College of Virginia, Virginia Commonwealth University, Richmond, VA 23298. Tel.: (804) 828-0389; Fax: (804) 828-8700.

include ischemia,[12] pressure or volume overload,[13] and treatment with heavy metals such as cadmium[14] as well as drugs such as vasopressin or angiotensin[15] and isoproterenol.[16]

Stress also induces the translocation of a specific form of HSP 70 from the cytoplasm of the nucleus.[17] Protective effects of HSP 70s are mediated by their binding to malfolded proteins which may protect these proteins from further denaturation and thus prevent the formation of large and damaging protein aggregates.[7,18] In addition, HSP 70 may rearrange folding towards a more normal configuration. It has been postulated that HSP 70 may destin irreversibly denatured proteins to removal by protein degradation.[19] HSP 70 isoforms therefore either protect or repair proteins in critical cellular structures during or after a noxious stress. It is also interesting to note that HSP 70s are ATP binding proteins.[20] Release of HSP 70 from malfolded proteins requires the energy derived from splitting of ATP, and some of this chemical energy may also be used for the refolding process.[21]

Regulation of HSP 70 Gene Expression

The stress-induced increases of HSP 70 are triggered by protein denaturation.[22] Stress increases transcription of the HSP 70 gene, and increases HSP 70 mRNA in contrast to a marked decrease in the synthesis of other proteins.[23] The increased transcription, which presents the major mechanism of increase of HSP 70 levels, is mediated by binding of oligomeric heat shock factor (HSF) to cis acting regions of HSP 70 genes, the so-called heat shock element (HSE).[24] FIGURE 1 illustrates the diversity of transcriptional control elements within a heat-inducible human HSP 70 gene.[25] At least two different HSFs occur in mammalian cells.[26,27] In *S. cerevisiae*, HSF is a nuclear protein that is bound constitutively to the HSE.

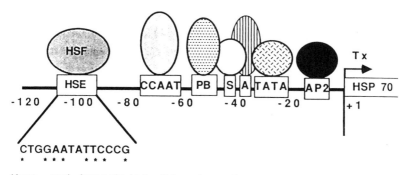

Heat- and hypoxia-inducible element

FIGURE 1. Transcriptional control elements of a human HSP 70 gene. The 5′ flanking region of this gene contains binding sites for a number of transcription factors including TFIID (TATA), AP2, ATF (A) and Ap1 (S), as well as CCAAT and purine-rich box (PB) motifs). The heat shock element (HSE) is required for activation of the promoter by thermal stress and hypoxia. Mutations in bases (indicated by an *asterisk*) disrupt the function of HSE. (From Williams & Benjamin.[25] Reprinted by permission from *Molecular Biology and Medicine*.)

The transcriptional activation function of the protein is masked in unstressed cells, but is activated by heat shock. The mechanism of this activation may involve temperature-dependent phosphorylation of HSF.[28,29] However, in insect, avian and mammalian cells, HSF is present within unstressed cells in a form that does not bind the HSE. During heat stress, transcriptional activation accompanies HSF binding to the HSE.[30–33] HSP 70 is also regulated posttranslationally. The half life of HSP 70 mRNA was found to increase 10-fold with heat shock in HeLa cells.[34] At the translational level, feedback inhibition of HSP 70 synthesis occurs in response to the level of unbound HSP 70.[35–39]

Free Radicals and Heat Shock Proteins

Mediators of inflammation such as tumor necrosis factor[40] and endotoxin polysaccharide increase the activity of myocardial antioxidant enzymes and induce a state of tolerance to the issue injury produced by hyperoxia or reperfusion.[41–44] These mediators are known to increase the generation of reactive oxygen species derived from activated neutrophils in the inflammatory sites. Also, preconditioning of the heart by repeated brief periods of occlusion with intermittent reperfusion improves myocardial salvage after prolonged ischemia[45] and induces translation of HSP 70.[46] Since oxygen-derived free radicals are generated during ischemia/reperfusion injury in the heart,[47] we hypothesized that bursts of free radicals generated by ischemic preconditioning might trigger an increased expression of HSP 70. We tested the ability of reduced oxygen species such as superoxide anion and hydrogen peroxide, or singlet oxygen to directly induce gene expression of HSP 70 in the rat heart.[48]

Experimental Model

A Langendorff's perfused rat heart preparation was used in these studies. Following anesthetization, the hearts were excised and then cannulated via the aorta and retrogradely perfused at a constant perfusion pressure equivalent to 100 cm H_2O. All hearts were initially perfused with modified Krebs-Henseleit (K-H) buffer at 37°C, containing (in mM) NaCl 118.5, $NaHCO_3$ 25.0, KCl 3.2, $MgSO_4$ 1.19, $CaCl_2$ 1.25, KH_2PO_4 1.2 and glucose 11.1 and was bubbled with 95%/5% O_2/CO_2 mixture. The pH was maintained at 7.4. After the heart began spontaneous contraction, a small incision was made in the left atrium. A latex balloon, connected to a pressure transducer via a polyethylene cannula, was inserted through the left atrium and mitral valve into the left ventricle. The balloon was filled with enough water to increase the end diastolic pressure to approximately 5 mmHg. The transducer was connected to a multichannel polygraph (Grass). Care was taken to maintain the temperature of heart at 37°C by enclosing in a double jacketed chamber. Coronary flow was measured by timed collections of the effluent.

Free oxygen radicals were generated by xanthine oxidase acting on 100 μM xanthine as a substrate. The hearts were equilibrated for a period of 30 min prior to perfusion with generators of activated oxygen species or hydrogen peroxide. Following 15 min of perfusion with oxygen radical generators, the hearts were perfused with K-H buffer for 30 min. At the end of this protocol, the hearts were taken from the Langendorff apparatus and frozen in liquid nitrogen. The experimental groups were: 1. control (buffer only), 2. xanthine

(100 μM), 3. xanthine oxidase (0.09 U/ml), 4. xanthine (100 μM) plus xanthine oxidase (0.09 U/ml), and 5. hydrogen peroxide (100 μM). Singlet oxygen was generated by photoexcitation of the light-sensitive dye rose bengal in the heart.[11] Following equilibration for 30 min, three groups of hearts were studied: (a) K-H buffer only, (b) perfusion with 250 nM rose bengal for 15 min without illumination and (c) continuously perfused with rose bengal and illuminated for 15 min. All groups were switched back to K-H buffer and allowed to recover for an additional 30 min. Because rose bengal is a photosensitive dye, all experiments in this group were carried out in the dark. For ischemia/reperfusion studies, the hearts were subjected to 30 min of global ischemia by clamping the aortic cannula. The ischemic period was followed by 20 min of reperfusion. In separate experiments, superoxide dismutase (30 U/ml) was administered in the perfusion buffer.

Oxidants and Myocardial Dysfunction

TABLE 1 shows the effects of perfusion with xanthine, xanthine oxidase, xanthine plus xanthine oxidase, and hydrogen peroxide on developed pressure at 5 min after infusion and at the end of the recovery period (30 min after discontinuation of free radical generating solutions). Perfusion with either xanthine oxidase or xanthine alone did not result in a significant difference in developed pressure when compared to control hearts at 5 min or at the end of the recovery period. A highly significant decrease in developed pressure was observed following perfusion with xanthine/xanthine oxidase at 5 min after infusion. At the end of a 30-min recovery period, the developed pressure in the xanthine/xanthine oxidase group remained significantly lower. Similarly, hearts perfused with 100 μM hydrogen peroxide demonstrated a significant depression in developed pressure during the infusion period, which also continued until the end of the recovery period. No significant changes in developed pressure were observed by perfusion with rose bengal (without illumination) (TABLE 1). However, developed pressure dropped significantly to $40.8 \pm 6.6\%$ of control values at 5 min after illumination and recovered to $58.4 \pm 6.7\%$ at the end of the recovery period. Xanthine or xanthine oxidase alone were without any significant effect on coronary flow during the infusion period as well as at the end of the recovery period when compared to control values. With xanthine plus xanthine oxidase a significant reduction in coronary flow ($p < 0.05$) was observed (TABLE 1). Hydrogen peroxide caused a transient significant increase in coronary flow during the infusion period ($p < 0.01$). However, the coronary flow was found to be significantly decreased at the end of the recovery period. With rose bengal perfusion without illumination, no significant changes in coronary flow were observed. However, coronary flow significantly declined to $60.7 \pm 5.5\%$ of control, and recovered significantly to $70.5 \pm 3.7\%$ at the end of the recovery period.

Normothermic global ischemia for 30 min caused a rapid decrease of the ventricular developed pressure, and within 6–8 min the hearts stopped contracting completely. Parallel to the loss of mechanical activity an increase in resting tension was also observed. The developed pressure and coronary flow were 60 ± 8 and $80 \pm 5\%$ (means $\pm$ SE) respectively of control in ischemic-reperfused hearts. A significant improvement of ventricular pressure was observed following reperfusion with SOD ($82 \pm 4\%$, $p < 0.05$) but no significant improvement in coronary flow was observed (FIG. 2).

TABLE 1. Effect of Oxygen Radicals, Hydrogen Peroxide and Singlet Oxygen on Developed Pressure and Coronary Flow in Isolated Perfused Rat Heart[a]

Experimental Group	Developed Pressure during Infusion (% of Baseline)	Coronary Flow during Infusion (% of Baseline)	Developed Pressure at the End of Recovery Period (% of Baseline)	Coronary Flow at the End of Recovery Period (% of Baseline)
Control	94.6 ± 2.09	87.93 ± 1.6	77.19 ± 2.5	77.19 ± 2.47
Xanthine (100 μM)	91.68 ± 2.41	91.30 ± 1.7	79.7 ± 2.4	78.77 ± 2.9
Xanthine oxidase (0.09 U/ml)	85.35 ± 6.3	87.64 ± 2.0	73.8 ± 3.2	83.8 ± 2.77
Xanthine (100 μM) + xanthine oxidase (0.09 U/ml)	35.87 ± 13.0*	75.99 ± 6.4*	15.20 ± 7.6*	67.18 ± 2.8*
Hydrogen peroxide (100 μM)	56.01 ± 5.91*	122.77 ± 4.9*	54.85 ± 4.4*	62.99 ± 10*
Rose bengal, 250 nM without light	93.40 ± 7.20	90.50 ± 2.5	75.77 ± 5.4	81.50 ± 4.6
Rose bengal, 250 nM plus light	40.75 ± 6.60*Ÿ	60.70 ± 5.5*Ÿ	58.40 ± 6.7	70.50 ± 3.7*Ÿ

[a] The data on developed pressure and coronary flow represent measurements taken at 5 min after infusion of oxygen radical/singlet generating system of H_2O_2. The measurements at the end of the recovery period represent data at the end of 30 min after cessation of oxygen radical generators or H_2O_2. Control baseline developed pressure and coronary flow were 114.2 mmHg and 16.5 ml/min, respectively. The results are means ± SE of 4–6 independent experiments. * represents significant difference from controls ($p < 0.05$); Ÿ, significant difference from rose bengal (without light) perfused heart. (From Kukreja et al.[48] Reprinted by permission from the American Journal of Physiology.)

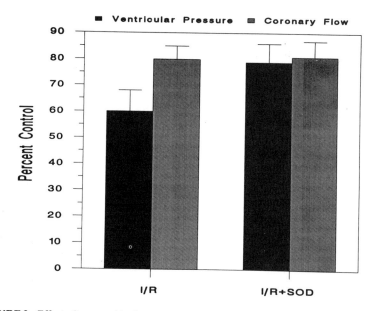

FIGURE 2. Effect of superoxide dismutase on developed pressure and coronary flow following 30 min of global ischemia and 20 min of reperfusion in isolated rat heart. Results represent means ± SE from 8 hearts. I/R, ischemia/reperfusion; IR + SOD, ischemia/reperfusion + superoxide dismutase. Control baseline developed pressure and coronary flow were 112 ± 3.2 mmHg and 15.2 ± 0.8 ml/min, respectively. * significantly different from I/R. (From Kukreja *et al.*[48] Reprinted by permission from the *American Journal of Physiology*.)

Oxygen Radicals, Ischemia/Reperfusion and HSP 70 mRNA

There was little or no HSP 70 message in the hearts perfused with K-H buffer, xanthine or xanthine oxidase alone (FIG. 3, lanes 1–3). However, xanthine plus xanthine oxidase caused a significant increase in the HSP 70 mRNA (lane 4). Densitometric analysis showed an over 13-fold increase in the density of this message. The combination of xanthine plus xanthine oxidase generates both superoxide and hydrogen peroxide, and in the presence of contaminant iron, can potentially generate hydroxyl radicals via Fenton's reaction. Since it was not clear which species was exactly responsible for the increase in mRNA we first examined the direct effect of exogenous hydrogen peroxide on HSP 70 gene expression. As shown in FIGURE 4, the HSP 70 message increased fivefold when isolated hearts were perfused with 100 μM hydrogen peroxide (lane 2). However, the combined effects of superoxide anion and hydrogen peroxide generated from xanthine plus xanthine oxidase were more pronounced (FIG. 1, lane 4) compared to the effects seen with hydrogen peroxide alone. Rose bengal in the absence of illumination does not generate singlet oxygen and thus did not increase HSP 70 message (FIG. 5, lane 2). The HSP 70 message increased 6–7-fold (FIG. 4, bottom) when rose bengal was illuminated, showing that singlet oxygen also induced expression (lane 3). Finally, we examined whether ischemia/reperfusion induced HSP 70 expression, and if this message could be diminished by superoxide dismutase. A significant increase (over 10-fold) of HSP mRNA was detected following ischemia/reperfusion. The message was diminished by superoxide dismutase, suggesting that superoxide was at least partially involved in the increase of HSP 70 mRNA during ischemia and reperfusion (FIG. 6, lane 3).

In general, the intensity of HSP 70 message appeared to be related to the severity of oxidative stress. HSP 70 message was not as strong with hydrogen

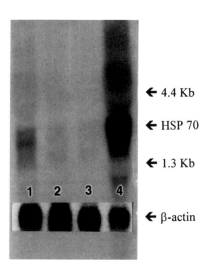

← 4.4 Kb

← HSP 70

← 1.3 Kb

← β-actin

FIGURE 3. Northern blot analysis showing direct increase in HSP 70 mRNA in isolated rat heart following perfusion with oxygen radicals generated from xanthine plus xanthine oxidase. Total cellular RNA was prepared from myocardial tissue, electrophoresced, transferred to nytran membrane and hybridized with ^{32}P-label HSP 70 probe. *Top*: lane 1, control; lane 2, 100 μM xanthine (X); lane 3, 0.09 U/ml xanthine oxidase (XO); and lane 4, xanthine (100 μM) plus xanthine oxidase (0.09 U/ml) (X + XO). Blots were stripped and rehybridized with β-actin cDNA probe. *Bottom*: transcript levels of HSP 70/β-actin measured by densitometer scanning of the autoradiogram bands. The results are means ± SE from 4 independent experiments. (From Kukreja et al.[48] Reprinted by permission from the *American Journal of Physiology*.)

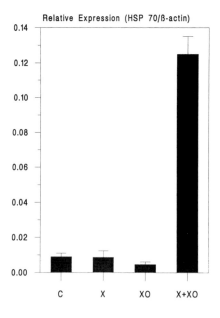

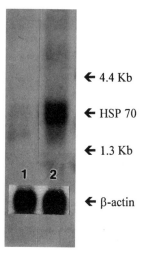

← 4.4 Kb

← HSP 70

← 1.3 Kb

← β-actin

FIGURE 4. Northern blot analysis showing increase in HSP 70 mRNA by 100 μM hydrogen peroxide in isolated rat heart. *Top*: lane 1, control; lane 2, hydrogen peroxide. *Bottom*: densitometer scanning of the autoradiogram bands. (From Kukreja *et al.*[48] Reprinted by permission from the *American Journal of Physiology*.)

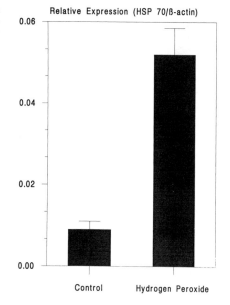

peroxide or irradiated rose bengal, and therefore the two bands were clearly differentiated. It was not clear whether the lower response of HSP 70 observed with irradiated rose bengal and hydrogen peroxide was due to lower oxidative stress or to the ability of each of these oxidants to produce differential response. While photoactivation of rose bengal results in the formation of singlet oxygen, superoxide is also formed,[49] which in the presence of contaminating iron could generate hydroxyl radical. Thus it is possible that low levels of hydroxyl radical generated from rose bengal induced lower response of HSP 70. In our study we obtained over 5-fold increase in HSP 70 with 100 μM hydrogen peroxide. Jornot and co-workers,[50] however, used higher concentrations of hydrogen peroxide (1 and 5 mM) for 15 min to observe expression of HSP 70 in human umbilical vein endothelial cells. On the other hand Lu *et al.*[51] were able to induce HSP 70 with

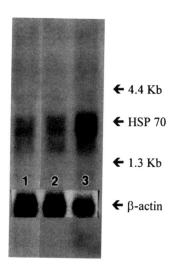

← 4.4 Kb

← HSP 70

← 1.3 Kb

← β-actin

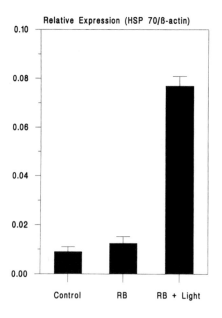

Relative Expression (HSP 70/ß-actin)

FIGURE 5. Northern blot analysis of HSP 70 mRNA of isolated hearts perfused with singlet generating system, rose bengal. *Top*: lane 1, control; lane 2, heart perfused with rose bengal without illumination (RB); lane 3, singlet oxygen generated from illuminated rose bengal (RB + light). *Bottom*: densitometer scanning of the autoradiogram bands. (From Kukreja *et al.*[48] Reprinted by permission from the *American Journal of Physiology*.)

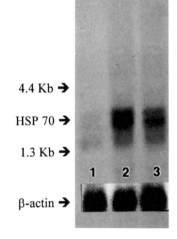

FIGURE 6. Northern blot showing HSP 70 mRNA following ischemia (Is) and reperfusion (Rep) with and without superoxide dismutase. *Top*: lane 1, control; lane 2, hearts subjected to ischemia/reperfusion; and lane 3, hearts subjected to ischemia/reperfusion in presence of SOD (30 U/ml). *Bottom*: densitometer scanning of the autoradiogram. (From Kukreja *et al.*[48] Reprinted by permission from the *American Journal of Physiology*.)

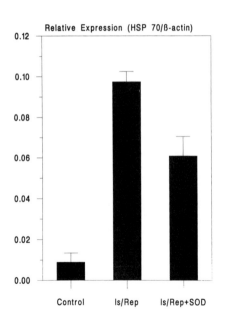

a relatively lower concentration of hydrogen peroxide (40 and 80 μM) in vascular endothelial cells. In the present studies, ischemia/reperfusion also increased HSP 70 mRNA which was decreased with superoxide dismutase, demonstrating that in addition to other unknown factors, free radicals were at least partially involved in inducing HSP 70 mRNA.

There is an extensive body of literature showing that free radicals generated during ischemia/reperfusion cause myocardial injury.[47] Cellular injury responsible for postischemic dysfunction has been ascribed to superoxide, hydrogen peroxide and the hydroxyl radical. Scavengers of free radicals such as superoxide dismutase, catalase or dimethylthiourea significantly enhance recovery of function following stunning of the myocardium.[52,53] Perfusion of isolated rat hearts with oxygen radical generating sources or hydrogen peroxide caused a significant reduction in myocardial contractility and ultrastructure damage.[54] Hearse et al.[55] showed that singlet oxygen generated from photosensitized rose bengal directly induced changes in the EKG such as inversion of the terminal portion of the T wave and prolongation of the Q-T interval. Direct exposure of isolated sarcoplasmic reticulum to singlet oxygen caused significant inhibition of activity as well as degradation of the Ca^{2+}-ATPase enzyme by fragmentation and polymerization.[56] Other sarcoplasmic reticulum proteins were also found to be degraded by singlet oxygen.

The exact mechanism for the increase in HSP 70 mRNA by free radicals or ischemia/reperfusion is not clear from these studies. However a number of possibilities exist. First, it is known that stress-induced increases in HSP 70 are triggered by protein denaturation.[22] the presence of denatured or damaged proteins within the cytoplasm may be a common feature of the signaling pathway by which diverse stresses mediate the activation of heat shock transcription factor. It has been shown that microinjection of denatured proteins directly lead to activation of heat shock transcription factor.[57] Thus it is quite possible that increases in mRNA by oxygen radicals may have been due to denaturation of proteins as a result of oxygen radical attack on subcellular components. Second, the changes in hemodynamics induced by oxygen radicals or ischemia/reperfusion may have directly triggered the increase of HSP 70 mRNA. Bauter et al.[58] reported that expression of c-*fos* and c-*myc* protooncogenes were both sequentially and transitorily increased when coronary flow (and/or pressure) was augmented. The increase in expression of these protooncogenes following changes in hemodynamics may directly induce HSP 70. Our data show that oxidants generated from various sources caused a significant reduction of ventricular developed pressure and coronary flow. Although speculative, it may be possible that changes in hemodynamics by oxidants or ischemia/reperfusion modulate expression of protooncogenes which could contribute to HSP 70 gene transcription. Third, during ischemia/reperfusion as well as perfusion with oxygen radicals, both ATP and creatine phosphate levels are reduced.[59,60] It has been postulated that the decrease in intracellular ATP content in cells under stress may be one of the triggers that leads to the induction of HSP 70 by reducing the pool of free HSP 70.[39] In these studies, the time course of induction of HSP 70 correlated closely with the amount of cellular damage and ATP depletion in the myocardial cell. On the other hand, Iwaki et al.[61] found that the induction of HSP 70 preceded the onset of cellular damage as measured by the release of cytoplasmic enzymes and preincorporated arachidonic acid. These authors concluded that cardiomyocytes were able to respond to hypoxia/reoxygenation and metabolic stress with increased HSP 70 production.

The increase of HSP 70 by oxygen radicals may have some interesting implications in preconditioning of the myocardium. For example, Murry et al.[62] proposed that oxygen radicals generated during brief periods of ischemia/reperfusion may actually contribute to a cardioprotective effect. This hyothesis was based on the observation that administration of superoxide dismutase and catalase partially blocked the ability of preconditioning to limit infarct size in dogs. Tritto et al.[63] preconditioned isolated rabbit hearts with free radicals by infusing xanthine/

xanthine oxidase and found a significant recovery of developed presure and coronary flow after ischemia and reperfusion. Thus antioxidants appear to limit the protective effects of repetitive ischemia and reperfusion, and free radical generation appears to trigger protection. Low dose infusion of hydrogen peroxide in lieu of sublethal ischemia precondition the heart *in situ*[64] against infarction. It is unlikely that free radicals induce protection via synthesis of HSP 70 during acute preconditioning of myocardium. However, recent studies suggest that a second window of protection along with synthesis of HSP 70 appears at 24 hours after preconditioning, which perhaps may last even longer.[46] It is quite possible that free radical-triggered HSP 70 synthesis may contribute to the second window of protection.

CONCLUSIONS

These results demonstrate that oxidant stress directly triggers an early increase in HSP 70 mRNA in the isolated perfused rat heart. A similar increase was observed during ischemia/reperfusion, and this message was diminished by superoxide dismutase, indicating that free radicals, particularly the superoxide anion, can contribute to an increase in HSP 70 mRNA. This is of great interest, because although free radicals may cause cell necrosis, low amounts of stress-induced oxygen species could actually be beneficial to the heart via induction of HSP 70. The significance of the oxygen radical-mediated increase in HSP 70 is not clear from our studies. It is, however, tempting to postulate that free radicals generated during ischemic preconditioning may mediate synthesis of stress proteins which may play a role in the second window of protection.

REFERENCES

1. GUNSALUS, I. C., T. C. PEDERSON & S. G. SLIGAR. 1975. Oxygenase-catalyzed biological hydroxylations. Annu. Rev. Biochem. **44:** 377–407.
2. DAS, D. K., R. M. ENGELMAN, H. OTANI, J. A. ROUSOU, R. H. BREYER & S. LEMESHOW. 1986. Effect of superoxide dismutase and catalase on myocardial energy metabolism during ischemia and reperfusion. Clin. Physiol. Biochem. **4:** 187–198.
3. OTANI, H., M. UMEMOTO, K. KAGAWA, Y. NAKAMURA, K. OMOTO, K. TANAKA, T. SATO, A. NONOYAMA & T. KAGAWA. 1986. Protection against oxygen-induced reperfusion injury of the isolated canine heart by superoxide dismutase and catalase. J. Surg. Res. **41:** 126–133.
4. NGUYEN, V. T., M. MORANGE & O. BENSAUDE. 1989. Protein denaturation during heat shock and related stress. *Escherichia coli* beta-galactosidase and Photoinus pyralis luciferase inactivation in mouse cells. J. Biol. Chem. **264:** 10487–10492.
5. ROTHMAN, J. E. 1989. Polypeptide chain binding proteins: catalysts of protein folding and related processes in cells. Cell **59:** 591–601.
6. PELHAM, H. R. B. 1986. Speculations on the functions of the major heat shock and glucose-regulated proteins. Cell **45:** 885–894.
7. PELHAM, H. R. B. 1986. Speculation on the functions of the major heat shock and glucose related proteins. Cell **46:** 959–961.
8. LANDRY, S. M. & L. M. GIERASCH. 1991. Recognition of nascent polypeptides for targeting and folding. Trends Biochem. Sci. **16:** 159–163.
9. MURAKAMI, H., D. PAIN & G. BLOBEL. 1987. 70-kD heat shock-related protein is one of at least two distinct cytosolic factors stimulating protein import into mitochondria. J. Cell Biol. **107:** 2051–2057.
10. ELLIS, J. 1987. Proteins as molecular chaperones. Nature (London) **328:** 378–379.
11. CURRIE, R. W. 1987. Effects of ischemia and perfusion temperature on the synthesis

of stress induced (heat shock) proteins in isolated and perfused hearts. J. Mol. Cell. Cardiol. **19**: 795–808.

12. HOWARD, G. & T. E. GEOGHEGAN. 1986. Altered cardiac tissue gene expression during acute hypoxic exposure. Mol. Cell. Biol. **69**: 155–160.

13. DELCAYRE, C., J. L. SAMUEL, F. MARROTHE, J. J. MESCADIER & L. RAPPAPORT. 1988. Synthesis of stress proteins in rat cardiac myocytes 2–4 days after imposition of hemodynamic overload. J. Clin. Invest. **82**: 460–468.

14. LOW, I., T. FRIEDRICH & W. SCHOEPPE. 1989. Synthesis of shock proteins in cultured fetal mouse myocardial cells. Exp. Cell Res. **180**: 451–459.

15. MOALIC, J. M., C. BAUTERS, D. HIMBERT, J. BERCOVICI, C. MOUAS, P. GUICHENEY, M. BAUDOIN-LEGRAS, L. RAPPAPORT, R. EMANOIL-RAVIER, V. MEZGER & B. SWYNGHEDAUW. 1989. Phenylepinephrine, vasopressin and angiotensin as determinants of heat shock protein gene expression in adult rat heart and aorta. J. Hypertens. **7**: 195–201.

16. WHITE, F. P. & S. C. WHITE. 1986. Isoproterenol induced myocardial necrosis is associated with stress protein synthesis in rat heart and thoracic aorta. Cardiovasc. Res. **20**: 512–515.

17. WELCH, W. J. & J. R. FERAMINSCO. 1984. Nuclear and nucleolar localization of the 72,000-dalton heat shock protein in heat shocked human mammalian cells. J. Biol. Chem. **259**: 4501–4513.

18. PALLEROS, D. R., W. J. WELCH & A. L. FINK. 1991. Interaction of hsp70 with unfolded proteins: effects of temperature and nucleotides on the kinetics of binding. Proc. Natl. Acad. Sci. USA **88**: 5719–5723.

19. CHIANG, H.-L., S. R. TERLECKY, C. P. PLANT & J. F. DICE. 1989. A role for a 70-kilodalton heat shock protein in lysosomal degradation of intracellular proteins. Science **246**: 382–385.

20. BELARDINELLI, L., J. LINDEN & R. BERNE. 1989. The cardiac effects of adenosine. Prog. Cardiovasc Dis. **32**: 73–97.

21. HOLL-NEUGEBAUER, B., R. RUDOLPH, M. SCHMIDT & J. BUCHNER. 1991. Reconstitution of heat shock effect *in vitro*: influence of GroE on the thermal aggregation of alpha-glucosidase from yeast. Biochemistry **30**: 11609–11614.

22. ANATHAN, J., A. L. GOLDBERG & R. VOELLMY. 1986. Abnormal proteins serve as eukaryotic stress signals and trigger the activation of heat shock genes. Science **232**: 522–524.

23. LINDQUIST, S. 1986. The heat-shock response. Annu. Rev. Biochem. **55**: 1151–1191.

24. XIAO, H., O. PERISIC & J. T. LIS. 1991. Cooperative binding of drosophila heat shock factor to arrays of conserved 5 bp unit. Cell **64**: 585–593.

25. WILLIAMS, R. S. & I. J. BENJAMIN. 1991. Stress proteins and cardiovascular disease. Mol. Biol. Med. **8**: 197–206.

26. RABINDRAN, S. K., G. GIORGI, J. CLOS & C. WU. 1991. Molecular cloning and expression of a human shock, HSF1. Proc. Natl. Acad. Sci. USA **88**: 6906–6910.

27. SCHUETZ, T. J., G. J. GALLO, L. SHELDON, P. TEMPST & R. E. KINGSTON. 1991. Isolation of a cDNA for HSF2: evidence for two heat shock factor genes in humans. Proc. Natl. Acad. Sci. USA **88**: 6911–6915.

28. SORGER, P. K. & R. B. PELHAM. 1988. Yeast heat shock factor is an essential DNA-binding protein that exhibits temperature-dependent phosphorylation. Cell **54**: 855–864.

29. SORGER, P. K., M. J. LEWIS & H. R. B. PELHAM. 1987. Heat shock factor is regulated differently in yeast and HeLa cells. Nature **329**: 81–83.

30. GOLDENBERG, C. J., Y. LUO, M. FENNA, R. BALER, R. WEINMANN & R. VOELLMY. 1988. Purified human factor activates heat shock promoter in a HeLa cell-free transcription system. J. Biol. Chem. **263**: 19734–19739.

31. LARSON, J. S., T. J. SCHUETZ & R. E. KINGSTON. 1988. Activation *in vitro* of sequence-specific DNA binding by a human regulatory factor. Nature (London) **335**: 372–376.

32. WU, C., S. WILSON, B. WALKER, I. DAWID, T. PAISLEY, V. ZIMARINO & H. UEDA. 1987. Purification and properties of *Drosophila* heat shock activator protein. Science **238**: 1247–1252.

33. ZIMARINO, V. & C. WU. 1987. Induction of sequence-specific binding of *Drosophila* heat shock activator protein without protein synthesis. Nature (London) **327:** 727–730.
34. THEODORAKIS, N. G. & R. I. MORIMOTO. 1987. Post-translational regulation of HSP 70 expression in human cells: effects of heat shock, inhibition of protein synthesis, and adenovirus infection on translation and mRNA stability. Mol. Cell. Biol. **7:** 4357–4368.
35. DIDOMENICO, B. J., G. E. BUUGAISKY & S. LINDQUIST. 1982. The heat shock response is self-regulated at both the transcriptional and post-translational levels. Cell **31:** 593–603.
36. YOST, H. J., R. B. PERERSEN & S. LINDQUIST. 1989. Post-transcriptional regulation of heat shock protein in *Drosophila*. *In* Stress Proteins in Biology and Medicine. R. Morimoto, A. Tissieres & C. Georgopoulos, Eds. 379–409. Cold Spring Harbor Laboratory Press. Cold Spring Harbor.
37. STONE, D. E. & E. A. CRAIG. 1990. Self-regulation of 70-kilodalton heat shock proteins in *Saccharomyces cerevisiae*. Mol. Cell. Biol. **10:** 1622–1632.
38. BALER, R., W. J. WELCH & R. VOELLMY. 1992. Heat shock gene regulation by nascent polypeptides and denatured proteins: HSP 70 as a potential autoregulatory factor. J. Cell. Biol. **117:** 1151–1159.
39. BECKMANN, R. P., M. LOVETT & W. J. WELCH. 1992. Examining the function and regulation of hsp70 in cells subjected to metabolic stress. J. Cell Biol. **6:** 1137–1150.
40. WONG, G. H. W. & D. V. GOEDDEL. 1988. Induction of manganese superoxide dismutase by tumor necrosis factor: possible protective mechanism. Science **242:** 941–943.
41. BROWN, J. M., M. A. GROSSO, G. J. TARADA, G. J. WHITMAN, A. BANERJEE, C. W. WHITE, A. H. HARKEN & J. E. REPINE. 1989. Endotoxin pretreatment increases endogenous myocardial catalase activity and decreases ischemia-reperfusion injury of isolated rat heart. Proc. Natl. Acad. Sci. USA **86:** 2516–2520.
42. SHIKI, Y., B. O. MEYRICK, K. L. BRIGHAM & I. M. BURR. 1987. Endotoxin increases superoxide dismutase in cultured bovine pulmonary endothelial cells. Am. J. Physiol. **252** (Cell. Physiol. **21**): C436–C440.
43. BROWN, J. M., C. W. WHITE, L. S. TERADA, M. A. GROSSO, P. F. SHANLEY, D. W. MULVIN, A. BANERJEE, G. J. R. WHITMAN, A. H. HARKEN & J. E. REPINE. 1990. Interleukin 1 pretreatment decreases ischemia/reperfusion injury. Proc. Natl. Acad. Sci. USA **87:** 5026–5030.
44. WHITE, C. W., P. GHEZZI, C. A. DINARELLO, S. A. CALDWELL, I. F. MCMURTRY & J. E. REPINE. 1987. Recombinant tumor necrosis factor/cachectin and interleukin 1 pretreatment decreases lung oxidized glutathione accumulation, lung injury, and mortality in rats exposed to hyperoxia. J. Clin. Invest. **79:** 1868–1873.
45. MURRY, C. E., R. B. JENNINGS & K. A. REIMER. 1986. Preconditioning with ischemia: a delay of lethal cell injury in ischemic myocardium. Circulation **74:** 1124–1136.
46. MARBER, M. S., D. S. LATCHMAN, J. M. WALKER & D. M. YELLON. 1993. Cardiac stress protein elevation 24 hours after brief ischemia or heat stress is associated with resistance to myocardial infarction. Criculation **88:** 1264–1272.
47. ZWEIER, J. L., J. T. FLAHERTY & M. L. WEISFELDT. 1987. Direct measurement of free radical generation following reperfusion of ischemic myocardium. Proc. Natl. Acad. Sci. USA **84:** 1404–1407.
48. KUKREJA, R. C., M. C. KONTOS, K. E. LOESSER, S. K. BATRA, Y. QIAN, C. J. J. GBUR, S. A. NASEEM, R. L. JESSE & M. L. HESS. 1994. Oxidant stress increases heat shock protein 70 mRNA in isolated perfused rat heart. Am. J. Physiol. **267:** H2213–H2219.
49. PACZKOWSKI, J., J. J. M. LAMBERTS, B. PACZKOWSKA & D. C. NECKERS. 1985. Photophysical properties of rose bengal and its derivatives. J. Free Radical Biol. Med. **17:** 485–499.
50. JORNOT, L., A. F. MIRAULT & A. F. JUNOD. 1991. Differential expression of hsp70 stress protein in human endothelial cells exposed to heat shock and hydrogen peroxide. Am. J. Respir. Cell. Mol. Biol. **5:** 265–275.
51. LU, D., N. MAULIK, I. I. MORARU, D. L. KREUTZER & D. K. DAS. 1994. Molecular adaptation of vascular endothelial cells to oxidative stress. Am. J. Physiol. **264:** C715–C722.

52. BOLLI, R., ZHU. WEI-XI, C. J. HARTLEY, L. H. MICHAEL, J. E. REPINE, M. L. HESS, R. C. KUKREJA & R. ROBERTS. 1987. Attenuation of dysfunction in the postischemic stunned myocardium by dimethylthiourea. Circulation **76**: 458–468.

53. JEROUDI, M. O., F. J. TRIANA, B. S. PATEL & R. BOLLI. 1990. Effect of superoxide dismutase and catalase, given separately, on myocardial "stunning." Am. J. Physiol. **259**: H889–H901.

54. MIKI, S., M. ASHRAF, S. SALKA & N. SPERELAKIS. 1988. Myocardial dysfunction and ultrastructural alterations mediated by oxygen metabolites. J. Mol. Cell. Cardiol. **20**: 1009–1024.

55. HEARSE, D. J., Y. KUSAMA & M. BERNIER. 1989. Rapid electrophysiological changes leading to arrhythmias in the aerobic rat heart: photosensitization studies with rose bengal-derived reactive oxygen intermediates. Circ. Res. **65**: 146–153.

56. KUKREJA, R. C., A. A. KEARNS, J. L. ZWEIER, P. KUPPUSAMY & M. L. HESS. 1991. Singlet oxygen interaction with Ca^{2+}-ATPase of cardiac sarcoplasmic reticulum. Circ. Res. **69**: 1003–1014.

57. KOZUTSUMI, Y., M. SEGAL, K. NORMINGTON, M. J. GETHING & J. SAMBROOK. 1988. The presence of malfolded proteins in the endoplasmic reticulum signals the induction of glucose-regulated proteins. Nature (London) **355**: 372–376.

58. BAUTERS, C., J. M. MOALIC, J. BERCOVICI, C. MOUAS, R. EMANOIL-RAVIER, S. SCHIAFFINO & B. SWYNGHEDAUW. 1988. Coronary flow as a determinant of c-myc and c-fos proto-oncogene expression in an isolated adult rat heart. J. Mol. Cell. Cardiol. **88**: 2018–2025.

59. ABD-ELFATTAH, A. S., M. E. JESSEN, S. A. HANAN, G. TUCHY & A. S. WECHSLER. 1990. Is adenosine 5'-triphosphate derangement or free-radical-mediated injury the major cause of ventricular dysfunction during reperfusion? Circulation **82**: IV-341–IV-350.

60. YTREHUS, K., R. MYKLEBUST & O. D. MJOS. 1986. Influence of oxygen radicals generated by xanthine oxidase in the isolated perfused rat heart. Cardiovasc. Res. **20**: 597–603.

61. IWAKI, K., S. H. CHI, W. H. DILLMANN & R. MESTRIL. 1993. Induction of HSP 70 in cultured rat neonatal cardiomyocytes by hypoxia and metabolic stress. Circulation **87**: 2023–2032.

62. MURRY, C. E., V. J. RICHARD, R. B. JENNINGS & K. A. REIMER. 1988. Preconditioning with ischemia: Is the protective effect mediated by free radical-induced myocardial stunning? Circulation **78**(Suppl. II): II-77.

63. TRITTO, I., G. AMBROSIO, P. P. ELIA, A. SCOGNAMIGLIO, P. CIRILLO & M. CHIARIELLO. 1992. Evidence that oxygen radicals may mediate preconditioning in isolated rabbit hearts (abstract). Circulation **86**: I-30.

64. PATHAK, S. K., Y. QIAN, M. L. HESS & R. C. KUKREJA. 1995. Hydrogen peroxide preconditions rabbit heart via activation of ATP-sensitive potassium channel (abstract). Circulation **92**: I-717.

Myocardial Adaptation, Stress Proteins, and the Second Window of Protection

MICHAEL S. MARBER[a,b] AND DEREK M. YELLON[c]

[b]The Department of Cardiology
St. Thomas's Hospital
London SE1 7EH, United Kingdom

[c]The Hatter Institute for Cardiovascular Studies
Division of Cardiology
University College London Medical School
Grafton Way
London WC1E 6DB, United Kingdom

INTRODUCTION

Ischemic heart disease is the most common single cause of death in the UK.[1] Patients often present with advanced disease with severe atherosclerotic stenoses within the coronary arteries and damage to the myocardium. Currently, the mainstay of treatment is to bypass or dilate such stenoses or to treat patients with thrombolytic drugs should one of the atherosclerotic plaques suffer an occlusive complication that results in acute myocardial infarction.[2] The mortality from acute myocardial infarction is inversely related to the amount of myocardial salvage by thrombolytic reperfusion;[2] therefore, agents that slow the rate of ischemic necrosis are very likely to save lives.[2]

One strategy to decrease the rate of myocardial necrosis is to understand the events that lead to cell death during ischemia and then to target appropriate interventions. Unfortunately, the key events leading to ischemic cell death are poorly understood.[3-6] However, the changes in the cellular milieu during ischemia and reperfusion[4] (notably, ATP depletion, free radical exposure and the accumulation of protons and sodium ions) are known to perturb protein structure.

Evidence is accumulating that alterations in the tertiary structure of key metabolic enzymes[5] and cytoskeletal proteins[6] may play a central role in myocardial ischemic injury. A family of proteins known as heat shock proteins (HSP) or stress proteins attenuate cell injury following denaturing stresses such as heat,[7] and are also capable of re-naturing and returning protein function *in vitro*.[8] The hypothesis was therefore formulated that stress proteins may be capable of protecting cells, including myocytes, from ischemic injury.[7] This hypothesis was supported by the initial studies of Currie *et al.*, which suggested that myocardial stress proteins, elevated by whole body heat stress, may protect the rat heart from ischemic injury.[9] Subsequent studies by independent investigators, including ourselves, have now confirmed these observations in other species and models of myocardial ischemic injury.[7,10,11]

[a] Tel.: 044-171-922-8191; Fax: 044-171-928-0658.

The purpose of this paper is to chart the progress of this interesting field from myocardial stress protein induction by whole body heat stress to induction by sublethal ischemia and the second window of protection.

Crosstolerance and Ischemic Induction of HSP 70i

Acquired thermotolerance describes the resistance to lethal thermal injury that follows sublethal temperature elevation.

The weight of evidence indicates that heat shock proteins, in particular inducible members of the HSP 70 family (HSP 70i), are involved in acquired thermotolerance.[12-16] The accepted dogma is that the first episode of sublethal temperature elevation results in HSP accumulation and that acquired tolerance is a result of this accumulation. A similar line of reasoning would suggest that if two different stresses induce HSPs, then pretreatment with one stress should protect against exposure to the second stress. This phenomenon does occur in certain situations and is known as crosstolerance.

The concept of crosstolerance was first suggested by the experiments performed by Li and Hahn (1978),[17] who found that a hamster cell line could be rendered resistant to both adriamycin and heat toxicity by pretreatment with ethanol. Subsequent studies have demonstrated similar findings but with very different stresses. For example; whole body heat stress in rats protects retinal pigment cells from light injury, protection being temporally related to HSP 70i induction;[18] heat stress protects against subsequent oxidative stress in a number of models;[19] heat-stressed human breast cancer cells are rendered resistant to doxorubicin, an effect that seems related to HSP 70i and HSP 27 cell content;[20] heat-stressed neuronal cells are resistant to the excitotoxic effects of glutamate, an effect dependent on protein synthesis and related to HSP 70i;[21,22] and in the mouse whole body heat stress induces HSP 70i in various organs and protects against death following exposure to endotoxin.[23]

Based upon the apparent central role of stress proteins in crosstolerance, crosstolerance to myocardial ischemia would require stress protein induction by ischemia.

Within the heart ischemia is known to induce HSP 70i. Dillmann et al.[24,25] first demonstrated HSP 71 m-RNA in tissue taken from ischemic (nonreperfused) canine myocardium, whilst White and White[26] found competent translation of HSP 70i in a different model of myocardial infarction. More recently Knowlton et al.[27] showed an induction of HSP 70i within rabbit myocardium following brief 5-min periods of ischemia with reperfusion, a finding confirmed by other investigators.[28] In addition, individual components of ischemia such as hypoxia or anoxia are capable of inducing HSP 70i.[29,30]

These observations suggest that pretreatments that increase myocardial HSP 70i content prior to ischemia may limit myocardial necrosis.

Whole Body Heat Stress and the Heart

A number of investigators have examined the responses of rabbit and rat myocardium to different stresses after whole body heat stress.

In experimental cardiology various models have been developed that allow the whole heart or portions of myocardium to be subjected to ischemia or components of ischemia. These models have different endpoints, and generally speaking findings cannot be extrapolated between one model or species and another. For the purpose of this review each model of ischemia is discussed separately.

The Isolated Retrogradely Perfused Heart and Global Ischemia

In this model the heart is retrogradely perfused with nutrients by cannulating the aorta above the coronary sinuses as described by Langendorff.[31] Ischemia is induced by either a reduction or cessation of aortic flow. On the return of normal aortic flow (reperfusion) contractile function, dysrhythmias and efflux of intracellular enzymes can be measured.[32]

Using this model Currie et al.[33] were the first to show that 24 hours after elevating the temperature of rats to 42°C for at least 15 min both cardiac HSP 70i and catalase activity were increased, whilst at this timepoint hearts became resistant to ischemia/reperfusion injury. Protection was measured in terms of increased postischemic contractile recovery with a dramatic reduction in postischemic creatine kinase efflux in heat stress compared to control hearts. These findings have been confirmed by Yellon's group and others in both the rat[34,35] and the rabbit.[36] Moreover, these authors[36] have observed improvements in additional parameters of protection in the heat-stressed rabbit heart postischemia. These include preservation of high energy phosphates, a reduction in oxidative stress during reperfusion (as measured by lower levels of oxidized glutathione) and significant preservation of mitochondrial function following ischemia.[36] There does, however, appear to be some species variation in the metabolic changes associated with protection following heat stress. In the rabbit, for example, elevated levels of high energy phosphates mirror the enhanced contractile activity of heat-stressed hearts during reperfusion.[36] In the rat, however, the enhanced contractile activity following ischemia in the heat-stressed groups is not associated with differences in high energy phosphate content between heat-stressed and control hearts.[35,37]

The protective effects of whole body heat stress have also been shown in the hypertrophied heart, which ordinarily has an increased susceptibility to ischemic injury. In the hypertrophied rat heart 24 hours after whole body heat stress preliminary evidence suggests that HSP 70i is induced, and ischemic dysrhythmias are diminished, whilst contractile function is enhanced.[38,39]

The pathophysiology underlying the genesis of dysrhythmias during ischemia or reperfusion differs from that underlying necrosis. For example, dysrhythmias occur with short episodes of ischemia not severe enough to cause necrosis, and dysrhythmias are attenuated by free-radical scavengers.[40,41] It is possible therefore that the mechanism(s) by which heat stress diminishes dysrhythmias differ from those by which it reduces infarction. After whole body heat stress, Mocanu et al. have shown[42] that late PBN adducts are reduced upon reperfusion of the isolated retrogradely perfused rat heart. This finding is in keeping with the observations above[36] and suggests that heat stress, like exogenous free-radical scavengers, may attenuate dysrhythmias by limiting the exposure of the myocardium to free-radicals.

The Isolated Retrogradely Perfused Heart and Regional Ischemia

The studies summarized to this point have demonstrated protection expressed in terms of myocardial contractility and metabolic state. Of perhaps more clinical relevance is the effect of whole body heat stress and HSP 70i induction on the amount of necrosis within the ischemic zone. When a volume of myocardial tissue is rendered ischemic (the risk zone) myocardial necrosis will occur after a certain duration of ischemia. As the ischemic time increases a larger and larger portion of the risk zone will necrose.[43] Most investigators therefore express the amount of necrosis/infarction for a given duration of ischemia as volume of necrosis divided by volume at risk.

Walker et al.[44] have examined infarct size after 45 minutes of regional ischemia in the buffer and blood perfused rabbit heart removed 24 hours after whole body heat stress. The purpose of this study was to investigate the reason for our negative findings with respect to infarct size reduction in vivo after myocardial HSP 70i induction by whole body heat stress[45] (see below). The design of this experiment allowed isolated rabbit hearts to be perfused either with buffer or with the blood from a support rabbit.[44] Infarct size was reduced by approximately 15% of the risk volume in heat-stressed hearts perfused with either buffer, or blood from a control support rabbit. However, when the support rabbit had been heat stressed this protection was lost. Our conclusions were that in certain circumstances "blood-borne factors" may interfere with the protection that follows heat stress[44] (see below for further discussion).

Similar protection against infarction was reported in a preliminary study. In the rat, infarct size was reduced following 37.5 minutes of ischemia, with protection being temporally related to elevated HSP 70i levels 24–96 hours after whole body heat stress.[46]

Alternative endpoints in this model are ischemia and reperfusion induced dysrhythmias. Steare and Yellon[47] have shown that 24 hours after whole body heat stress the isolated rat heart is resistant to dysrhythmias triggered by coronary ligation and reperfusion. In addition, in keeping with the findings of Currie's group,[33,48] Steare and Yellon[47] have also found that HSP 70i and catalase were induced by heat stress. The mechanism of protection in this model may be related to the reduction in free-radical generation after reperfusion of heat-stressed hearts.[42]

In Vitro Models of Simulated Ischemia

Ischemia consists of substrate deprivation and metabolite accumulation. Certain aspects of this complicated process can be simulated in vitro.

Papillary muscles can survive in an organ bath by simple diffusion of substrates and metabolites down their respective concentration gradients.[49] In this model some aspects of ischemia can be mimicked by removal of substrates; however, the large extracellular space prevents the accumulation of metabolites. When right ventricular papillary muscles were harvested from rabbits 24 hours after heat stress baseline contractile parameters were not altered.[50] However, when these muscles were subjected to a period of hypoxic superfusion without substrate injury occurred, but the amount of injury was less in muscles harvested from heat-stressed hearts. Moreover the degree of resistance to simulated ischemia was related to the HSP 70i content of "sister" papillary muscles from the same heart[50] (FIGS. 1, 2). Similar techniques have been used to subject cells in culture to simulated ischemia.

Mestril et al.[51] have transfected a myocyte-derived cell line (H9c2) with the human HSP 70i gene driven by the thymidine kinase promoter and obtained stable overexpression of HSP 70i. Cells overexpressing HSP 70i were more resistant to

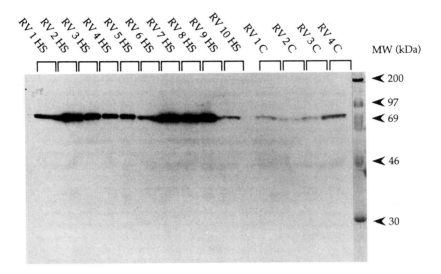

FIGURE 1. Western blot analysis of right ventricular papillary muscles probed with a monoclonal antibody directed against the inducible member of the 70 kDa stress protein family HSP 70i. The samples on the *left-hand side* of the blot (RV 1 HS to RV 10 HS) are of papillary muscles harvested from rabbit hearts 24 hours after whole body heat stress. The samples on the *right-hand side* of the blot (RV 1 C to RV 4 C) are of papillary muscles harvested from control hearts. (From Marber et al.[50] Reprinted by permission from the *Journal of Clinical Investigation.*)

simulated ischemia than either cells transfected with a gene coding for neomycin resistance or wild type cells. Ischemia was simulated by exposing H9c2 cells in a limited extracellular volume to an atmosphere without oxygen, thus allowing metabolite accumulation. Similarly, a muscle cell line transiently transfected so as to overexpress HSP 70i was resistant to metabolic inhibition and substrate deprivation designed to simulate ischemia with reperfusion.[52]

The In Situ Heart and Infarct Size

In this model a coronary artery is ligated to render a volume of myocardium ischemic and infarct size determined (see above).

Interestingly, in contrast to the *in vitro* studies above controversy surrounds the ability of whole body heat stress and HSP 70i induction to reduce infarct size *in vivo*. In the rabbit, we found that heat stress 24 hours prior to ischemia was unable to reduce infarct size following a 45-minute coronary occlusion[45] although protection was found in an identical model following a 30-minute occlusion by both Currie et al.[53] and ourselves.[28] A similar dependence of protection on the duration of coronary occlusion is seen in the rat. Donnelly and co-workers[54] have demonstrated a reduction in infarct size in the rat following a 35-minute, but not a 45-minute, coronary occlusion performed 24 hours after whole body heat stress. Moreover, in this model the reduction in infarct size, following a graded heat stress procedure, is related to the degree of stress protein induction.[55] The apparent

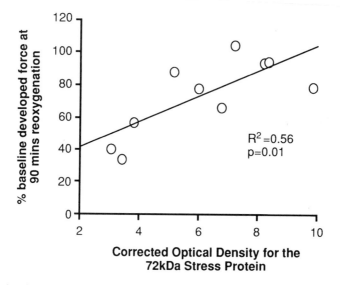

FIGURE 2. The relationship between papillary muscle HSP 70i content and posthypoxic contractile performance of the neighboring papillary muscles from the heat stress. Papillary muscle HSP 70i (72 kDa) content was measured by optical densitometry of samples RV 1 HS to RV 10 HS using the actin band of an identically loaded Coomasie stained gel to correct for differences in loading between samples. Papillary muscle developed force was measured 90 minutes after a 30-minute period of superfusion without metabolic substrates. The relationship between corrected optical density and papillary muscle contractile activity at 90 minutes of reoxygenation was determined using the Spearman rank correlation method. (From Marber *et al.*[50] Reprinted by permission from the *Journal of Clinical Investigation*.)

dependency of protection on the length of ischemic insult is difficult to explain. One possibility is that the protection conferred by heat stress is only moderate, and that as the severity of the ischemic insult increases the protection becomes less evident. A similar phenomenon occurs with ischemic preconditioning in dogs where a marked reduction in infarct size occurs with 60 minutes of coronary occlusion, but not with 90 minutes.[56] Another apparent anomaly is the fact that although infarct size in the rabbit is reduced after a 30-minute coronary occlusion performed 24 hours after whole body heat stress, no protection is seen at 40 hours after heat stress at a time when cardiac stress protein content is still increased.[53]

Other investigators have been able to demonstrate similar *in vivo* protection following hot blood cardioplegia of the pig heart.[57]

The cause for the discrepancy between *in vivo* and *in vitro* studies and between *in vivo* studies performed at different time intervals after heat stress is not clear. However, observations from our laboratory suggest that whole body heat stress may activate a blood-borne component that overrides the beneficial effect of cardiac stress protein induction (see above). It may be that whole body heat stress, although conferring myocardial protection, causes confounding physiological changes which have negative effects on infarct size. This is consistent with the finding that cytotoxic T cells directed against myocardial heat shock proteins are induced in rats by stresses that elevate myocardial HSP 70i content,[58] and that these cells are cytotoxic *in vitro* to heat-stressed myocytes from the same species.

In conclusion, there is no satisfactory explanation for the observations that the duration of recovery after heat stress and the length of the ischemic insult influence cardioprotection.

Heat Stress Proteins and Classical Ischemic Preconditioning

Acquired thermotolerance, where sublethal hyperthermia protects against subsequent lethal hyperthermia is similar in concept to ischemic preconditioning, with sublethal ischemia protecting against subsequent lethal ischemia.[59] One could speculate that stress proteins synthesized in response to the first brief episode of preconditioning ischemia protect the heart from subsequent ischemic injury.

In agreement with this idea Knowlton *et al.*[27] demonstrated that brief bursts

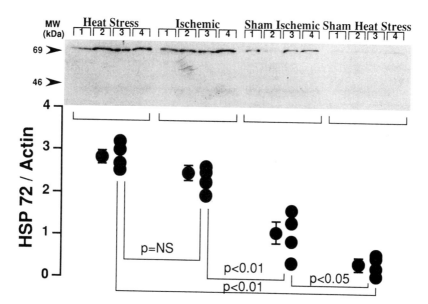

FIGURE 3. Densitometric assessment of Western blot loaded with 4 rabbit myocardial specimens from each group and probed against HSP 70i. Heat stress = whole body heat stress 24 hours before removing hearts. Ischemic = 4,5-min coronary ligations 24 hours before exising myocardial risk volume. Sham Ischemic and Sham Heat Stress are the corresponding control groups. The graded induction of HSP 70i (72 kDa) between groups seen after immunoblotting (*upper portion* of figure) becomes more obvious after densitometric assessment (*lower portion* of figure). On the basis of optical density ratios, heat stress and ischemic pretreatment resulted in a similar level of HSP 70i induction (2.8 ± 0.3 units v 2.5 ± 0.2 units, respectively). However, sham ischemia caused a greater induction than sham heat stress (1.0 ± 0.3 units v 0.3 ± 0.1 units, respectively). All comparisons were by ANOVA with a post-hoc Fischer's protected least significance difference test. (From Marber *et al.*[50] Reprinted by permission from *Circulation*.)

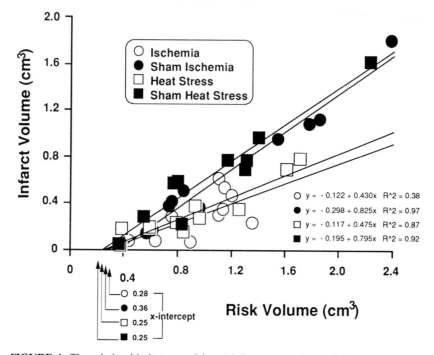

FIGURE 4. The relationship between risk and infarct zone volumes following 30 minutes of regional ischemia in each of the intervention groups of FIGURE 3. Risk zones were demarcated by the absence of fluorescent microspheres and infarct zones by absence of staining with triphenyltetrazolium. Both ischemic and heat stress pretreatments were associated with a significant reduction in the slope of the relationship between risk and infarct volume by ANCOVA. When these values are expressed in terms of infarct volume as a percentage of risk volume (I/R%) ischemia group = 28.8 ± 5.2 %, sham ischemia = 52.0 ± 5.2%, heat stress 32.8 ± 3.8%, sham heat stress 56.9 ± 6.5%. (From Marber *et al.*[50] Reprinted by permission from *Circulation*.)

of ischemia, such as those used in preconditioning protocols, can induce HSP 70i mRNA and protein accumulation. The mechanism by which stress proteins are induced by short episodes of ischemia may be secondary to the free-radical stress induced by reperfusion, since in the isolated rat heart stress protein induction following a 15-min infusion of xanthine plus xanthine oxidase is quantitatively similar to that induced by ischemia with reperfusion.[60] However, in both the study by Knowlton *et al.*[27] and work from our laboratory,[28] elevated levels of the HSP 70i protein were only manifest 2–24 hours after the ischemic insult (FIG. 3). In contrast the protective effect of preconditioning is lost approximately 1 hour after the initial brief ischemic episode.[62]

The involvement of stress protein in ischemic preconditioning has been further questioned by a study[63] which indicates that the protective effect of preconditioning can be observed under conditions where *de novo* protein synthesis has been almost entirely inhibited. Thus, it is unlikely that stress proteins are involved in classical ischemic preconditioning. However, the changes in mRNA coding for stress proteins indicate an adaptive response to ischemia which may predict a delayed protection dependent on stress protein synthesis.

The Second Window of Protection

Sublethal Ischemia and Delayed Protection against Infarction

The fact that stress protein induction by ischemia is not temporally related to classical ischemic preconditioning has prompted some investigators to examine whether the preconditioning ischemia is associated with a delayed, as well as an early phase of myocardial protection.[28,64]

We followed this line of reasoning and designed an experiment that examined myocardial HSP 70i and HSP 60 content following sublethal thermal and ischemic injuries. We adopted the protocol used by Knowlton[27] and subjected the *in vivo* rabbit myocardium to 4, 5-minute periods of regional ischemia separated by 10 minutes of reperfusion. After 24 hours this ischemic pretreatment increased myocardial HSP 70i content approximately 2–3-fold (FIG. 3). The HSP 70i accumulation was quantatively similar to that seen 24 hours after whole body heat stress in the rabbit, whilst induction of HSP 60 was greater with sublethal ischemia than with sublethal heat stress (FIG. 3).[28] We had shown previously in the rabbit that whole body heat stress resulted in myocardial protection. The question therefore was whether sublethal ischemia resulted in a similar response. Twenty-four hours after both sublethal ischemia and whole body heat stress, the volume of infarction expressed as a percentage of the volume at risk of infarction was reduced to approximately 50% of that seen in respective controls (FIG. 4). Since the protocol used to trigger the protection was identical to those known to trigger classical, short lived, preconditioning we termed the protection we saw the second window of protection or SWOP.[28,74]

Protective effects following sublethal ischemia were also seen in another study with a different underlying hypothesis. Hori and colleagues[64] had noted that 24 hours after 4, 5-minute coronary artery occlusions the activity of the mitochondrial form of superoxide dismutase was increased within the dog myocardium. This group hypothesized that a change in the activity of this enzyme within an organelle that is both a target and a source of superoxide anion generation during ischemia and reperfusion may result in protection. This hypothesis was confirmed in the dog utilizing a protocol virtually identical to that described above. The reduction in infarction 24 hours after sublethal ischemia was also approximately 50%.[64]

FIGURE 5. Cell injury in stably transfected H9c2 cell lines after simulated ischemia. Colony survival assay of H9c2 cells and stably transfected cell lines H9/NEO (neomycin expression vector only containing cell line) and H9/hHSP 70/1 (human HSP 70 overexpressing cell line) after simulated ischemia. Cells were replated and cultured for 7–9 days. The number of surviving colonies was normalized to untreated H9c2 cells. Results are from 6 independent experiments (*$p < 0.05$). (From Mestril *et al.*[93] Reprinted by permission from the *Journal of Clinical Investigation*.)

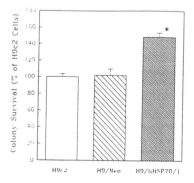

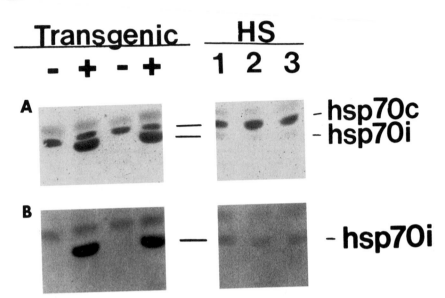

FIGURE 6. Western blot analysis of HSP 70i in hearts from mice with and without an HSP 70i transgene. Western blot of samples prepared from hearts harvested from transgene gene positive, transgene negative and mice after whole body heat stress. The samples are probed with a polyclonal (panel A) and a monoclonal (panel B) antibody recognizing HSP 70. In both panels, lanes from left to right, − denotes transgene negative, + denotes transgene positive and 1, 2 and 3 are samples from transgene negative mice harvested 8 to 24 hours after heat shock. *Panel A.* The primary polyclonal antibody recognizes constitutive (HSP 70c) and inducible (HSP 70i) forms of the 70-kDa heat shock protein. Hsp70c runs above HSP 70i. A strong HSP 70i signal is seen in the hearts of transgene positive mice and no signal is seen in transgene negative litter mates. The signal is present, but weak, in hearts harvested from transgene negative mice after heat stress (HS). *Panel B.* The primary monoclonal antibody recognizes only the HSP 70i band, the upper band is a nonspecific signal. The immunoreactive staining confirms that the pattern seen with the polyclonal antibody is indeed due to HSP 70i rather than a degradation product of HSP 70c. (From Marber *et al.*[96] Reprinted by permission from the *Journal of Clinical Investigation.*)

In conjunction with Cohen and Downey's group, we have also undertaken a study of delayed protection in a novel conscious animal model of coronary occlusion.[65] In rabbits pretreated with 4, 5-minute cycles of ischemia we observed a significant reduction of infarction after 24 hours. Interestingly, the incidence of ventricular fibrillation (VF) during a 30-min coronary occlusion was also reduced in preconditioned rabbits compared with controls, a reduction that we had not previously noted in our anesthetized rabbit model.[28,66] The attenuation of lethal arrhythmias during the second window of protection is consistent with the antiarrhythmic effects reported by Vegh *et al.*[67] (see below).

Studies Related to the Second Window of Protection

A number of investigators have described delayed myocardial protection following interventions which with hindsight may have induced myocardial ischemia.

For example Vegh and colleagues[67] demonstrated an intra- and postischemic antiarrythmic effect 24 hours after rapid pacing *in vivo* in the dog. Similarly Banerjee and colleagues[68] were able to show that postischemic contractility was enhanced in the rat 24 hours after parenteral nonadrenaline. In addition noradrenaline pretreatment resulted in an increased myocardial HSP 70i content at 24 hours.[68]

More recently the second window of protection was also documented in concious swine with postischemic myocardial contractility rather than infarct size as the endpoint.[69] Bolli and colleagues[69] were able to demonstrate in conscious pigs that 10 2-minute coronary occlusions increased myocardial HSP 70i content and nuclear localization within the risk zone. The increase in HSP 70i was associated with resistance to myocardial stunning 48 and 72 hours after repetitive ischemia. Myocardial antioxidant status was not measured.

Signalling in the Second Window of Protection

There is a wealth of evidence implicating adenosine receptors in classical ischemic preconditioning. The scheme proposed by Downey[70] is that adenosine formed as a consequence of ATP breakdown during the first brief period of ischemia, acts locally on a subclass of adenosine receptors (A_1 or A_3). Thus, the ischemic trigger can be replaced by briefly exposing the heart to either adenosine or a number of its analogues both *in vitro* and *in vivo*,[71,72] whilst preconditioning is abolished if an adenosine antagonist is present during the first brief period of ischemia.[71,72] The adenosine receptors are coupled to various effectors and second messenger systems, and it is as a consequence of the activation of these pathways that tolerance to ischemia is enhanced.

Our initial investigation of the signalling pathway(s) that might be involved in the development of the delayed protection following ischemic preconditioning examined the possibility that adenosine receptor activation was also a trigger for the second window in the rabbit.[66] We showed that the delayed protection was abolished if 8-(p-sulphophenyl)theophylline (8-SPT), an adenosine A_1 and A_2 receptor antagonist, was given during the preconditioning protocol. In addition substituting a selective adenosine A_1 agonist, 2-chlorocyclopentyladenosine (CCPA), for preconditioning we found a significant reduction in infarct size at 24 hours.[66]

Moreover we have shown that classical preconditioning and the second window of protection have other signalling pathways in common, since PKC activation

FIGURE 7. Myocardial, infarct and risk volume and normalized infarct size after 20 minutes of global ischemia in hearts from mice with and without an HSP 70i transgene. Hearts were reperfused for 30 or 120 minutes. Transgene negative, n = 12; transgene positive, n = 15. *Bars* represent one standard error of the mean. *$p \leq 0.05$, **$p \leq 0.01$. (From Marber *et al.*[96] Reprinted by permission from the *Journal of Clinical Investigation*.)

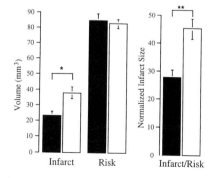

seems essential to both.[73] The current hypothesis therefore is that in classical preconditioning PKC activation results in the phosphorylation of a target that is either directly or indirectly protective. Whilst in the second window of protection preconditioning PKC activation orchestrates a change in gene expression that is ultimately responsible for delayed protection.[74]

Clinical Implication of the Second Window of Protection

It is perhaps not surprising that the intense research activity surrounding experimental preconditioning has kindled the interest of clinicians. Studies designed to subject the human heart to controlled sublethal ischemia suggest that short-term adaptation exists.[75] Unfortunately a major limitation of these prospective intervention studies is the need to use a surrogate endpoint that does not involve irreversible myocardial injury.

More recently a number of investigators began to examine the influence that spontaneous preinfarction angina may have on spontaneous subsequent infarction.[76–79] The rationale for this approach is that in the human the sensation of angina is thought to be secondary to the accumulation of sufficient interstitial adenosine to activate A_1 receptors on cardiac nerve endings.[80] Therefore, angina is also likely to be an indication of myocyte A_1 receptor activation. Hence angina may be followed both by classical preconditioning and the second window of protection. Is there any evidence that this is the case?

Studies in the prethrombolysis era did not consistently show that preinfarction angina had a favorable influence upon postinfarction mortality and left ventricular function.[81,82] There were numerous difficulties with these studies including the absence of thrombolytic reperfusion and adequate control for differences that exist between patients with and without preinfarction angina. In recent studies these difficulties were overcome with a detailed clinical history and coronary angiography in the acute phase of infarction.[76–79] In these studies preinfarction angina was associated with a limitation of infarct size and an improvement of in-hospital outcome. Patients recruited for 2 of these studies had episodes of angina within 48[76] or 24[77] hours of the index acute myocardial infarct. In patients with angina within 24 hours, the mean time interval between the last episode of angina and the onset of infarction was 11.2 hours.[77] It is likely that this time interval was even greater in the study recruiting patients with angina within 48 hours of infarction. Since the benefits of classical preconditioning in animals and probably humans lasts only for 60 minutes, it is likely that the advantages seen in these studies[76,77] correspond not to the classical preconditioning phenomenon but rather to the second window of protection.[83]

Negative Studies

Although there are a number of studies supporting the concept of a second window of protection there are others that do not. For example, Donnelly et al.[54] compared the protective benefit of heat stress with 24 hours of recovery to 20 minutes of ischemia with 8 hours of reperfusion. Following a subsequent 35-minute occlusion in the rat, heat stress pretreatment reduced infarct size, whilst ischemic pretreatment did not. However, as heat stress resulted in a more marked HSP 70i accumulation, the authors concluded[54] that ischemic pretreatment failed to protect because of insufficient stress protein accumulation.

Tanaka and colleagues[84] using a rabbit model similar but by no means identical to that described by ourselves[28] have failed to show a reduction of infarction 24 hours after 4 5-minute coronary artery occlusions. These investigators demonstrated HSP 70 accumulation qualitatively by immunohistochemistry but not quantitatively by Western blotting or ELISA. In view of the findings reported by Donnelly[54] the amount of HSP 70 accumulation is clearly critical to the protection and a lesser accumulation, as may have occurred in the Tanaka study,[84] may not be protective.

Mechanisms of Cardiac Protection

Thermal and Ischemic Conditioning

All studies using heat to elevate HSP 70i result in a large number of physiological perturbations which may in themselves have cardioprotective properties. For example, Currie's group[37,48] have shown that heat stress also increases the endogenous levels of the antioxidant enzyme catalase, whilst Hori and colleagues have demonstrated sublethal ischemia also induces superoxide dismutase.[64] The picture is further complicated by the findings of Currie's group which suggest that inactivating catalase with 3-AT (3-aminotriazole) results in an abolition of the protective effect normally observed at 24 and 48 hours after heat stress.[48,85] In agreement with such a mechanism, we have observed a reduction in the levels of oxidized glutathione in the coronary effluent following ischemia/reperfusion in heat-stressed rabbit hearts[36] and a reduction in PBN adducts during reperfusion of heat-stressed rat hearts.[42] These observations[36,42] have two possible explanations, the first is that antioxidant defences are increased following heat stress, so that free-radical scavenging is enhanced whilst free-radical production is unchanged; the second is that the changes occurring during ischemia are reduced following heat stress, so that there is less mitochondrial uncoupling and catecholamine accumulation, and hence less free-radical production.

The relative contributions of catalase, superoxide dismutase and HSP 70i to the myocardial protection that follows whole body heat stress and sublethal ischemia are uncertain. Although the evidence from Currie's group suggests that inhibiting catalase with 3-AT abolishes protection[48,85,86] the picture is complicated. For example Steare et al.[47] found that although 3-AT inhibits catalase it paradoxically reduces (rather than potentiates) reperfusion dysrhythmias in heat-stressed hearts. Similarly, Mocanu et al.[42] have shown that 3-AT reduces, rather than increases free-radical production in reperfused isolated rat hearts. In the same species other investigators using 3-AT have failed to abolish the enhanced postischemic contractile function seen in heat-stressed hearts. Further studies are required to more precisely delineate the role of the increases in catalase and superoxide dismutase seen following heat stress and sublethal ischemia.

Other evidence suggests that stress proteins may be able to limit myocardial damage independent of an antioxidant effect. Two reports suggest that the injury occurring during the calcium paradox can be influenced by procedures that cause stress protein synthesis.[87,88] The precise mode by which the calcium paradox damages the heart is a matter of controversy, but free-radical production is probably not involved[89] suggesting the protection does not depend upon increases in myocardial antioxidants. It is thought that during the period of low calcium exposure changes occur in the structural proteins of the myocyte so as to increase fragility, and, on calcium repletion, the return of contractile activity causes myocyte mechanical disruption.[90] A similar process involving cytoskeletal disruption may also occur during ischemia.[91] Heat stress proteins are known to alter the physical properties of actin and desmin,[90] and this interaction may prevent cytoskeletal disruption[92] and reduce calcium overload injury.

Recently more direct evidence became available that conclusively demonstrates that manipulating HSP 70i content can alter myocardial resistance to ischemia.

HSP 70i Transgenic Studies

The studies described above provide circumstantial evidence linking myocardial stress proteins to enhanced ischemic resistance. The drawback being that when a physiological stress is used to induce myocardial stress proteins, other alterations occur within the myocardium that make it difficult to ascribe any protection to changes within stress protein content. Therefore, conclusive proof that stress proteins are protective within the myocardium requires an intervention that specifically increases stress protein content without causing other alterations.

In vitro standard DNA transfection techniques have been used to generate stable cell lines that overexpress HSP 70i. These cell lines are then subjected to simulated ischemia. Studies of this type in an embryonic heart-derived and skeletal muscle-derived cell line suggest that HSP 70i is cytoprotective[94,95] (FIG. 5). The disadvantage of studies of this type is the need to use dividing cells which clearly must differ appreciably from terminally differentiated cardiac myocytes.

More recently transgenic mouse lines have been constructed where HSP 70i is expressed constitutively within the myocardium[96-98] (FIG. 6). In a study that we performed in collaboration with Dillmann and Mestril, we were able to conclusively demonstrate that hearts harvested from mice heterozygote for a rat HSP 70i transgene were more resistant to ischemia than hearts harvested from transgene negative litter mates.[96] The enhanced resistance to ischemia was manifest both as enhanced postischemic contractility and a decrease in infarct size[96] (FIG. 7). Moreover in transgene positive hearts HSP 70i levels were markedly elevated without any change in catalase activity.[96]

These studies[96-98] provide the most direct evidence currently available that HSP 70i is at least partially responsible for the protection that follows whole body heat stress and sublethal ischemia.

CONCLUSIONS

The weight of evidence presented suggests that HSP 70i increases the resistance of the heart to ischemia and may offer an endogenous route to myocardial protection. Such a route represents an obvious pathway for therapeutic intervention. It is hoped that by such methods it may eventually be possible to benefit the patient by exploiting the protective mechanisms that may already exist within their own heart.

REFERENCES

1. OPCS, Office of Population Census and Surveys. 1991. Mortality Statistics: Cause. Series DH2, no. 17. HMSO. London.

2. McMurray, J. & A. Rankin. 1994. Treatment of myocardial infarction, unstable angina, and angina pectoris. Br. Med. J. **309:** 1343–1350.
3. Marber, M. S. 1994. Stress proteins and myocardial protection. Clin. Sci. **86:** 375–381.
4. Allen, D. G. & C. H. Orchard. 1987. Myocardial contractile function during ischemia and hypoxia. Circ. Res. **60:** 153–168.
5. Pauly, D. F., K. A. Kirk & J. B. McMillin. 1991. Carnitine palmitoyltransferase in cardiac ischemia. A potential site for altered fatty acid metabolism. Cir. Res. **68:** 1085–1094.
6. Ganote, C. & S. Armstrong. 1993. Ischaemia and the myocyte cytoskeleton: review and speculation. Cardiovasc. Res. **27:** 1387–1403.
7. Yellon, D. M. & M. S. Marber. 1994. Hsp70 in myocardial ischaemia. Experientia: **50:** 1075–1084.
8. Weich, H., J. Buchner, R. Zimmermann & U. Jakob. 1992. Hsp90 chaperones protein folding *in vitro*. Nature **358:** 169–170.
9. Currie, R. W., M. Karmazyn, M. Kloe & K. Mailer. 1988. Heat shock response is associated with enhanced postischaemic ventricular recovery. Circ. Res. **63:** 543–549.
10. Marber, M. S., D. S. Latchman, J. M. Walker & D. M. Yellon. 1993. Cardiac stress protein elevation 24 hours after brief ischemia or heat stress is associated with resistance to myocardial infarction. Circulation **88:** 1264–1274.
11. Minowada, G. & W. J. Welch. 1995. Clinical implications of the stress response. J. Clin. Invest. **95:** 3–12.
12. Gerner, E. W. & M. J. Scheider. 1975. Induced thermal resistance in HeLa cells. Nature **256:** 500–502.
13. Currie, R. W., B. M. Ross & T. A. Davis. 1990. Induction of the heat shock response in rats modulates heart rate, creatine kinase and protein synthesis after a subsequent hyperthermic treatment. Cardiovasc. Res. **24:** 87–93.
14. Johnston, R. N. & B. L. Kucey. 1988. Competitive inhibition of HSP 70 gene expression causes thermosensitivity. Science **242:** 1551–1554.
15. Li, G. C., L. Li, Y. Liu, J. Y. Mak, L. Chen & W. M. F. Lee. 1991. Thermal response of rat fibroblasts stably transfected with the human 70 kDa heat shock protein-encoding gene. Proc. Natl. Acad. Sci. USA **88:** 1681–1685.
16. Riabowol, K. T., L. A. Mizzen & W. J. Welch. 1988. Heat shock is lethal to fibroblasts microinjected with antibodies against HSP 70. Science **242:** 433–436.
17. Li, G. C. & G. M. Hahn. 1978. Ethanol-induced tolerance to heat and adriamycin. Nature **274:** 669–701.
18. Barbe, M. F., M. Tytell, D. J. Gower & W. J. Welch. 1988. Hyperthermia protects against light damage in the rat retina. Science **241:** 1817–1820.
19. Polla, B. S., N. Mili & S. Kantengwa. 1991. Heat shock and oxidative injury in human cells. *In* Heat Shock. B. Maresca & S. Lindquist, Eds. 279–290. Springer-Verlag. Berlin.
20. Ciocca, D. R., A. W. Fuqua, S. Lock-Lim, D. O. Toft, W. J. Welch & W. L. McGuire. 1992. Response of human breast cancer cells to heat shock and chemotherapeutic drugs. Cancer Res. **53:** 3648–3654.
21. Lowenstein, D. H., P. H. Chan & M. F. Miles. 1991. The stress protein response in cultured neurones: characterization and evidence for a protective role in excitotoxicity. Neuron **7:** 1053–1060.
22. Rordorf, G., W. J. Koroshetz & J. V. Bonventre. 1991. Heat shock protects cultured neurons from glutamate toxicity. Neuron **7:** 1043–1051.
23. Hotchkiss, R., I. Nunnally, S. Lindquist, J. Taulien, G Perdrizet & I. Karl. 1993. Hyperthermia protects mice against the lethal effects of endotoxin. Am. J. Physiol. **265:** R1447–R1457.
24. Dillmann, W. H., H. B. Mehta, A. Barrieux, B. D. Guth, W. E. Neeley & J. Ross. 1986. Ischemia of the dog heart induces the appearance of a cardiac mRNA coding for a protein with migration characteristics similar to heat-shock/stress protein 71. Circ. Res. **59:** 110–114.

25. MEHTA, H. B., B. K. POPOVICH & W. H. DILLMAN. 1988. Ischemia induces changes in the level of mRNAs coding for stress protein 71 and creatine kinase M. Circ. Res. **63:** 512–517.
26. WHITE, F. P. & S. WHITE. 1986. Isoproterenol induced myocardial necrosis is associated with stress protein synthesis in rat heart and thoracic aorta. Cardiovasc. Res. **20:** 512–515.
27. KNOWLTON, A. A., P. BRECHER & C. S. APSTEIN. 1990. Rapid expression of heat shock protein in the rabbit after brief cardiac ischemia. J. Clin. Invest. **87:** 139–147.
28. MARBER, M. S., D. S. LATCHMAN, J. M. WALKER & D. M. YELLON. 1993. Cardiac stress protein elevation 24 hours after brief ischemia or heat stress is associated with resistance to myocardial infarction. Circulation **88:** 1264–1274.
29. HOWARD, G. & T. E. GEOGHEGAN. 1986. Altered cardiac tissue gene expression during acute hypoxic exposure. Mol. Cell. Biochem. **69:** 155–160.
30. TUIJL, M. J., P. M. VAN BERGEN EN HENEGOUWEN, R. VAN WIJK & A. J. VERKLEIJ. 1991. The isolated neonatal rat-cardiomyocyte used as an *in vitro* model for "ischemia." II. Induction of the 68 kDa heat shock protein. Biochim. Biophys. Acta **1091:** 278–284.
31. LANGENDORFF, O. 1995. Untersushungen am überlebenden Saugethierherzen. Pflugers Arch. **61:** 291–332.
32. OPIE, L. H. 1992. Cardiac metabolism emergence, decline and resurgence. Part I. Cardiovasc. Res. **26:** 721–733.
33. CURRIE, R. W., M. KARMAZYN, M. KLOC & K. MAILER. 1988. Heat shock response is associated with enhanced postischemic ventricular recovery. Circ. Res. **63:** 543–549.
34. AMRANI, M., N. J. ALLEN, J. O'SHEA, J. CORBETT, M. J. DUNN, S. TADJKARIMI, S. THEODOROPOULOS, J. PEPPER & M. H. YACOUB. 1993. Role of catalase and heat shock protein on recovery of cardiac endothelial and mechanical function after ischaemia. Cardioscience **4:** 193–198.
35. PASINI, E., A. CARGNONI, R. FERRARI, M. S. MARBER, D. S. LATCHMAN & D. M. YELLON. 1991. Heat stress and oxidative damage following ischemia and reperfusion in the isolated rat heart (abstract). Eur. Heart J. **12**(Suppl.): 306.
36. YELLON, D. M., E. PASINI, A. CARGNONI, M. S. MARBER, D. S. LATCHMAN & R. FERRARI. 1992. The protective role of heat stress in the ischemic and reperfused rabbit myocardium. J. Mol. Cell. Cardiol. **24:** 895–907.
37. CURRIE, R. W. & M. KARMAZYN. 1990. Improved post-ischemic ventricular recovery in the absence of changes in energy metabolism in working rat hearts following heat shock. J. Mol. Cell. Cardiol. **22:** 631–636.
38. CORNELUSSEN, R. N., L. H. SNOECKX, L. G. DE BRUIN, G. J. VAN DER VUSSE & R. S. RENEMAN. 1993. Hyperthermic preconditioning improves ischemia tolerance in the hypertrophied and non-hypertrophied rat heart (abstract). J. Mol. Cell. Cardiol. **25**(Suppl. I): S56.
39. SNOECKX, L. H., R. N. CORNELUSSEN, G. J. VAN DER VUSSE & R. S. RENEMAN. 1993. Post-ischemic electrical stability in the heat-shocked hypertrophied and non-hypertrophied rat heart (abstract). J. Mol. Cell. Cardiol. **25**(Suppl. I): S56.
40. OPIE, L. H. 1989. Reperfusion injury and its pharmacological modification. Circulation **80:** 1049–1062.
41. YELLON, D. M. & J. M. DOWNEY. 1990. Current research views on myocardial reperfusion and reperfusion injury. Cardioscience **1:** 89–98.
42. MOCANU, M. M., S. E. STEARE, M. C. EVANS, J. H. NUGENT & D. M. YELLON. 1993. Heat stress attenuates free radical release in isolated perfused rat heart. Free Radical. Biol. Med. **15:** 459–463.
43. REIMER, K. A. & R. B. JENNINGS. 1979. The "wavefront phenomenon" of myocardial ischemic cell death. II. Transmural progression of necrosis within the framework of ischemic bed size (myocardium at risk) and collateral flow. Lab. Invest. **40:** 633–644.
44. WALKER, D. M., E. PASINI, S. KUCUKOGLU, M. S. MARBER, E. ILIODROMITIS, R. FERRARI & D. M. YELLON. 1993. Heat stress limits infarct size in the isolated perfused rabbit heart. Cardiovasc. Res. **27:** 962–967.

45. YELLON, D. M., E. ILIODROMITIS, D. S. LATCHMAN, D. M. VAN WINKLE, J. M. DOWNEY, F. M. WILLIAMS & T. J. WILLIAMS. 1992. Whole body heat shock fails to limit infarct size in the reperfused rabbit heart. Cardiovasc. Res. **26:** 342–346.
46. LOESSER, K. E., A. K. VINNIKOVA, Y. Z. QIAN, M. L. HESS, R. L. JESSE & R. C. KUKREJA. 1992. Protection of ischemia/reperfusion injury by heat stress in rats (abstract). Circulation **86**(Suppl. I): I-557.
47. STEARE, S. E. & D. M. YELLON. 1993. The protective effect of heat stress against reperfusion arrhythmias in the rat. J. Mol. Cell. Cardiol. **25:** 1471–1481.
48. KARMAZYN, M., K. MAILER & R. W. CURRIE. 1991. Acquisition and decay of heat shock enhanced post-ischemic ventricular recovery. Am. J. Physiol. **259:** H424–H431.
49. PARADISE, N. F., J. L. SCHMITTER & J. M. SURMITIS. 1981. Criteria for adequate oxygenation of isometric kitten papillary muscle. Am. J. Physiol. **241:** H348–H353.
50. MARBER, M. S., J. M. WALKER, D. S. LATCHMAN & D. M. YELLON. 1994. Myocardial protection following whole body heat stress in the rabbit is dependent on metabolic substrate and is related to the amount of the inducible 70 kiloDalton heat stress protein. J. Clin. Invest. 93. In press.
51. MESTRIL, R., S-H. CHI, R. SAYEN, K. O'REILLY & W. H. DILLMANN. 1994. Expression of inducible stress protein 70 in rat heart myogenic cells confers protection against simulated ischaemia-induced injury. J. Clin. Invest. **93:** 759–767.
52. WILLIAMS, R. S., J. A. THOMAS, M. FINA, Z. GERMAN & I. J. BENJAMIN. 1993. Human heat shock protein 70 (HSP 70) protects murine mouse cells from injury during metabolic stress. J. Clin. Invest. **92:** 503–508.
53. CURRIE, R. W., R. M. TANGUAY & J. G. KINGMA. 1993. Heat-shock response and limitation of tissue necrosis during occlusion/reperfusion in rabbit hearts. Circulation **87:** 963–971.
54. DONNELLY, T. J., R. E. SIEVERS, F. L. J. VISSERN, W. J. WELCH & C. L. WOLFE. 1992. Heat shock protein induction in rat hearts. A role for improved myocardial salvage after ischemia and reperfusion? Circulation **85:** 796–778.
55. HUTTER, M. M., R. E. SIEVERS, V. BARBOSA & C. L. WOLFE. 1994. Heat-shock protein induction in rat hearts. A direct correlation between the amount of heat-shock protein induced and the degree of myocardial protection. Circulation **89:** 355–360.
56. NAO, B. S., T. B. MCCLANAHAN, M. A. GROH, R. J. SCHOTT & K. P. GALLAGHER. 1990. The time limit of effective ischemic preconditioning in dog (abstract). Circulation **82**(Suppl. III): 271.
57. LIU, X., R. M. ENGELMAN, I. I. MORARU, J. A. ROUSOU, J. E. FLACK, D. W. DEATON, N. MAULIK & D. K. DAS. 1992. Heat shock. A new approah for myocardial preservation in cardiac surgery. Circulation **86**(Suppl. II): II-358–II-363.
58. HUBER, S. A. 1992. Heat-shock protein induction in adriamycin and picornavirus-infected cardiocytes. Lab. Invest. **67:** 218–224.
59. MARBER, M. S., D. M. WALKER & D. M. YELLON. 1994. Ischaemic preconditioning. Br. Med. J. **308:** 1–2.
60. KUKREJA, R. C., M. C. KONTOS, K. E. LOESSER, S. K. BATRA, Y-Z. QUIAN, C. J. GBUR, S. A. NASEEM, R. L. JESSE & M. L. HESS. 1994. Oxidant stress increases heat shock protein 70 mRNA in isolated perfused rat heart. Am. J. Physiol. **36:** H2213–H2219.
61. KUCUKOGKU, S., E. ILIODROMITIS, D. VAN WINKLE, J. DOWNEY, M. MARBER, R. HEADS & D. M. YELLON. 1991. Protection by ischaemic preconditioning appears independent of stress protein synthesis (abstract). J. Mol. Cell. Cardiol. **23**(Suppl. V): S73.
62. VAN WINKLE, D. M., J. THORNTON & J. M. DOWNEY. 1991. Cardioprotection from ischaemic preconditioning is lost following prolonged reperfusion in the rabbit. Coron. Artery Dis. **2:** 613–619.
63. THORNTON, J. D., S. STRIPLIN, G. S. LIU, A. SWAFFORD, W. H. STANLEY, D. M. VAN WINKLE & J. M. DOWNEY. 1990. Inhibition of protein synthesis does not block myocardial protection afforded by preconditioning. Am. J. Physiol. **259:** H1822–H1825.

64. KUZUYA, T., S. HOSHIDA, N. YAMASHITA, H. FUIJI, H. OE, M. HORI, T. KAMADA
    & M. TADA. 1993. Delayed effects of sublethal ischemia on the acquisition of toler-
    ance to ischemia. Cir. Res. **72:** 1293–1299.
65. YANG, X-M., G. F. BAXTER, D. M. YELLON, J. R. FLETCHER, J. M. DOWNEY &
    M. V. COHEN. 1995. Second window of protection in conscious rabbits (abstract).
    J. Mol. Cell. Cardiol. Supplement in press.
66. BAXTER, G. F., M. S. MARBER, V. C. PATEL & D. M. YELLON. 1994. Adenosine
    receptor involvement in a delayed phase of myocardial protection 24 hours after
    ischemic preconditioning. Circulation **90:** 2993–3000.
67. VEGH, A., J. G. PAPP & J. R. PARRATT. 1994. Prevention by dexamethasone of the
    marked antiarrhythmic effects of preconditioning induced 20 hours after rapid cardiac
    pacing. Br. J. Pharmacol. **113:** 1081–1082.
68. MENG, X., J. M. BROWN, L. AO, M. B. MITCHELL, A. BANERJEE & A. H. HARKEN.
    1993. Norepinephrine induces late cardiac protection preceded by oncogene and
    heat shock protein overexpression (abstract). Circulation **88**(Suppl.): I-633.
69. SUN, J-Z., X-L. TANG, A. A. KNOWLTON, S-W. PARK, Y. QIU & R. BOLLI. 1995.
    Late preconditioning against myocardial stunning. An endogenous protective mecha-
    nism that confers resistance to postischemic dysfunction 24 h after brief ischemia
    in conscious pigs. J. Clin. Invest. **95:** 388–403.
70. COHEN, M. V. & J. M. DOWNEY. 1993. Ischaemic preconditioning: can the protection
    be bottled? The Lancet **341:** 6.
71. LIU, G. S., J. THORNTON, D. M. VAN WINKLE, A. W. H. STANLEY, R. A. OLSSON
    & J. M. DOWNEY. 1991. Protection against infarction afforded by precondition-
    ing is mediated by A1 adenosine receptors in rabbit heart. Circulation **84:** 350–356.
72. ARMSTRONG, S. & C. E. GANOTE. 1994. Adenosine receptor specificity in precondition-
    ing of isolated rabbit cardiomyocytes: evidence of A_3 receptor involvement. Cardio-
    vasc. Res. **28:** 1049–1056.
73. BAXTER, G. F., F. M. GOMA & D. M. YELLON. 1995. Involvement of protein kinase
    C in the delayed cytoprotection following sublethal ischaemia in rabbit myocardium.
    Br. J. Pharmacol. **115:** 222–224.
74. YELLON, D. M. & G. F. BAXTER. 1995. A "second window of protection" or delayed
    preconditioning phenomenon: future horizons for myocardial protection? J. Mol.
    Cell. Cardiol. **27:** 1023–1034.
75. DEUTSCH, E., M. BERGER, W. G. KUSSMAUL, J. W. HIRSHFELD, H. C. HERRMANN
    & W. K. LASKEY. 1990. Adaptation to ischemia during percutaneous transluminal
    coronary angioplasty: clinical hemodynamic and metabolic features. Circulation
    82: 2044–2051.
76. KLONER, R. A., T. SHOOK, K. PRYZKLENK, V. G. DAVIS, L. JUNIO, R. V. MATTHEWS,
    S. BURSTEIN, M. GIBSON, K. W. POOLE, C. P. CANNON, C. H. MCCABE & E.
    BRAUNWALD. 1995. Previous angina alters in-hospital outcome in TIMI-4. A clinical
    correlate to preconditioning? Circulation **91:** 37–47.
77. OTTANI, F., M. GALVANI, D. FERRINI, F. SORBELLO, P. LIMONETTI, D. PANTIOLI
    & F. RUSTICALI. 1995. Prodromal angina limits infarct size. A role for ischemic
    preconditioning. Circulation **91:** 291–297.
78. NAKAGAWA, Y., H. ITO, M. KITAKAZE, H. KUSUOKA, M. HORI, T. KUZUYA & Y.
    HIGAHINO. 1995. Effect of angina pectoris on myocardial protection in patients with
    reperfused anterior wall myocardial infarction: retrospective clinical evidence of
    "preconditioning." J. Am. Coll. Cardiol. **25:** 1076–1083.
79. ANZAI, T., T. YOSHIKAWA, Y. ASAKURA, A. SUMIHISA, T. MEGURO, M. AKAISHA,
    H. MITAMURA, S. HANDA & S. OGAWA. 1994. Effect on short-term prognosis and
    left ventricular function of angina pectoris prior to first Q-wave anterior wall acute
    myocardial infarction. Am. J. Cardiol. **74:** 755–759.
80. GASPARDONE, A., F. CREA, F. TOMAI, F. VERSACI, M. IAMELE, G. GIOFFRÈ, L.
    CHIARIELLO & P. A. GIOFFRÈ. 1995. Muscular and cardiac adenosine-induced pain
    is mediated by A_1 receptors. J. Am. Coll. Cardiol. 251–257.
81. BEHAR, S., H. REICHER-REISS & E. ALLMADER. 1992. The prognostic significance of
    angina pectoris preceding the occurrence of a first acute myocardial infarction in
    4166 consecutive hospitalized patients. Am. Heart. J. **123:** 1481–1486.

82. MULLER, D. W., E. J. TOPOL, R. M. CALIFF, K. N. SIGMON, L. GORMAN, B. S. GEORGE, D. J. KEREIAKES, K. L. LEE & S. G. ELLIS. 1990. Relationship between antecedent angina pectoris and short-term prognosis after thrombolytic therapy for acute myocardial infarction. Thrombolysis and angioplasty in myocardial infarction (TAMI) study group. Am. Heart J. **119:** 224–231.

83. MARBER, M. S., G. F. BAXTER & D. M. YELLON. 1995. Prodromal angina limits infarct size. A role for ischaemic preconditioning. Circulation **92:** 1061–1062.

84. TANAKA, M., H. FUJIWARA, K. YAMASAKI, M. MIYAMAE, R. YOKOTA, K. HASEGAWA, T. FUJIWARA & S. SASYAMA. 1994. Ischemic preconditioning elevates cardiac stress protein but does not limit infarct size 24 or 48 h later in rabbits. Am. J. Physiol. **267:** H1476–H1482.

85. CURRIE, R. W. 1987. Effects of ischemia and perfusion temperature on the synthesis of stress induced (heat shock) proteins in isolated and perfused rat hearts. J. Mol. Cell. Cardiol. **19:** 795–808.

86. KINGMA, J. G., R. W. CURRIE, D. SIMARD & R. J. ROULEAU. 1993. Contribution of catalase to hyperthermia-mediated protection in rabbits after ischaemia-reperfusion (abstract). Circulation **88:** I-568.

87. MARBER, M. S., J. M. WALKER & D. M. YELLON. 1993. Heat stress attenuates a sub-maximal calcium paradox. J. Mol. Cell. Cardiol. **25:** 1119–1126.

88. MEERSON, F. Z., I. U. MALYSHEV, Y. V. ARKHIPENKO & V. I. VOVK. 1991. Adaptive increase in the resistance of the heart to calcium paradox (abstract). J. Mol. Cell. Cardiol. **23**(Suppl. V): S162.

89. FERRARI, R., C. CECONI, S. CURELLO, A. CARGNONI & T. J. C. RUIGROK. 1989. No evidence of oxygen free radical-mediated damage during the calcium paradox. Basic Res. Cardiol. **84:** 396–403.

90. ALTSCHULD, R. A., C. E. GANOTE, W. G. NAYLER & H. M. PIPER. 1991. Editorial comment: What constitutes the calcium paradox? J. Mol. Cell. Cardiol. **23:** 765–776.

91. STEENBERG, C., M. L. HILL & R. B. JENNINGS. 1987. Cytoskeletal damage during myocardial ischemia: changes in vinculin immunofluorescence staining during total *in vitro* ischemia in canine heart. Circ. Res. **60:** 478–486.

92. BENNARDINI, F., A. WRZOSEK & M. CHIESI. 1992. Alpha B-crystallin in cardiac tissue. Association with actin and desmin filaments. Circ. Res. **71:** 288–294.

93. MESTRIL, R, S-H. CHI, M. R. SAYEN, K. O'REILLY & W. H. DILLMANN. 1994. Expression of inducible stress protein 70 in rat heart myogenic cells confers protection against simulated ischemia-induced injury. J. Clin. Invest. **93:** 759–767.

94. WILLIAMS, R. S., J. A. THOMAS, M. FINA, Z. GERMAN & I. J. BENJAMIN. 1993. Human heat shock protein 70 (HSP 70) protects murine cells from injury during metabolic stress. J. Clin. Invest. **92:** 503–508.

95. HEADS, R. J., D. M. YELLON & D. S. LATCHMAN. 1995. Differential cytoprotection against heat stress or hypoxia following expression of specific stress protein genes in myogenic cells. J. Mol. Cell. Cardiol. **27:** 1669–1678.

96. MARBER, M. S., R. MESTRIL, S-H. CHI, M. R. SAYEN, D. M. YELLON & W. G. DILLMANN. 1995. Overexpression of the rat inducible 70 kiloDalton heat stress protein in a transgenic mouse increases the resistance of the heart to ischemic injury. J. Clin. Invest. **95:** 1446–1456.

97. RADFORD, N. B., M. FINA, I. J. BENJAMIN, R. W. MOREADITH, K. H. GRAVES, P. ZHAO, S. GAVVA, A. D. SHERRY, C. R. MALLOY & R. S. WILLIAMS. 1994. Enhanced functional and metabolic recovery following ischemia in intact hearts from HSP 70 transgenic mice (abstract). Circulation **90:** I-G.

98. PLUMIER, J. C. L., B. M. ROSS, R. W. CURRIE, C. E. ANGELIDIS, H. KAZLARIS, G. KOLLIAS & G. N. PAGOULATOS. 1995. Transgenic mice expressing the human heat shock protein 70 have improved post-ischemic myocardial recovery. J. Clin. Invest. **95:** 1854–1860.

Complete Stunning in Hypertrophied Guinea Pig Heart

Defects in Sarcolemmal Calcium Influx[a]

ARVINDER K. DHALLA, NEELAM KHAPER, AND
PAWAN K. SINGAL[b]

Division of Cardiovascular Sciences
St. Boniface General Hospital Research Centre
and
Department of Physiology
Faculty of Medicine
University of Manitoba
Winnipeg, Canada

INTRODUCTION

Myocardial stunning, one of the postischemic dysfunctions, has been defined as a prolonged but reversible depression in contractile function on reperfusion of a portion of the left ventricle subjected to brief periods of ischemia.[1] The important and essential aspect of this definition is that contractile function is eventually completely reversible with prolonged reperfusion. The phenomenon of myocardial stunning was first recognized in an animal model in the mid-seventies.[2] Subsequently, it was confirmed in various clinical settings where it was suspected to contribute to left ventricular dysfunction associated with ischemic heart disease.[1,3] Myocardial stunning has now been documented in many different animal models including dog,[4,5] rabbit,[6] pig,[7] ferret[8] and rat[9] hearts under various experimental conditions. It is to be noted that in these ischemia-reperfusion studies on myocardial segments or whole hearts, some contractile function was always noted upon reperfusion thus demonstrating so called "partial stunning."

Properties of many fundamental mechanisms are altered in a hypertrophied heart. Stable hyperfunctional hypertrophied hearts subsequent to pressure overload were found to be more resistant to a brief ischemic stress.[10] This increased resistance of the hypertrophied heart was attributed to increased endogenous activities of antioxidant enzymes.[10,11] However, in other studies ischemic injury has been shown to cause more abnormalities in hypertrophied hearts as compared to normal hearts.[12-14] Although systolic function, subsequent to low-flow ischemia was found to be comparable in the sham and hypertrophied rat hearts,[13] diastolic

[a] This study was supported by the Medical Research Council Group Grant in Experimental Cardiology (PKS). Dr. Dhalla was supported by a studentship from the Manitoba Health Research Council and is now a post-doctoral fellow of the Medical Research Council. Ms. Khaper was supported by a student fellowship from the University of Manitoba.

[b] Address for correspondence: Dr. Pawan K. Singal, R 3022, St. Boniface General Hospital, Research Centre, 351 Tache Ave., Winnipeg, Manitoba, Canada, R2H 2A6. Tel.: (204) 235-3416; Fax: (204) 233-6723.

function was found to be more sensitive to the ischemic insult. Furthermore, hypertrophied dog hearts with normal pump function were more tolerant to ischemia-reperfusion injury than hearts with mechanical pump failure.[15] Some of the discrepancies may have been due to the animal model and/or functional stage of hypertrophy.

The present study was undertaken to examine the ischemic tolerance of hyper-functional hypertrophied guinea pig hearts without any signs of failure. Data show for the first time that a brief period of ischemia followed by reperfusion results in "complete stunning" in the hypertrophied heart and this ischemic episode also unmasked a potential "sarcolemmal defect" in these hearts. It is suggested that reduced availability of Ca^{2+} through Ca^{2+} channels as well as Na^+-Ca^{2+} exchange across sarcolemma may play an important role in the observed phenomenon of complete stunning.

MATERIALS AND METHODS

Induction of Hypertrophy

Heart hypertrophy due to a chronic pressure overload was induced in male guinea pigs weighing 250 ± 25 g by narrowing the ascending aorta to a cross section area of about $3.6 \ mm^2$ as described previously.[16] Briefly, animals were anesthetized with methohexital sodium (35 mg/kg i.p.). The ascending aorta was dissected free and a loosely constricting band was placed around it just above the coronary ostia. Positive pressure ventilation was provided to the animals during the operation. The chest was closed after putting on the band and antibiotic powder (Cicatrin: Wellcome Burrows) was applied topically. Animals were given injections of bupernorphine (0.04 mg/kg i.m.) every 8–12 hours for 3 days. Sham-operated animals were treated in an identical manner except that no constriction around the aorta was placed. After the surgery, banded and sham-operated guinea pigs were randomized and later used in the study.

Hemodynamic Measurements

Animals were anesthetized with methohexital (35 mg/kg i.p.), and a miniature pressure transducer catheter (model PR 249, Millar Instruments, Houston, TX) was inserted through the right carotid artery and then advanced into the left ventricle. Heart rate, left ventricular systolic pressure (LVSP), left ventricular end-diastolic pressure (LVEDP), maximal rate of rise and fall of left ventricular pressure ($\pm$ dP/dt), and aortic pressures were recorded on a precalibrated multi-channel dynograph (Beckman Instruments, Fullerton, CA). Aortic pressures were measured proximal to the constriction. All hemodynamic measurements were taken 15 minutes after catheterization when a steady state was reached. After the hemodynamic measurements, hearts were excised and used for perfusion studies. Wall thickness of the left ventricle was measured in heart slices, midway between the apex and the base, with the ocular micrometer at four randomly selected diametric points.

Heart Perfusions

Hypertrophic and sham-operated animals were sacrificed 10 weeks after the surgery and their hearts were rapidly excised, weighed and placed in oxygenated buffer solution. The hearts were mounted on a steel cannula and perfused in a retrograde fashion through the coronary arteries at a constant flow rate of 8 ml/min in Langendorff mode. The flow rate was maintained by a peristaltic pump and was found to be adequate to sustain contractile function in sham as well as hypertrophied hearts for more than 1 hr. The perfusion buffer was a modified Krebs-Henseleit (KH) solution containing (mM) NaCl, 120; $NaHCO_3$, 25.4; KCl, 4.8; KH_2PO_4, 1.2; $MgSO_4$, 0.86; $CaCl_2$, 1.25 and glucose 11.0 (pH 7.4). The buffer solution was continuously gassed with a mixture of 95% O_2–5% CO_2. The temperature of the entire perfusion system was maintained at 37°C. The hearts were trimmed of all atrial material and electrically paced with bipolar platinum electrodes attached to the ventricular muscle. Supramaximal stimuli of 1.5 msec duration were delivered at the rate of 240 pulses/min. Myocardial contractile force was recorded by using a (FT03) force displacement transducer attached by a hook ligature to the apex of the heart. A resting tension of 2.0 gm was applied to all hearts to achieve an optimal baseline length-tension relationship. Hearts were made ischemic for 5 min by stopping the flow and reperfused for 20 min by starting the flow again. After each experiment hearts were analyzed for total myocardial Ca^{2+} and Na^+ content.

For studying the effects of different interventions, hypertrophied hearts were reperfused with buffer containing low Ca^{2+} (0.65 mM), high Ca^{2+} (2.5 mM), low Na^+ (35 and 60 mM), isoproterenol (50 and 100 μM), Bay K8644 (0.1, 1.0 and 10 μM) and amiloride (0.17, 0.6 and 1.2 mM). In order to ensure that every heart showed stunning and also to test its reversibility, reperfusion with buffer containing different interventions was started after 5 min reperfusion with normal buffer. Low Na^+ buffer solutions were prepared by adjusting osmolarity with choline chloride giving final concentrations of Na^+ at 35 or 60 mM.[17]

Cation Content

At the end of each experimental perfusion, the coronaries were flushed with 8 ml of ice-cold Dowex (50 W) treated sucrose (0.35 M)-HEPES (5 mM) buffer, pH 7.4, to wash out the extracellular fluid. Perfusion of hearts with 8 ml of ice-cold buffer has been reported to remove all the extracellular cations and the contents thus monitored are believed to reflect principally intracellular cations.[18,19] After flushing, the hearts were removed from the perfusion apparatus, and visible connective tissue was removed. Hearts were dried and digested in 1 : 10 volumes of an acid mixture containing 70% perchloric acid and 70% nitric acid in equal volumes. Lucite tubes containing heart homogenate-acid mixture were incubated at 40°C in a shaking water bath. The digestion was continued until the solution was no longer turbid. The acid extract was then analyzed for Na^+ and Ca^{2+} content using atomic absorption spectrometer (Perkin-Elmer, 2380). Lanthanum chloride (1%) was added to the samples as well as to known standards to minimize interference by contaminating phosphates. Cation standards were processed in a manner similar to heart samples so that they contained amounts of acid equivalent to that of the samples.

Chemicals and Data Analysis

Amiloride hydrochloride and isoproterenol were purchased from the Sigma Chemical Co., St. Louis, MO. Bay K8644 was purchased from Calbiochem Co.,

CA. All other reagents were of analytical grade. Statistical differences between control and experimental values were evaluated by the Student t test and analysis of variance followed by Bonferroni's post-hoc tests and a p value of 0.05 was taken to show a significant difference.

RESULTS

Assessment of Hypertrophy and Heart Function

Cardiac hypertrophy as well as hemodynamic function were assessed at 10 weeks after the surgery and these data are shown in TABLE 1. Ten weeks of aortic constriction resulted in about 44% and 52% increase in ventricular weight and ventricular to body weight ratio, respectively, in banded animals as compared to the sham control. Left ventricle wall thickness in the banded animals was increased by 34%. Both aortic, systolic and diastolic pressures in the hypertrophied animals as compared to their sham controls were higher by 30%. Left ventricular systolic pressure was increased by 81% at 10 weeks postoperation while no significant change was seen in left ventricular end-diastolic pressure in any of the banded animals. This was accompanied by 21% increase in $+$ dP/dt while $-$ dP/dt remained unchanged. None of the animals in the hypertrophy group showed any clinical signs of heart failure, e.g., dyspnea, enlarged abdomen (ascites) and cynosis of the limbs and ear lobes.

TABLE 1. Data on Heart Hypertrophy and Hemodynamic Function in Guinea Pigs after 10 Weeks of Aortic Banding[a]

	Sham	Hypertrophic
Body wt (gm)	692 ± 27	658 ± 16
Ventricle wt (gm)	1.6 ± 0.1	2.3 ± 0.11**
V.W./B.W. × 10³	2.3 ± 0.04	3.5 ± 0.05**
LV wall thickness (mm)	4.4 ± 0.04	5.9 ± 0.25**
Heart rate	265 ± 18	277 ± 12
Aortic systolic press. (mmHg)	73.8 ± 1.8	95.1 ± 1.5**
Aortic diastolic press. (mmHg)	57.5 ± 3.1	74.7 ± 2.1**
LV systolic press. (mmHg)	75.1 ± 1.3	136.1 ± 2.1**
LV end diastolic press. (mmHg)	3.1 ± 1.2	5.2 ± 0.8
LV + dP/dt (mmHg/sec)	3900 ± 150	4740 ± 264*
LV − dP/dt (mmHg/sec)	3000 ± 142	2700 ± 195

[a] B.W., body weight; V.W., ventricular weight; LV, left ventricle; $+$ dP/dt and $-$ dP/dt represent the positive and negative first derivatives of LV systolic pressure. Values are mean ± SE from 5–6 experiments. *p <0.05; **p < 0.01, significantly different from sham.

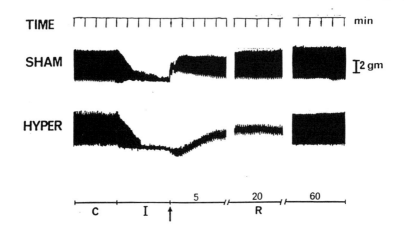

FIGURE 1. A typical recording showing the effects of 5 min ischemia (I) and 60 min reperfusion (R) on sham and hypertrophied guinea pig hearts. C refers to control perfusion. Time scale is shown on *top* and force calibration on the *right*. Segments numbered 5, 20 and 60 represent reperfusion time in minutes. *Arrow* marks the beginning of reperfusion.

Ischemia-Reperfusion Studies

Isolated perfused hearts, after a stable contractile function for 10–15 min, were subjected to global ischemia for 5 min followed by reperfusion for 20 min. A typical recording of ischemia-reperfusion induced changes in the developed force and resting tension in control and hypertrophic hearts is shown in FIGURE 1. The contractile force prior to ischemia-reperfusion (I-R) was normalized to 100% for each heart, and percentage recovery of mechanical function was determined by comparing the contractile activity of each heart after I-R with its own preischemic value (FIG. 2). Within 2–3 min of ischemia, the force declined to near zero without any change in resting tension in both sham and hypertrophied hearts.

On reperfusion, however, a differential effect was noted in the two groups. There was almost complete recovery of developed force within 20 min of reperfusion in sham hearts (FIG. 2A). There was an early transient rise in resting tension which returned to control levels (FIG. 2B). Hypertrophied hearts on the other hand showed no recovery of the mechanical activity within 20 min of reperfusion and resting tension increased to 250% of control values (FIG. 2B). With a continued reperfusion, hypertrophied hearts also recovered their contractile function near control values within 40–60 min. Recovery of the contractile function in these hearts was sudden and about $98 \pm 5\%$.

In order to understand the mechanism of this stunning, hypertrophied hearts made ischemic for 5 min and reperfused for 5 min with normal buffer showing no force recovery (stunned hearts), were exposed to different perfusion conditions known to modify Ca^{2+} influx across the sarcolemma. Data from these experiments are shown in TABLE 2. Reperfusion with buffer containing low Ca^{2+} (0.62 mM) had no effect on the mechanical recovery. With high Ca^{2+} (2.5 mM), occasional arrhythmic activity was noted but a sustained contractile function did not recover. Addition of isoproterenol at 100 μM in the reperfusion buffer resulted in an immediate recovery of contractile activity. This complete recovery of mechanical activity was also accompanied by a decline in resting tension. Lower concentration of isoproterenol (50 μM) had no beneficial effect on stunning. Perfusing the stunned hearts with Bay K8644 (0.1, 1.0 and 10 μM), and L-type calcium channel agonist, did not have any beneficial effect on stunning at any concentration used in the study.

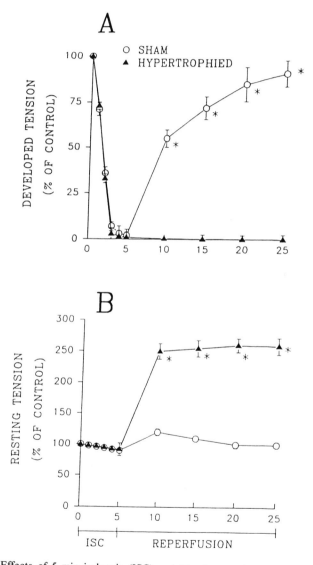

FIGURE 2. Effects of 5 min ischemia (ISC) and 20 min reperfusion on the developed force **(A)** and resting tension **(B)** in sham and hypertrophied guinea pig hearts. *p <0.05 significantly different from sham hearts. Values are percent of preischemic control. Mean ± SE of 6–8 experiments.

TABLE 2. Effects of Different Reperfusion Conditions on Recovery of
Developed Force in the Stunned Hypertrophied Hearts[a]

Perfusion Conditions	% Developed Force at Different Times of Reperfusion		
	5 min	10 min	15 min
Low Ca (0.62 mM)	stunned	stunned	stunned
High Ca (2.5 mM)	stunned	stunned	stunned
Isoproterenol (50 μm)	stunned	stunned	stunned
Isoproterenol (100 μm)	106 ± 18	96 ± 16	100 ± 5
Bay K8644 (0.1–10 μM)	stunned	stunned	stunned
Low Na (35 mM)	106 ± 4	66 ± 3	66 ± 5
Low Na (60 mM)	118 ± 15	108 ± 11	100 ± 2
Amiloride (0.17 mM)	stunned	stunned	stunned
Amiloride (0.17 mM) + low Na (60 mM)	70 ± 9	96 ± 6	101 ± 3
Amiloride (0.6 mM) + low Na (60 mM)	65 ± 10	66 ± 5	73 ± 100
Amiloride (1.2 mM) + low Na (60 mM)	stunned	stunned	stunned

[a] Hypertrophied hearts were made globally ischemic for 5 min followed by reperfusion
for 5 min which caused stunning. These stunned hearts were exposed to different conditions
for a further 15 min. Values are mean ± SE of 5–7 experiments.

Since low Na^+ containing buffer has been shown to have a positive inotropic
effect in isolated hearts by increasing Ca^{2+} entry through Na^+-Ca^{2+} exchange, we
perfused the stunned hearts with buffer containing low Na^+ (35 mM and 60 mM).
Both concentrations of low Na^+ were able to reverse the process of stunning
(TABLE 2). A biphasic effect on contractile force was seen with 35 mM Na^+
solution. Almost a 100% recovery in force was evident within the first 5 min of
perfusion which lasted for 3–4 min. The force then gradually declined to 66% and
remained at that level. At 60 mM Na^+, a sustained 100% recovery in the contractile
function from stunning was observed (TABLE 2). Resting tension declined to normal
at both concentrations of low Na^+.

In order to further examine the role of Na^+-Ca^{2+} exchange, hearts were perfused with amiloride, a nonspecific inhibitor of Na^+ exchange. Inclusion of amiloride in the perfusion medium in different concentrations (0.17 mM, 0.6 mM,
1.2 mM) had no beneficial effect on mechanical function. However, at 0.6 mM,
amiloride induced some arrhythmic activity. Effects of these concentrations of
amiloride were also studied in the presence of low Na^+. Since 60 mM concentration
of low Na^+ had more stable and pronounced effect, this concentration was used
in all experiments with amiloride and these data are shown in TABLE 2. These
hearts were first reperfused for 5 min with buffer containing only amiloride. The
stunned hearts were then switched to the buffer containing amiloride and low
Na^+. At 0.17 mM concentrations, amiloride delayed the recovery of contractile
function but by 10 min of reperfusion, recovery with low Na^+ (60 mM) was
complete. At higher concentration (0.6 mM) of amiloride, positive inotropic effect
of low Na^+ was partially blocked, i.e., increase in developed force averaged
between 65–73% instead of a complete recovery. Raising the amiloride concentration to 1.2 mM completely blocked the effect of low Na^+ and there was no
mechanical recovery (TABLE 2).

Cation Content

At the end of each experiment, hearts were analyzed for myocardial Na^+ and Ca^{2+} contents. It is pointed out that the washout procedure used in this study has been shown to minimize the contamination from the extracellular compartment.[18,19] Since it is difficult to rule out the small contamination from the extracellular compartment, we have chosen to express our results as myocardial, rather than intracellular, cation contents. Sodium and calcium contents of sham control and hypertrophied hearts perfused with the normal buffer for 40 min were found to be comparable (TABLE 3). Sham hearts made ischemic for 5 min and reperfused for 20 min showed no significant change in their cation contents. However, calcium content of the hypertrophied stunned hearts was significantly decreased whereas sodium content was increased.

Stunned hearts perfused with low or high calcium buffer did not show any change in their cation contents (TABLE 4). In isoproterenol (100 μM) perfused hearts, there was no change in sodium content; however, calcium content was increased significantly as compared to stunned hearts. Lower concentrations of isoproterenol (50 μM) had no effect on the cation contents. Bay K8644, at all concentrations did not influence the myocardial calcium or sodium concentration in stunned hearts. Perfusion with 35 mM Na^+ buffer normalized both Na^+ and Ca^{2+} values whereas 60 mM Na^+ perfusion increased calcium levels significantly. With low Na^+ plus amiloride (0.1 mM), sodium values were comparable to sham control hearts, whereas calcium content was significantly higher. In hearts reperfused with 0.6 mM amiloride and 60 mM Na^+, myocardial sodium and calcium levels were not significantly different from sham control hearts. Upon reperfusion with 1.2 mM amiloride + 60 mM Na^+, myocardial sodium values were significantly higher and calcium content was below the levels seen in sham control hearts.

DISCUSSION

Data in the present study make three important points: 1) It shows for the first time that a hypertrophied guinea pig heart undergoes "complete stunning" on reperfusion after a brief (5-min) episode of ischemia; 2) This complete stunning is fully reversible by interventions which improve myocardial Ca^{2+} content with or without the normalization of the myocardial Na^+ content; and 3) Hypertrophied hearts, in spite of sustaining a better hemodynamic function *in vivo*, suffer from

TABLE 3. Myocardial Cation Content in Isolated Perfused Sham and Hypertrophied Guinea Pig Hearts[a]

Animal Group	Na^+ (μmol/gm dry wt)	Ca^{2+} (μmol/gm dry wt)
Perfusion with normal buffer for 40 min		
Sham	145 ± 6.7	5.4 ± 0.4
Hyper	161 ± 6.6	5.7 ± 0.3
5 min ischemia (I) and 20 min reperfusion (R)		
Sham	153 + 3.1	5.3 ± 0.3
Hyper	252 ± 5.3*	3.4 ± 0.3*

[a] Values are mean ± SE from 6–8 experiments. *p <0.01, significantly different from sham.

TABLE 4. Cation Content of Stunned Hypertrophic Myocardium Subsequent to 5-Min Ischemia + 5-Min Reperfusion + 15-Min of Further Perfusion with Different Interventions[a]

Intervention	Na$^+$ (μmol/gm dry wt)	Ca^{2+} (μmol/gm dry wt)
Stunned heart	252 ± 5.3	3.4 ± 0.3
High Ca (2.5 mM)	254 ± 13.4*	4.4 ± 0.3*
Low Ca (0.62 mM)	239 ± 12.1*	4.1 ± 0.5*
Isoprot. (50 μM)	240 ± 6.2	4.2 ± 0.4*
Isoprot. (100 μM)	237 ± 5.8*	7.3 ± 0.2*†
Bay K (0.1 μ μM)	267 ± 6.3*	4.2 ± 1.2
Bay K (1.0 μM)	273 ± 15.8*	4.1 ± 1.0
Bay K (10 μM)	293 ± 10.4*	4.5 ± 0.8
Low Na (60 mM)	157 ± 4.1†	7.2 ± 0.3*†
Low Na (35 mM)	160 ± 5.3†	5.8 ± 0.4†
Amiloride (0.17 mM) + low Na (60 mM)	144 ± 6.9†	6.4 ± 0.4*†
Amiloride (0.6 mM) + low Na (60 mM)	161 ± 5.3†	4.9 ± 0.6
Amiloride (1.2 mM) + low Na (60 mM)	304 ± 6.2*	3.9 ± 0.5*

[a] Values are mean ± SE from 6–8 experiments. †p <0.05, significantly different from stunned hearts; *p <0.05, significantly different from sham control hearts.

a potential defect in sarcolemmal calcium influx which is unmasked by an exposure to a brief ischemic stress. Although a defect in calcium influx across the sarcolemma is shown to explain depressed contractile function in the stunned hypertrophied heart, the possibility of the other subcellular abnormalities such as reduced sensitivity of filaments to calcium and/or problem at the sarcoplasmic reticulum level are not ruled out.

We do not know whether the mechanism of "complete stunning" in hypertrophied heart is similar to stunning in normal myocardium where it has been suggested that depression in mechanical activity occurs due to abnormal Ca^{2+} handling by the cell which results in Ca^{2+} overload.[20] In this regard, reperfusion of the stunned myocardium with low Ca^{2+} containing buffer was reported to result in a better recovery.[8] However, in the present study, low Ca^{2+} did not have any beneficial effect on the phenomenon of stunning. This is consistent with the hypothesis that Ca^{2+} overload in the stunned myocardium, if present, may be transient and occurs only in the very early part of reperfusion, following which there may be a normalization of Ca^{2+} transients or even a relative Ca^{2+} deficiency.[9] A significant decrease in the myocardial Ca^{2+} content in stunned hearts was also noted in the present study. In this regard, administration of Ca^{2+} from outside has been shown to improve contractile function of the stunned myocardium to preischemic levels.[5] Since increasing extracellular Ca^{2+} did not have any beneficial effect on the mechanical function in our study, it is possible that mechanisms by which Ca^{2+} enters the cell may be disrupted in the stunned hypertrophied heart. This is further substantiated by the observation that high extracellular Ca^{2+} did not influence myocardial Ca^{2+} content in these hearts.

Here it should be pointed out that our baseline values for myocardial Na$^+$

content (145–304 μmoles/gm wet wt) in guinea pigs were relatively higher than those reported for other species.[18] This may not be due to the poor washing of the vascular space as myocardial Ca^{2+} content values in our study were within the range.[18] Higher Na^+ content may have been due to binding of this cation at some unspecified site. At any rate baseline cation content in the hypertrophied heart was not different from sham control hearts. It is important to point out that measurement of total cation contents of sodium and calcium as done in this study is limited in discerning changes in different intracellular pools represented by different subcellular organelles. However, the pharmacological approach followed in this study does point out a defect in sarcolemmal calcium influx.

Isoproterenol, a β-adrenergic agonist, which increases intracellular Ca^{2+} by phosphorylation of Ca^{2+} channels via cAMP-dependent protein kinase, was able to recover the hearts from stunning. Beneficial effects of other inotropic agents on stunned myocardium have also been shown by many other investigators.[21–23] On the other hand, Bay K8644, a dihydropyridine (DHP) receptor agonist, was unable to reverse the phenomenon of stunning. It should be noted that although Bay K8644 increases Ca^{2+} channel activity by the same magnitude as isoproterenol, the mechanism of action of the two is very different.[24] Bay K8644 increases Ca^{2+} concentration by promoting a pattern of gating characterized by long openings and short closings thereby increasing the activity of channels already open. Isoproterenol, on the other hand, brings into play the activity of Ca^{2+} channels that were otherwise inactive. Unlike β-adrenergic agents, DHP receptor agonists do not increase c-AMP levels in heart cells.[25] Moreover, enhancement of Ca^{2+} current by Bay K8644 has been shown to be additive with the increase produced by β-adrenergic stimulation, thus confirming different sites and/or mechanisms of action for these two agents.[24] This may suggest that a greater number of Ca^{2+} channels in the hypertrophied stunned heart become inactive during the oxidative stress of ischemia-reperfusion and the defect is corrected by β-adrenergic stimulation. Since isoproterenol also increases calcium movements across the sarcoplasmic reticulum, the involvement of sarcoplasmic reticulum in this stunning cannot be ruled out.

Positive inotropic action of low Na^+ perfusion has been suggested to be mediated by increased Ca^{2+} influx through Na^+-Ca^{2+} exchanger in the sarcolemma.[17] Calcium entry through Na^+-Ca^{2+} exchange itself has been shown to induce appreciable contractions and this calcium influx can also induce calcium release from sarcoplasmic reticulum.[26] In the present study, perfusion with low Na^+ (60 mM) was able to recover the hearts from stunning and the effect was stable and sustained for a long time. Cation data also suggests that perfusion with low Na^+ lowered the myocardial Na^+ content and increased Ca^{2+} content above control levels. Furthermore amiloride, a nonspecific inhibitor of the exchanger, abolished the beneficial effect of low Na^+ in a dose-dependent manner. At lower concentration (0.17 mM), amiloride was not able to block the inotropic effect of low Na^+, which may be due to the fact that at this concentration, amiloride mainly blocks Na^+-H^+ exchange.[27] At higher doses, amiloride has been reported to block Na^+-Ca^{2+} exchange in guinea pig atrial muscle[28] and in beef heart sarcolemmal vesicles.[29] At a higher dose of amiloride, beneficial effect of low Na^+ was completely blocked suggesting that the Ca^{2+} entering through Na^+-Ca^{2+} exchange is able to restore contractile function. Recently it was shown that removal of Na^+ ions also modulates Ca^{2+} channel phosphorylation via cAMP-dependent protein kinase,[30] raising the possibility that low Na^+ and isoproterenol may share a common mechanism.

Depletion of adenine nucleotide pool and their slow replacement with time,[1,31] decreased efficiency of energy utilization and impaired sensitivity of myofilaments towards Ca^{2+} [8,32] have also been suggested to explain the phenomenon of stunning. Increase in resting tension in the stunned hearts may be a result of depletion of ATP levels. However, recent studies demonstrated a dissociation between postischemic ATP levels and recovery of function in stunned hearts and showed that ATP levels are decreased very modestly in stunned hearts.[6,33] Since intracellular calcium was increased above normal levels with low Na^+ as well as isoproterenol, reversal of the stunning may have resulted from above normal levels of calcium compensating for any decreased sensitivity of myofilaments towards calcium. Although the possibility of decreased Ca^{2+} sensitivity of myofilaments as a mechanism of stunning is indicated by these data, force recovery did require Ca^{2+} influx across the sarcolemma suggesting it to be a primary event. This issue needs to be addressed further in detail by doing a force-calcium relationship study or by subcellular fractionation of cardiac tissue at various time intervals to determine the subcellular changes in the hypertrophied vs control hearts.

Oxygen free radicals have also been suggested to be involved in the mechanism of stunning,[34] and in this regard hypertrophied hyperfunctional rat hearts were reported to be less vulnerable to oxidative stress due to oxygen radicals,[35] hypoxia-reoxygenation[36] and ischemia reperfusion.[10] This increased tolerance to various oxidative stress conditions has been attributed to the increase in endogenous antioxidant enzyme activities.[10,11,14,37] Hypertrophied guinea pig hearts in the present study exhibited a better *in vivo* hemodynamic function and are reported to contain higher endogenous antioxidants and redox state.[38] Despite the higher antioxidant levels at this stage, occurrence of stunning suggests a potential defect with respect to sarcolemmal Ca^{2+} influx, which was unmasked by the ischemic stress.

Reduced tolerance of the guinea pig hypertrophied heart to ischemia reperfusion in this study may appear to be inconsistent with earlier findings in rat hypertrophied hearts.[10,35,36] However, this stage of hypertrophy in guinea pigs may represent either an early event in the pathogenesis of heart failure and/or it may denote unavailability of antioxidants at some critical site in the sarcolemma. With respect to the former possibility, clinical signs of heart failure in this animal model begin to appear at about 15 weeks of the postsurgery period[16] suggesting a borderline compensated stage of hypertrophy at 10 weeks. Abnormalities in energy metabolism, excitation-contraction coupling, β-adrenergic receptors and structural changes in myofilaments have also been suggested to contribute in the shift from heart hypertrophy to heart failure.[39,40] The sarcolemmal defect suggested by our study, however, does not preclude any of these mechanisms, and the defect may in fact lead to other abnormalities, and ultimately congestive heart failure at a later stage.[16,41]

In conclusion, this study reports complete stunning in hypertrophied guinea pig hearts subjected to brief ischemic stress, which also unmasks a latent defect in sarcolemmal calcium influx. Although impairment in sarcolemmal influx through the Ca^{2+} channels as well as Na^+-Ca^{2+} exchanger is suggested to be a primary event, reduced myofilament sensitivity to Ca^{2+} is also indicated.

SUMMARY

Isolated sham control as well as hypertrophied guinea pig hearts were subjected to global ischemia and reperfusion. Developed force declined to zero during 5 min of ischemia without any significant change in resting tension in both sham control and hypertrophied hearts. Upon reperfusion, control hearts showed nearly complete recovery of developed force within 20 min, whereas hypertrophied hearts during this time showed no contractile function, *i.e.*, "a complete stunning" was observed. A continued reperfusion of the stunned hypertrophied hearts ultimately resulted in complete recovery of force within 40–60 min. Data on myocardial cation content showed a relative calcium deficiency in the stunned hearts (3.4 μmol/gm dry wt) as compared to sham control hearts (5.3 μmol/gm dry wt). Stunning could be reversed sooner by isoproterenol (100 μm), and low Na^+ (35 and 60 mM) perfusion. Recovery of contractile function by low Na^+ was blocked by amiloride (0.17–1.2 mM) in a dose-dependent manner. Perfusion with Bay K8644 (0.1–10 μM) as well as low (0.62 mM) and high (2.5 mM) extracellular calcium concentrations failed to reverse stunning. The pharmacological interventions that were able to reverse the stunning condition also increased the myocardial calcium content. Although the possibilities of a sarcoplasmic reticulum dysfunction and/or reduced sensitivity of myofilaments are not excluded, data suggest that a defect in calcium influx across the sarcolemma is an important factor in "complete stunning." It is suggested that this "potential sarcolemmal defect" in the hypertrophied heart, which is unmasked by the ischemic stress, may also represent an early abnormality in the pathogenesis of heart failure.

REFERENCES

1. BRAUNWALD, E. & R. A. KLONER. 1982. The stunned myocardium: prolonged, postischemic ventricular dysfunction. Circulation **66**: 1146–1149.
2. HEYNDRICKX, G. R., R. W. MILLARD, R. J. MCRITCHIE, P. R. MAROKO & S. F. VATNER. 1975. Regional myocardial functional and electrophysiological alterations after brief coronary artery occlusion in conscious dogs. J. Clin. Invest. **56**: 978–985.
3. PATEL, B., R. A. KLONER, K. PRZYKLENK & E. BRAUNWALD. 1988. Post ischemic myocardial "stunning": a clinically relevant phenomenon. Ann. Intern. Med. **108**: 626–628.
4. BOLLI, R., B. S. PATEL, C. J. HARTLEY, J. I. THORNBY, M. O. JEROUDI & R. ROBERTS. 1989. Nonuniform transmural recovery of contractile function in the "stunned" myocardium. Am. J. Physiol. **257**: H375–H385.
5. ITO, B. R., H. TATE, M. KOBAYASHI & W. SCHAPER. 1987. Reversibly injured, postischemic canine myocardium retains normal contractile reserve. Circ. Res. **616**: 834–846.
6. AMBROSIO, G., W. E. JACOBUS, C. A. BERGMAN, H. F. WEISMAN & L. C. BECKER. 1987. Preserved high energy phosphate metabolic reserve in globally "stunned" hearts despite reduction of basal ATP content and contractility. J. Mol. Cell. Cardiol. **19**: 953–964.
7. LIEDTKE, A. J., L. DE MAISON, A. M. EGGLESTON, L. M. CHOEN & S. H. NELLIS. 1988. Changes in substrate metabolism and effects of excess fatty acids in reperfused myocardium. Circ. Res. **62**: 535–542.
8. KUSUOKA, H., Y. KORETSUN, V. P. CHACKO, M. L. WEISFELDT & E. MARBAN. 1990. Excitation-contraction coupling in postischemic myocardium: Does failure of activator Ca^{2+} transients underline stunning? Circ. Res. **66**: 1268–1276.
9. DU TOIT, E. F. & L. H. OPIE. 1992. Modulation of severity of reperfusion stunning in the isolated rat heart by agents altering calcium flux at onset of reperfusion. Circ. Res. **70**: 960–967.
10. KIRSHENBAUM, L. A. & P. K. SINGAL. 1993. Increase in endogenous antioxidant enzymes protects the heart against reperfusion injury. Am. J. Physiol. **265**: H484–H493.
11. GUPTA, M. & P. K. SINGAL. 1989. Higher antioxidant capacity during chronic stable heart hypertrophy. Circ. Res. **64**: 398–406.

12. ANDERSON, P. G., M. F. ALLARD, G. D. THOMAS, S. P. BISHOP & S. B. DIGERNESS. 1990. Increased ischemic injury but decreased hypoxic injury in hypertrophied rat hearts. Circ. Res. **67:** 948–959.

13. EBERLI, F. R., C. S. APSTEIN, S. NGOY & B. H. LORELL. 1992. Exacerbation of left ventricular diastolic dysfunction by pressure-overload hypertrophy: modification by specific inhibition of cardiac angiotensin converting enzyme. Circ. Res. **70:** 931–943.

14. SINK, J. D., G. L. PELLON, W. D. CURRIE, R. C. HILL, C. O. OLSEN, R. N. JONES & A. S. WECHSLER. 1981. Response of hypertrophied myocardium to ischemia: correlation with biochemical and physiological parameters. J. Thorac. Cardiovasc. Surg. **81:** 865–872.

15. GAASCH, W. H., M. R. ZILE, P. K. HOSHINO, E. O. WEINBERG, B. S. RHODES & C. S. APSTEIN. 1990. Tolerance of hypertrophied heart to ischemia studies in compensated and failing dog hearts with pressure overload hypertrophy. Circulation **81:** 1644–1653.

16. RANDHAWA, A. K. & P. K. SINGAL. 1992. Pressure overload induced cardiac hypertrophy with and without dilation. J. Am. Coll. Cardiol. **20:** 1569–1575.

17. LANGER, G. A., L. M. NUDD & N. V. RICCHIUTI. 1976. The effect of sodium deficient perfusion on calcium exchange in cardiac tissue culture. J. Mol. Cell. Cardiol. **8:** 321–328.

18. ALTO, L. E. & N. S. DHALLA. 1979. Myocardial cation contents during induction of calcium paradox. Am. J. Physiol. **237** (Heart. Circ. Physiol. **6**): H713–H719.

19. MENG, H. P., B. B. LONSBERRY & G. N. PIERCE. 1991. Influence of perfusate pH on the postischemic recovery of cardiac contractile function: involvement of sodium-hydrogen exchange. J. Pharmacol. Exp. Ther. **2583:** 772–777.

20. KUSUOKA, H., J. K. PORTERFIELD, H. F. WEISMAN, M. L. WEISFELDT & E. MARBAN. 1987. Pathophysiology and pathogenesis of stunned myocardium: depressed Ca^{2+} activation of contraction as a consequence of reperfusion-induced cellular calcium overload in ferret hearts. J. Clin. Invest. **79:** 950–961.

21. BECKER, L. C., J. H. LEVINE, A. F. DiPAULA, T. GUARNIERI & T. AVERSANO. 1986. Reversal of dysfunction in postischemic stunned myocardium by epinephrine and postextrasystolic potentiation. J. Am. Coll. Cardiol. **73:** 580–589.

22. ELLIS, S. G., J. WYNNE, E. BRAUNWALD, C. I, HENSCHKE, T. SANDOR & R. A. KLONER. 1984. Response of reperfusion-salvaged, stunned myocardium to inotropic stimulation. Am. Heart J. **107:** 13–19.

23. MERCIER, J. C., U. LANDO, K. KANMATSUSE, K. NINOMIYA, S. MEERBAUM, M. C. FISHBEIN, H. J. C. SWAN & W. GANZ. 1982. Divergent effects of inotropic stimulation on the ischemic and severely depressed reperfused myocardium. Circulation **66:** 397–400.

24. TSIEN, R. W., B. P. BEAN, P. HESS, J. B. LANSMAN, B. NILIUM & M. C. NOWYCKY. 1986. Mechanisms of calcium channel modulation by β-adrenergic agents and dihydropyridine calcium agonists. J. Mol. Cell. Cardiol. **18:** 691–710.

25. KOKUBUM, S. & H. REUTER. 1984. Dihydropyridine derivatives prolong the open state of Ca channels in cultured cardiac cells. Proc. Natl. Acad. Sci. USA **81:** 4824–4827.

26. BERS, D. M., D. M. K. CHRISTENSEN & T. X. NGUYEN. 1988. Can Ca^{2+} entry via Na^+-Ca^{2+} exchange directly activate cardiac muscle contractions? J. Mol. Cell. Cardiol. **20:** 405–414.

27. KARMAZYN, M. 1988. Amiloride enhances postischemic ventricular recovery: possible role of Na^+-H^+ exchange. Am. J. Physiol. **255** (Heart Circ. Physiol. **24**): H608–H615.

28. KENNEDY, R. H., J. R. BERLIN, Y. C. NG, T. AKERA & T. M. BRODY. 1986. Amiloride: effects on myocardial force of contraction, sodium pump and Na^+/Ca^{2+} exchange. J. Mol. Cell. Cardiol. **18:** 177–188.

29. FLOREANI, M. & S. LUCIANI. 1984. Amiloride: relationship between cardiac effects and inhibition of Na^+/Ca^{2+} exchange. Eur. J. Pharmacol. **105:** 317–322.

30. BLAKE, C. W. & W. G. WIER. 1992. Modulation of L-type calcium channels by sodium ions. Proc. Natl. Acad. Sci. USA **89:** 4417–4421.

31. REIMER, K. A., M. L. HILL & R. B. JENNINGS. 1981. Prolonged depletion of ATP and of the adenine nucleotide pool due to delayed resynthesis of adenine nucleotides

following reversible myocardial ischemic injury in dogs. J. Mol. Cell. Cardiol. **13:** 229–239.

32. HOFMANN, P. A., W. P. MILLER & R. L. MOSS. 1993. Altered calcium sensitivity of isometric tension in myocyte-sized preparations of porcine postischemic stunned myocardium. Circ. Res. **72:** 50–56.

33. PRZYKLENK, K. & R. A. KLONER. 1988. Effect of verapamil on postischemic "stunned" myocardium: importance of the timing of treatment. J. Am. Coll. cardiol. **11:** 614–623.

34. BOLLI, R. 1990. Mechanism of myocardial "stunning." Circulation **823:** 723–738.

35. SINGAL, P. K., M. GUPTA & A. K. RANDHAWA. 1991. Reduced myocardial injury due to exogenous oxidants in pressure induced heart hypertrophy. Basic Res. Cardiol. **86:** 273–282.

36. KIRSHENBAUM, L. A. & P. K. SINGAL. 1992. Antioxidant changes in heart hypertrophy: significance during hypoxia-reoxygenation injury. Can. J. Physiol. Pharmacol. **7010:** 1330–1335.

37. DHALIWAL, H., L. A. KIRSHENBAUM, A. K. RANDHAWA & P. K. SINGAL. 1991. Correlation between antioxidant changes during hypoxia and recovery upon reoxygenation. Am. J. Physiol. **261:** H632–H638.

38. DHALLA, A. K. & P. K. SINGAL. 1994. Antioxidant changes in hypertrophied and failing guinea pig hearts. Am. J. Physiol. **266** (Heart Circ. Physiol. **35**): H1280–H1285.

39. DHALLA, N. S., P. K. DAS & G. P. SHARMA. 1978. Subcellular basis of cardiac contractile failure. J. Mol. Cell. Cardiol. **10:** 363–385.

40. NEWMAN, W. H. 1983. Biochemical, structural and mechanical defects of the failing myocardium. Pharmacol. Ther. **22:** 215–247.

41. SIRI, F. M., C. NORDIN, S. M. FACTOR, E. SONNELICK & R. AROUSON. 1989. Compensatory hypertrophy and failure in gradual pressure-overload guinea pig heart. Am. J. Physiol. **257:** H1016–H1024.

Late Ischemic Preconditioning Is Mediated in Myocytes by Enhanced Endogenous Antioxidant Activity Stimulated by Oxygen-Derived Free Radicals[a]

XIAOLIN ZHAI, XIAOBO ZHOU, AND
MUHAMMAD ASHRAF[b]

Department of Pathology and Laboratory Medicine
University of Cincinnati Medical Center
Cincinnati, Ohio

INTRODUCTION

Ischemic preconditioning refers to the reduction of infarct size resulting from prolonged and severe myocardial ischemia by one or more preceding short episodes of ischemia and reperfusion.[1,2] However, the protective effect disappears in 2 or 3 hours,[2] but reappears after 24 hours, which is called late preconditioning.[3-6] The mechanism of this unique protection is not known. Some studies[3,4,6] suggest that the late phase of ischemic preconditioning is due to synthesis of stress proteins and antioxidant enzymes. Marber *et al.*[4] found that both ischemic and heat stress pretreatment elevate myocardial heat shock proteins and are associated with a reduction of infarct size. Yamashita *et al.*[6] demonstrated a direct association between Mn SOD induction and acquisition of tolerance to ischemia at a late phase of preconditioning in myocytes. Although these data suggest that the initial preconditioning stimuli (ischemia, hypoxia, etc.) can lead to the synthesis of these proteins that are of primary importance in the acquisition of tolerance to subsequent ischemia, it is unclear which component is responsible for the late protection.

Active oxygen-derived free radicals, such as $\cdot O_2^-$, have been shown to be generated during ischemia and reperfusion.[7,8] The reactive oxygen species play a role in ischemic injury.[9,10] Although the excessive amount of free radicals is believed to be toxic, mild oxidative stress might be beneficial to myocardium.[11] We therefore determined that late preconditioning is mediated by endogenous antioxidant defenses enhanced by oxygen-derived free radicals. The results of this study demonstrate that oxygen radicals during the initial preconditioning stimulate increased activity of Mn SOD, which contributes to the late cardioprotection of preconditioning.

[a] This work was supported by National Institutes of Health Research Grant HL 23597.

[b] Address for correspondence: Muhammad Ashraf, Ph.D., Department of Pathology and Laboratory Medicine, University of Cincinnati, Cincinnati, OH 45267-0529. Tel.: (513) 558-0145; Fax: (513) 558-2289.

156

METHODS

Materials

Collagenase type II was bought from Worthington Biochemical Corp., laminin from Collaborative Research Inc., medium 199 from Gibco BRL, and xanthine, xanthine oxidase, and allopurinol from Sigma Chemical Co. All animals received humane care according to the guidelines of the animal care committee of The University of Cincinnati, which is accredited by the American Association of Laboratory Animal Care.

Cell Culture

Adult Sprague-Dawley rats were anesthetized by injection of 60 mg/kg pentobarbital IP and anticoagulated with heparin sodium (100 IU/100 g IV). Hearts were rapidly excised and perfused for 5 minutes in the Langendorff mode with minimum essential medium that was gassed with 95% O_2/5% CO_2 at 37°C. Hearts were then perfused with the same medium plus 0.1% collagenase and 0.1% albumin for about 30 minutes. Hearts were removed and minced. The suspension was filtered through 200 μm mesh and centrifuged slowly. The pellet was resuspended in the medium containing 1% albumin and 1 mmol/L calcium, and cells were allowed to settle at 37°C. After that, the cell pellet was resuspended in medium 199 containing 10% calf serum, 2 mmol/L glutamine, 100 μg/mL streptomycin, and 100 U/mL penicillin. A total of 4×10^6 to 5×10^6 cells were obtained from each heart. The percentage of viable myocytes (rod shaped and beating) was >95% in each preparation. Approximately 2.4×10^5 viable cells were plated in 60-mm laminin-coated dishes and incubated overnight in an incubator.

Anoxia and Reoxygenation

Myocytes were exposed to anoxia in a chamber (Forma 1025 Anaerobic System). Cells were washed three times with anoxic Tyrode's solution containing (mmol/L): NaCl 125, KCl 2.6, KH_2PO_4 1.2, $MgSO_4$ 1.2, $CaCl_2$ 1.0, and HEPES 25, pH 7.4, bubbled with 100% N_2. Cells were rendered anoxic at 37°C in 3 mL anoxic Tyrode's solution per dish. O_2 content of the air inside the chamber was <0.1% throughout experiments. After anoxia, myocytes were reoxygenated in a CO_2 water jacketed incubator with a humidified atmosphere of 95% air/ 5% CO_2.

Experimental Protocol

Myocytes were randomized into six groups. All groups were performed in four replicates (n = 4 per group). Myocytes in normal control (Group 1) were continuously incubated in aerobic solutions for the duration of experiments. Myocytes in anoxic control (Group 2) were aerobically incubated for 24 hours and 20 minutes before they were subjected to 60 minutes of anoxia followed by 60 minutes of reoxygenation. Myocytes in late preconditioning (Group 3) were preconditioned with two cycles of 5 minutes of anoxia and 5 minutes of reoxygenation. These myocytes were allowed to recover in medium 199 in an incubator. After 24 hours of incubation, cells were subjected to 60 minutes of anoxia followed by 60 minutes of reoxygenation. Myocytes in Group 4 were treated similar to Group 3, except that a xanthine oxidase inhibitor (1 μmol/L allopurinol) was added to the Tyrode's solution during the preconditioning period. In Group 5, myocytes were preconditioned with exogenous $\cdot O_2^-$, *i.e.*, two cycles of 5 minutes of incubation with the Tyrode's solution containing 100 μmol/L xanthine and 0.05 U/mL xanthine oxidase[11] and 5 minutes of incubation without xanthine and xanthine oxidase. In Group 6, myocytes were treated similar to Group 5, except that 1 μmol/L allopurinol was added to the Tyrode's solution during the preconditioning period.

The supernatant in dishes was collected at specific periods for measurement of $\cdot O_2^-$ and LDH. Cells were harvested at the end of reoxygenation after longer anoxia for SOD, malondialdehyde, cell viability, and morphological changes.

Measurement of $\cdot O_2^-$

$\cdot O_2^-$ was quantified by monitoring SOD-inhibitable cytochrome *c* reduction as described by us previously.[9] The results were expressed as nanomoles per milligram protein.

Measurement of SOD Activity

SOD activity was determined by its inhibitory action on $\cdot O_2^-$-dependent reduction of ferricytochrome *c* by xanthine-xanthine oxidase.[12] Ice cold Tris-sucrose buffer containing 0.25 mol/L sucrose, 10 mmol/L Tris-HCl, 1 mmol/L EDTA, and 0.5 mmol/L dithiothreitol was used to homogenize myocytes followed by centrifugation at 1000 g for 15 minutes. The supernatant was centrifuged at 10 000 g for 20 minutes to obtain the mitochondrial pellet that was used as a source of Mn SOD. The supernatant was again centrifuged at 105 000 g for 1 hour. The supernatant was used to assay Cu/Zn SOD. The final concentrations in the assay medium (1 mL) were 100 mmol/L cytochrome *c*, 100 mmol/L hypoxanthine, 10 mmol/L Tris-HCl, and 70 μg enzyme protein. The reaction was initiated by addition of 8 mU xanthine oxidase. SOD activity was determined from a standard curve, which was obtained by running with commercial standard SOD. SOD activity was expressed as units per milligram protein.

Measurement of Myocyte Protein Content

A Sigma assay kit was used to measure protein content. Myocytes were mixed with 2 mL of 6% cold perchloric acid. The cell suspension was heated at 70°C for 20 minutes, and then centrifuged at 1000 g for 20 minutes. The pellet was dissolved in 2 mL of 0.1N NaOH solution, and was cooled for 20 minutes, after which it was centrifuged at 1000 g for 20 minutes. The absorbance of supernatant was measured by brilliant blue G reaction with protein at 595 nm.

Measurement of LDH

Spectrophotometric assay of LDH was performed with a Sigma assay kit, and the activity of LDH was expressed as units per milligram protein.

TABLE 1. Amount of Superoxide Anion (nmol/mg protein) Produced in Experimental Groups[a]

Groups (n = 4 per Group)	Baseline	Preconditioning	Reoxygenation
Normal control	0.48 ± 0.07	—	0.52 ± 0.05
Anoxic control	0.49 ± 0.06	0.51 ± 0.04	3.47 ± 0.12
Late PC with anoxia	0.51 ± 0.05	1.65 ± 0.08*	0.78 ± 0.07*
Late PC with anoxia + allopurinol	0.49 ± 0.08	0.55 ± 0.06	2.93 ± 0.09
Late PC with exogenous $\cdot O_2^-$	0.50 ± 0.06	1.42 ± 0.11*	0.93 ± 0.08*
Late PC with exogenous $\cdot O_2^-$ + allopurinol	0.52 ± 0.07	0.57 ± 0.08	3.08 ± 0.07

[a] Baseline and preconditioning readings were taken before and after preconditioning sequences. Reoxygenation reading was made at the end of 60 minutes of reoxygenation after 60 minutes of anoxia. *$p < 0.05$ versus anoxic control. PC indicates preconditioning.

Measurement of Lipid Peroxidation

Thiobarbituric acid reactive compounds (TBAR) were measured as previously described,[13] which was a sensitive index of lipid peroxidation. Myocytes were homogenized in 1.15% KCl solution. After that, 0.1 mL of the homogenate was mixed with 0.4 mL of 8.1% sodium dodecyl sulfate, 3 mL of 20% acetic acid, and 3 mL of 0.8% thiobarbituric acid, followed by boiling for 15 minutes. After cooling, 1 mL of distilled water was added, and the sample was extracted with 5 mL of butanol/pyridine. The optical density of the upper organic layer was read at 532 nm. TBAR formation was expressed as nanomoles per milligram protein.

Evaluation of Cell Viability and Cell Morphology

Myocytes were treated with 0.1% trypan blue, and were viewed under a phase-contrast microscope.[8] Dead cells were permeable to trypan blue, whereas viable cells excluded the dye. The percentage of these cells was calculated.

Statistical Analysis

Statistical analysis was based on guidelines described by Wallenstein *et al.*[14] All data were expressed as mean ± SEM. A one-way ANOVA was first carried out to test for any differences between mean values. When a significant F value was obtained, comparisons between individual means of groups were performed by a Student-Newman-Keuls test. A difference of $p < 0.05$ was considered significant.

RESULTS

Measurement of Superoxide Anion

Cytochrome c reduction represents $\cdot O_2^-$ in various experimental groups, and is summarized in TABLE 1. Immediately after preconditioning with anoxia or exogenous $\cdot O_2^-$, cytochrome c reduction was significantly higher than that in the anoxic control. Allopurinol reduced the amount of cytochrome c reduction in preconditioning. After 24 hours, the amount of $\cdot O_2^-$ was produced significantly less in myocytes preconditioned with anoxia or exogenous $\cdot O_2^-$, as compared with the anoxic control. There was a significant increase in $\cdot O_2^-$ production in the myocytes treated with allopurinol.

SOD Activity

Mn SOD activity in different groups after reoxygenation is shown in FIGURE 1. Longer anoxia resulted in reduced activity of Mn SOD in anoxic control (0.38 ± 0.06 U/mg protein, $p < 0.05$ versus normal control) after 24 hours, whereas activity of Mn SOD increased significantly in late preconditioned myocytes (3.25 ± 0.15 U/mg protein) and in preconditioned myocytes with exogenous $\cdot O_2^-$ (2.27 ± 0.10 U/mg protein, $p < 0.05$ versus anoxic control). On the contrary, the increase in Mn SOD activity induced by preconditioning was considerably blocked by allopurinol, a xanthine oxidase inhibitor. Cu/Zn SOD activity remained the same among groups after longer anoxia (data not shown).

LDH Release

The LDH release in various experimental groups is given in FIGURE 2. LDH release was markedly reduced in late preconditioned myocytes (0.209 ± 0.018 U/

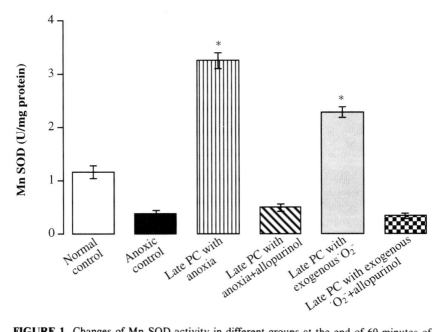

FIGURE 1. Changes of Mn SOD activity in different groups at the end of 60 minutes of reoxygenation after 60 minutes of anoxia. *$p < 0.05$ versus anoxic control, n = 4 per group, PC indicates preconditioning.

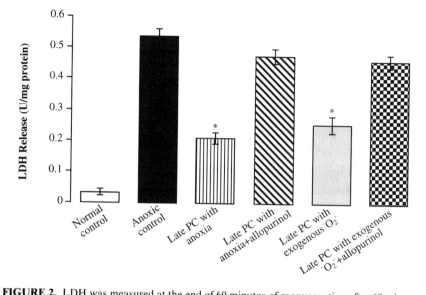

FIGURE 2. LDH was measured at the end of 60 minutes of reoxygenation after 60 minutes of anoxia. *p <0.05 versus anoxic control, n = 4 per group. PC indicates preconditioning.

mg protein) and in myocytes preconditioned with exogenous $\cdot O_2^-$ (0.255 ± 0.027 U/mg protein), compared with anoxic control (0.537 ± 0.024 U/mg protein). Allopurinol completely blocked the protective effect of preconditioning on LDH release.

Cell Viability

FIGURE 3 depicts cell viability at the end of reoxygenation in different groups. After 24 hours, the percentage of viable cells declined to 26.3 ± 2.5% in the anoxic control. When myocytes were preconditioned by brief repeated anoxia or by exogenous $\cdot O_2^-$, the survival rate of myocytes subjected to longer anoxia increased significantly after 24 hours (68.7 ± 3.3% and 61.6 ± 2.3%, respectively). On the contrary, the survival rate was completely reduced in preconditioned myocytes treated with allopurinol.

TBAR Formation

TBAR formation in experimental groups is illustrated in FIGURE 4. TBAR formation was 0.726 ± 0.035 nmol/mg protein in the anoxic control and was significantly reduced after 24 hours in myocytes preconditioned with anoxia or with exogenous $\cdot O_2^-$ (0.331 ± 0.025 and 0.401 ± 0.024 nmol/mg protein, p <0.05 versus anoxic control). Allopurinol completely abolished the reduction of TBAR formation by preconditioning.

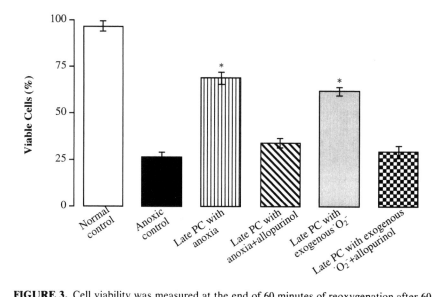

FIGURE 3. Cell viability was measured at the end of 60 minutes of reoxygenation after 60 minutes of anoxia. *p <0.05 versus anoxic control, n = 4 per group, PC indicates preconditioning.

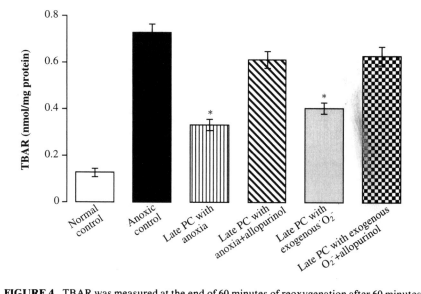

FIGURE 4. TBAR was measured at the end of 60 minutes of reoxygenation after 60 minutes of anoxia. *p < 0.05 versus anoxic control, n = 4 per group, PC indicates preconditioning.

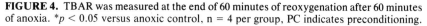

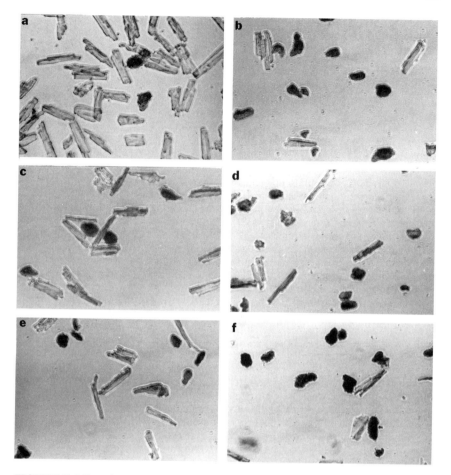

FIGURE 5. Microphotographs (magnification ×200) were taken at the end of 60 minutes of reoxygenation after 60 minutes of anoxia. (a) Normal control: most cells are elongated and rod shaped forms that excluded trypan blue stain. (b) Anoxic control: many cells are rounded and stained positively. (c) Late preconditioning significantly reduced the number of round and stained myocytes. (d) Late preconditioning and allopurinol: the number of rod shaped cells is decreased, suggesting that the beneficial effect of preconditioning disappeared in the presence of allopurinol during repetitive transient anoxia. (e) The number of normal cells is similar to anoxic preconditioning. (f) Late preconditioning with exogenous $\cdot O_2^-$ and allopurinol: the number of rod shaped cells is decreased.

Cell Morphology

Morphological features of myocytes in different groups are shown in FIGURE 5. The myocytes in the normal control group maintained their elongated rod shape and excluded trypan blue. Cells were rounded up in the anoxic control group. The typical rod shaped pattern was preserved in preconditioned myocytes, and the number of rounded myocytes was significantly reduced. The beneficial effect of preconditioning was not observed in the presence of allopurinol during the initial preconditioning period.

DISCUSSION

The aim of this study was to determine whether oxygen-derived radicals enhanced endogenous antioxidant activity to protect myocardium against ischemic or hypoxic injury in late preconditioning. Reoxygenation of ischemic hearts has been associated with increased lipid peroxidation,[10,15] suggesting that oxygen free radicals contribute to cellular injury during ischemia and reperfusion. It is therefore likely that the intracellular antioxidant defenses would be a potential candidate for the late protection initiated by ischemic preconditioning. The results reported here clearly demonstrate that (1) brief repetitive episodes of anoxia led to the production of free radicals such as $\cdot O_2^-$, (2) initial mild oxidative stress caused by those oxygen species in turn decreased subsequent anoxic injury by increasing endogenous antioxidant defenses, and (3) exogenous $\cdot O_2^-$ mimicked repetitive anoxia to enhance endogenous antioxidant defenses, which were associated with late protection initiated by ischemic preconditioning.

Ischemic preconditioning has been extensively studied in whole hearts. Recently, studies showed that preconditioning can also be induced in isolated myocytes. Armstrong and Ganote[16] developed an ischemic slurry method to stimulate ischemia in isolated rabbit myocytes instead of low oxygen tension in glucose-free medium. In this model, the role of adenosine and protein kinase C in early preconditioning was studied.[16] Another report showed that hypoxic preconditioning of isolated rat myocytes induces tolerance to hypoxia 24 hours after preconditioning.[6] In the present study, two cycles of 5 minutes of anoxia followed by 5 minutes of reoxygenation preconditioned myocytes against a subsequent longer anoxia 24 hours later. This protection was associated with increased Mn SOD activity, decreased $\cdot O_2^-$ production, reduced enzyme leakage, decreased lipid peroxidation, increased cell viability, and well-preserved cell structure. These studies strongly suggest that preconditioning can be induced in isolated myocytes against anoxic injury 24 hours after repetitive short episodes of anoxia.

As early at 1992, Tritto et al.[17] showed that exposure of isolated rabbit hearts to a low, nontoxic dose of oxygen radicals produced by xanthine and xanthine oxidase mimicked the beneficial effects of ischemic preconditioning. The present study also showed that exogenous $\cdot O_2^-$ could act similarly to brief repeated anoxia to trigger the late preconditioning, which was associated with increased Mn SOD activity. Thus, oxygen-derived free radicals besides being toxic may be beneficial to hearts at low levels by inducing preconditioning.

Although preconditioning is a very powerful endogenous mechanism of myocardial protection, one of its major limitations is that it lasts only up to two hours. However, myocardium becomes tolerant to longer ischemia after 24 hours. This is called late preconditioning. The exact time course of late preconditioning remains unknown. Recent data showed that a 50% reduction in infarct size is seen 48 hours after preconditioning and may last up to 72 hours.[18] In a conscious pig model, Sun et al.[5] found that late preconditioning is present 24 hours after the first sequence of coronary occlusions, but it can be extended for an additional 24 hours by a repeated sequence of occlusions. However, it dissipates within 10 days after the last exposure to ischemia. Thus, unlike early preconditioning, late preconditioning can last several days. This characteristic of late preconditioning makes it more attractive in the clinical setting. Unfortunately, the mechanisms of late preconditioning are less understood. It is most likely that the induction of cardioprotective proteins, including stress proteins[4] and endogenous antioxidant enzymes,[6,11] may play a significant role in late preconditioning. Preconditioning with brief repeated ischemia significantly decreased infarct size after a 90-minute occlusion performed 24 hours after preconditioning. This protective effect was associated with a significant increase in myocardial Mn SOD, glutathione peroxidase and reductase.[3] Our results were in general agreement with the latter study that $\cdot O_2^-$ generated by brief repeated anoxia induced increased activity of Mn SOD, which was associated with reduced $\cdot O_2^-$ production and reduced cell injury 24 hours after preconditioning. When myocytes were treated with allopurinol, a xanthine oxidase inhibitor, during the initial preconditioning phase, the beneficial effects of repetitive anoxia were abolished. Similarly, late protection by exogenous $\cdot O_2^-$ was also lost. Taken together, these data provide strong evidence that oxygen radicals produced by short repetitive anoxia served as a strong stimulant of the endogenous antioxidant defense system, which was associated with late protection of preconditioning.

In addition to Mn SOD, endogenous antioxidant defense systems may also include catalase, another antioxidant enzyme. Induction of catalase is observed in swine hearts preconditioned by repeated short ischemia and reperfusion.[19] Thus, catalase could be a part of endogenous antioxidant defenses enhanced by initial oxidative stress of ischemic preconditioning, though it was not tested in the present study. Recently, considerable attention was focused on the role of stress proteins, another group of cardioprotective proteins, in late preconditioning. Marber *et al.*[4] reported that a "second window of protection" of ischemic preconditioning was associated with induction of heat shock proteins. This was further explored by Kukreja *et al.*,[20] who have shown that oxygen species such as exogenous $\cdot O_2^-$, hydrogen peroxide, or singlet oxygen can trigger an increased expression of heat shock protein 70 in isolated rat hearts. Therefore, synthesis of stress proteins might occur as a result of initial oxidative stress of ischemic preconditioning.

Adenosine released during initial ischemia is another component of early preconditioning.[21] However, its role in late preconditioning is conflicting. A recent study[22] showed that the late protection in the rabbit could be blocked by administration of 8-(*p*-sulphophenyl) theophylline, a nonspecific adenosine A_1 receptor blocker, showing a common pathway of both early and late preconditioning. In contrast, another study[5] demonstrated that a sequence of brief coronary occlusions activates an unknown endogenous cardioprotective mechanism, not mediated by adenosine receptors, which increase the resistance of the myocardium to stunning 24 hours later.

In conclusion, the present results provide evidence that oxygen-derived free radicals caused by brief repetitive anoxia enhance endogenous antioxidant defenses that appear to be responsible for the late protection of preconditioning. Further work is needed to explore potential mechanisms underlying induction of endogenous antioxidant defenses.

SUMMARY

The primary objective of the study was to test the hypothesis that oxygen radical during initial anoxia stimulate endogenous antioxidant activity in late preconditioning in myocytes. Isolated rat myocytes were preconditioned in one group with two cycles of 5 minutes of anoxia and 5 minutes of reoxygenation and in another group with exogenous superoxide anion ($\cdot O_2^-$) generated by reaction of xanthine oxidase with xanthine. Myocytes were kept for 24 hours, after which they were exposed to 60 minutes of anoxia and 60 minutes of reoxygenation. Preconditioned myocytes exhibited decreased LDH release, reduced malondialdehyde formation, increased cell viability, and well-preserved cell structure. $\cdot O_2^-$ production was increased in myocytes immediately after treatment with repetitive anoxia (1.65 $\pm$ 0.08 nmol/mg protein) or exogenous $\cdot O_2^-$ (1.42 $\pm$ 0.11 nmol/mg protein). Allopurinol, a xanthine oxidase inhibitor, abolished $\cdot O_2^-$ production during the initial preconditioning period. Twenty-four hours later, Mn SOD activity declined in anoxic control myocytes (0.38 $\pm$ 0.06 U/mg protein), whereas it increased significantly in myocytes preconditioned with repetitive anoxia (3.25 $\pm$ 0.15 nmol/mg protein) or with exogenous $\cdot O_2^-$ (2.27 $\pm$ 0.10 nmol/mg protein). The increase in Mn SOD activity and myocardial protective effects observed in preconditioned myocytes were totally blocked by allopurinol. These results indicate that oxygen radicals generated during the initial preconditioning period activate endogenous antioxidant defense (increased Mn SOD activity) 24 hours later, which contributes to the late cardioprotection of preconditioning.

REFERENCES

1. DOWNEY, J. M. 1992. Trends Cardiovasc. Med. 2: 170–176.
2. MURRY, C. E., V. J. RICHARD, R. B. JENNINGS & K. A. REIMER. 1991. Am. J. Physiol. 260: H796–H804.
3. HOSHIDA, S., T. KUZUYA, N. FUJI, N. YAMASHITA, H. OE, M. HORI, K. SUZUKI, N. TANIGUCHI & M. TADA. 1993. Am. J. Physiol. 264: H33–H39.
4. MARBER, M. S., D. S. LATCHMAN, J. M. WALKER & D. M. YELLON. 1993. Circulation 88: 1264–1272.
5. SUN, J. Z., X. L. TANG, A. KNOWLTON, S. W. PARK, Y. QIU & R. BOLLI. 1995. J. Clin. Invest. 95: 388–403.
6. YAMASHITA, N., M. NISHIDA, S. HOSHIDA, T. KUZUYA, M. HORI, N. TANIGUCHI, T. KAMADA & M. TADA. 1994. J. Clin. Invest. 94: 2193–2199.
7. ZWEIER, J. L. 1988. J. Bio. Chem. 263: 1353–1357.
8. KHALID, M. A. & M. ASHRAF. 1993. Circ. Res. 72: 725–736.
9. MIKI, S., M. ASHRAF, S. SALKA & N. SPERELAKIS. 1988. J. Mol. Cell. Cardiol. 20: 1009–1024.
10. BOLLI, R. 1990. Circulation 82: 723–738.
11. ZHOU, X. B., X. L. ZHAI & M. ASHRAF. 1996. Circulation 93: 1177–1184.
12. DAS D. K., R. M. ENGELMAN & Y. KIMURA. 1993. Cardiovasc. Res. 27: 578–584.
13. TAKEMURA, G., T. ONODERA & M. ASHRAF. 1994. J. Mol. Cell. Cardiol. 26: 441–454.
14. WALLENSTEIN, S., C. L. ZUKER & J. L. FLEISS. 1980. Circ. Res. 47: 1–9.
15. KIRSHENBAUM, L. A., T. P. THOMAS, A. K. RANDHAWA & P. K. SINGAL. 1992. Mol. Cell. Biochem. 111: 25–31.
16. ARMSTRONG, S. & C. E. GANOTE. 1995. Cardiovasc. Res. 29: 647–652.
17. TRITTO, I., G. AMBROSIO, P. P. ELIA, A. SCOGNAMINGLIO, P. CIRILLO & M. CHIARIELLO. 1992. Circulation 86: I-30 (abstract).
18. YELLON, D. M. & G. F BAXTER. 1995. J. Mol. Cell. Cardiol. 27: 1023–1034.
19. DAS, D. K., M. R. PRASAD, D. LU & R. M. JONES. 1992. Cell. Mol. Biol. 38: 739–749.
20. KUKREJA, R. C., M. C. KONTOS, K. E. LOESSER, S. K. BATRA, Y. QIAN, C. J. GBUR, JR., S. A. NASEEM, R. L. JESSE & M. L. HESS. 1994. Am. J. Physiol. 267: H2213–H2219.
21. LIU, G. S., J. THORNTON, D. M. VAN WINKLE, A. W. H. STANLEY, R. A. OLSSON & J. M. DOWNEY. 1991. Circulation 84: 350–356.
22. BAXTER, G. F., M. R. PHARMS, M. S. MARBER, V. C. PATEL & D. M. YELLON. 1994. Circulation 90: 2993–3000.

Windows for HSP 70[a]

LUC H. E. H. SNOECKX,[b] RICHARD CORNELUSSEN,
ROBERT S. RENEMAN, AND GER J. VAN DER VUSSE

Cardiovascular Research Institute Maastricht (CARIM)
Department of Physiology
University of Limburg
Maastricht, The Netherlands

INTRODUCTION

It is now widely accepted that the induction of heat-shock proteins (HSPs) in the heart can confer protection against an ischemic insult and accompanying reperfusion damage.[1-3] Indeed, following an initial (over)expression of HSPs in cardiac tissue, reperfusion after a period of global ischemia is characterized by a significantly improved global left ventricular hemodynamic performance, a diminution of the duration of postischemic arrhythmias, and a reduced loss of intracellular enzymes compared to nontreated controls.[4-7] In models with regional ischemia in which stress pretreatment of the heart leads to overexpression of HSPs, infarct size as related to the area at risk has been shown to be diminished.[8-12] Tissue necrosis was found to be limited and regional contractile function to be improved significantly. As such, hyperthermic pretreatment also prevents myocardial stunning.[13]

By far the most striking inducible heat-shock protein during increased cellular stress is a member of the HSP 70 family, *i.e.*, HSP 72.[14,15] To ascertain a causal relationship between the amount of induced protein and the concomitant protection, several investigators studied isolated cells transfected with HSP 72.[16-18] By this technique unwanted influences of secondary phenomena related to the applied form of pretreatment (for example, heat shock, endotoxin, or amphetamines) could be excluded. In these cells and in even more sophisticated models, like transgenic mice, it was confirmed that increased intracellular levels of the HSP 72 protein are indeed associated with a better resistance to stressful events and with an improved postischemic functional recovery.[19,20] As such these experiments strengthened earlier observations in intact animals that the degree of postischemic improvement is related to the amount of HSP 72 protein induced in cardiac tissue.[21,22]

Although all these data provided strong evidence that the improvement of postischemic performance is related to the amount of the HSP 72 protein present in the tissue, it is still unclear whether the protein itself is responsible for the protection or that the protein activates secondary mechanisms yielding the protective effect. This question is difficult to answer, since the inhibition of the expression of the HSP 72 protein itself also would prevent the protection by secondary

[a] Supported by grants from the Dutch Heart Foundation (Grant No. 92.057) and the European Community (Grant No. BMH1-CT-1171).

[b] Address for correspondence: LHEH Snoeckx, PhD, Cardiovascular Research Institute Maastricht (CARIM), Department of Physiology, University of Limburg, P.O. Box 616, NL-6200 MD Maastricht, The Netherlands. Tel.: 043-3881203; Fax: 043-3671028.

mechanisms to occur. Moreover the inhibition of associated phenomena has not led to unequivocal results. For instance, it was demonstrated that the overexpression of HSP 72 in heat-shocked rat hearts is associated with a higher activity of the hydroxyl scavenging enzyme catalase,[4,7,23,24] the activity of which can be blocked by pretreatment with the drug 3-amino-1,2,4-triazole.[23,25,26] Some investigators reported that the improvement of postischemic mechanical recovery could be abolished completely after pretreatment with this compound,[25,26] while others only found an inhibiting effect on the heat shock-associated postischemic improvement of total coronary vasodilatory capacity but not on the mechanical recovery of the left ventricle.[23] Although it is still unclear how specific aminotriazole is in blocking the effects of catalase, these results support the hypothesis that the HSP 72 protein is not solely responsible for the acquired increased ischemia tolerance, on the condition that aminotriazole has no effect on the activity of the HSP 72 protein itself.

Although the evidence is overwhelming that heat-shock proteins can provide cardioprotection, there are circumstances under which the beneficial effects are absent. In the present survey these circumstances will be discussed and some illustrative examples, indicating that the heat shock-related cardioprotection can only be appreciated under some but not all experimental conditions, will be presented. In other words, there are several windows for optimal protection by heat shock-induced HSP 72 (over)expression.

The Dependency on Time after Induction of HSP 72

Preliminary data obtained in *in vitro* perfused rat hearts indicate that heat shock exerts a triphasic effect on the subsequent tolerance to an ischemic insult.[28] If heat shock precedes the ischemic period by only 60 min, postischemic mechanical recovery is significantly less than in nontreated control hearts. However, during a period of 90–420 min after heat shock the depressant effect disappears and postischemic mechanical performance in heat-shocked and control hearts is completely comparable. Only 24 hours after heat shock a significant improvement of postischemic functional recovery has been observed. These findings indicate that directly or indirectly heat shock exerts a negative effect on left ventricular performance immediately following heat shock. The nature of this depressant effect is unknown but could be due to excessive destabilization or denaturation of intracellular proteins as a consequence of the superimposition of two consecutive stresses, *i.e.*, heat shock and ischemia. It is conceivable that the HSP 72 protein is not yet present in high enough amounts within one hour following heat shock, although it has been shown by several investigators that the HSP 72 protein is an early gene product and can be detected in myocardial tissue within 3 hours following transient increased stress.[14,15,27] On the other hand, since there is an obvious (over)expression of the HSP 72 protein within a few hours after heat shock, it is surprising that the ischemia tolerance is only improved 24 hours after the stress period.[26,28] This obvious discrepancy between presence of the HSP 72 protein in the cardiac tissue and the absence of protection could be a consequence of different intracellular locations of the interacting molecules or to secondary mechanisms which take more time to be activated. Besides, it cannot be excluded that paracrine effects are also involved, being a consequence of HSP 72-mediated exocytosis of active compounds.

In line with the discrepancy between HSP 72 protein presence and absence of protection during the early phase following heat shock is the observation of

Currie and colleagues that infarct size in rabbit hearts could not be limited anymore when ischemia was applied 40 hours following heat shock, although the HSP 72 protein was still present in the tissue in substantial amounts.[10] Therefore, a better understanding of the interaction of the HSP 72 protein with other proteins within the first 3 days following heat shock is needed to elucidate the discrepancy between the presence of the HSP 72 protein and its cardioprotective effect occurring at certain moments during the posthyperthermic period. The above mentioned observations provide clear evidence for the presence of a time-window for the efficacy of heat shock-mediated cardioprotection.

The Dependency on the Duration of the Ischemic Period

In recent years some interesting information was presented regarding the effects of variable durations of the regional or global ischemic period on heat shock-mediated cardioprotection. For instance, in rabbits under *in vivo* circumstances hyperthermic pretreatment was associated with a significant reduction in infarct size as related to the area at risk following a 30-min period of regional global ischemia.[10,11] However, Yellon and colleagues reported earlier that following hyperthermic pretreatment infarct size of the heart could not be reduced compared to that in nontreated control hearts following a period of regional ischemia of 45 min.[29] This obvious absence of protection was probably not due to differences in or a lack of induction of HSP 72[27] so that it is likely that in this case the absence or presence of heat shock-mediated protection is determined by a rather narrow time-window. It also indicates that every additional minute between 30 and 45 min of ischemia is critical for the final metabolic and functional outcome of the compromised tissue. It is of interest to note that also in other animal models, like the rat, a comparable window of protection has been reported. Indeed, twenty-four hours after hyperthermic treatment a temporary *in vivo* coronary occlusion for 30 and 45 min was followed by improved salvage of tissue and absence of any beneficial effect, respectively.[9]

However, the time dependency of heat shock-mediated protection is also affected by the experimental circumstances. Unlike the *in vivo* circumstances as discussed above, in an *in vitro* study in the isolated rabbit heart, using cristalloid buffers or erythrocyte-supplemented cristalloid buffers, it has been reported that after a 45-min period of regional ischemia infarct size could successfully be reduced by earlier hyperthermic treatment.[8] The explanation which has been forwarded for this obvious contradictory observation is that the *in vivo* and *in vitro* perfusion circumstances differ substantially. It has been suggested that circulating whole blood contains elements which adversely affect the beneficial effects of heat shock.[8] Another indication that *in vivo* and *in vitro* circumstances differ substantially comes from observations in the global ischemic *in vitro* perfused heart model. We and others studied isolated cristalloid-perfused rat hearts, in which hyperthermic pretreatment failed to improve postischemic mechanical recovery when the ischemic time interval was too short.[30] In our laboratory we compared the postischemic functional recovery in isolated heat-shocked rat hearts (TABLE 1). Postischemic functional recovery after a 30-min ischemic period was compared with that after 45 min of global ischemia. During reperfusion following 30 min ischemia mechanical recovery was comparable in heated and nonheated hearts, while after 45 min ischemia pretreated hearts showed a significantly better mechanical function than the control hearts. These observations suggest that a certain degree of ischemic or reperfusion damage must be present before heat-shock

TABLE 1. Preischemic and Postischemic Mechanical Performance in Isolated Ejecting Rat Hearts 24 h after Normothermic (Control) or Hyperthermic (Heat Shock) Treatment[a]

	30-min Low-Flow Ischemia			45-min Global Ischemia		
	CO (ml/min)	dP/dt_{max} (kPa/s)	dP_{lv} (kPa)	CO (ml/min)	dP/dt_{max} (kPa/s)	dP_{lv} (kPa)
Control		(n = 7)			(n = 6)	
Preischemic	63 ± 13†	579 ± 85	10.5 ± 1.1	82 ± 11	559 ± 104	9.7 ± 1.1
Postischemic	51 ± 14	483 ± 53†	9.6 ± 0.9†	49 ± 13	371 ± 53	7.7 ± 0.8
% recovery	80 ± 11†	84 ± 5†	91 ± 3†	57 ± 10	70 ± 5	80 ± 1
Heat shock		(n = 6)			(n = 6)	
Preischemic	74 ± 10	587 ± 74	11.1 ± 1.2	84 ± 11	587 ± 157	10.5 ± 0.7
Postischemic	68 ± 12	506 ± 68	10.4 ± 0.9	64 ± 7*	476 ± 143*	9.1 ± 1.1*
% recovery	90 ± 5	87 ± 5	93 ± 2	77 ± 8*	80 ± 7*	87 ± 4*

[a] In an isolated ejecting heart preparation, hearts were allowed to eject against a pressure head of 8 kPa and were filled at a preload of 1.3 kPa. Left ventricular pressure was measured through a fluid-filled catheter via the left ventricular apex. Hearts were electrically paced at 300 beats per min. CO: cardiac output; dP/dt_{max}: positive maximal first derivative of the left ventricular pressure; dP_{lv}: left ventricular developed pressure. Heat shock was applied by hyperthermic treatment of the animals at 42°C for 15 min 24 h earlier. Number of investigated hearts is indicated above each group. Data are presented as mean values ± SD. *: significantly different from the values in the corresponding control group; †: significantly different from the values in the 45-min global ischemia group.

proteins can effectively provide protection to the heart. So, although identical periods of ischemia were applied as in the above mentioned *in vivo* models of regional ischemia, completely opposite results were obtained. All these experimental observations have to be taken into account to evaluate the dependency of the degree of protection on the duration of ischemia, but support the hypothesis of the presence of an ischemia duration window for heat shock-mediated cardioprotection.

The Dependency on the Load Imposed on the Heart

In hearts isolated from animals heat-shocked 24 hours earlier, we and others have shown that the afterload level imposed upon the heart is determinant for the presence or absence of improvement of postischemic mechanical function.[31,32] In our laboratory we investigated left ventricular contractile function at various afterloads in hearts isolated from hyperthermic pretreated rats before and after a 45-min period of global ischemia. The data are presented in FIGURE 1. When during the preischemic period afterload was increased above 13.3 kPa heat-shocked hearts performed significantly less than control hearts. Postischemically, the beneficial effects of hyperthermic pretreatment on mechanical performance can be appreciated when the hearts ejected against low afterloads. Stroke work, although compromised, was on the average 60% higher in heat-shocked than in control hearts. In contrast, at high afterload, this favorable effect had completely disappeared. The mechanism behind this afterload dependency is not completely clear, but the experimental findings suggest that the contractile proteins in the cardiomyocytes can only operate under certain (optimal) circumstances. It is not clear whether this is due to a nonspecific phenomenon linked to the heat shock procedure, to destabilization of the contractile proteins, to a limited availability of calcium for contraction, or to the use of a cristalloid solution to perfuse the heart. Again, a discrepancy between *in vivo* and *in vitro* circumstances appears, since in the heat-shocked heart under *in vivo* circumstances maximal (regional) recruitable stroke work is not hampered.[13] It should be emphasized, however, that in this situation extrapolations were made from regional contractile responses to a decrease in preload, and not from increases in afterload, as in our study.[31]

It is known that the pressure-overloaded hypertrophied heart functions at higher than normal afterload levels. Besides, it has been recognized that this type of heart is more vulnerable to damage induced by ischemia and/or reperfusion than the nonhypertrophied heart.[33] As such, protection of this type of heart during cardiac surgery has been a continuing problem for cardiac surgeons. In this particular case heat shock-mediated protection could meet the demands for a more optimal protection, since we and others found that the hypertrophied heart keeps its full capabilities to increase the expression of heat-shock proteins upon enhanced stress (unpublished results).[34] Thus it was tempting to investigate whether the hypertrophied heart could also be protected against ischemic damage by the prior induction of HSP 72 expression. Therefore, we performed a study on hypertrophied hearts (30% increase in heart weight to body weight ratio), isolated from rats heat-shocked 24 hours earlier. Ischemia tolerance in these hearts could be improved dramatically.[7] In addition, during both the preischemic and postischemic perfusion period coronary flow was significantly higher in the pretreated than in the control hearts. Even more important is the observation in the pretreated hypertrophied hearts that myocardial blood flow was more homogeneously distributed and that subendocardial no-reflow was prevented.

In earlier studies, we found that the functional recovery of the hypertrophied left ventricle can be improved by increasing postischemic perfusion pressure.[35]

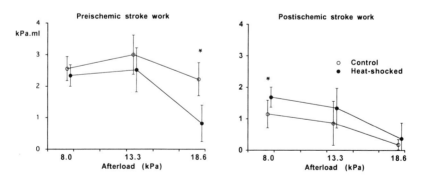

FIGURE 1. Preischemic and postischemic left ventricular stroke work [stroke volume (ml) × left ventricular systolic pressure (kPa)] in isolated rat hearts (n = 7 in both groups), ejecting against different afterload levels, varying between 8 and 18.6 kPa. Hearts were perfused with a cristalloid buffer and the left atrium was filled at a constant atrial pressure of 1.3 kPa. The buffer contained among others 2.25 mM $CaCl_2$ and 11 mM glucose. All hearts were paced at a frequency of 300 beats/min. Heat-shocked hearts were isolated from rats, hyperthermically pretreated 24 h earlier. *: significantly different from the corresponding values in the control group.

Because of the dependency of heat shock-mediated protection on afterload level (see above) heat-shocked hypertrophied hearts were reperfused after a period of ischemia at afterloads up to 18 kPa. In contrast to nonhypertrophied hearts, in which the beneficial effects of heat-shock pretreatment are completely absent at this afterload level, in hypertrophied hearts the improvement of postischemic mechanical performance was sustained, and significantly higher recovery values were found than in nontreated hypertrophied hearts. These observations again point to a specific dependency of heat shock-mediated cardioprotection on the loading conditions of each type of heart.

The Dependency on the Concentration of Circulating Calcium

The intracellular calcium homeostasis in the heat-shocked heart has not yet been studied in detail, but some evidence has been presented that calcium homeostasis is disturbed during the postischemic reperfusion period. This alteration has been ascribed to be associated with the beneficial effects of heat shock on membrane stability, since less calcium has been found in the mitochondria of reperfused heat-shocked hearts and heat-shocked hearts seem to be more resistant to a submaximal calcium paradox.[6,36]

We approached the eventual existing relationship between calcium homeostasis and hyperthermic pretreatment by challenging isolated ejecting rat hearts temporarily with various extracellular calcium concentrations during both the preischemic and postischemic perfusion periods 24 hours after heat shock.[37] As shown in FIGURE 2, under preischemic circumstances left ventricular stroke work was comparable in heat-shocked and control hearts at extracellular calcium levels ranging between 1.25 and 3 mM. However, at the lowest calcium concentration, i.e., 0.63 mM, heat-shocked hearts performed significantly less than the respective

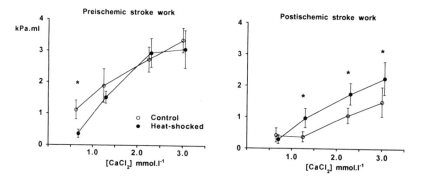

FIGURE 2. Preischemic and postischemic stroke work [stroke volume (ml) × left ventricular systolic pressure (kPa)] in isolated rat hearts (n = 7 in both groups) perfused with a cristalloid buffer in which the extracellular calcium concentration was temporarily varied in 4 consecutive steps between 0.63 and 3 mM. The diastolic aortic pressure was held constant at 8 kPa, a level known to have no negative effects on the left ventricular performance of the heat-shocked heart. All hearts were paced at a frequency of 300 beats/min. Hearts were isolated from rats, hyperthermically or normothermically pretreated 24 h earlier. *: significantly different from the corresponding values in the control group.

control hearts. A comparable phenomenon was observed during reperfusion following a 45-min global ischemia period. At extracellular calcium concentrations above 1.25 mM, stroke work in the heat-shocked hearts was significantly higher compared to that in control hearts, reflecting the beneficial effects of heat shock on postischemic mechanical performance. However, at the lowest calcium concentration, identical stroke work values in both groups of hearts were attained indicating that the beneficial effects of heat shock strongly depend on the interstitial calcium concentration. These findings strongly suggest the existence of a calcium-dependent window of heat shock-mediated cardioprotection.

The Dependency on Age and Condition of the Cardiac Tissue

In the search for the effectiveness of heat shock-mediated cardioprotection, the age of the heart should be considered. In view of the therapeutical application possibilities of this technique in cardiac patients, it is obvious that a substantial number of patients will be in the older age class. A complicating factor is that the cardiac tissue probably will not be in optimal condition, and function will be compromised. In animal experiments such circumstances are difficult to mimic. The age-related expression of HSP 72 has been documented only in healthy cardiac tissue. In rat hearts it was found that the induction of HSP 72 following heat stress decreases during aging.[34,39,40] In other studies performed on isolated cells, it was also observed that the ability to express heat-shock proteins decreases with age.[41-43] However, the age-related decrease in HSP 70 expression might be organ-specific. For instance, in heat-shocked hepatocytes isolated from young and old rats, identical HSP 70 transcript levels were found.[44] As mentioned these results were obtained in healthy tissue, whereas data on for instance infarcted or failing hearts lack completely. The difficulty in obtaining conclusive data in this domain is reflected in a study performed on patients undergoing coronary bypass surgery.[38] In these hearts the HSP 72 protein levels were found to be already high before any surgical manipulation of the heart, probably reflecting the activated stress response of the compromised cardiac tissue. However, since in this study no attempt was made to correlate the levels of expression to the patient's age, the range of which was between 4 and 71 years, conclusions on the age-dependency of HSP 72 expression are difficult to make. So, more detailed studies on healthy and/or failing human heart tissue of different ages will be needed to assess the significance of a possible age-related window for HSP 72 induction in cardiac tissue for applicability in the clinical setting.

CONCLUSIONS

During the last decade, the potential of stress-induced expression of heat-shock proteins for the protection of the ischemic heart has been studied extensively. The attractive side of this type of protection is that it involves an intrinsic defense mechanism of the heart, which seems to be present even in compromised tissues. However, since it is still unclear what the precise molecular mechanisms for induction of heat-shock proteins into the cardiac tissue are and how these proteins, once induced, confer cardioprotection, the level of protection is still difficult to control. Under certain circumstances, protection can even be absent, at least when mechanical performance is taken as a measure for cardiac function. The windows in which the heat shock-mediated cardioprotection can be appreciated are determined, among others, by the time lag between hyperthermic pretreatment and the ischemic insult, by the duration of the ischemic episode, by the afterload imposed upon the heart during reperfusion following ischemia, by the chosen experimental conditions, and by the calcium concentration present in the extracellular fluid during the postischemic reperfusion period. Moreover, the age of the hearts may also be a factor influencing the efficacy of heat shock-mediated protection. Within the clinical setting all these findings have to be taken into account when this pretreatment is considered to enhance the ischemic tolerance of the heart. Furthermore, in order to obtain better insight into the circumstances under which cardioprotection can be achieved more detailed studies on the interactions of inducible heat-shock proteins with other molecules and/or cardiac cellular structures are needed.

REFERENCES

1. MESTRIL, R. & W. DILLMANN. 1995. Heat shock proteins and protection against myocardial ischemia. J. Mol. Cell. Cardiol. **27:** 45–52.
2. MARBER, M. 1994. Stress proteins and myocardial protection. Clin. Sci. **86:** 375–381.
3. YELLON, D. M. & D. S. LATCHMAN. 1992. Stress proteins and myocardial protection. J. Mol. Cell. Cardiol. **24:** 113–124.
4. CURRIE, R., M. KARMAZYN, M. KLOC & K. MAILER. 1988. Heat-shock response is associated with enhanced post-ischemic recovery. Circ. Res. **63:** 543–549.
5. STEARE, S. & D. YELLON. 1993. The protective effect of heat stress against reperfusion arrhythmias in the rat. J. Mol. Cell. Cardiol. **25:** 1471–1481.
6. YELLON, D., E. PASINI, A. CARGNONI, M. MARBER, D. LATCHMAN & R. FERRARI. 1992. The protective role of heat stress in the ischaemic and reperfused rabbit myocardium. J. Mol. Cell. Cardiol. **24:** 895–907.
7. CORNELUSSEN, R., W. SPIERING, J. WEBERS, L. DE BRUIN, R. RENEMAN, G. VAN DER VUSSE & L. SNOECKX. 1994. Heat shock improves the ischemic tolerance of the hypertrophied rat heart. Am. J. Physiol. **267:** H1941–H1947.
8. WALKER, D., S. KUCUKOGLU, M. MARBER, E. ILIODROMITES, R. FERRARI & D. YELLON. 1993. Heat stress limits infarct size in the isolated perfused rat heart. Cardiovasc. Res. **27:** 962–967.
9. DONNELLY, T., R. SIEVERS, F. VISSERN, W. WELCH & C. WOLFE. 1991. Heat-shock protein induction in rat hearts. A role for improved myocardial salvage after ischemia and reperfusion. Circulation **85:** 769–778.
10. CURRIE, R. W., R. M. TANGUAY & J. J. KINGMA. 1993. Heat-shock response and limitation of tissue necrosis during occlusion/reperfusion in rabbit hearts. Circulation **87:** 963–971.
11. MARBER, M. S., D. S. LATCHMAN, J. M. WALKER & D. M. YELLON. 1993. Cardiac stress protein elevation 24 hours after brief ischemia or heat stress is associated with resistance to myocardial infarction. Circulation **88:** 1264–1272.
12. KUZUYA, T., A. HOSHIDA, N. YAMASHITA, H. FUJI, H. OE, M. HORI, T. KAMADA & M. TADA. 1993. Delayed effects of sublethal ischemia on the acquisition of tolerance to ischemia. Circ. Res. **72:** 1293–1299.
13. ROBINSON, B., T. MORITA, D. TOFT & J. MORRIS. 1995. Accelerated recovery of postischemic stunned myocardium after induced expression of heat shock protein (HSP 70). J. Thorac. Cardiovasc. Surg. **109:** 753–764.
14. SNOECKX, L. H., F. CONTARD, J. L. SAMUEL, F. MAROTTE & L. RAPPAPORT. 1991. Expression and cellular distribution of heat-shock and nuclear oncogene proteins in rat hearts. Am. J. Physiol. H1443–H1451.
15. CURRIE, R. W. & R. M. TANGUAY. 1991. Analysis of RNA for transcripts for catalase and SP71 in rat hearts after *in vivo* hyperthermia. Biochem. Cell Biol. **69:** 375–382.

16. SANDERS WILLIAMS, R., J. THOMAS, M. FINA, Z. GERMAN & I. BENJAMIN. 1993. Human heat-shock protein 70 (HSP 70) protects murine cells from injury during metabolic stress. J. Clin. Invest. **92:** 503–508.
17. HEADS, R., D. LATCHMAN & D. YELLON. 1994. Stable high level expression of a transfected human HSP 70 gene protects a heart-derived muscle cell line against thermal stress. J. Mol. Cell. Cardiol. **26:** 695–699.
18. MESTRIL, R., S. CHI, M. SAYEN, K. O'REILLY & W. DILLMANN. 1994. Expression of inducible stress protein 70 in rat heart myogenic cells confers protection against simulated ischemia-induced injury. J. Clin. Invest. **93:** 759–767.
19. MARBER, M., R. MESTRIL, S-H. CHI, M. SAYEN, D. YELLON & W. DILLMANN. 1995. Overexpression of the rat inducible 70-kD heat stress protein in a transgenic mouse increases the resistance of the heart to ischemic injury. J. Clin. Invest. **95:** 1446–1456.
20. PLUMIER, J., B. ROSS, R. CURRIE, C. ANGELIDIS, H. KAZLARIS, G. KOLLIAS & G. PAGOULATOS. 1995. Transgenic mice expressing the human heat shock protein 70 have improved post-ischemic myocardial recovery. J. Clin. Invest. **95:** 1854–1860.
21. HUTTER, M. M., R. E. SIEVERS, V. BARBOSA & C. L. WOLFE. 1994. Heat-shock protein induction in rat hearts. A direct correlation between the amount of heat-shock protein induced and the degree of myocardial protection. Circulation **89:** 355–360.
22. MARBER, M. S., J. M. WALKER, D. S. LATCHMAN & D. M. YELLON. 1994. Myocardial protection after whole body heat stress in the rabbit is dependent on metabolic substrate and is related to the amount of the inducible 70-kD heat stress protein. J. Clin. Invest. **93:** 1087–1094.
23. AMRANI, M., J. O'SHEA, J. CORBETT, M. DUNN, S. TADJKARIMI, S. THEODOROPOULOS, J. PEPPER & M. YACOUB. 1993. Role of catalase and heat shock protein on recovery of cardiac endothelial and mechanical function after ischemia. Cardioscience **4:** 193–198.
24. STEARE, S. & D. YELLON. 1994. Increased endogenous catalase activity caused by heat stress does not protect the isolated rat heart against exogenous hydrogen peroxide. Cardiovasc. Res. **28:** 1096–1101.
25. BROWN, J., M. GROSSO, L. TERADA, G. WHITMAN, A. BANERJEE, C. WHITE, A. HARKEN & J. REPINE. 1989. Endotoxin pretreatment increases indogenous myocardial catalase activity and decreases reperfusion injury of isolated rat hearts. Proc. Natl. Acad. Sci. USA **86:** 2516–2520.
26. KARMAZYN, M., K. MAILER & R. CURRIE. 1990. Acquisition and decay of heat-shock-enhanced post-ischemic ventricular recovery. Am. J. Physiol. **259:** H424–H431.
27. KNOWLTON, A., P. BRECHER & C. APSTEIN. 1991. Rapid expression of heat shock protein in the rabbit after brief cardiac ischemia. J. Clin. Invest. **87:** 139–147.
28. CORNELUSSEN, R., M. VORK, G. VAN DER VUSSE, R. RENEMAN & L. SNOECKX. 1995. Time-related effects of heat stress on cardiac protection against ischemia and reperfusion in the isolated rat heart. Pflügers Arch. (Eur. J. Physiol.) **430:** R20.
29. YELLON, D. M., E. ILIODROMITIS, D. S. LATCHMAN, W. D. VAN, J. M. DOWNEY, F. M. WILLIAMS & T. J. WILLIAMS. 1992. Whole body heat stress fails to limit infarct size in the reperfused rabbit heart. Cardiovasc. Res. **26:** 342–346.
30. CURRIE, R. W. & M. KARMAZYN. 1990. Improved post-ischemic ventricular recovery in the absence of changes in energy metabolism in working rat hearts following heat-shock. J. Mol. Cell. Cardiol. **22:** 631–636.
31. CORNELUSSEN, R., L. DE BRUIN, G. VAN DER VUSSE & L. SNOECKX. 1994. Is the post-ischemic heat-shock mediated protection of the hypertrophied rat heart perfusion pressure dependent? *In* ISHR European Section Meeting, Copenhagen (Denmark). S. Hannso & K. Kjeldsen, Eds. 559–563. Monduzzi Editore. Bologna, Italy.
32. WALL, S., H. FLISS & B. KORECKY. 1993. Role of catalase in myocardial protection against ischemia in heat shocked rats. Mol. Cell. Biochem. **129:** 187–194.
33. SNOECKX, L., G. VAN DER VUSSE, W. COUMANS, P. WILLEMSEN & R. RENEMAN. 1993. Differences in ischemia tolerance between hypertrophied hearts of adult and aged spontaneously hypertensive rats. Cardiovasc. Res. **27:** 874–881.
34. BONGRAZIO, M., L. COMINI, G. GAIA, T. BACHETTI & R. FERRARI. 1994. Hypertension, aging, and myocardial synthesis of heat shock protein 72. Hypertension **24:** 620–624.

35. SNOECKX, L., G. VAN DER VUSSE, F. VAN DER VEEN, W. COUMANS & R. RENEMAN. 1989. Recovery of hypertrophied rat hearts after global ischemia and reperfusion at different perfusion pressures. Pflügers Arch. **413:** 303–312.

36. MARBER, M. S., J. M. WALKER, D. S. LATCHMAN & D. M. YELLON. 1993. Attenuation by heat stress of a submaximal calcium paradox in the rabbit heart. J. Mol. Cell. Cardiol. **25:** 1119–1126.

37. CORNELUSSEN, R., G. VAN DER VUSSE, R. RENEMAN & L. SNOECKX. 1996. Inability of the heat-shocked to adjust its preischemic and postischemic performance to variable loading conditions. J. Mol. Cell. Cardiol. **28:** 291–298.

38. MCGRATH, L., M. LOCKE, M. CANE, C. CHEN & C. IANUZZO. 1995. Heat shock protein (HSP 72) expression in patients undergoing cardiac operations. J. Thorac. Cardiovasc. Surg. **109:** 370–376.

39. NITTA, Y., K. ABE, M. AOKI, I. OHNO & S. ISOYAMA. 1994. Diminished heat shock protein 70 mRNA induction in aged rats after ischemia. Am. J. Physiol. **267:** H1795–H1803.

40. LUCE, M. & V. CRISTOFALO. 1992. Reduction in heat shock gene expression correlates with increased thermosensitivity in senescent human fibroblasts. Exp. Cell Res. **202:** 9–16.

41. PAHLAVANI, M., M. HARRIS, S. MOORE, R. WEINDRUCH & A. RICHARDSON. 1995. The expression of heat shock protein 70 decreases with age in lymphocytes from rats and rhesus monkeys. Exp. Cell Res. **218:** 310–318.

42. EFFROS, R., X. ZHU & R. WALFORD. 1994. Stress response of senescent T-lymphocytes: reduced cHSP 70 is independent of the proliferative block. J. Gerontol. **49:** B65–B70.

43. FARGNOLI, J., T. KUNISADA, A. FORNACE, E. SCHNEIDER & N. HOLBROOK. 1990. Decreased expression of heat shock protein 70 mRNA and protein after heat shock treatment in cells of aged rats. Proc. Natl. Acad. Sci. USA **87:** 846–850.

44. HEYDARI, A., C. CONRAD & A. RICHARDSON. 1995. Expression of heat shock genes in hepatocytes is affected by age and food restriction in rats. J. Nutr. **125:** 410–418.

The Role of Protein Kinase C in Ischemic Preconditioning

MAHIKO GOTO, MICHAEL V. COHEN, AND
JAMES M. DOWNEY[a]

Departments of Physiology and Medicine
University of South Alabama
College of Medicine
Mobile, Alabama 36688

INTRODUCTION

Ischemic preconditioning is a phenomenon whereby a brief period of ischemia renders the myocardium resistant to infarction from a subsequent ischemic insult. Preconditioning was first reported by Murry *et al.* in 1986.[1] They demonstrated that preconditioning the dog heart with four brief periods of ischemia caused the heart to tolerate a subsequent ischemic insult with only a fraction of the infarction realized in nonpreconditioned hearts. Since then, numerous studies have been done to elucidate the mechanism of preconditioning. While the exact mechanism remains unknown, much evidence has accumulated from this[2,3] and other[4,5] laboratories that protein kinase C plays an important role.

Adenosine Receptor Antagonists Block the Protection of Ischemic Preconditioning

The first insight into preconditioning's mechanism came when we found that adenosine receptor stimulation could also trigger the protection associated with ischemic preconditioning.[6] Open-chest anesthetized rabbits experienced 30 minutes of regional ischemia and 180 minutes of reperfusion. One of 2 antagonists, 8-(*p*-sulfophenyl)theophylline (SPT) or *N*-[2-(dimethylamino)ethyl]*N*-methyl-4-(2,3,6,7-tetrahydro-2,6-dioxo-1,3-dipropyl-1*H*-purine-8-yl)benzosulfonamide (PD 115,199), was given 20 minutes prior to the 30-minute ischemia. FIGURE 1 reveals that in the untreated group $38.9 \pm 4.2\%$ of the ischemic risk zone infarcted, while preconditioning with 5 minutes of regional ischemia and 10 minutes of reflow prior to the same 30-min ischemic insult caused infarcts to be much smaller ($7.8 \pm 1.8\%$) ($p < 0.001$ vs control). Pretreatment with SPT or PD 115,199 had no significant effect on infarct size in nonpreconditioned hearts, but the protection afforded by preconditioning disappeared when hearts were pretreated with either antagonist.

[a] Address for correspondence: James M. Downey, Ph.D., Department of Physiology, MSB 3024, University of South Alabama, College of Medicine, Mobile, AL 36688. Tel.: 334-460-6818; Fax: 334-460-6464.

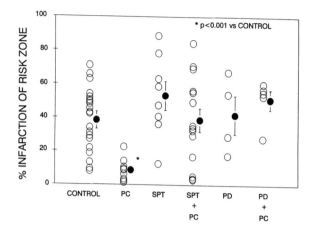

FIGURE 1. Infarct size normalized as a percentage of the risk zone appears on the *vertical axis. Open symbols* represent individual animals and *closed symbols* are means and standard error for the groups. PC, preconditioned; SPT, 8-(*p*-sulfophenyl)theophylline; PD, *N*-[2-(dimethylamino)ethyl]*N*-methyl-4-(2,3,6,7-tetrahydro-2,6-dioxo-1,3-dipropyl-1*H*-purine-8-yl)benzosulfonamide (PD 115,199). Both adenosine receptor blockers, SPT and PD 115,199, blocked protection of preconditioning. (From Liu *et al.*[6] Reprinted by permission from *Circulation.*)

Adenosine Agonists Can Mimic Ischemic Preconditioning

We hypothesized that endogenous adenosine released during the brief ischemia was the initiator of preconditioning. If that hypothesis were correct, it was reasoned that exposure to exogenous adenosine should protect the heart equally as well as exposure to ischemia. We first tried to infuse adenosine intravenously as a substitute for preconditioning.[6] A dose of 1 mg/min produced profound hypotension and further increases in dose were not tolerated by the animals. Infarct size in this group was $44.0 \pm 8.3\%$, indicating that this dose of adenosine was not sufficient to protect the myocardium from infarction. The inability of intravenous adenosine to protect was probably due to a failure to achieve a sufficient concentration of adenosine in the myocardium to induce a preconditioning effect. Adenosine deaminase quickly degrades adenosine in the blood which would further limit the amount of adenosine that actually gets into the myocardium. This suggestion was supported by the absence of cardiac slowing, a known A_1-mediated cardiac effect of adenosine, in these rabbits treated with intravenous adenosine.

To eliminate the systemic side effect, we decided to infuse adenosine directly into the coronary arteries. Because intracoronary infusions are difficult in the *in situ* heart, a blood-perfused, isolated heart model was used to test the adenosine hypothesis. The hearts were perfused with circulating oxygenated blood from a support rabbit and electrically paced to avoid adenosine-mediated bradycardia. The hearts underwent 45 minutes of regional ischemia followed by 120 minutes of reperfusion. The results appear in FIGURE 2. Infarct size in the control group averaged $32.1 \pm 4.1\%$, whereas that in preconditioned hearts was significantly smaller at $7.8 \pm 1.7\%$. In a third group, adenosine was infused directly into the coronary perfusate for 5 minutes at a total dose of 1.4 mg. The infusion was then

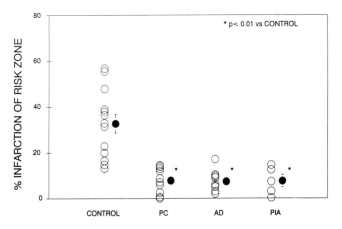

FIGURE 2. Infarct size for four isolated rabbit heart groups. PC, preconditioned; AD, adenosine; PIA, N^6-1-(phenyl-2R-isopropyl)-adenosine. Intracoronary infusion of adenosine or PIA was equipotent with ischemic preconditioning in protecting the isolated blood-perfused rabbit heart from infarction. (From Liu *et al.*[6] Reprinted by permission from *Circulation*.)

stopped for 10 minutes to simulate the period of reperfusion. The third panel of FIGURE 2 reveals that intracoronary adenosine significantly protected the heart, to the same degree as ischemic preconditioning.

The Adenosine A_1 Receptor Is Involved in Preconditioning

In an attempt to determine which adenosine receptor subtype is involved in the protection of preconditioning, we tested the A_1 selective analogue N^6-1-(phenyl-2R-isopropyl)-adenosine (PIA). The fourth panel of FIGURE 2 shows that PIA also protected the heart when infused at a total dose of 26.6 μg over 5 minutes followed by 10 minutes of drug-free washout. This dose of PIA was chosen because it lengthened the P-R interval, an adenosine A_1 effect, but had no effect on the coronary resistance, an adenosine A_2 effect. Thus, an A_1 selective agonist was equipotent with ischemic preconditioning.

There has been verification of the adenosine theory of preconditioning in rabbit,[7] pig,[8,9] and dog[10] and human cardiomyocytes.[11] Interestingly, adenosine receptor blockade does not block protection from preconditioning in rat heart.[12,13]

Protein Kinase C Activation Is an Important Step

Recent studies from this[2,3] and other[4,5] laboratories have shown that protein kinase C (PKC) plays an important role in ischemic preconditioning. Adenosine A_1 receptors in tissues including guinea pig myocardium have been reported to cause phospholipase C activation.[14–18] Phospholipase C activity leads to the production of two second messengers, diacylglycerol (DAG) and inositol trisphosphate. DAG is an activator of PKC.[19–21] PKC modifies proteins within the cell by phosphorylating them. Therefore, we tested the proposal that activation of PKC by A_1 receptor stimulation is an important step leading to protection.

To test this hypothesis, either of two inhibitors of PKC, staurosporine (50 μg/kg) or polymyxin B (24 mg/kg), was administered as a bolus to *in vivo* rabbits 5 minutes prior to the 30-minute ischemia.[2] In all rabbits regional ischemia was followed by 180 minutes of reperfusion. PC groups were preconditioned with 5 minutes of ischemia and 10 minutes of reperfusion. Regional ischemia in nonpreconditioned hearts treated with staurosporine or polymyxin B resulted in $40.5 \pm 2.8\%$ and $42.0 \pm 7.0\%$ infarction of the risk zone, respectively (FIG. 3). Both inhibitors, however, blocked protection in preconditioned hearts with $36.2 \pm 2.7\%$ and $40.9 \pm 2.5\%$ of the risk zone infarcted, respectively.

Staurosporine inhibits PKC by interacting with the ATP-binding site, but its specificity for PKC is poor.[22] On the other hand, polymyxin B acts at the lipid regulatory site of PKC and has no known effect against other kinases.[23] Furthermore, a subsequent study from this laboratory[24] showed that chelerythrine, which competitively inhibits the phosphate acceptor and reportedly has very high selectivity for PKC,[25] also abolished the protective effect of ischemic preconditioning. Taken together these results strongly support a role for PKC in ischemic preconditioning.

We tested whether activation of PKC with 1-oleoyl-2-acetyl glycerol (OAG) or 4β-phorbol 12-myristate 13-acetate (PMA) could mimic ischemic preconditioning in buffer-perfused isolated hearts. All hearts underwent 30 minutes of regional ischemia and 120 minutes of reperfusion. Exposure of hearts to either OAG (10 nmol/min) or PMA (0.01 nmol/min) for 5 minutes followed by 10 minutes of washout prior to the 30 minutes of ischemia significantly limited infarct size ($11.7 \pm 3.3\%$ and $5.9 \pm 1.2\%$, respectively) (FIG. 4). Because PKC activity is required for the preconditioned heart to be protected and because pretreatment with PKC

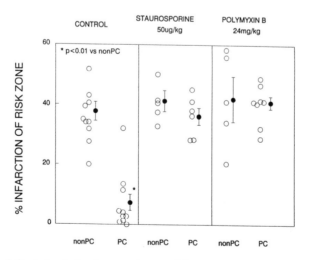

FIGURE 3. Infarct size in *in vivo* experiments. PC, preconditioned. Both protein kinase C inhibitors staurosporine and polymyxin B abolished protection from ischemic preconditioning. (From Ytrehus *et al.*[2] Reprinted by permission from the *American Journal of Physiology*.)

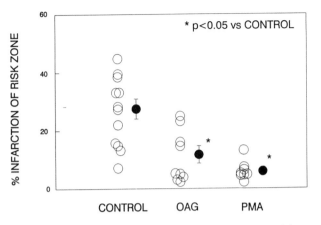

FIGURE 4. Infarct size in isolated heart experiments. OAG, 1-oleoyl-2-acetyl glycerol; PMA, 4β-phorbol 12-myristate 13-acetate. Pretreatment with OAG or PMA protected the heart. (From Ytrehus *et al.*[2] Reprinted by permission from the *American Journal of Physiology.*)

activators mimic preconditioning, we concluded that PKC is an important step in the mechanism of preconditioning.

The Translocation Theory of Ischemic Preconditioning

One of the striking characteristics of ischemic preconditioning is that the myocardium can somehow remember that it has been preconditioned. The myocardium enters the preconditioned state once it is exposed to brief ischemia, and it stays in that state for about one hour.[26,27] Similarly, exposure to adenosine causes protection even when the adenosine is allowed to wash out prior to the onset of ischemia.[6] The mechanism of this "memory" has not been determined, but we have hypothesized that it may be related to PKC. The most obvious explanation would be phosphorylation of a protective protein which persisted for about one hour. When the phosphate was removed, the heart would revert back to a nonprotected state.

The data, however, do not support the phosphorylation theory of memory. Note that protection from ischemic preconditioning was blocked by the PKC inhibitors even though they were administered late in the reflow phase after the end of the preconditioning ischemia (FIG. 3). That would indicate that the phosphorylation step that is being blocked must be occurring during the 30-minute ischemic period rather than during the preceding 5-minute preconditioning ischemia. Furthermore, we found that in isolated hearts staurosporine had no effect on the protection of ischemic preconditioning when it was included in the perfusate only before and during the preconditioning ischemia and then allowed to wash out prior to the 30-minute period of ischemia. Staurosporine, however, completely blocked protection when administered just prior to the sustained ischemia.[3,28] These results suggest that phosphorylation of protein is not necessary during the preconditioning ischemia, but that protection requires phosphorylation of protein to occur during the long ischemia.

That observation led us to propose an alternative hypothesis, the translocation theory of preconditioning. One of the peculiarities of PKC is that it must first translocate from the cytosol to the membranes before it can be activated. Translocation can be relatively slow and is thought to account for the delayed response often seen with PKC activation, since most of the kinase resides in the cytosol of the quiescent cell. Strasser et al.[29] reported that translocation of PKC from the cytosolic to the particulate fraction of the heart occurred in acute myocardial ischemia in the rat. Moreover, Yuan et al.[20] reported that in rat ventricle translocation induced by phorbol dibutyrate was complete only after 10 minutes, a time course which is very compatible with the kinetics of ischemic preconditioning.

We propose that adenosine receptor activation during ischemic preconditioning initiates translocation of PKC into the membrane as is shown in FIGURE 5 and once PKC has translocated it stays in the membrane for about 1 hour. During the second occlusion renewed binding of agonist to the adenosine receptor would reactivate PKC which would already be in place, thus permitting kinase activity to begin immediately. If the protein responsible for protection must be phosphorylated in the first few minutes of ischemia to realize protection then the delay caused by the translocation step would prevent the critical phosphorylation from occurring in nonpreconditioned myocardium. Such a delay would be absent in preconditioned myocardium since PKC is already in the membrane and phosphory-

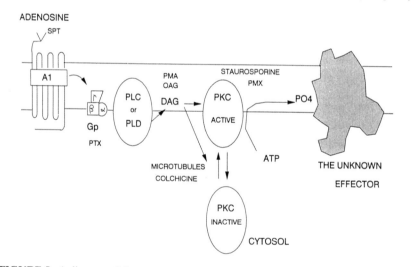

FIGURE 5. A diagram of the proposed intracellular signaling system used in preconditioning. In the first ischemic period adenosine populates A_1 receptors. Adenosine receptors couple to phospholipase C through a pertussis toxin-sensitive G protein. The DAG produced by the lipase causes cytosolic protein kinase C to translocate slowly into the membranes where it can be activated. Because of the delay required for translocation, little protein is phosphorylated. PKC remains in the membranes during reperfusion. In the second ischemic period repopulation of adenosine receptors reactivates the pathway. Since translocation has already occurred, an unidentified protein is phosphorylated early in ischemia resulting in protection. PTX, pertussis toxin; PMX, polymyxin B; PMA, phorbol myristate acetate; OAG, oleoyl acetyl glycerol; SPT, 8-(p-sulfophenyl)theophylline—all either activators or antagonists of preconditioning.

lation could proceed immediately after the onset of the second ischemia. The translocation theory then states that the only difference between preconditioned and nonpreconditioned myocardium is that the former has PKC translocated into the membrane at the onset of the sustained ischemia.

Microtubules have been shown to be involved in translocation. We also found that disrupting microtubules with colchicine blocked the protective effect of preconditioning, further supporting the translocation theory.[3] Direct proof of the translocation theory has been difficult to obtain. The reason is that there are many isoforms of PKC in the heart[30] and each has a different translocation pattern.[31] Any one of these could be responsible for the protection, and technical problems have so far prevented quantification of individual isoform movements in rabbit heart.

Agents That Activate PKC Can Precondition the Heart

The translocation theory predicts that any agent that activates PKC should also trigger protection. For example, the α_1-adrenergic receptor is known to couple to PKC in the myocyte.[30,32-36] We tested whether phenylephrine (PE), an α_1 agonist, could precondition isolated hearts.[37] Infarction was produced by 30 minutes of regional ischemia. PE (0.1 μM) was infused for 5 minutes, followed by a 10-minute drug-free interval before the prolonged ischemia. This brief infusion of PE was able to protect the heart, and this protective effect could be abolished by the PKC inhibitor, polymyxin B (50 μM). Thus we concluded that α_1-adrenergic receptors can precondition the heart with involvement of PKC activation.

Similarly we examined the roles of angiotensin AT_1[38] and bradykinin B_2[39] receptors, which have also been shown to activate PKC.[40-45] Either angiotensin II (100 mM) or bradykinin (400 nM) was infused for 5 minutes prior to the 30-minute ischemia. As expected, both agents significantly limited infarction and the protection again could be blocked by a PKC inhibitor, polymyxin B (50 μM). The protection from angiotensin II was abolished by an AT_1 receptor blocker, losartan, and that from bradykinin by a B_2 receptor antagonist, HOE 140, indicating that both AT_1 and B_2 receptors indeed triggered the protection.

Multiple Agonists Activate PKC to Trigger Ischemic Preconditioning

Agonists binding to the adenosine A_1,[6,7] adrenergic α_1,[37] angiotensin AT_1,[38] and bradykinin B_2[39,46] receptors infused in lieu of ischemia can all trigger preconditioning. Furthermore, endogenous agonists to all these receptors are released to some extent during ischemia. Thus we must ask if any other than adenosine acts to mediate ischemic preconditioning? Adenosine receptor blockers can block protection from ischemic preconditioning with a single 5-minute coronary occlusion in rabbit hearts,[6,7] whereas α_1-adrenergic antagonists[37,47] cannot. Hence not enough endogenously produced adrenergic agonist is released during a 5-minute period of ischemia in rabbit hearts to stimulate sufficient α_1-receptors and trigger the protection of ischemic preconditioning. However, when we tried to precondition isolated rabbit hearts with 10 minutes of hypoxia we found that the adenosine receptor blocker SPT could not block that protection. Only when we combined SPT with an α_1-receptor blocker was protection from hypoxia blocked.[48] Thus, under conditions of hypoxia enough norepinephrine was released to participate in the protection. In the rat heart α_1 stimulation appears to be much more important than adenosine.[49]

Next we tested whether bradykinin B_2 receptor activation is involved in the mechanism of ischemic preconditioning. A B_2 receptor antagonist HOE 140 was administered intravenously to anesthetized rabbits.[39] All rabbits underwent 30 minutes of regional ischemia followed by 180 minutes of reperfusion. In the PCx1 group hearts were subjected to 5 minutes of ischemia and 10 minutes of reperfusion before 30 minutes of ischemia. The PCx4 group was preconditioned with four cycles of 5-minute ischemia/10-minute reperfusion. The HOE group received HOE 140 (26 μg/kg) 30 minutes before the 30-minute ischemia. In the HOE + PCx1 and HOE + PCx4 groups, the same dose of HOE 140 was given 15 minutes before the ischemic preconditioning protocol. This dose of HOE 140 was shown to completely abolish the transient hypotensive effect of bradykinin for up to 2 hours. The infarct size data are shown in FIGURE 6. Thirty minutes of regional ischemia produced 36.7 ± 2.6% infarction of the risk zone in the control group, whereas preconditioning with one cycle of ischemia/reperfusion dramatically reduced infarct size to 10.2 ± 2.2%. Preconditioning with four cycles also significantly limited infarct size (6.4 ± 2.2%). HOE 140 alone had no effect on infarct size (40.6 ± 5.3%), but it completely abolished the protective effect of one-cycle ischemic preconditioning (34.1 ± 1.6%). However, when the hearts were preconditioned by four cycles of ischemia/reperfusion, HOE 140 failed to block protection (10.7 ± 3.5%).

Because blockade of either bradykinin B_2[39] or adenosine[6] receptors could abort the protection of one-cycle ischemic preconditioning, we proposed that preconditioning with 5 minutes of ischemia, which itself is very close to the threshold of protection,[26,50] does not produce enough bradykinin or adenosine

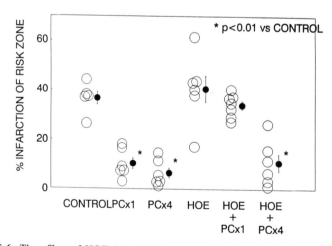

FIGURE 6. The effect of HOE 140 (HOE) on protection from ischemic preconditioning (PC). Both one (PCx1) and four cycles of PC (PCx4) were protective. HOE by itself did not affect infarct size. HOE was able to block the protection of one cycle of PC (HOE + PCx1). However, if the ischemic stimulus were reinforced with four cycles of PC, then HOE could no longer abort the protection (HOE + PCx4). (Modified from Goto *et al.*[39])

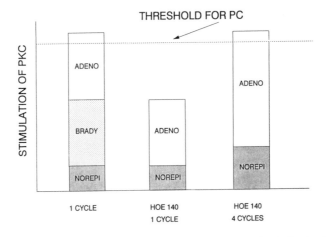

FIGURE 7. Scheme suggesting that a threshold of protein kinase C (PKC) stimulation must be reached before ischemic preconditioning (PC) can protect the heart. One cycle of PC releases multiple agonists, of which at least two (adenosine [ADENO] and bradykinin [BRADY]) play major roles in triggering protection by having additive effects on PKC stimulation such that the hypothesized threshold is exceeded. However, BRADY receptor blockade with HOE 140 will remove the BRADY component of PKC stimulation, thus resulting in subthreshold PKC stimulation and absence of protection. But if the ischemic stimulus is reinforced with four cycles of PC, additional release of ADENO and other agonists can adequately compensate for the absent BRADY and result in sufficient PKC stimulation to exceed the threshold level. NOREPI indicates norepinephrine. (From Goto et al.[39] Reprinted by permission from *Circulation Research*.)

separately for either one to precondition the heart. Rather, their combined effect appears to be required before enough PKC stimulation occurs to reach the threshold for protection. As shown in FIGURE 7 blockade of either the bradykinin or the adenosine component would prevent that threshold from being reached. However, when the preconditioning stimulus was intensified with four cycles, bradykinin blockade was no longer able to abort protection. We propose that repeated episodes of ischemia simply increased the duration of adenosine receptor stimulation to attain the threshold level even when bradykinin receptors were blocked.

We do not know what other stimuli to PKC may also participate along with bradykinin and adenosine. Angiotensin AT_1 receptors may play a role in ischemic preconditioning.[51] Blockade of endothelin-1 receptors does not abolish protection from ischemic preconditioning in the isolated rabbit heart,[52] suggesting that this agonist plays a minor role. Free radicals produced by reperfusion after a 5-minute period of ischemia can activate PKC directly. Indeed, free radical scavengers block protection from a single cycle of preconditioning[53] but not from multiple cycles.[54] Thus, free radicals may also have an important physiological role in this response. These studies reveal that the pathway for triggering preconditioning is very redundant, which apparently insures that this adaptation will occur should the heart experience ischemia. They also reveal that interspecies differences are to be expected. Different agonists may well predominate in different species.

Interruption of Glucose Uptake Can Also Trigger Ischemic Preconditioning

Recently we noted that isolated rabbit hearts could be preconditioned by transient perfusion with perfusate devoid of glucose.[55] Our first assumption was that the metabolic deficit simply caused ATP catabolism and adenosine production. This protection could be blocked by polymyxin B (50 μM), a protein kinase C inhibitor, but not by the adenosine receptor inhibitor SPT, suggesting that the mechanism was similar to that of ischemic preconditioning but did not involve adenosine receptors. Adding 20 mM pyruvate to the glucose-containing buffer for 15 minutes prior to ischemia inhibited glycolysis without incurring a metabolic deficit because pyruvate is a preferred substrate over glucose. This again preconditioned the hearts. Every time that glucose uptake was inhibited the heart was put into a preconditioned state. These results suggested that the heart could be preconditioned by simply blocking glucose uptake transiently. When we infused pyruvate into the blood of open-chest rabbits, however, no protection was seen. One difference between the blood-perfused and the isolated Krebs buffer-perfused hearts is that the former derives only a small fraction of its energy from glucose metabolism and as a result has a low rate of glucose uptake. These data would suggest that interruption of glucose uptake would only trigger protection in a heart in which glucose uptake was substantial to begin with. To test that theory we added to the perfusate acetate (1 mM), which increases the rate of tricarboxylate-cycle turnover. As predicted, neither omission of glucose nor addition of pyruvate caused protection in hearts perfused with buffer containing acetate. We concluded that inhibition of glycolysis can precondition the heart by activation of PKC, but only if lipid substrates are absent.

Workers should be cautioned that addition of pyruvate can unexpectedly precondition the isolated heart. That can give the appearance that pyruvate is cardioprotective, but unfortunately the observation cannot be extrapolated to the clinical setting.

Phospholipase D Couples Adenosine Receptors to PKC

One of the most vexing problems with the PKC hypothesis of preconditioning is the issue of whether adenosine receptors couple to PKC. For technical reasons few studies attempt measurements of PKC activity in response to receptor stimulation. Rather, most investigators measure the release of inositol phosphate, a product of phospholipase C (PLC) activation. Indeed, the amount of PLC activity resulting from adenosine receptor stimulation is modest at best,[14] while others have claimed that adenosine does not couple to PLC.[56,57] Recently we investigated whether phospholipase D (PLD) might be activated by A_1 adenosine receptors. Phospholipase D (PLD) hydrolyzes phosphatidylcholine rather than phosphatidylinositol and in so doing does not produce inositol phosphate. The lipid product from PLD is phosphatidic acid rather than diacylglycerol. The phosphatidic acid is subsequently converted to diacylglycerol by a phosphohydrolase.

PLD activity in the heart can be measured by its ability to effect the transphosphatidylation reaction. In that reaction labeled alcohol such as butanol is added to the perfusate and PLD performs a base exchange with endogenous phospholipids leaving labeled phosphatidylbutanol in the tissue.[58] We perfused rabbit hearts with ^{14}C-butanol and measured the amount of labeled phosphatidylbutanol formed. Preconditioning increased PLD activity 90% above baseline. Furthermore, a 20-minute exposure to PIA caused a similar 78% increase in PLD activity.[59] PLD-derived diacylglycerol appears to be physiologically significant. When PLD was activated by sodium oleate in the isolated rabbit heart model, infarction decreased from 30.4 ± 2.2% of the risk zone in untreated hearts to 15.1 ± 2.0%. Furthermore, 100 μM propranolol, which is a potent inhibitor of the phosphohydrolase,[58] completely blocked protection from both traditional preconditioning and PIA pretreatment in the isolated myocyte preparation.[59] Therefore, we propose that PLD may serve to couple adenosine receptors to PKC in the heart.

CONCLUSION

These studies strongly suggest that PKC activation plays an important role in the infarct-limiting effect of ischemic preconditioning. However, the overall mechanism of how PKC activation protects the ischemic heart remains unknown. We do not know what isoform of PKC is activated and what protein is phosphorylated by PKC. If the mechanism can be fully understood, we will be able to use a safe and efficient drug to precondition patients with coronary artery disease in lieu of ischemia.

REFERENCES

1. MURRY, C. E., R. B. JENNINGS & K. A. REIMER. 1986. Preconditioning with ischemia: a delay of lethal cell injury in ischemic myocardium. Circulation 74: 1124–1136.
2. YTREHUS, K., Y. LIU & J. M. DOWNEY. 1994. Preconditioning protects ischemic rabbit heart by protein kinase C activation. Am. J. Physiol. 266: H1145–H1152.
3. LIU, Y., K. YTREHUS & J. M. DOWNEY. 1994. Evidence that translocation of protein kinase C is a key event during ischemic preconditioning of rabbit myocardium. J. Mol. Cell. Cardiol. 26: 661–668.
4. SPEECHLY-DICK, M. E., M. M. MOCANU & D. M. YELLON. 1994. Protein kinase C: its role in ischemic preconditioning in the rat. Circ. Res. 75: 586–590.
5. BUGGE, E. & K. YTREHUS. 1995. Ischaemic preconditioning is protein kinase C dependent but not through stimulation of α adrenergic or adenosine receptors in the isolated rat heart. Cardiovasc. Res. 29: 401–406.
6. LIU, G. S., J. THORNTON, D. M. VAN WINKLE, A. W. H. STANLEY, R. A. OLSSON & J. M. DOWNEY. 1991. Protection against infarction afforded by preconditioning is mediated by A₁ adenosine receptors in rabbit heart. Circulation 84: 350–356.
7. TSUCHIDA, A., T. MIURA, T. MIKI, K. SHIMAMOTO & O. IIMURA. 1992. Role of adenosine receptor activation in myocardial infarct size limitation by ischaemic preconditioning. Cardiovasc. Res. 26: 456–461.
8. SCHWARZ, E. R., M. MOHRI, S. SACK & M. ARRAS. 1991. The role of adenosine and its A₁-receptor in ischemic preconditioning. Circulation 84(Suppl. II): II-191. Abstract.
9. VAN WINKLE, D. M., G. L. CHIEN, R. A. WOLFF, B. E. SOIFER, K. KUZUME & R. F. DAVIS. 1994. Cardioprotection provided by adenosine receptor activation is abolished by blockade of the K$_{ATP}$ channel. Am. J. Physiol. 266: H829–H839.
10. AUCHAMPACH, J. A. & G. J. GROSS. 1993. Adenosine A₁ receptors, K$_{ATP}$ channels, and ischemic preconditioning in dogs. Am. J. Physiol. 264: H1327–H1336.
11. IKONOMIDIS, J. S., T. SHIRAI, R. D. WEISEL, B. DERYLO, V. RAO, C. I. WHITESIDE, D. A. G. MICKLE & R-K. LI. 1995. "Ischemic" or adenosine preconditioning of human ventricular cardiomyocytes is protein kinase C dependent. Circulation 92(Suppl. I):I-12. Abstract.
12. LIU, Y. & J. M. DOWNEY. 1992. Ischemic preconditioning protects against infarction in rat heart. Am. J. Physiol. 263: H1107–H1112.
13. LI, Y. & R. A. KLONER. 1993. The cardioprotective effects of ischemic 'preconditioning' are not mediated by adenosine receptors in rat hearts. Circulation 87: 1642–1648.

14. Kohl, C., B. Linck, W. Schmitz, H. Scholz, J. Scholz & M. Tóth. 1990. Effects of carbachol and $(-)$-N^6-phenylisopropyladenosine on myocardial inositol phosphate content and force of contraction. Br. J. Pharmacol. **101:** 829–834.
15. Schiemann, W. P., D. P. Westfall & I. L. O. Buxton. 1991. Smooth muscle adenosine A_1 receptors couple to disparate effectors by distinct G proteins in pregnant myometrium. Am. J. Physiol. **261:** E141–E150.
16. Spielman, W. S., K-N. Klotz, L. J. Arend, B. A. Olson, D. G. LeVier & U. Schwabe. 1992. Characterization of adenosine A_1 receptor in a cell line (28A) derived from rabbit collecting tubule. Am. J. Physiol. **263:** C502–C508.
17. Schwiebert, E. M., K. H. Karlson, P. A. Friedman, P. Dietl, W. S. Spielman & B. A. Stanton. 1992. Adenosine regulates a chloride channel via protein kinase C and a G protein in a rabbit cortical collecting duct cell line. J. Clin. Invest. **89:** 834–841.
18. Stiles, G. L. 1992. Adenosine Receptors. J. Biol. Chem. **267:** 6451–6454.
19. Kishimoto, A., Y. Takai, T. Mori, U. Kikkawa & Y. Nishizuka. 1980. Activation of calcium and phospholipid-dependent protein kinase by diacylglycerol, its possible relation to phosphatidylinositol turnover. J. Biol. Chem. **255:** 2273–2276.
20. Yuan, S., F. A. Sunahara & A. K. Sen. 1987. Tumor-promoting phorbol esters inhibit cardiac functions and induce redistribution of protein kinase C in perfused beating rat heart. Circ. Res. **61:** 372–378.
21. Capogrossi, M. C., T. Kaku, C. R. Filburn, D. J. Pelto, R. G. Hansford, H. A. Spurgeon & E. G. Lakatta. 1990. Phorbol ester and dioctanoylglycerol stimulate membrane association of protein kinase C and have a negative inotropic effect mediate by changes in cytosolic Ca^{2+} in adult rat cardiac myocytes. Circ. Res. **66:** 1143–1155.
22. Tamaoki, T. 1991. Use and specificity of staurosporine, UCN-01, and calphostin C as protein kinase inhibitors. Methods Enzymol. **201:** 340–347.
23. Casnellie, J. E. 1991. Protein kinase inhibitors: probes for the functions of protein phosphorylation. Adv. Pharmacol. **22:** 167–205.
24. Liu, Y., M. V. Cohen & J. M. Downey. 1994. Chelerythrine, a highly selective protein kinase C inhibitor, blocks the antiinfarct effect of ischemic preconditioning in rabbit hearts. Cardiovasc. Drugs Ther. **8:** 881–882.
25. Herbert, J. M., J. M. Augereau, J. Gleye & J. P. Maffrand. 1990. Chelerythrine is a potent and specific inhibitor of protein kinase C. Biochem. Biophys. Res. Commun. **172:** 993–999.
26. Van Winkle, D. M., J. D. Thornton, D. M. Downey & J. M. Downey. 1991. The natural history of preconditioning: cardioprotection depends on duration of transient ischemia and time to subsequent ischemia. Coron. Artery Dis. **2:** 613–619.
27. Miura, T., T. Adachi, T. Ogawa, T. Iwamoto, A. Tsuchida & O. Iimura. 1992. Myocardial infarct size-limiting effect of ischemic preconditioning: its natural decay and the effect of repetitive preconditioning. Cardiovasc. Pathol. **1:** 147–154.
28. Yang, X-M., J. R. Fletcher, J. M. Downey & M. V. Cohen. 1995. The long ischemia is the critical time for kinase activity during ischemic preconditioning. J. Mol. Cell. Cardiol. **27:** A157. Abstract.
29. Strasser, R. H., R. Braun-Dullaeus, H. Walendzik & R. Marquetant. 1992. α_1-Receptor-independent activation of protein kinase C in acute myocardial ischemia: mechanisms for sensitization of the adenylyl cyclase system. Circ. Res. **70:** 1304–1312.
30. Bogoyevitch, M. A., P. J. Parker & P. H. Sugden. 1993. Characterization of protein kinase C isotype expression in adult rat heart: protein kinase C-ε is a major isotype present, and it is activated by phorbol esters, epinephrine, and endothelin. Circ. Res. **72:** 757–767.
31. Mitchell, M. B., X. Meng, L. Ao, J. M. Brown, A. H. Harken & A. Banerjee. 1995. Preconditioning of isolated rat heart is mediated by protein kinase C. Circ. Res. **76:** 73–81.
32. Okumura, K., T. Kawai, H. Hashimoto, T. Ito, K. Ogawa & T. Satake. 1988. Sustained diacylglycerol formation in norepinephrine-stimulated rat heart is associated with α_1-adrenergic receptor. J. Cardiovasc. Pharmacol. **11:** 651–656.

33. KAKU, T., E. LAKATTA & C. FILBURN. 1991. α-Adrenergic regulation of phosphoinositide metabolism and protein kinase C in isolated cardiac myocytes. Am. J. Physiol. **260:** C635–C642.

34. TALOSI, L. & E. G. KRANIAS. 1992. Effect of α-adrenergic stimulation on activation of protein kinase C and phosphorylation of proteins in intact rabbit hearts. Circ. Res. **70:** 670–678.

35. FEDIDA, D., A. P. BRAUN & W. R. GILES. 1993. α_1-Adrenoceptors in myocardium: functional aspects and transmembrane signaling mechanisms. Physiol. Rev. **73:** 469–487.

36. TERZIC, A., M. PUCÉAT, G. VASSORT & S. M. VOGEL. 1993. Cardiac α_1-adrenoceptors: an overview. Pharmacol. Rev. **45:** 147–175.

37. TSUCHIDA, A., Y. LIU, G. S. LIU, M. V. COHEN & J. M. DOWNEY. 1994. α_1-Adrenergic agonists precondition rabbit ischemic myocardium independent of adenosine by direct activation of protein kinase C. Circ. Res. **75:** 576–585.

38. LIU, Y., A. TSUCHIDA, M. V. COHEN & J. M. DOWNEY. 1995. Pretreatment with angiotensin II activates protein kinase C and limits myocardial infarction in isolated rabbit hearts. J. Mol. Cell. Cardiol. **27:** 883–892.

39. GOTO, M., Y. LIU, X-M. YANG, J. L. ARDELL, M. V. COHEN & J. M. DOWNEY. 1995. Role of bradykinin in protection of ischemic preconditioning in rabbit hearts. Circ. Res. **77:** 611–621.

40. SADOSHIMA, J-I. & S. IZUMO. 1993. Signal transduction pathways of angiotensin II-induced c-*fos* gene expression in cardiac myocytes *in vitro*: roles of phospholipid-derived second messengers. Circ. Res. **73:** 424–438.

41. FU, T., Y. OKANO, M. HAGIWARA, H. HIDAKA & Y. NOZAWA. 1989. Bradykinin-induced translocation of protein kinases C in neuroblastoma NCB-20 cell: dependence on 1,2-diacylglycerol content and free calcium. Biochem. Biophys. Res. Commun. **162:** 1279–1286.

42. MURRAY, M. A., D. D. HEISTAD & W. G. MAYHAN. 1991. Role of protein kinase C in bradykinin-induced increases in microvascular permeability. Circ. Res. **68:** 1340–1348.

43. BASCANDS, J-L., C. PECHER, G. BOMPART, J. RAKOTOARIVONY, J. L. TACK & J-P. GIROLAMI. 1994. Bradykinin-induced *in vitro* contraction of rat mesangial cells via a B_2 receptor type. Am. J. Physiol. **267:** F871–F878.

44. DIXON, B. S., R. V. SHARMA, T. DICKERSON & J. FORTUNE. 1994. Bradykinin and angiotensin II: activation of protein kinase C in arterial smooth muscle. Am. J. Physiol. **266:** C1406–C1420.

45. TIPPMER, S., U. QUITTERER, V. KOLM, A. FAUSSNER, A. ROSCHER, L. MOSTHAF, W. MÜLLER-ESTERL & H. HÄRING. 1994. Bradykinin induces translocation of the protein kinase C isoforms α, ε, and ζ. Eur. J. Biochem. **225:** 297–304.

46. WALL, T. M., R. SHEEHY & J. C. HARTMAN. 1994. Role of bradykinin in myocardial preconditioning. J. Pharmacol. Exp. Ther. **270:** 681–689.

47. THORNTON, J. D., J. F. DALY, M. V. COHEN, X-M. YANG & J. M. DOWNEY. 1993. Catecholamines can induce adenosine receptor-mediated protection of the myocardium but do not participate in ischemic preconditioning in the rabbit. Circ. Res. **73:** 649–655.

48. COHEN, M. V., R. S. WALSH, M. GOTO & J. M. DOWNEY. 1995. Hypoxia preconditions rabbit myocardium via adenosine and catecholamine release. J. Mol. Cell. Cardiol. **27:** 1527–1534.

49. BANERJEE, A., C. LOCKE-WINTER, K. B. ROGERS, M. B. MITCHELL, E. C. BREW, C. B. CAIRNS, D. D. BENSARD & A. H. HARKEN. 1993. Preconditioning against myocardial dysfunction after ischemia and reperfusion by an α_1-adrenergic mechanism. Circ. Res. **73:** 656–670.

50. MIURA, T. & O. IIMURA. 1993. Infarct size limitation by preconditioning: its phenomenological features and the key role of adenosine. Cardiovasc. Res. **27:** 36–42.

51. DIAZ, R. J., R. SANDHU & G. J. WILSON. 1995. Participation of angiotensin II receptors in ischemic preconditioning. J. Mol. Cell. Cardiol. **27:** A43. Abstract.

52. WANG, P., K. P. GALLAGHER, J. M. DOWNEY & M. V. COHEN. 1996. Pretreatment

with endothelin-1 mimics ischemic preconditioning against infarction in isolated rabbit heart. J. Mol. Cell. Cardiol. **28:** 579–588.

53. TANAKA, M., H. FUJIWARA, K. YAMASAKI & S. SASAYAMA. 1994. Superoxide dismutase and *N*-2-mercaptopropionyl glycine attenuate infarct size limitation effect of ischaemic preconditioning in the rabbit. Cardiovasc. Res. **28:** 980–986.

54. IWAMOTO, T., T. MIURA, T. ADACHI, T. NOTO, T. OGAWA, A. TSUCHIDA & O. IIMURA. 1991. Myocardial infarct size-limiting effect of ischemic preconditioning was not attenuated by oxygen free-radical scavengers in the rabbit. Circulation **83:** 1015–1022.

55. GOTO, M., A. TSUCHIDA, Y. LIU, M. V. COHEN & J. M. DOWNEY. 1995. Transient inhibition of glucose uptake mimics ischemic preconditioning by salvaging ischemic myocardium in the rabbit heart. J. Mol. Cell. Cardiol. **27:** 1883–1894.

56. HOLLINGSWORTH, E. B., R. A. DE LA CRUZ & J. W. DALY. 1986. Accumulations of inositol phosphates and cyclic AMP in brain slices: synergistic interactions of histamine and 2-chloroadenosine. Eur. J. Pharmacol. **122:** 45–50.

57. SCHACHTER, J. B. & B. B. WOLFE. 1992. Cyclic AMP differentiates two separate but interacting pathways of phosphoinositide hydrolysis in the DDT$_1$-MF$_2$ smooth muscle cell line. Mol. Pharmacol. **41:** 587–597.

58. MORARU, I. I., L. M. POPESCU, N. MAULIK, X. LIU & D. K. DAS. 1992. Phospholipase D signaling in ischemic heart. Biochim. Biophys. Acta **1139:** 148–154.

59. COHEN, M. V., Y. LIU, G. S. LIU, P. WANG, C. WEINBRENNER, G. A. CORDIS, D. K. DAS & J. M. DOWNEY. 1996. Phospholipase D plays a role in ischemic preconditioning in rabbit heart. Circulation. (In press.)

Preconditioning Potentiates Molecular Signaling for Myocardial Adaptation to Ischemia[a]

DIPAK K. DAS,[b] NILANJANA MAULIK,
TETSUYA YOSHIDA, RICHARD M. ENGELMAN,[c]
AND YOU-LI ZU[d]

Cardiovascular Division
Departments of Surgery and [d]Physiology
University of Connecticut School of Medicine
Farmington, Connecticut
and
[c]Department of Surgery
Baystate Medical Center
Springfield, Massachusetts

INTRODUCTION

Recent years have witnessed the development of a novel concept for myocardial preservation based on the fact that the enhancement of the endogenous cellular defense system provides each cell with new protein synthesis and thereby the means to protect itself when it is more susceptible to injury. Using this concept, it has been shown that preconditioning of heart by repeated stunning can delay the onset of further irreversible injury,[1,2] or even reduce the subsequent postischemic ventricular dysfunction[3–6] and incidence of ventricular arrhythmias.[7,8] Our laboratory has demonstrated that repeated ischemia, distinguished from a single ischemic insult, can reduce subsequent ischemia reperfusion injury[3,4] and postischemic ventricular fibrillation.[7] Such myocardial preservation by repeated short-term reversible ischemia leads to the development of the concept of stress adaptation. Consequently, new ideas of preconditioning have been developed which include adenosine,[9] potassium channel opening,[10] α_1-receptor,[11,12] oxidative stress,[13–15] hypoxia[16,17] and drug.[18,19]

Myocardial protection by ischemic preconditioning has opened a new horizon, and this concept is now believed to be one of the most powerful state-of-the-art techniques for the myocardial protection. Now recognized as a specific phenomenon, this is believed to occur via an endogenous protective mechanism.

The precise mechanism of ischemic preconditioning is far from clear. It is generally believed that ischemic preconditioning occurs in two different steps: (i) early effect (short-term adaptation) triggered between seconds to minutes, which

[a] This study was supported by NIH Grants HL 22559 and HL 34360, a Grant-in-Aid from the American Heart Association, as well as a grant from the Donaghue Medical Research Foundation.

[b] Correspondence: Dipak K. Das, Ph.D., Cardiovascular Division, Department of Surgery, University of Connecticut School of Medicine, Farmington, CT 06030-1110. Tel: (203) 679-3687; Fax: (203) 679-2451.

is likely to be mediated by the release of some endogenous compound(s) such as catecholamines and adenosine, and may last up to 1–2 hr (ischemic preconditioning); and late effect (long-term adaptation) which may occur after several hours and may last days to months. The long-term adaptation is believed to be mediated by the transcription of genes and their subsequent translation into proteins, and has been termed myocardial adaptation to ischemia.[20,21]

It remains, however, to establish the biochemical, cellular and molecular link between the early events of ischemic preconditioning and the late events of adaptation. Very recently, a role of protein kinase C in ischemic preconditioning was suggested. A short-term ischemia as well as ischemia followed by reperfusion were previously shown to translocate and activate protein kinase C.[22] Furthermore, both α_1-receptor stimulation and Ca^{2+} ion can translocate and activate protein kinase C.[23,24] Given the fact that both α_1-receptor activation and intracellular Ca^{2+} overloading are the manifestations of ischemia/reperfusion injury, it was not surprising when ischemic preconditioning consisting of repeated ischemia and reperfusion was also found to translocate and activate protein kinase C.[25,26] Interestingly, it has long been known that protein kinase C can activate the transcription of genes.[27] Indeed, many genes were found to be activated in the preconditioned myocardium.[28–32] Thus, protein kinase C, which is activated as a result of the events controlled by endogenous compounds (viz., α_1-receptor, adenosine, diacylglycerol), can be instrumental for gene expression leading to the translation into proteins. This uniqueness of protein kinase C led us to believe that this kinase could be the molecular link between ischemic preconditioning and myocardial adaptation.[20,21]

The results of a number of recent studies from our laboratory led us to believe that protein kinase C may not be the ultimate link between ischemic preconditioning and myocardial adaptation. These include the abundance of MAP kinase-activated protein (MAPKAP kinase 2) in heart, rapid activation of MAPKAP kinase 2 by stresses including heat stress, oxidative stress and ischemia/reperfusion, and most importantly, that it is MAPKAP kinase 2, and not protein kinase C that can phosphorylate small heat shock proteins, HSP 25/HSP 27, which are also activated by ischemic preconditioning. The objective of this study was, therefore, to re-examine the molecular link between ischemic preconditioning and ultimate adaptation to ischemia. In this study, we demonstrate for the first time that activation of protein tyrosine kinase is coupled with the activation of phospholipase D in ischemic preconditioning. Inhibition of tyrosine kinase results not only in the inhibition of phospholipase D, but also abolishes preconditioning-mediated activation of protein kinase C, MAP kinase and MAPKAP kinase 2. Finally, our studies demonstrate that induction of the expression of antioxidant genes are vital for adaptive modification, and transfection of mice with glutathione peroxidase (GSH-Px) gene supports this notion.

MATERIALS AND METHODS

Isolated Perfused Rat Heart Preparation for Intracellular Signaling Study

Sprague-Dawley male rats of approximately 350 gm body weight were anesthetized with intraperitoneal pentobarbital (80 mg/kg). After intravenous administration of heparin (500 IU/kg), the chests were opened, and the hearts were rapidly excised and mounted on a non-recirculating Langendorff perfusion apparatus. Retrograde perfusion was established at a pressure of 100 cm H_2O with oxygenated normothermic Krebs-Henseleit bicarbonate (KHB) buffer with the following ion concentrations (in mM): 118.0 NaCl, 24.0 NaHCO$_3$, 4.7 KCl, 1.2 KH$_2$PO$_4$, 1.2 MgSO$_4$, 1.7 CaCl$_2$, and 10.0 glucose. The KHB buffer had been previously equilibrated with 95% O$_2$/5% CO$_2$, pH 7.4 at 37°C. The experiments were divided into two groups. The experimental group received 100 μM genistein (Sigma Chemical, St. Louis, MO), a tyrosine kinase inhibitor, supplemented with KHB buffer for 10 min while the control group was perfused with buffer alone. The heart was preconditioned by subjecting to 5 min of ischemia by terminating the coronary flow followed by 10 min of reperfusion. The process was repeated four times.[3] The pulmonary vein was then cannulated and the Langendorff perfusion discontinued for subsequent working heart perfusion as described previously.[16] It was essentially a left-heart preparation in which oxygenated KHB at 37°C enters the cannulated pulmonary vein and left atrium at a filling pressure of 17 cm H$_2$O. The perfusion fluid then passes to the left ventricle from which it is spontaneously ejected through the aortic cannula against a pressure of 100 cm H$_2$O. The working hearts were perfused for 5 min for stabilization. Normothermic ischemia was induced for 30 min by terminating the left atrial flow which was followed by 30 min of reperfusion. The experiments were terminated prior to genistein treatment (baseline), after preconditioning, and after ischemia and reperfusion. Heart biopsies were frozen in liquid nitrogen for subsequent analysis of phospholipase D, protein kinase C, MAP kinases, and MAPKAP kinase 2. The release of creatine kinase (CK) was estimated in the perfusate buffer.

To examine the effects of genistein on myocardial functions, aortic flow and developed pressure were measured. The aortic flow was monitored using a calibrated rotameter while the developed pressure was determined as the difference between aortic end-systolic and aortic end-diastolic pressure measured through an on-line aortic pressure transducer. The data were recorded and analyzed in real time using the Cordat II data acquisition, analysis, and presentation system (Data Integrated Scientific Systems, Pinckney, MI; Triton Technologies, Inc., San Diego, CA).

To estimate phospholipase D activity, hearts were perfused with the buffer containing 250 μCi [1-^{14}C]-butanol (NEN, Boston, MA (4 mCi/mmol) (final concentration of butanol was 20 mM) prior to any treatment and preconditioning.[33] Biopsies were frozen in liquid nitrogen for subsequent assay for ^{14}C-phosphatidylbutanol.

Isolated Mouse Hearts from Control and GSH-Px Gene Transfected Mice

Mouse genomic clones for the cellular glutathione peroxidase (GSHPx-1) were initially isolated from a bacteriophage FIX II genomic library, prepared with DNA of 129/SVJ mouse (Stratagene, La Jolla, CA), by hybridization screening with a corresponding rat cDNA clone. A 5.3-kb SacI genomic fragment containing the entire mouse GSHPx-1 gene including approximately 2.0 kb of 5′ flanking sequence was used in microinjecting into fertilized mouse eggs derived from B6C3F1 × B6C3F1 mating according to the methods described by Hogan *et al.*[34] Two lines of transgenic mice carrying extra copies of the mouse GSHPx-1 gene were generated. The transgenic line Tg[MGP]-41 was used in this study.

Mice were randomly divided into two groups: transgenic-overexpressing GSHPx-1 and nontransgenic control. They were anesthetized with an intraperitoneal injection of sodium pentobarbital (200 mg/kg) and intravenous heparin sodium (500 U/kg) administered at the same time to prevent intravascular coagulation of blood. The heart was excised immediately after thoracotomy, and placed in cold perfusion buffer. The aorta was cannulated, and the heart was perfused by retrograde Langendorff method. The perfusion was maintained with Krebs-Henseleit bicarbonate buffer (KHB: composed of (in mM) NaCl, 118; $NaHCO_3$, 24; KCl, 4.7; KH_2PO_4, 1.2; $MgSO_4$, 1.2; $CaCl_2$ 1.7; and glucose 10) and gassed with 95% O_2 and 5% CO_2, pH 7.4 at 37°C, at a constant perfusion pressure of 80 cm H_2O. A small incision was made at the main trunk of the pulmonary artery to drain coronary effluent. The effluent was collected for one minute before ischemia, after ischemia and during reperfusion and stored at -20°C for subsequent measurement of creatine kinase (CK).

A 4-0 silk suture on a round bodied needle was passed through the apex of the heart and attached to the apex which in turn was attached to a force transducer. The heart rate (HR), force developed by the heart (DF) and first derivative of developed force (dF/dT) were recorded. Data of myocardial contractile function were recorded and analyzed in real time using the Cordat II data acquisition, analysis, and presentation system[16] (Data Integrated Scientific Systems, Pinckney, MI; Triton Technologies, Inc, San Diego, CA).

After stabilization, preischemic baseline contractile function was measured. The heart underwent 30 min ischemia under normothermia by clamping the aortic cannula, followed by 20 min reperfusion. Coronary flow was calculated before ischemia and at 20 min of reperfusion by quantifying the release of coronary effluent over one min.

CK release from the heart was estimated in the perfusate collected from the heart before ischemia, and at 1, 5, 10, 15 and 20 min after reperfusion using a CK assay kit obtained from Sigma Chemical Company (St. Louis, MO). The enzyme activity was expressed as units/ml perfusate.

Myocardial infarct size was determined by methods described previously by Marber et al.[37] with the following modifications. At the end of reperfusion, a 10% (wt/vol) solution of triphenyl tetrazolium in phosphate buffer (Na_2HPO_4 88 mM, NaH_2PO_4 1.8 mM) was infused into a side arm of the aortic cannula until the myocardium stained deep red. The heart was then excised, weighed and stored at -70°C.

For infarct size determination, frozen hearts were sliced perpendicularly to the long axis from apex to base in 0.8-mm-thick sections. Sections were then fixed in 2% paraformaldehyde. Thin mouse heart cross sections were placed between two cover slips and digitally imaged using an IBM-compatible PC and a Microtek ScanMaker 600z, a 600 dot per inch, flat-bed, full color scanner. The cross section was imaged at the maximum scaling and dot resolution that the scanner would allow. The digitized image was stored in Adobe TIFF file format by the software package, PhotoStyler, v.1.0.3, by U-Lead Systems, Inc. For analysis of infarct areas, some enhancement of the image was necessary at times to more clearly visualize the areas of staining by Corel Photo-Paint 4.0 (Corel Inc.). Corel was also used to mark the stained areas. To quantitate the areas of interest in pixels, a NIH Image 5.1 (a public-domain software package) was used. The entire area of risk was quantified in pixels using the computer software, and the measured infarct areas were compared to the entire area at risk in a blinded fashion.

Estimation of Phospholipase D

The frozen biopsies were homogenized and extracted with chloroform/methanol mixture.[33] Phospholipds were separated by thin layer chromatography on silica gel K6 plates using the organic phase of 2,2,4-trimethylpentane/ethyl acetate/ acetic acid/H_2O (6:11:2:9, v/v) as solvent. The phosphatidylbutanol band was identified by co-chromatography of authentic standard. The band was scraped off into a tube and radioactivity quantitated using a liquid scintillation counter.

Enzymatic Assay of Protein Kinase C, MAP Kinases, and MAPKAP Kinase 2

Approximately 0.3–0.4 gm of heart biopsy was placed in a measured volume of ice-cold Tris-sucrose buffer that contained 0.35 M sucrose, 10 mM Tris-HCl, pH 7.5, 1 mM EDTA, 0.5 mM DTT and 0.1 mM PMSF. The tissue was homogenized with a Polytron homogenizer, and the resulting homogenate was centrifuged at 15,000 g for 20 min. The supernatant was used for the estimation of protein kinase C, MAP kinases and MAPKAP kinase 2. Protein concentration was determined with a BCA protein assay kit (Pierce, Rockville, IL). For protein kinase C assay, 15 μg protein/15 μl were used from each sample in duplicate and added to 30 μl of final volume of kinase reaction mixture containing kinase buffer (20 mM Tris-HCl, pH 7.4, 1 mM EDTA, 50 mM KCl and 1 mM DTT), synthetic peptide substrate (M.W. 2342) (Upstate Biotechnology Inc., Lake Placid, NY), 40 μM [γ-^{32}P] ATP (4.4 × 10^3 cpm/pmol), phosphatidylserine (20 μg/ml), phorbol-12-myristate 13-acetate (2 μg/ml) and 1.6 mM $CaCl_2$. The reaction was allowed to proceed for 15 min at 30°C. The amount of [^{32}P] incorporation into the peptide was analyzed by a liquid scintillation counter.

To examine MAPKAP kinase 2, a synthetic peptide substrate derived from the amino acid residues 1–13 of glycogen synthase N-terminals (KKPLNRTLS-VASLPG-amide) was used.[35] Kinase assay was initiated by adding 15 μg of supernatant protein to a 40-μl reaction mixture containing 20 mM HEPES, pH 7.3, 10 mM $MgCl_2$, 1 mM EGTA, 5 μM sodium ortho-vanadate, 5 μM okadaic acid, 2 mM DTT, 20 μM H-7, 40 μM [γ-^{32}P] ATP (4.4 × 10^3 cpm/pmol), and 40 μM substrate peptide. The reaction was allowed to proceed for 10 min at 30°C. The amount of [^{32}P] incorporation into the peptide was analyzed by a liquid scintillation counter. MAP kinase activity was assessed using myelin basic protein as substrate under the same conditions as MAPKAP kinase 2 assay.

Statistical Analysis

The results are expressed as the mean ± standard error of the mean. An F-test was carried out first to compare variance between groups. Differences between groups were analyzed by a two-tailed unpaired Student's *t* test. A *p* value <0.05 was considered statistically significant.

RESULTS

Effects of Preconditioning on Myocardial Performance

For rats, we studied the left ventricular performances of the normal hearts after preconditioning and ischemia/reperfusion, and compared the results with those of genistein-treated hearts. Heart rate was not affected by preconditioning or by ischemia/reperfusion. Genistein had no effect on the heart rate. DP,

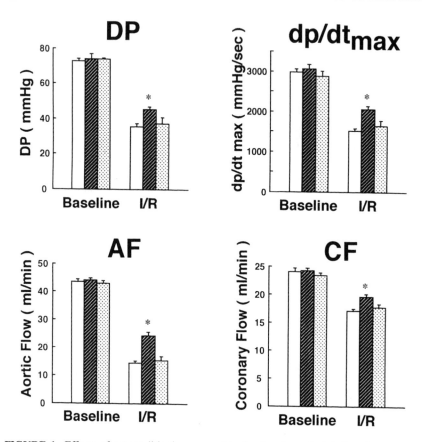

FIGURE 1. Effects of preconditioning on ventricular functions. Isolated rat hearts were perfused in the presence or absence of 100 μM genistein. Hearts were then subjected to preconditioning (4 × PC) followed by 30 min of ischemia and 30 min of reperfusion as described in Methods. Myocardial functions were obtained in real time using the Cordat II data acquisition, analysis, and presentation system. □ control, ▨ preconditioned, ▨ genistein. *p <0.05 compared to control.

dp/dt$_{max}$, AF CF—all remained unchanged after preconditioning (FIG. 1). These parameters were significantly lowered after ischemia/reperfusion in both groups. However, the values were significantly higher compared to the non-preconditioned control group. The beneficial effects of preconditioning were completely abolished in genistein-treated hearts.

Effects of Preconditioning on Phospholipase D

Phospholipase D activity was increased by 50% after ischemic preconditioning (TABLE 1). The enzyme activity was further increased after 30 min of ischemia followed by 30 min of reperfusion. Genistein had no effect on phospholipase D

TABLE 1. Effects of Ischemic Preconditioning on the Activities of Phospholipase D, Protein Kinase C, MAP Kinase and MAPKAP Kinase 2

	Phospholipase D (μmol/min/gm)		Protein Kinase C ($\times 10^3$ cpm)		MAP Kinase ($\times 10^4$ cpm) Relative Activities		MAPKAP Kinase 2 ($\times 10^4$ cpm)	
	Baseline	I/R	Baseline	I/R	Baseline	I/R	Baseline	I/R
Control	90 ± 5	$125 \pm 4^{**}$	6 ± 0.4	$7 \pm 0.5^{**}$	4.2 ± 0.4	$6.1 \pm 0.5^{**}$	2.9 ± 0.34	$5.7 \pm 0.3^{**}$
Preconditioned	$185 \pm 10^{*}$	$225 \pm 8^{*}$	$8.2 \pm 0.5^{*}$	$10.1 \pm 0.6^{*}$	$8.4 \pm 0.5^{*}$	$9.8 \pm 0.4^{*}$	$9.3 \pm 0.4^{*}$	$12.4 \pm 0.4^{*}$
Genistein	$115 \pm 7^{***}$	$145 \pm 5^{***}$	$6.9 \pm 0.6^{***}$	$8.1 \pm 0.5^{***}$	$5.9 \pm 0.5^{***}$	$6.9 \pm 0.5^{***}$	4.9 ± 0.4	$7.7 \pm 0.5^{***}$

* $p < 0.05$ compared to control; ** $p < 0.05$ compared to baseline; *** $p < 0.05$ compared to preconditioned.

in the normal heart (data not shown), but it inhibited the preconditioning and ischemia/reperfusion-mediated enhancement of the activities.

Effects of Preconditioning on Protein Kinase C, MAP Kinases and MAPKAP Kinase 2

The activities of protein kinase C, MAP kinases as well as MAPKAP kinase 2 were enhanced significantly after preconditioning (TABLE 1). They were further activated after ischemia and reperfusion. For example, protein kinase C was stimulated by 37% after preconditioning, and further stimulated by another 23% after ischemia and reperfusion. About 17% enhancement of activity was also observed in the control group after ischemia/reperfusion. Much higher stimulation was observed for MAP kinases and MAPKAP kinase 2 activities. Preconditioning stimulated MAP kinases by 100% while MAPKAP kinase 2 was activated by 221% over the baseline levels. Ischemia/reperfusion further stimulated these activities. The tyrosine kinase inhibitor, genistein, inhibited the activation of kinases.

Myocardial Performance

For mouse, heart rates were not different between control and GPHPx-1 transgenic groups throughout the study, suggesting that overexpression of GSHPx-1 had no effects on heart rates. Developed force (DF) defined as [peak systolic force − diastolic force] during the reperfusion was significantly higher for the transgenic hearts (TABLE 2). Postischemic myocardial ischemic recovery was expressed as a percentage of preischemic baseline DF. Prior to ischemia, there was no difference in DF between the two groups (TABLE 2). After 5 min of reperfusion, DF in the transgenic group was 68 ± 7% compared to 46 ± 8% for nontransgenic hearts. This trend was maintained throughout reperfusion such that at 20 min of reperfusion, the DF in the transgenic mouse group was 87 ± 3% compared to 59 ± 8% for the nontransgenic group. df/dt_{max} followed a similar pattern as shown in TABLE 2. There was no difference in $+df/dt_{max}$ before ischemia. Significantly higher recovery of df/dt_{max} occurred throughout reperfusion. These results demonstrate that transgenic mouse hearts showed significantly greater myocardial contractile recovery than nontransgenic control mouse during postischemic reperfusion. We also measured the coronary flow during the experiments. Coronary flow was not different between the two groups at any point. FIGURE 1 shows the coronary flow of two groups of hearts at baseline and at 20 min of reperfusion.

Creatine kinase release from the heart (TABLE 2) which reflects cellular injury or tissue necrosis and membrane permeability, was only about 5 units/ml for either group prior to ischemia. After ischemia CK release was increased for both groups, but amount of release was much smaller for transgenic mouse hearts. For example, at 1 min of reperfusion CK release was 20.0 ± 5.0 units/ml for transgenic mice as compared to 44.0 ± 8.2 units/ml for nontransgenic controls. Amount of CK release was lowered as the duration of reperfusion progressed. At 10 min of reperfusion, CK release amounted to 7.2 ± 1.8 units/ml for transgenic mouse heart compared to 16.0 ± 3.6 units/ml ($p < 0.05$) for nontransgenic controls. There was no difference in the amount of CK release between the two groups at 15 min and 20 min of reperfusion.

Infarct size for each heart was expressed as: (Σ infarct area of each slice/Σ total ventricular area of each slice) $\times$ 100. Global ischemia for 30 minutes demon-

TABLE 2. Comparison of Performance between Control and GSHPx-1 Transgenic Mice[a]

	DF (% of Baseline)		dF/dt (% of Baseline)		CK (U/l)		Infarct Size (% of Total Risk Area)	
	Control	Transgenic	Control	Transgenic	Control	Transgenic	Control	Transgenic
Baseline	100	100	100	100	5.9 ± 1.1	5 ± 0.9		
R-1					44 ± 8.2	20 ± 5.0*		
R-5	46 ± 8	68 ± 7*	48 ± 10	73 ± 5				
R-10	48 ± 7	78 ± 4*	51 ± 9	79 ± 4*	16 ± 3.6	7.2 ± 1.8*		
R-15	53 ± 8	85 ± 4*	57 ± 10	86 ± 6*	9.1 ± 2.8	6 ± 1.7		
R-20	59 ± 8	87 ± 3*	69 ± 9	95 ± 7*	6.5 ± 1.5	5.2 ± 0.8	8.3 ± 1.0	3.7 ± 0.83*

[a] Isolated perfused hearts from control and transgenic mice were made ischemic for 30 min followed by 20 min of reperfusion. Recovery of DF, dF/dt were measured at 5 (R-5), 10 (R-10), 15 (R-15), and 20 (R-20) min of reperfusion. Coronary effluents were withdrawn at 1 (R-1), 10, 15, and 20 min of reperfusion to measure CK release. Infarct size was determined at the end of the experiment. * $p < 0.05$ compared to nontransgenic control hearts.

strated a different pattern of staining from regional lethal ischemia. Myocardial infarcted tissue was scattered throughout the ventricle in each heart from both groups. The white area that was not stained by triphenyl tetrazolium indicated irreversible ischemic injury. The mean value of infarct size in the transgenic group was significantly smaller than that in the control group ($3.7 \pm 0.83\%$ versus $8.3 \pm 1.0\%$, $p < 0.05$) (TABLE 2). Our results indicated that transgenic mice with overexpressed GSHPx-1 had significantly decreased myocardial necrosis.

DISCUSSION

The results of this study demonstrate for the first time that ischemic preconditioning triggers protein tyrosine phosphorylation in heart. The stimulation of tyrosine kinase is linked with the activation of phospholipase D, because preconditioning-mediated enhancement of phospholipase D was inhibited by the blocker of tyrosine kinase, genistein. Inhibition of tyrosine kinase also attenuated the activation of MAP kinases, MAPKAP kinase 2 and protein kinase C, further suggesting the existence of a phospholipase D-mediated signaling pathway in the ischemic myocardium.

The results also support our previous hypothesis that phospholipase D plays a major role in cell signaling in ischemic heart.[33] Phospholipase D hydrolyzes the phosphate ester bond of the head group that converts the phospholipids, especially, phosphatidylcholine into phosphatidic acid and free head group alcohol generating the second messenger, diacylglycerol. The intermediate compound, phosphatidic acid, may itself be a second messenger product, but its precise role in signal transduction is not known. Diacylglycerol serves as the major cofactor for the translocation and activation of protein kinase C. In turn, protein kinase C may trigger MAP kinase pathway leading to the activation of MAPKAP kinase 2.

The precise role of MAPKAP kinase 2 in heart is not known. However, the abundance of its expression in heart (TABLE 3) suggests a regulatory role of this

TABLE 3. Amount of 3.3 kb and 4.8 kb mRNAs of MAPKAP Kinase 2 in Human Tissues (Relative to Skeletal Muscle)[a]

	4.8 kb mRNA	3.3 kb mRNA
Skeletal muscle	100	100
Heart	82	69
Kidney	55	59
Brain	35	17
Liver	31	36
Lung	27	22
Placenta	16	15
Pancreas	12	29

[a] Human multiple tissue Northern blot (hMTN obtained from ClonTech Laboratories, Inc., New York) containing mRNAs from various organs were hybridized with a synthetic oligonucleotide probe corresponding to amino acid residues 344 to 353 in the C-terminal region of human MAPKAP kinase 2.[50] Northern analysis revealed two mRNA species of MAPKAP kinase 2 with sizes of 4.8 and 3.3 kb. The highest amount was detected in the skeletal muscle with the second highest in the heart tissue. Results are expressed as activities relative to skeletal muscle, which was set as 100%.

kinase. Stresses such as heat stress, oxidant stress, and ischemia/reperfusion can rapidly induce the activation of MAPKAP kinase 2 in myocardial cells (TABLE 4). More interestingly, results from our recent study indicated that it is MAPKAP kinase 2, and not protein kinase C, that could directly phosphorylate the small heat shock protein such as HSP 25 derived from rat heart (unpublished results). Activation of heat shock and antioxidant proteins have been shown to be instrumental for the adaptation of heart to ischemic stress.[13–15,28,36–38] It is tempting to speculate that MAPKAP kinase 2 may be the cellular link between preconditioning (early adaptation) and ultimate adaptation (FIG. 2).

The kinases including protein kinase C and MAPKAP kinase 2 as well as other kinases are likely to induce expression of a variety of genes, presumably at the transcription level. The synthesis of stress proteins such as oxidative stress and heat shock proteins, as well as those genes that are related to growth factors, appears to be regulated at the same transcriptional level.[27] All major membrane signal transduction mechanisms lead to at least one effector link capable of selective phosphorylation of proteins. However, the involvement of such kinase activity (C kinase, A kinase, G kinase, Ca^{2+}-CaM kinase, MAP kinase, a.s.o.) in modulation of gene expression is also dependent to a large extent on the availability of specific target molecules. Thus, the time course of stress stimulus and the number and sequence of signaling pathways activated ultimately determines the observed pattern of specific myocardial gene expression.

Interestingly, when myocardial cells are subjected to acute stress such as ischemia/reperfusion, oxidative stress and hyperthermia, they readily react by inducing genes encoding antioxidant enzymes and related proteins in addition to other stress proteins. In most cases, mRNA for catalase is transcribed in mammalian heart after being subjected to a stress insult.[39] In addition, increased expression of Mn-SOD mRNA has also been documented in the heart. Mn-SOD constitutes one of the major cellular defense mechanisms against the toxic effects of the superoxide radical. Repeated ischemia and reperfusion was associated with the enhancement of the antioxidant defense system. It was shown that repeated ischemia (four times 5 min of ischemia each separated by 10 min of reperfusion, 4 × PC) enhanced the expression of catalase and Mn-SOD genes.[3] Interestingly, 4 × PC showed a relatively higher amount of the expression of these genes compared to those present in the 1 × PC (5 min of ischemia followed by 10 min of reperfusion) hearts. We also observed enhanced peroxisomal catalase activity after 60 min of reperfusion following repeated ischemia and reperfusion. In addition, glutathione peroxidase, glutathione reductase and Mn-SOD activities were also higher in the 4 × PC hearts after 60 min of reperfusion compared to those in 1 × PC and control hearts, suggesting that these enzymes could have been modulated by the stress induced by repeated ischemia and reperfusion. The development of oxygen adaptation has been related to an increase in enzyme activities such as glucose-6-phosphate dehydrogenase, glutathione peroxidase, as well as catalase and SOD.[40,41] Oxidative stress induced by cytokines such as IL-1, IL-6, or TNF can induce the expression of mRNA levels of Mn-SOD in human hepatoma cells.[42] Oxidative stress induced by endotoxin, IL-1 and IL-6 also increased the Mn-SOD mRNA levels in rat liver.[43] SOD plays a key role in protection against oxygen radicals, and SOD gene expression is highly induced during stress. Recently our laboratory showed that oxidative stress induced by IL-1α caused the enhancement of several antioxidant enzymes in rat heart including catalase, Cu/Zn-SOD, Mn-SOD, glutathione peroxidase and glucose-6-phosphate dehydrogenase.[13–15] Oxidative stress is likely to shift the cellular redox equilibrium towards the oxidized status. Surprisingly, the expression of the Cu/Zn-SOD gene is induced

TABLE 4. Effects of Different Stresses on MAPKAP Kinase 2 Activities of Heart[a]

Time after the Stress (min)	Baseline	Relative MAPKAP Kinase 2 Activity ($\times 10^4$ cpm)					
		0	2	5	10	20	30
Ischemic preconditioning	2.9 ± 0.34	$12.4 \pm 0.47^*$	4.1 ± 0.63	5.9 ± 0.34	$9.2 \pm 0.81^*$	$7.3 \pm 0.72^*$	$12.0 \pm 1.1^*$
Heat shock	3.0 ± 0.52	3.3 ± 0.45	3.5 ± 0.55	$8.7 \pm 0.80^*$	$11.9 \pm 1.2^*$	$10.2 \pm 0.91^*$	5.0 ± 0.30
Oxidative stress	2.9 ± 0.45	2.8 ± 0.61					$8.8 \pm 0.63^*$

[a] Ischemic preconditioning was achieved by inducing 5 min of ischemia followed by 10 min of reperfusion, repeated four times ($4 \times$ PC) as described in the Methods section. Heat shock was produced by perfusing the heart with KHB buffer at 42.5°C for 10 min. Oxidative stress was induced by perfusing the heart with OH· generating system for 10 min.

* $p < 0.05$ compared to baseline.

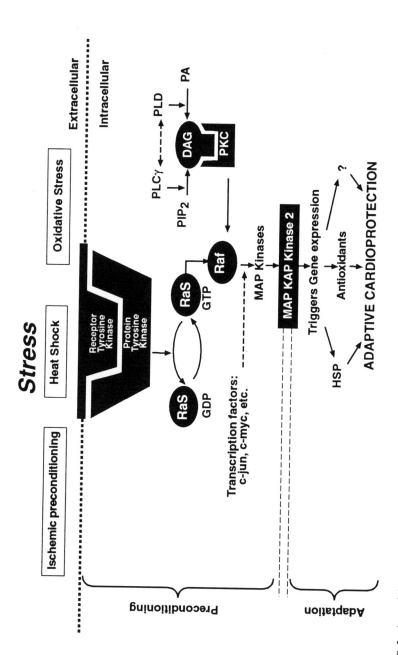

FIGURE 2. A model supported by our results. The figure indicates the existence of a tyrosine kinase–phospholipase D–MAPKAP kinase 2 signal transduction pathway in the preconditioned heart. MAPKAP kinase 2 is shown as the molecular link between the preconditioning and adaptation.

by sulfhydryl antioxidants such as reduced glutathione, cysteine, and dithiothreitol. It seems likely, therefore, that reduced GSH directly acts as an antioxidant and
simultaneously activates the Cu/Zn-SOD gene during oxidative stress. Another
antioxidative enzyme, glutathione S-transferase (GST) was recently found to be
transcriptionally regulated by oxidative stress induced by reactive oxygen intermediates.[44] The authors speculated that the gene product of primary GR target genes
directly or indirectly affects the redox state of the cell. A recent study from our
laboratory demonstrated activation of SOD when an isolated in situ pig heart was
subjected to heat shock by warm blood cardioplegia.[36] In contrast, Currie and
Tanguay found no detectable change in mRNA for catalase after heat shock or
during the recovery following the heat shock.[39] However, they demonstrated an
increase in catalase enzyme activity at 24 h and 48 h after the induction of heat
shock response. The authors concluded that catalase activity is either translation-
ally or posttranslationally regulated. These studies suggested that heat shock
enhances the cellular antioxidative defense system. Thus, the stimulation of SOD
and catalase could reflect a mechanism of myocardial adaptation to the stress.
While it is tempting to speculate that stress-mediated stimulation of antioxidant
enzymes is instrumental in the enhanced postischemic functional recovery of
heart, further study is required to confirm such a possibility.

The expression of catalase, glutathione reductase, and a novel alkyl hydroperoxide reductase is believed to be controlled by a positive regulator, OxyR.[45] OxyR
is homologous to the LYSR-Nod D family of bacterial regulatory proteins and
binds to the promoters of OxyR-regulated genes. The oxidized form of the OxyR
protein activates transcription of OxyR-regulated genes in vitro, thereby suggesting
that oxidation of the OxyR protein brings about a conformational change by
which OxyR senses as well as transduces an oxidative stress signal to RNA
polymerase II.[46]

Constitutive cellular protection against acute stress can be provided by various
intracellular antioxidants such as glutathione, α-tocopherol, ascorbic acid, β-caro-
tene, etc., and antioxidant enzymes that include superoxide dismutase (SOD),
catalase, and glutathione (GSH) peroxidase. These cellular compounds reduce/
eliminate the oxidative stress by directly quenching the reactive oxygen species
before they damage vital cellular components and, therefore, can be considered
as part of the first line of defense against the external stress. Often, because of
the inadequacy of the intracellular antioxidants or due to the presence of an
increased amount of oxidative stress, the reactive oxygen species may reach their
targets that include nucleic acid, protein, and lipids.[47] This results in the injury
to the cellular components causing DNA strand breaks, protein degradation, and
lipid peroxidation. Mammalian cells are also protected by a second line of defense
system consisting of several lipolytic and proteolytic enzymes, proteases, phospholipases, etc. which are involved in the systematic recognition and removal
of the injured cellular components. In view of the increasing evidence for the
involvement of cellular oxidation and oxidative stress in various pathophysiological conditions of heart disease, especially ischemic heart disease, it is of considerable interest to examine whether myocardial cells possess an inducible pathway
for the antioxidant defense. The signal transduction pathways by which various
stress signals are translated into oxidative stress leading to the modulation of
antioxidants/antioxidant enzymes are likely to be different, but the induction
of the expression of their mRNAs and/or the increased translation of mRNA
accumulation as a result of changes at the level of RNA transcription or stability
seem to be the most plausible mechanism. This could lead to the synthesis of
proteins involved in cellular protection or repair of injury. These phenomena

Ischemia/Reperfusion

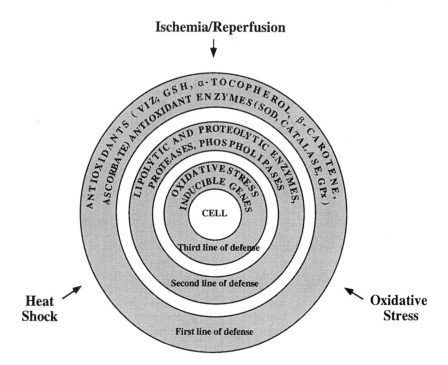

FIGURE 3. A model demonstrating myocardial defense against ischemia/reperfusion, heat shock and oxidative stress. The induction of gene expression is shown as the third line of defense.

related to specific gene expression could be viewed as a third line of defense, and may reflect the ultimate adaptive responses (FIG. 3).

To test our hypothesis that cellular antioxidant enzymes indeed constitute the cellular defense against acute stress, we studied myocardial ischemia reperfusion injury in transgenic mice overexpressing the cellular glutathione peroxidase (GSHPx-1). Glutathione peroxidase is a key enzyme in the antioxidant defense system which catalyzes the reduction of organic hydroperoxides and H_2O_2 in a reaction that involves reduced glutathione (GSH):

$$ROOH + 2GSH \rightarrow GSSG + ROH + H_2O \tag{i}$$

$$H_2O_2 + 2GSH \rightarrow GSSG + 2H_2O \tag{ii}$$

This enzyme performs three essential functions in the heart: (i) converts H_2O_2 into H_2O, thus removing any excessive H_2O_2 that may be formed by the action of oxygen free radicals; (ii) converts peroxidized fatty acids that are formed during lipid peroxidation into hydroxy fatty acids; (iii) reverses the oxidation of protein sulfhydryl groups. The presence of GSHPx is particularly important for maintaining the structural and functional integrity of the cytosolic and mitochondrial compartments. Catalase is also capable of removing H_2O_2, but its presence in relatively low amounts in the heart (only 1–2% as compared to liver), especially in the mitochondrial and cytosolic compartments (>90% catalase is present in peroxisomes) where free radicals are generated, makes it of lesser importance compared to GSH-peroxidase. The amount of GSH-peroxidase in the hearts and livers of several species including mice, rats and dogs are comparable.[48] The presence of a higher GSHPx activity may be vital for the heart to survive the attack of reactive oxygen species that are produced in the ischemic reperfused myocardium. The results of our study clearly demonstrated increased resistance of transgenic GSHPx-1 overexpressed mouse hearts to ischemia reperfusion injury compared to those of nontransgenic controls. Transgenic mouse hearts showed improved postischemic ventricular recovery as evidenced by increased DF and df/dt_{max}. Relatively less tissue injury was also reflected in the lesser amount of CK release. Furthermore, and more importantly, the area of infarction in the postischemic myocardium of the transgenic mice was smaller compared to those of nontransgenic mice. Taken together, these results clearly demonstrate the important role of GSHPx enzyme in myocardial protection.

In summary, although our understanding of myocardial adaptation to stress is far from complete, there cannot be any doubt that such adaptation occurs in two distinct phases: early adaptation also known as preconditioning, a rapid short-lived phenomenon likely to be mediated by signal transduction process; and late adaptation believed to occur by the regulation of gene expression. The results of this study implicate that ischemic preconditioning rapidly activates the tyrosine kinase-phospholipase D signaling pathway resulting in the activation of protein kinase C, MAP kinases and MAPKAP kinase 2. MAPKAP kinase 2 seems to be situated at the crossroad of signal transduction and gene expression, suggesting that this kinase may be the molecular link between preconditioning and adaptation processes.

Antioxidants seem to play an important role in the constitution of the intracellular defense that is triggered by preconditioning.[49] Once the particular set of genes expressed as a consequence of preconditioning/adaptation are identified and their beneficial or detrimental role in the resistance of myocardial cells to further ischemic insult is known, there are a number of powerful new therapeutical approaches which can be envisaged based on this information. In the first place, it is most important to establish the exact intracellular signaling link between the membrane events and gene expression. Preconditioning-mediated second messengers can be generated by pharmacological manipulations independent of (prior to) ischemic episodes, and thus protective gene expression can be induced. On the other hand, it is possible to selectively alter the information encoded by genes through cell transformation by site-directed mutagenesis, which can be directed either to induce continuous expression of a useful (protective) intracellular protein, or to induce expression of an unfunctional product (in case the expressed protein appears to be detrimental). However, while these manipulations require the use of cultured cells for transformation experiments and are thus more difficult to extend to *in vivo* practical purposes, some new techniques were recently established which allow insertion of known and altered genes into the cells. Due to these and other recent technological breakthroughs, which bring gene therapy from the realm of speculation into reality, our ultimate goal will be to use our body's own intracellular defense system to protect the myocardium from ischemic heart disease.

ACKNOWLEDGMENTS

The transgenic mice used in this study were obtained from Dr. Y-S. Ho.

REFERENCES

1. MURRY, C. E., V. J. RICHARD, K. A. REIMER & R. B. JENNINGS. 1990. Ischemic preconditioning slows energy metabolism and delays ultrastructural damage during a sustained ischemic episode. Circ. Res. **66:** 913–931.

2. LI, G. C., J. A. VASQUES, K. P. GALLAGHER & B. R. LUCCHESI. 1990. Myocardial protection with preconditioning. Circulation **82:** 609–619.

3. DAS, D. K., R. M. ENGELMAN & Y. KIMURA. 1993. Molecular adaptation of cellular defences following preconditioning of the heart by repeated ischemia. Cardiovasc. Res. **27:** 578–584.

4. FLACK, J. E., Y. KIMURA & R. M. ENGELMAN. 1991. Preconditioning the heart by repeated stunning improves myocardial salvage. Circulation **84**(Suppl. V): 369–374.

5. SCHOTT, R. J., S. ROHMANN, E. R. BRAUN & W. SCHAPER. 1990. Ischemic preconditioning reduces infarct size in swine myocardium. Cir. Res. **66:** 1133–1142.

6. MEERSON, F. Z. 1991. Adaptation to stress and its cardioprotective effects in stress, ischemic, and reperfusion damage. *In* Adaptive Protection of the Heart. 127–153. CRC Press. Boca Raton, FL.

7. TOSAKI, A., G. A. CORDIS, P. SZERDAHELYI, R. M. ENGELMAN & D. K. DAS. 1994. Effects of preconditioning on reperfusion arrhythmias, myocardial functions, formation of free radicals, and ion shifts in isolated ischemic/reperfused rat hearts. J. Cardiovasc. Pharmacol. **23:** 365–373.

8. LAWSON, C. S., D. J. O. COLTART & D. J. HEARSE. 1992. Ischemic preconditioning and protection against reperfusion-induced arrhythmias, reduction in vulnerability or delay in onset? Studies in the isolated blood perfused rat heart. Eur. Heart J. **13:** 2334.

9. LIU, G. S., J. THORNTON, D. M. VAN WINKLE, A. W. H. STANLEY, R. A. OLSSON & J. M. DOWNEY. 1991. Protection against infarction afforded by preconditioning is mediated by A1-adenosine receptors in rabbit hearts. Circulation **84:** 350–356.

10. GROSS, G. A. & AUCHAMPACH. 1992. Blockade of ATP-sensitive potassium channels prevents myocardial preconditioning in dogs. Circ. Res. **70:** 223–233.

11. TOSAKI, A., D. T. ENGELMAN, R. M. ENGELMAN & D. K. DAS. 1995. Alpha-1 adrenergic receptor agonist-induced preconditioning in isolated working rat hearts. J. Pharmacol. Exp. Ther. **273:** 689–694.

12. BANERJEE, A., C. LOCKE-WINTER, K. B. ROGERS, M. B. MITCHELL, D. D. BENSARD, E. C. BREW, C. B. CAIRNS & A. H. HARKEN. 1993. Transient ischemia preconditions against subsequent cardiac ischemia reperfusion injury by an alpha-1 adrenergic mechanism. Circ. Res. **73:** 656–670.

13. MAULIK, N., R. M. ENGELMAN, Z. WEI, D. LU, J. A. ROUSOU & D. K. DAS. 1993. Interleukin-1α preconditioning reduces myocardial ischemia reperfusion injury. Circulation **88**(Part II): 387–394.

14. MAULIK, N., M. WATANABE, D. T. ENGELMAN, R. M. ENGELMAN & D. K. DAS. 1995. Oxidative stress adaptation improves postischemic ventricular recovery. Mol. Cell. Biochem. **144:** 67–74.

15. MAULIK, N., M. WATANABE, D. ENGELMAN, R. M. ENGELMAN, V. E. KAGAN, E. KISIN, V. TYURIN, G. A. CORDIS & D. K. DAS. 1995. Myocardial adaptation to ischemia by oxidative stress induced by endotoxin. Am. J. Physiol. **269:** C907–C916.

16. ENGELMAN, D. T., M. WATANABE, R. M. ENGELMAN, J. A. ROUSOU, E. KISIN, V. E. KAGAN, N. MAULIK & D. K. DAS. 1995. Hypoxic preconditioning preserves antioxidant reserve in the working rat heart. Cardiovasc. Res. **29:** 133–140.

17. SHIZUKUDA, Y., T. IWAMOTO, R. T. MALLET & H. F. DOWNEY. 1993. Hypoxic preconditioning attenuates stunning caused by repeated coronary artery occlusions in dog heart. Cardiovasc. Res. **27:** 559–564.

18. MAULIK, N., Z. WEI, X. LIU, R. M. ENGELMAN, J. A. ROUSOU & D. K. DAS. 1994. Improved postischemic ventricular functional recovery by amphetamine is linked with its ability to induce heat shock. Mol. Cell. Biochem. **137:** 17–24.

19. MAULIK, N., R. M. ENGELMAN, Z. WEI, X. LIU, J. A. ROUSOU, J. FLACK, D. DEATON & D. K. DAS. 1995. Drug-induced heat shock improves post-ischemic ventricular recovery after cardiopulmonary bypass. Circulation **92**(Suppl. II): 381–388.

20. DAS, D. K., I. I. MORARU, N. MAULIK & R. M. ENGELMAN. 1994. Gene expression during myocardial adaptation to ischemia and reperfusion injury. Ann. N.Y. Acad. Sci. **723:** 292–307.

21. DAS, D. K. 1993. Ischemic preconditioning and myocardial adaptation to ischemia. Cardiovasc. Res. **27:** 2077–2079.

22. PRASAD, M. R. & R. M. JONES. 1992. Enhanced membrane protein kinase C activity in myocardial ischemia. Basic Res. Cardiol. **87:** 19–26.

23. HENRICH, C. J. & P. C. SIMPSON. 1988. Differential acute and chronic response of protein kinase C in cultured neonatal rat heart myocytes to α1-adrenergic and phorbol ester stimulation. J. Mol. Cell. Cardiol. **20:** 1081–1085.

24. FEARON, C. W. & A. H. TASHJIAN. 1985. Thyrotropin-releasing hormone induces redistribution of protein kinase C in GH4C1 rat pituitary cells. J. Biol. Chem. **260:** 8366–8371.

25. YTREHUS, K., Y. LIU & J. M. DOWNEY. 1994. Preconditioning protects ischemic rabbit heart by protein kinase C activation. Am. J. Physiol. **266:** H1145–H1152.

26. MITCHELL, M. B., X. MENG, J. BROWN, A. H. HARKEN & A. BANERJEE. 1995. Preconditioning of isolated rat heart is mediated by protein kinase C. Circ. Res. **76:** 73–81.

27. NISHIZUKA, Y. 1986. Studies and perspectives of protein kinase C. Science **233:** 305–312.

28. MAULIK, N., H. S. SHARMA & D. K. DAS. 1996. Induction of the haem oxygenase gene expression during the reperfusion of ischemic rat myocardium. J. Mol. Cell. Cardiol. **28:** 1261–1270.

29. DAS, D. K., N. MAULIK & I. I. MORARU. 1995. Gene expression in acute myocardial stress. Induction by hypoxia, ischemia, reperfusion, hyperthermia, oxidative stress. J. Mol. Cell. Cardiol. **27:** 181–193.

30. BRAND, T., H. S. SHARMA, K. E. FLEISCHMANN, D. J. DUNCKER, E. O. MCFALLA, P. D. VERDOUW & W. SCHAPER. 1992. Proto-oncogene expression in porcine myocardium subjected to ischemia and reperfusion. Circ. Res. **71:** 1351–1360.

31. DAS, D. K. & N. MAULIK. 1995. Cross talk between heat shock and oxidative stress inducible genes during myocardial adaptation to ischemia. *In* Cell Biology of Trauma. J. J. Lemasters & C. Oliver, Eds. 193–212. CRC Press. Boca Raton, FL.

32. HEADS, R. J., D. S. LATCHMAN & D. M. YELLON. 1995. Differential stress protein mRNA expression during early ischemic preconditioning in the rabbit heart and its relationship to adenosine receptor function. J. Mol. Cell. Cardiol. **27:** 2133–2148.

33. MORAU, I. I., L. M. POPESCU, N. MAULIK, X. LIU & D. K. DAS. 1992. Phospholipase D signaling in ischemic heart. Biochim. Biophys. Acta **1139:** 148–154.

34. HOGAN, B. F., B. F. CONSTANTINI & E. LACY. 1986. Manipulating the Mouse Embryo. Cold Spring Harbor Laboratory. Cold Spring Harbor, NY.

35. ZU, Y-L., Y. AI, A. GILCHRIST, R. I. SHA'AFI, D. K. DAS & C-K. HUANG. Heat shock, oxidative stress, or phorbol ester stimulate activation of MAPKAP kinase 2 and HSP 25 phosphorylation in rat cardiac myocytes. Communicated.

36. LIU, X., R. M. ENGELMAN, I. I. MORARU, J. A. ROUSOU, J. E. FLACK, D. W. DEATON, N. MAULIK & D. K. DAS. 1992. Heat shock: a new approach for myocardial preservation in cardiac surgery. Circulation **86**(Suppl. II): 358–363.

37. MARBER, M. S., R. MESTRIL, S-H. CHI, R. SAYEN, D. M. YELLON & W. H. DILLMAN. 1995. Overexpression of the rat inducible 70-kD heat stress protein in a transgenic mouse increases the resistance of the heart to ischemic injury. J. Clin. Invest. **95:** 1446–1456.

38. PLUMIER, J. C. L., B. M. ROSS, R. W. CURRIE, C. E. ANGELIDIS, H. KAZLARIS, G. KOLLIAS & G. N. PAGOULATOS. 1995. Transgenic mice expressing the human heat shock protein 70 have improved post-ischemic myocardial recovery. J. Clin. Invest. **95:** 1854–1860.

39. CURRIE, R. W. & R. M. TANGUAY. 1991. Analysis of RNA for transcripts for catalase and SP71 in rat hearts after *in vivo* hyperthermia. Biochem. Cell Biol. **69:** 375–382.

40. LU, D. & D. K. DAS. 1993. Induction of differential heat shock gene expression in heart, lung liver, brain and kidney by a sympathomimetic drug, amphetamine. Biochem. Biophys. Res. Commun. **192:** 808–812.

41. LU, D., N. MAULIK, I. I. MORARU, D. L. KREUTZER & D. K. DAS. 1993. Molecular adaptation of vascular endothelial cells to oxidative stress. Am. J. Physiol. **264:** C715–C722.
42. ONO, M., H. KOHDA, T. KAWAGUCHI, M. OHHIRA, C. SEKIYA, M. NAMIKI, A. TAKE-YASU & N. TANIGUCHI. 1992. Induction of Mn-SOD by TNF, IL-1, and IL-6 in human hepatoma cells. Biochem. Biophys. Res. Commun. **182:** 110–1107.
43. VISNER, G. A., S. E. CHESROWN, J. MONNIER, U. S. RYAN & H. S. NICK. 1992. Regulation of Mn-SOD: IL-1 and TNF induction in pulmonary artery and microvascular endothelial cells. Biochem. Biophys. Res. Commun. **188:** 453–462.
44. FLOMERFELT, F. A., M. M. BRIEHL, D. R. DOWD, E. S. DIEKEN & R. L. MIESFELD. 1993. Elevated glutathione S-transferase gene expression is an early event during steroid-induced lymphocyte apoptosis. J. Cell. Physiol. **154:** 573–581.
45. TARTAGLIA, L. A., G. STORZ & B. N. AMES. 1989. Identification and molecular analysis of oxyR-regulated promoters important for the bacterial adaptation to oxidative stress. Mol. Biol. **210:** 709–719.
46. STORZ, G., L. A. TARTAGLIA & B. N. AMES. 1990. The OxyR regulon. Antonie Van Leeuwenhoek **58:** 157–161.
47. DAS, D. K. & R. M. ENGELMAN. 1990. Mechanism of free radical generation during reperfusion of ischemic myocardium. *In* Oxygen Radicals: Systemic Events and Disease Processes. D. K. Das & W. B. Essman, Eds. 97–121. Karger. Basel.
48. KANTER, M. W., R. L. HAMLIN, D. V. UNVERFERTH, H. W. DAVIS & A. J. MEROLA. 1985. Effect of exercise training on antioxidant enzymes and cardiotoxicity of doxorubicin. J. Appl. Physiol. **59:** 1298–1303.
49. DAS, D. K. & N. MAULIK. 1994. Evaluation of antioxidative effectiveness in ischemia reperfusion tissue injury. Methods Enzymol. **233:** 601–610.

Exploration of the Possible Roles of Phospholipase D and Protein Kinase C in the Mechanism of Ischemic Preconditioning in the Myocardium[a]

YVONNE E. G. ESKILDSEN-HELMOND,[b]
BEN C. G. GHO,[c] KAREL BEZSTAROSTI,[b]
DICK H. W. DEKKERS,[b] LOE KIE SOEI,[c]
HAN A. A. VAN HEUGTEN,[b] PIETER D. VERDOUW,[c]
AND JOS M. J. LAMERS[b]

[b]Department of Biochemistry
and
[c]Experimental Cardiology, Thorax Center
Cardiovascular Research Institute COEUR
Faculty of Medicine & Health Sciences
Erasmus University Rotterdam
P.O. Box 1738
3000 DR Rotterdam, The Netherlands

INTRODUCTION

Brief periods of acute myocardial ischemia protect the heart against subsequent episodes of prolonged ischemia.[1] This endogenous phenomenon, first described by Murry et al.,[2] is known as ischemic preconditioning and has been demonstrated in a wide variety of species such as the rat,[3] dog,[4] rabbit[5] and pig.[6,7] For a number of reasons, the occurrence of ischemic preconditioning in the clinical setting has not yet been demonstrated convincingly, but evidence is accumulating that it occurs in situations such as angina preceding an acute myocardial infarction and percutaneous transluminal coronary angioplasty.[8–10] In addition to limiting infarct size caused by prolonged ischemia,[3–7] preconditioning improves the recovery of function after reperfusion and reduces ventricular arrhythmias during ischemia and/or after reperfusion.[3,11,12] The protective state afforded by ischemic preconditioning lasts for about 2 hours.[13,14] In addition to brief episodes of total coronary occlusion, several other stimuli can mimic ischemic preconditioning, as recently reviewed by Kloner et al.[15] Partial coronary artery stenosis without reperfusion, hypoxia, stretch, catecholamines, rapid pacing and certain pharmacological interventions are such preconditioning-like stimuli.[7,10,15]

Extensive studies have been undertaken to elucidate the mechanism(s) by which transient ischemia protects the myocardium. Liu et al.[16] took the first

[a] This work was supported by Grant No. 900-516-146 from the Netherlands Organization for Scientific Research (NWO) and Grant No. 95.103 from The Netherlands Heart Foundation.

important step towards revealing the possible mechanism(s) of ischemic preconditioning, by describing the role of adenosine in mediating the phenomenon. Since then, results obtained by experiments with specific agonists and antagonists have shown that activation of K^+_{ATP} channels,[17] α_1-adrenergic[18,19]- and muscarinic[20,21] agonists, bradykinin,[22,23] angiotensin II,[24] A_1 adenosine agonists[16,25,26] and protein kinase C (PKC) activators[19,27–29] might be other endogenous mediators of preconditioning. At present, a unifying hypothesis for preconditioning proposes that these endogenous ligands such as A_1 adenosine-, α_1-adrenergic- and muscarinic agonists, bradykinin and angiotensin II initiate an intracellular pathway by acting via G-protein-coupled receptors, which leads to activation of phospholipase C-β.[15,19,24,27–30] Subsequently, modulation of the latter enzyme changes levels of the second messengers inositol-1,4,5-trisphosphate ($Ins(1,4,5)P_3$) and 1,2-diacylglycerol ($(1,2)DAG$).[30] The mechanism by which these messengers act is by direct or indirect activation of the Ca^{2+}-dependent and/or Ca^{2+}-independent PKC isoenzymes and Ca^{2+}-calmodulin-dependent protein kinase (CaM-PK). Activated PKC isoforms and/or CaM-PK then phosphorylate specific proteins that ultimately lead to the cardioprotective effect. The rate of dephosphorylation of these specific phosphoproteins by phosphoprotein phosphatases likely determines the period in which the protective state is maintained. A recent report describes that in superfused human right atrial trabeculae undergoing simulated ischemia the mechanism(s) of preconditioning may indeed act via PKC and rely on the activation of the K^+_{ATP} channel as the final effector.[31] This supports the evidence, obtained by whole cell patch-clamp or whole cell voltage-clamp of isolated rabbit ventricular myocytes, that the ATP-sensitive K^+ current is activated by a PKC-mediated phosphorylation. The potentiation of the K^+_{ATP} current by PKC provides an explicit basis for current paradigms of ischemic preconditioning.[32,33]

In this report we will first briefly review the evidence derived from experiments using specific activators and blockers and enzymatic measurements that PKC plays a key role in the intracellular mechanism of preconditioning. The latter may be valid for all species despite the variability of the endogenous extracellular triggers. We will also present evidence derived from studies using an *in situ* porcine model that supports the PKC hypothesis for preconditioning. Until now the possible phospholipid sources of the PKC activator $(1,2)DAG$ during preconditioning have been scarcely explored. For several of the postulated endogenous mediators of cardioprotection such as α_1-adrenergic-, A_1 adenosine and muscarinic agonists and angiotensin II it has been shown that in myocardium these stimuli activate not only phospholipase C-β but also phospholipase D (PLD).[34–39] Furthermore, Moraru *et al.*[40] provided direct evidence of membrane PLD stimulation induced by reversible ischemia in the isolated perfused rat heart. Considerable emphasis has been put on the fact that administration of the potent PKC activator phorbol myristate acetate (PMA), mimics preconditioning-like protection.[15,19,27–29,33] This finding may indicate the involvement of PLD in ischemic preconditioning.

Translocation of PKC: a Possible Key Event during Ischemic Preconditioning

Most studies assessing the role of PKC in ischemic preconditioning have used an indirect pharmacological approach. For instance, several groups of investigators attempted to block the cardioprotective effect of a brief antecedent ischemia episode by administration of PKC inhibitors such as polymyxin B,[19,23,24,27,41,42] staurosporine,[23,27,29,43] 1-(5-isoquinolinesulfonyl)-2-methylpiperazine (H-7),[33,41] chelerythrine,[28,31,42,44] and calphostin-C,[45,46] before the onset of the prolonged period of ischemia. However, H-7, staurosporine and polymyxin B are not very selective for PKC compared with cyclic AMP-dependent protein kinase, CaM-PK or tyrosine kinase.[47] In contrast, chelerythrine[48] and calphostin C[49] are more specific inhibitors of PKC with high potencies. For instance, calphostin C acts on the regulatory domain of PKC, which is distinct from other protein kinases and calphostin C therefore induces a more specific inhibition than other PKC inhibitors. PKC inhibitors, such as staurosporine and H-7, acting on the catalytic domain of PKC, carry a high degree of sequence homology with other protein kinases and thus lack a high specificity for PKC. In addition, it is unknown whether these inhibitors effectively block all PKC isoenzymes. Molecular cloning techniques have revealed that PKC exists in at least 10 isoforms with distinct substrate proteins.[50-53] These isoforms may have different sensitivities towards the PKC inhibitors. In this respect it is important to note that Przyklenk et al.[41] found that neither H-7 nor polymyxin B attenuated preconditioning in an in situ canine model, which contrasts the results of the numerous reports[19,23,24,27-29,42,44-46] in which it was shown that PKC inhibitors abolished the protection by ischemic preconditioning. In contrast, the PKC inhibitors H-7 and polymyxin B produced the opposite effect: they further limited infarct size, suggesting inhibition of PKC protected the canine heart during sustained ischemia.[41] Differences in PKC isoform expression may provide an explanation for the disparity among dog, rabbit, rat and pig models. Myocardial expression of PKC isoforms is still poorly character-ized, and it is quite feasible that not all PKC isoforms are expressed in the different species. For example, the Ca^{2+}-dependent PKC-α is the most abundant form of PKC in bovine heart,[54] whereas in adult rat ventricular myocytes, the Ca^{2+}-independent isoform PKC-ε was abundantly present and PKC-α could not be detected.[29,55] These differences in isoform expression may be important because (i) the isoforms differ in their extent of activation by Ca^{2+}, (1,2)DAG and phorbol-esters (ii) distinct isoforms of PKC are thought to translocate to distinct intracellu-lar sites (e.g., sarcolemma, sarcoplasmatic reticulum, myofibrils and the perinu-clear region) and phosphorylate distinct proteins[41,56] and (iii) different isoforms of PKC may mediate different cellular functions.

The second approach used to evaluate the role of PKC in preconditioning is to activate PKC by phorbolester (e.g., PMA),[33,42] or other (1,2)DAG analogs such as oleyl acetyl-glycerol (OAG),[41] 1,2-dioctanoyl sn-glycerol (DOG)[31] and 1-stearoyl-2-arachidonoyl glycerol (SAG).[29] Unlike (1,2)DAG, which is rapidly degraded, phorbolesters are not metabolized and are associated with sustained PKC activation and pathological changes.[29] Occupancy of the regulatory site of PKC by (1,2)DAG analogs induces intracellular PKC translocation. This partition mechanism is characterized by increased affinity of PKC for acid membrane phospholipids, such as phosphatidylserine and increased activation. Thus, regula-tor-induced translocation and activation of PKC may be inseparable events, since occupation of the regulatory domain in PKC removes an N-terminal inhibitory (pseudosubstrate) sequence from its close juxtaposition to the catalytic site.[29] Binding of (1,2)DAG to the conventional Ca^{2+}-dependent cPKC's (PKC-α, -β and -γ) increases their affinity for Ca^{2+}.[50-53] Recently, the nPKC's (PKC-δ, -ε, -η, and -θ), which are directly activated by (1,2)DAG without the need of Ca^{2+}, were discovered.[50-53] Several studies have demonstrated that activation of PKC by PMA or other (1,2)DAG analogs mimics preconditioning.[28,29,31] Such findings suggest that the mechanism of preconditioning in the rat and rabbit involves activation of PKC.

A third strategy to examine the role of PKC in preconditioning is by directly measuring the translocation of PKC in response to repeated brief ischemia. The translocation from cytosolic to organellar compartments is believed to be a marker for activation of PKC. Translocation can be measured by direct visualization of PKC by (*i*) immunofluorescence staining of dissected myocardium, (*ii*) quantification of the distribution of PKC activity in subcellular fractions (isolated from myocardial homogenates) detected by measurement of Ca^{2+}- and/or (1,2)DAG-dependent ^{32}P incorporation from γ-^{32}P-labelled ATP into histone III-S or PKC isoenzyme-specific substrate peptide and (*iii*) immunoblot analysis using PKC isoenzyme-specific antibodies tested on subcellular fractions isolated from myocardial homogenates. At present, in only a few studies has one of these last approaches been used to investigate the role of PKC in ischemic preconditioning. Weinbrenner *et al.*[57] showed that α, β, ε and ζ are the prominent isoforms of PKC in the rat heart which, except for the β-form, is similar to what has been observed in cultured neonatal[38] and adult rat cardiomyocytes.[58] Weinbrenner *et al.*[57] also showed that a brief period of ischemia, caused a rapid translocation of the Ca^{2+}-independent subtypes (δ, ε and ζ) and the Ca^{2+}-dependent subtype α to the membrane. Prolonged ischemia led to the induction of Ca^{2+}-independent forms of PKC-δ and -ε in the cytosol. Immunohistofluorescence studies of Mitchell *et al.*[29] showed translocation of the PKC-δ isoform to the sarcolemma following transient ischemia or α_1-adrenergic stimulation. In addition, transient ischemia resulted in PKC-ε translocation to the nucleus.[29] These results demonstrate activation of PKC with both transient ischemia and α_1-adrenergic agonist stimulation and suggest that the PKC-δ and -ε isoforms may be involved in ischemic preconditioning in the rat.

Immunohistofluorescence detection does not distinguish between active and inactive PKC. Przyklenk *et al.*[41] used a probe that binds to activated PKC (*i.e.*, a bisindolylmaleimide PKC inhibitor yielded fluorescent through conjugation to fluorescein) and could not show a difference in the amount or distribution of PKC fluorescence before and after preconditioning in the canine model by using this new and sensitive technique.[41] To obtain quantitative information regarding the amount and subcellular distribution of PKC in control versus preconditioned myocardium, additional experiments were performed in which the incorporation of ^{32}P from γ-^{32}P-labelled ATP into the threonine group of PKC-specific peptide was measured.[41] Subtle, but significant increases in PKC activity in the particulate fraction in all dogs after 10 min of sustained occlusion compared with those sacrificed immediately after 5 min episodes of preconditioning ischemia or no intervention appeared.[41] However, there was no trend towards a difference in the amount of distributed PKC between control and preconditioned groups at any time point.[41] Using the same method of PKC analysis Vogt *et al.*[59] described a modest 10 to 20% redistribution of PKC from the cytosol to the particulate fraction in *in vivo* pig hearts subjected to 10 min of sustained coronary occlusion.[59]

Does PKC Play a Role in Ischemic Preconditioning in Porcine Myocardium?

Although there is now considerable evidence that PKC activation may be involved in the mechanism leading to ischemic preconditioning, its role is not yet entirely clear as there is also conflicting evidence that inhibition of PKC may be beneficial in pig.[59] Using an *in situ* porcine model, we tested the hypothesis that translocation of PKC enzyme activity towards PKC-specific substrates (histone III-S and ε-peptide) and immunoreactivity of some major PKC isoforms (PKC-α,

TABLE 1. PKC Activity in Cytosolic and Particulate Fractions Isolated from Homogenized Biopsies Excised at 15 Min Reperfusion from the LADCA-(Preconditioned) and LCXCA-(Control) Perfused Beds of the Left Ventricle from Anesthetized Open-Chest Pigs[a]

| | Histone III-S[b] | | Peptide-ε[b] | |
	Basal	Ca^{2+} and (1,2)DAG-Stimulated	Basal	(1,2)DAG-Stimulated
LADCA				
Cytosolic	95 ± 11	232 ± 30	117 ± 11	36 ± 9
Particulate	56 ± 6	38 ± 8[c]	51 ± 9	−4 ± 5
LCXCA				
Cytosolic	86 ± 8	170 ± 5	111 ± 13	36 ± 8
Particulate	63 ± 4	8 ± 3	38 ± 3	−3 ± 1

[a] Pigs underwent a 10-min occlusion of the LADCA.[6,7] After 15 min reperfusion, transmural needle biopsies (1–3 mg) were taken from the LADCA-(preconditioned) and LCXCA-(control) perfused beds of the left ventricle, and immediately frozen in liquid nitrogen. Frozen tissue samples were homogenized at −80°C in 150 μl buffer containing 5 mM EGTA, 2 mM EDTA, 100 mM NaF, 200 μM PMSF, 2 μM leupeptine, 5 mM dithiothreitol in 25 mM TrisHCl (pH 7.4) using a dismembrator (Micro Dismembrator of Braun). After thawing the samples were centrifuged for 30 min at 48000 g in a JA 20 rotor (Beckman centrifuge J-2-21). The obtained supernatants (cytosolic fractions) were stored overnight at −80°C. The sediments were resuspended in homogenizing buffer and also stored overnight at −80°C. Before the PKC assay, the particulate fraction was solubilized in 0.5 mM EGTA, 2 mM EDTA, 2 mM PMSF, 10 mM β-mercaptoethanol, 0.5% (w/v) leupeptine, 0.3% (v/v) Triton X-100 in 20 mM TrisHCl (pH 7.5). PKC was assayed in both the cytosolic and particulate fractions in 100 μl reaction medium containing 5 mM MgCl$_2$, 10 μM β-mercaptoethanol, 0.25% (w/v) bovine serum albumin, 200 nM okadaic acid, 0.05% (w/v) histone III-S 10 μM γ-^{32}P-ATP (50–100 cpm/pmol), 20 mM TrisHCl (pH 7.5) with 2.5 mM CaCl$_2$ and an ultrasonified mixture of 0.016% (w/v) phosphatidylserine (PS) and with or without 0.004% (w/v) (1,2)DAG. When the phosphorylation of the ε-peptide was measured, the reaction mixture did not contain Ca^{2+} but instead of histone III-S 30 μM ε-peptide. The assay mixture was preincubated at 30°C for 2 min and the reactions were started with fractionated tissue sample and stopped after 5 min by the addition of ice-cold 200 μl 25% (w/v) trichloric acetic acid (TCA) plus 20 μl 1% (w/v) bovine serum albumin. Thereafter the mixture is millipore filtrated, the filters are four times washed with ice-cold 10% TCA and counted by liquid scintillation.

[b] Activities are expressed as pmol incorporated ^{32}P · mg protein^{-1} · min^{-1}.

[c] p <0.05 versus the particulate fraction from the LCXCA (control) bed.

-ε, -δ and -ζ) from the cytosol to the membrane fraction (a rough particulate and sarcoplasmatic reticulum), could play a role in ischemic preconditioning. Experiments were performed with four open-chest anesthetized pigs in which the proximal left anterior descending coronary artery (LADCA) was occluded for 10 min followed by reperfusion, a standard protocol to induce ischemic preconditioning.[7] Needle biopsies from the LADCA (preconditioned) perfused bed and from the normally perfused left circumflex coronary artery (LCXCA) bed were taken at 15 min reperfusion, a time point at which the postischemic myocardium is preconditioned.[7] The homogenized biopsies were centrifuged to obtain a supernatant (the cytosolic fraction) and a sediment (the particulate fraction). PKC activity was assayed in both fractions using γ-^{32}P-labelled ATP and histone III-S as peptidic substrate. As shown in TABLE 1, Ca^{2+} and (1,2)DAG stimulated PKC activity with histone III-S as substrate was significantly higher in the cytosolic as well as particulate fractions isolated from the LADCA-perfused myocardium (precondi-

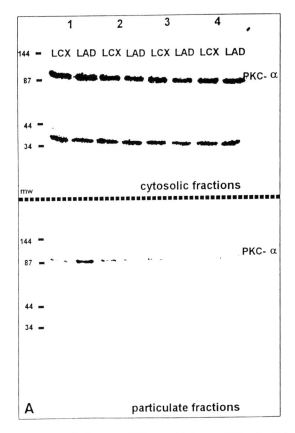

FIGURE 1. Immunoreactivity images of Western blots on which subcellular fractions isolated from biopsies taken from the LADCA and LCXCA beds of pigs were separated. (For
details of the experimental protocol and the isolation procedure of cytosolic and particulate
fractions from myocardial needle biopsies, see TABLE 1.) The immunoblot analysis is carried
out on the same needle biopsies of which results are shown in TABLE 1. Parts **(A)** and **(B)**
show, respectively, the PKC-α and PKC-ε obtained with cytosolic and particulate fractions
from the LCX and the LAD beds. Immunoblotting was carried out essentially as described.[61]
Rabbit polyclonal antibodies for PKC-α, -δ, -ε and -ζ were purchased from Santa Cruz
Biotechnology (Santa Cruz, CA). Chemiluminescence images of the blots are shown, ob-
tained by applying the ECL™ Western Blotting Kit and BioRad's Imaging Screen-CH in
the Molecular Phosphor Imaging System (GS-525).

tioned) than from the LCXCA (control) region of the left ventricle, whereas the
basal activities were the same. The peptide-ε was also used because it was previously shown that histone III-S is very poorly phosphorylated by PKC-ε,[60] which
in our hands turned out to be one of the major PKC isoforms in porcine myocardium
(FIG. 1). We observed significant (1,2)DAG-stimulated activities towards the
ε-peptide in the cytosolic fractions, but none in the particulate fraction. Based
upon our PKC-ε immunoreactivity measurements (FIG. 1) this was an unex-
pected finding.

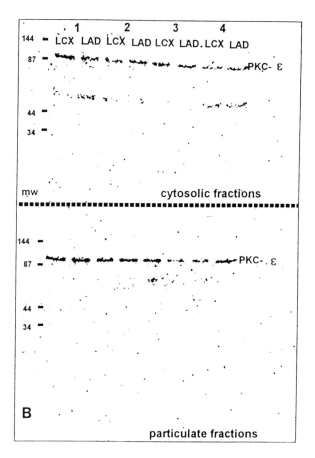

FIGURE 1. (*Continued*)

The cytosolic and particulate fractions were also examined by immunoblot analysis using rabbit polyclonal antibodies specific for PKC-α, -δ, -ε and -ζ isotypes. This analysis revealed significant levels of expression of the Ca^{2+}-independent isotype PKC-ε, which was detected as a band of 90–97-kDa molecular mass (FIG. 1B), while PKC-α was also abundantly present (FIG. 1A). The appearance of both bands could be blocked by addition of PKC-isopeptide demonstrating the specificity of detection. PKC-δ and -ζ were virtually undetectable using the rabbit polyclonal antibodies. The latter results, however, do not prove that PKC-δ and -ζ isoenzymes are not present in porcine myocardium, because it is possible that the polyclonal rabbit antibodies are not suitable for Western blot detection of PKC-δ and -ζ. The immunoreactivity expressed as chemiluminescence counts, determined by applying the ECL™ Western Blotting Kit and BioRad's Imaging Screen-CH in the Molecular Phosphor Imaging System, revealed no differences between the biopsies of the LADCA (preconditioned) and LCXCA (control) beds of the left ventricle (results not shown). These results indicate that neither the

(Ca^{2+} and (1,2)DAG)-stimulated histone III-S kinase activities of the cytosolic nor those of the particulate fractions are reflected by relative changes in immunoreactivities (FIG. 1). Moreover, in the particulate fraction we found relatively more PKC-ε immunoreactivity than in the cytosolic fraction (respectively, 903 ± 104 and 529 ± 38 chemiluminescence counts in biopsies taken from the LCXCA bed), whereas the particulate PKC activity determined with ε-peptide as substrate was not detectable (TABLE 1). The immunofluorescence results suggest that the amount of subcellular distribution of PKC-α and -ε was not altered in the LADCA (preconditioned) region compared to the LCXCA (control region). However, it could be argued that this detection method is not suitable for distinguishing between active and inactive PKC isoenzymes. Nevertheless, using histone III-S as substrate for determining total (Ca^{2+} and (1,2)DAG)-dependent PKC activity, increased activity was found in the cytosolic as well as in the particulate fractions isolated from the LADCA (preconditioned) compared with the LCXCA (control) bed of the ventricle. Therefore, by using these methods we were unable to discriminate between the occurrence of ischemia-induced expression of PKC isoenzymes or ischemia-induced translocation from the cytosolic to the particulate fraction. The results demonstrate activation of cytosolic and membrane-bound PKC with transient ischemia in the LADCA bed compared with the normally perfused LCXCA bed and suggest that PKC might be involved in preconditioning in the pig. However, it should be kept in mind that the presented PKC data were obtained at only one time point. In order to prove that intracellular redistribution and activation of PKC is an important mechanism for the reduction of infarct size, the endogenous target proteins for PKC should be known. Comparing the time courses of phosphorylation of these target proteins on their serine or threonine residues by the PKC isoenzymes and their subsequent dephosphorylation with the gradual appearance and decay of protection during transient ischemia followed by reperfusion, is essential before a potential role of PKC as intracellular mediator of ischemic preconditioning can be accepted.

Exploration of the Possible Role of PLD in PKC-Mediated Preconditioning

The PKC hypothesis for ischemic preconditioning suggests that endogenous ligands such as A_1 adenosine-, α_1-adrenergic and muscarinic agonists, bradykinin and angiotensin II initiate an intracellular pathway resulting in stimulating PLC-β via G-coupled receptors ultimately leading to (1,2)DAG activation of Ca^{2+}-dependent and Ca^{2+}-independent PKC-isoenzymes. Many of the postulated endogenous ligands can also activate PLD. Lindmar *et al.*[62] were the first to show that muscarinic receptors, stimulated by carbachol, were coupled to PLD in the perfused chicken heart. Examining isolated subcellular membranes from rat ventricular myocardium, Panagia *et al.*[63] showed indeed that an active PLD is bound to the sarcolemmal membranes. However, a drawback of the PLD analysis in cell-free preparations is that PLD activity can only be detected in the presence of surfactants such as oleate[64] but not by stimulation with agonists. Angiotensin II activates PLD via the AT_1-receptor present in intact rat cardiomyocytes.[65] Cardiomyocytes, prelabelled with [^{3}H]myristic acid showed a rapid increase in [^{3}H]phosphatidic acid ([^{3}H]PtdOH) within minutes after stimulation by angiotensin II and the [^{3}H]PtdOH accumulation persisted thereafter for more than 30 minutes, suggesting that the [^{3}H]PtdOH was derived from [^{3}H]myristoyl-phosphatidylcholine ([^{3}H]myristoyl-PtdCho). However, [^{3}H]PtdOH could also be produced by PtdCho-hydrolysis catalyzed by PtdCho-specific PLC and subsequent phosphorylation of (1,2)DAG catalyzed by DAG kinase. Both reactions could also explain the early [³H](1,2)DAG response. However, in the presence of a diacylglycerol kinase inhibitor, accumulation of [³H]PtdOH persisted. The latter finding proved that PLD must be responsible for angiotensin II-stimulated [³H]PtdOH production in the cultured cardiomyocytes.[65] The PtdOH formed can also be separated from other phospholipids by thin layer chromatography (TLC) and the stained spot quantified by photodensitometry. This method was recently employed by Hong-ping et al.,[66] who examined the response of adult rabbit ventricular myocytes to stimulation by noradrenaline and endothelin-1. In the latter study it was also demonstrated that exogenously added PtdOH stimulated the production of inositol-phosphates (InsP$_n$). Because the presence of exogenous PtdOH activated PLC-β, it was assumed by these authors that this second messenger is the activator of PLC-β following PLD activation.[66] It is possible that PtdOH is produced from (1,2)DAG via phosphorylation when PLC-β is stimulated by muscarinic agonists, endothelin-1, angiotensin II or α_1-adrenergic agonists. Newly formed PtdOH could then function as a positive feedback mechanism for PLC-β via increased PtdIns(4,5)P$_2$ hydrolysis. PLD most likely also produces PtdOH, which serves as an alternative pathway by which agonists could activate PLC-β-mediated cleavage of PtdIns(4,5)P$_2$.[67] However, the coupling function of PtdOH between PLD and PLC-β, postulated in this study, is in contrast to most other reports, were PtdOH is believed to primarily originate from PLD action and will subsequently be transformed to (1,2)DAG. PLD activity can also be detected by measuring the formation of free choline in the extracellular medium, using incubation of cardiac tissue or isolated and cultured cardiomyocytes, or the medium by which the heart is perfused. We measured choline formation in cultured cardiomyocytes, of which endogenous PtdCho was first prelabelled with [³H]choline followed by a short incubation in an unlabelled choline-containing medium. In these cardiac myocytes, [³H]choline production increased above control cells between 20 and 40 min after endothelin-1 and increased markedly between 10 and 20 min after PMA stimulation (results not shown). These late responses suggest that PLD is involved in the hydrolysis of PtdCho and that direct PKC stimulation by PMA can lead to PLD activation. These results are consistent with our measurements using the PLD-catalyzed transphosphatidylation assay (see below).

In general, the reason for the relatively late discovery of the existence of receptor-coupled PLD was the established route of agonist-dependent (1,2)DAG production by hydrolysis of phosphatidylinositol-4,5-bisphosphate (PtdIns(4,5)P$_2$) by PLC-β as well as the fact that the observed increase of PtdOH in many cells following receptor stimulation was thought to result from the rapid action of DAG-kinase on (1,2)DAG.[68] However, it has been reported that the formation of (1,2)DAG was dissociated in time from the generation of InsP$_n$,[69] often to the extent that (1,2)DAG is formed in the complete absence of Ins(1,4,5)P$_3$ accumulation.[30,39,70] PLC-β hydrolyzes the glycerophosphate ester in PtdIns(4,5)P$_2$ to form (1,2)DAG and Ins(1,4,5)P$_3$. PLD cleaves on the other side of the phosphoryl linkage to form PtdOH and the free base mostly from PtdCho and subsequently PtdOH is hydrolyzed by PtdOH-hydrolase to (1,2)DAG. The concentration in the cell of PtdCho is usually about 100 times higher than PtdIns(4,5)P$_2$ concentration. The continuous production of (1,2)DAG could be of major importance for the maintenance of activation of specific PKC isoenzymes involved in the mechanism of ischemic preconditioning. Furthermore, several nonmyocardial studies (see for instance Ref. 71) indicate that (1,2)DAG formed in the early transient phase of receptor stimulation predominantly contains fatty acids present in the PtdIns(4,5)P$_2$ pool (stearate, 18:0 and arachidonate, 20:4n-6), whereas in the later phase of

TABLE 2. Activation of PLC-β and PLD by Agonists in Cultured Rat Cardiomyocytes[a]

	[^{14}C]PtdEth Formation[b]		[^{3}H]InsP$_n$ Formation[c]	
	10 min	40 min	10 min	40 min
Control	0.053 ± 0.003	0.037 ± 0.012	4.34 ± 0.41	4.09 ± 0.53
Phenylephrine (10^{-5} M)	0.041 ± 0.001	0.042 ± 0.004	6.63 ± 0.67[d]	16.07 ± 0.76[d]
Endothelin-1 (10^{-8} M)	0.115 ± 0.003[d]	0.221 ± 0.079[d]	11.96 ± 0.39[d]	38.45 ± 2.06[d]
Angiotensin II (10^{-7} M)	0.067 ± 0.017	0.058 ± 0.000[d]	5.21 ± 0.52	6.62 ± 0.30[d]
PMA (10^{-6} M)	0.272 ± 0.115[d]	0.528 ± 0.065[d]	3.71 ± 0.51	4.64 ± 0.63

[a] Neonatal rat ventricular myocytes were cultured as previously described.[38,73] Briefly, ventricles from newborn, 2-day-old Wistar strain rats were minced and myocytes were isolated by 8 subsequent trypsinization steps at 30°C. Nonmyocytes were removed by differential preplating and myocytes were seeded at 150.000 cells/cm^2. Cells were grown in DMEM : M199 (4 : 1) supplemented with 5% fetal calf and 5% horse serum. After 24 hr, medium was changed to serum-free DMEM : M199, which was changed every 48 hr thereafter. Experiments were routinely performed 5–7 days after isolation of the cells. PLD activities were determined by measuring the production of [^{14}C]PtdEth in the presence of 0.5% ethanol in cardiomyocytes that were prelabelled for 48 hr with [^{14}C]palmitic acid. After the incubation with agonists the cellular lipids were extracted and [^{14}C]PtdEth was separated from other phospholipids by TLC. PLC-β activities were determined by measuring the production of [^{3}H]InsP$_n$ in cardiomyocytes that were prelabelled for 48 hr with [^{3}H]Ins. The [^{3}H]InsP$_n$ were separated from [^{3}H]Ins and [^{3}H]glycerophosphoinositol by column chromatography on a Dowex AG 1-X8 as previously described.[74] The values represent the mean ± SEM and are expressed as % of the total incorporated [^{14}C]palmitic acid[b] or [^{3}H]Ins.[c]
[d] p <0.05 versus control (respectively, n = 2[b] and n = 8[c]).

receptor stimulation it contains more saturated fatty acids typically found in PtdCho.[71] In line with these findings it can be expected that distinction in the molecular species of (1,2)DAG is responsible for the time-dependent differences in pattern of activation of PKC isoenzymes, which are often seen after stimulation with different agonists.[30,37–39,72] Recently, we observed a difference in fatty-acid composition, mainly in the 16 : 0 and 20 : 4n-6 of the (1,2)DAG formed comparing 10- and 40-min stimulation by endothelin-1 of cardiomyocytes (results not shown). These results indicate that after a 10-min stimulation (1,2)DAG originates mainly from PtdIns(4,5)P$_2$ and after 40 min from PtdCho.

The PLD-catalyzed transphosphatidylation assay (the formation of phosphatidylalcohol through a base exchange reaction of PtdCho with an alcohol such as ethanol or butanol) can be used to unmask the operation of the PLD pathway.[39,66,72] Accordingly, we determined the rate of [^{14}C]PtdEth formation in the presence of 0.5% ethanol in cardiomyocytes prelabelled with [^{14}C]palmitic acid. The [^{14}C]PtdEth formation was, respectively, 5.9-, 1.6- and 14.2-fold increased by 40 min of stimulation with, respectively, 10^{-8} M endothelin-1, 10^{-7} M angiotensin II and 10^{-6} M PMA (TABLE 2). α_1-Adrenergic stimulation, however, had no effect on PLD. These results were in agreement with those obtained by measuring [^{3}H]choline production from [^{3}H]choline prelabelled cardiomyocytes (see above). On the other hand, phenylephrine, endothelin-1 and angiotensin II markedly stimulated (respectively, 3.9-, 9.4- and 1.6-fold) PLC-β in these cells (TABLE 2). As expected, PMA had no significant effect on InsP$_n$ production. Unpublished results from our own laboratory showed also that the activation of PLD does not begin earlier than 10 min after agonist addition. In contrast, we found that the agonist-induced activation of PLC-β is very fast.[70,74,75] Also taking into account the strong activation of PLD by PMA, it is likely that the activation of PLD is a secondary response to PLC-β.

Until now, the question whether PtdIns(4,5)P$_2$ hydrolysis *per se* is sufficient for PLD activation or if it only has modulatory effects on receptor-coupled PLD activation, has not been addressed. The unequivocal proof for GTP-binding protein regulation of receptor-mediated PtdCho-hydrolysis must await appropriate reconstitution studies as were done with PtdIns(4,5)P$_2$ specific PLC.[39] One possible explanation forwarded for the receptor-coupled activation of both PLD and PLC is that a single receptor GTP-binding protein complex couples both effector enzymes and that this coupling is perhaps regulated by PKC.[76] However, this is highly unlikely due to the fact that PLC-β-G$_q$ is pertussis toxin insensitive, in contrast to the pertussis toxin inhibition of PLD activity.

Because PMA appeared to be very effective in inducing PtdCho-hydrolysis by PLD in cardiomyocytes, it became interesting to comparatively investigate the translocation of PKC isoenzymes to the membranes during agonist and PMA stimulation in these cells. Therefore, we measured the translocation of two PKC isotypes α and ε that were readily detectable in the cardiomyocytes, using immunoblot analysis as was shown by Clerk et al.[77] Endothelin-1 caused a very rapid and sustained disappearance of PKC-ε but not of PKC-α from the cytosol (FIG. 2). Since the PKC-ε levels in the membrane fraction reaches almost the detection level (results not shown), the translocation of PKC-ε to the membrane was not always visible. PMA (10^{-7} M), however, caused a rapid, sustained and clearly detectable translocation of PKC-α as well as -ε. It is important to note that minimal proportions of PKC-α and -ε are associated with the membrane fraction in the cardiomyocytes under unstimulated conditions (FIG. 2).

Mitchell et al.,[29] showed in rat heart that the PKC-δ and PKC-ε were translocated through transient ischemic stimulation. Since the initial PLC-β response

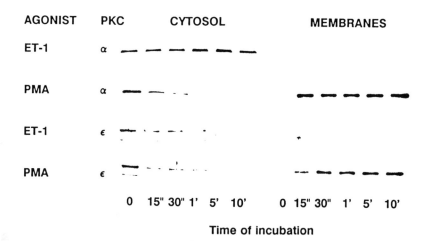

FIGURE 2. Immunoblots of the time course of distribution of PKC-α and PKC-ε between cytosol and membrane fraction after exposure of cardiomyocytes to endothelin-1 (10^{-8} M) (ET-1) and PMA (10^{-7} M). Cultured cardiomyocytes were incubated with either PMA or endothelin-1 under the conditions given in TABLE 2. The cell lysis, cell fractionation and immunoblot analysis of subcellular fractions was performed as previously described.[38]

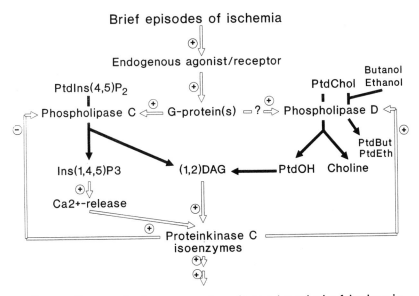

FIGURE 3. Interrelationships between PLC-β and PLD pathways that are possibly involved in the mechanism of ischemic preconditioning. *Open* and *closed arrows* refer to, respectively, stimulatory (+) or inhibitory actions (−) and chemical reactions. See text for further explanation.

usually is accompanied by increases in Ca^{2+} and (1,2)DAG and followed by a prolonged increase of (1,2)DAG with no rise in Ca^{2+}, the observed translocation of PKC-δ and PKC-ε is more likely due to the secondary PLD activation. The gradual decay of protection takes hours after the ischemic event, which is more in agreement with the involvement of PLD than PLC in the mechanism of ischemic preconditioning. The question remains, however, whether PLD indeed is activated by ischemia. In perfused rat heart, prelabelled with [^{14}C]arachidonic acid, ischemia (30 min)-reperfusion (30 min) induced a significant increase in the amount of [^{14}C]arachidonic acid incorporated into PtdOH and (1,2)DAG.[40] Recently, it was shown that brief episodes of ischemia induced increased endothelin-1 secretion in the perfused rat heart.[78] Thus on the basis of these findings endothelin-1 can be added to the list of potential endogenous mediators of cardioprotection such as α_1-adrenergic-, A_1 adenosine and muscarinic agonists and angiotensin II. A role for G-proteins in the PLD activation independent of PLC-β and PKC activation has been suggested but is not generally assumed (FIG. 3).[79]

It seems more likely that the PLD activation by the agonists, endogenously formed during ischemia, is initiated by G-coupled–PLC-β-derived (1,2)DAG that activates PKC isoenzymes (FIG. 3). By switching to PtdCho as source for (1,2)DAG the cardiomyocyte is able to maintain increased levels of (1,2)DAG for a prolonged period of time, which is expected to lead to changes in the molecular species of (1,2)DAG required for a distinct pattern of activation of PKC isoenzymes.

REFERENCES

1. DOWNEY, J. M. 1992. Ischemic preconditioning: nature's own cardioprotective intervention. Trends Cardiovasc. Med. **2:** 170–176.
2. MURRY, C. E. & R. B. JENNINGS. 1986. Preconditioning with ischemia: a delay of lethal cell injury in ischemic myocardium. Circulation **74:** 1124–1136.
3. LIU, Y. & J. M. DOWNEY. 1992. Ischemic preconditioning protects against infarction in rat heart. Am. J. Physiol. **263:** H1107–H1112.
4. LI, G. C., J. A. VASQUEZ, K. P. GALLAGHER & B. R. LUCCHESI. 1990. Myocardial protection with preconditioning. Circulation **82:** 609–619.
5. URABE, K., T. M. MIURA, T. I. IWAMOTO, T. OGAWA, M. GOTO, J. SAKAMOTO & O. IIMURA. 1993. Preconditioning enhances myocardial resistance to post-ischaemic myocardial stunning via adenosine receptor activation. Cardiovasc. Res. **27:** 657–662.
6. SCHOTT, R. J., S. ROHMAN, E. R. BRAUN & W. SCHAPER. 1990. Ischemic preconditioning reduces infarct size in swine myocardium. Circ. Res. **66:** 1122–1142.
7. KONING, M. M. G., L. A. J. SIMONIS, S. DE ZEEUW, S. NIEUKOOP, S. POST & P. D. VERDOUW. 1994. Ischaemic preconditioning by partial occlusion without intermittent reperfusion. Cardiovasc. Res. **28:** 1146–1151.
8. KLONER, R. A. & D. YELLON. 1994. Does ischemic preconditioning occur in patients? J. Am. Coll. Cardiol. **24:** 1133–1142.
9. LAWSON, C. S. 1994. Does ischemic preconditioning occur in the human heart? Cardiovasc. Res. **28:** 1461–1466.
10. VERDOUW, P. D., B. C. G. GHO & D. J. DUNCKER. 1995. Ischaemic preconditioning: is it clinically relevant? Eur. Heart J. **16:** 1169–1176.
11. SHIKI, K. & D. J. HEARSE. 1987. Preconditioning of ischemic myocardium: reperfusion-induced arrhythmias. Am. J. Physiol. **253:** H1470–H1476.
12. VEGH, A., S. KOHMARI, L. SZEKERES & J. R. PARRATT. 1992. Antiarrhythmic effects of preconditioning in anaesthetized dogs and rats. Cardiovasc. Res. **26:** 487–495.
13. LAWSON, C. S. & J. M. DOWNEY. 1993. Preconditioning: state of the art myocardial protection. Cardiovasc. Res. **27:** 542–550.
14. LI, Y., P. WHITTAKER & R. A. KLONER. 1992. The transient nature of the effect of ischemic preconditioning on myocardial infarct size and ventricular arrhythmia. Am. Heart J. **123:** 346–353.
15. KLONER, R. A., K. PRZYKLENK, P. WHITTAKER & S. HALE. 1995. Editorial. Preconditioning stimuli and inadvertent preconditioning. J. Mol. Cell. Cardiol. **27:** 743–747.
16. LIU, G. S., J. THORNTON, D. M. VAN WINKLE, A. W. H. STANLEY, R. A. OLSSON & J. W. DOWNEY. 1991. Protection against infarction afforded by preconditioning is mediated by A_1 adenosine receptors in rabbit heart. Circulation **84:** 350–356.
17. GROSS, G. J. & J. A. AUCHAMPACH. 1992. Blockade of ATP-sensitive potassium channels prevents myocardial preconditioning in dogs. Circ. Res. **70:** 223–233.
18. BANERJEE, A., C. LOCKE-WINTER, K. B. ROGERS, M. B. MITCHELL, E. C. BREW, C. B. CAIRNS, D. D. BENSARD & A. H. HARKEN. 1993. Preconditioning against myocardial dysfunction after ischemia and reperfusion by an α-adrenergic mechanism. Circ. Res. **73:** 656–670.
19. TSUCHIDA, A., Y. LIU, G. S. LIU, M. V. COHEN & J. M. DOWNEY. 1994. α_1-Adrenergic agonists precondition rabbit ischemic myocardium independent of adenosine by direct activation of protein kinase C. Circ. Res. **75:** 576–585.
20. THORNTON, J. D., G. S. LIU & J. M. DOWNEY. 1993. Pretreatment with pertussis toxin blocks the protective effects of preconditioning: evidence for a G-protein mechanism. J. Mol. Cell. Cardiol. **25:** 311–320.
21. YAO, Z. & G. J. GROSS. 1993. Acetylcholine mimics ischemic preconditioning via a glibencamide-sensitive mechanism in dogs. Am. J. Physiol. **264:** H2221–H2225.
22. PARRATT, J. R. 1994. Protection of the heart by ischemic preconditioning mechanisms and possibilities for pharmacological exploitation. Trends Pharmacol. Sci. **15:** 19–25.
23. GOTO, M., Y. LIU, X-M. YANG, J. L. ARDELL, M. V. COHEN & J. M. DOWNEY. 1995. Role of bradykinin in protection of ischemic preconditioning in rabbit heart. Circ. Res. **77:** 611–621.

24. LIU, Y., A. TSUCHIDA, M. V. COHEN & J. M. DOWNEY. 1995. Pretreatment with angiotensin II activates protein kinase C and limits myocardial infarction in isolated rabbit hearts. J. Mol. Cell. Cardiol. **27:** 883–892.

25. HALE, S. L., S. D. BELLOWS, H. HAMMERMAN & R. A. KLONER. 1993. An adenosine A_1 receptor agonist, R-(-)-N-E_2 phenylisopropyl-adenosine (PIA) acts as a therapeutic preconditioning-mimetic agent in rabbits. Cardiovasc. Res. **27:** 2140–2145.

26. TOOMBS, C. F., D. S. McGAE, W. E. JOHNSON & J. VINTON-JOHANSON. 1992. Myocardial protective effects of adenosine: infarct size reduction with pretreatment and continued receptor stimulation during ischemia. Circulation **86:** 986–994.

27. YTREHUS, K., Y. LIU & J. M. DOWNEY. 1993. Preconditioning protect the ischemic rabbit heart by protein kinase C activation. Am. J. Physiol. **266:** H1145–H1152.

28. SPEECHLY-DICK, M. E., M. M. MOCANU & D. M. YELLON. 1994. Protein kinase C. Its role in ischemic preconditioning in the rat. Circ. Res. **75:** 586–590.

29. MITCHELL, M. B., X. MENG, L. AO, J. M. BROWN, A. H. HARKEN & A. BANERJEE. 1995. Preconditioning of isolated rat heart is mediated by protein kinase C. Circ. Res. **76:** 73–81.

30. DE JONGE, H. W., H. A. A. VAN HEUGTEN & J. M. J. LAMERS. 1995. Review. Signal transduction by the phosphatidylinositol cycle in myocardium. J. Mol. Cell. Cardiol. **27:** 93–106.

31. SPEECHLY-DICK, M. E., G. J. GROVER & D. M. YELLON. 1995. Does ischemic preconditioning in the human involve protein kinase C and the ATP-dependent K^+ channel? Studies of the contractile function after simulated ischemia in an atrial *in vivo* model. Circ. Res. **77:** 1030–1035.

32. LIU, G. S., W. D. GAO, B. O'ROURKE & E. MARBAN. 1995. Synergistic potentiation of ATP-sensitive potassium current by protein kinase C and adenosine: implications for ischemic preconditioning. Circulation **92:** I-251.

33. HU, K., D. DUAN & S. NATTEL. 1995. Protein kinase C-mediated activation of ATP-sensitive potassium current—the missing link in ischemic preconditioning. Circulation 92(Suppl. I): I-251.

34. LINDMAR, R., K. LÖFFELHOLZ & J. SANDMAN. 1988. On the mechanism of muscarinic hydrolysis of choline phospholipids. Biochem. Pharmacol. **37:** 4689–4695.

35. KURZ, T. & R. A. WOLF. 1993. Phosphatidic acid stimulates inositol 1,4,5-triphosphate production in adult cardiac myocytes. Circ. Res. **72:** 701–706.

36. SADOSHIMA, J. & S. IZUMO. 1993. Signal transduction pathways of angiotensin II induced c-fos gene expression in cardiac myocytes *in vitro*. Circ. Res. **73:** 424–438.

37. LAMERS, J. M. J., H. W. DE JONGE, V. PANAGIA & H. A. A. VAN HEUGTEN. 1993. Receptor mediated signalling pathways acting through membrane phospholipid hydrolysis in cardiomyocytes. Cardioscience **4:** 121–131.

38. LAMERS, J. M. J., Y. E. G. ESKILDSEN-HELMOND, A. M. RESINK, H. W. DE JONGE, K. BEZSTAROSTI, H. S. SHARMA, H. A. A. VAN HEUGTEN. 1995. Endothelin-1-induced phospholipase C-β and D and protein kinase C isoenzyme signalling leading to hypertrophy in rat cardiomyocytes. J. Cardiovasc. Pharmacol. **26**(Suppl. 3): S100–S103.

39. ESKILDSEN-HELMOND, Y. E. G., H. A. A. VAN HEUGTEN & J. M. J. LAMERS. 1996. Regulation and functional significance of phospholipase D in myocardium. Mol. Cell. Biochem. In press.

40. MORARU, I. I., L. M. POPESCU, N. MAULIK, X. LIU & D. K. DAS. 1992. Phospholipase D signalling in ischemic heart. Biochim. Biophys. Acta **1139:** 148–154.

41. PRZYKLENK, K., M. A. SUSSMAN, B. Z. SIMKHOVICH & R. A. KLONER. 1995. Does ischemic preconditioning trigger translocation of protein kinase C in the canine model. Circulation **92:** 1546–1557.

42. BUGGE, E. & K. YTREHUS. 1995. Ischemic preconditioning is protein kinase C dependent but not through stimulation of α-adrenergic or adenosine receptors in the isolated rat heart. Cardiovasc. Res. **29:** 401–406.

43. LIU, Y., K. YTREHUS & J. M. DOWNEY. 1994. Evidence that translocation of protein kinase C is a key event during ischemic preconditioning of rabbit myocardium. J. Mol. Cell. Cardiol. **26:** 661–668.

44. LIU, Y., M. V. COHEN & J. M. DOWNEY. 1994. Chelerythrine, a highly selective protein kinase C inhibitor, blocks the anti-infarct effect of ischemic preconditioning in rabbit hearts. Cardiovasc. Drugs Ther. **8:** 881–882.
45. LI, Y. & R. A. KLONER. 1995. Does protein kinase C play a role in ischemic preconditioning in rat hearts? Am. J. Physiol. **268:** H426–H431.
46. ARMSTRONG, S., J. M. DOWNEY & C. E. GANOTE. 1994. Preconditioning of isolated rabbit cardiomyocytes: induction by metabolic stress and blockade by the adenosine antagonist SPT and calphostin C, a protein kinase C inhibitor. Cardiovasc. Res. **28:** 72–77.
47. TAMAOKI, T. 1991. Use and the specificity of staurosporine, UCN-01, and calphostin C as protein kinase inhibitors. Methods Enzymol. **201:** 340–347.
48. HERBERT, J. M., J. M. AUGEREAU, J. GLEYE & J. P. MAFFRAND. 1990. Chelerythrine is a potent and specific inhibitor of protein kinase C. Biochem. Biophys. Res. Commun. **172:** 993–999.
49. KOBAYASHI, E., H. NAKANO, M. MORIMOTO & T. TAMAOKI. 1989. Calphostin C (UCN-1028C), a novel microbial compound, is a highly potent and specific inhibitor of protein kinase C. Biochem. Biophys. Res. Commun. **159:** 548–553.
50. HUG, H. & T. F. SARRE. 1990. Protein kinase C isoenzymes: divergence in signal transduction? Biochem. J. **291:** 329–343.
51. NAKAMURA, S. & Y. NISHIZUKA. 1994. Lipid mediators and PKC activation for the intracellular signalling network. J. Biochem. **115:** 1029–1034.
52. STEINBERG, S. F., M. GOLDBERG & V. O. RYBIN. 1995. Protein kinase C isoform diversity in the heart. J. Mol. Cell. Cardiol. **27:** 141–153.
53. HARRINGTON, E. O. & J. A. WARE. 1995. Diversity of the protein kinase C gene family. Implications for cardiovascular disease. Trends Cardiovasc. Med. **5:** 193–198.
54. ALLEN, B. G. & S. KATZ. 1991. Isolation and characterization of the calcium and phospholipid-dependent protein kinase (protein kinase C) subtypes from bovine heart. Biochemistry **30:** 4334–4343.
55. RYBIN, V. O. & S. F. STEINBERG. 1994. Protein kinase C isoform expression and regulation in the developing heart. Circ. Res. **74:** 299–309.
56. MOCHLY-ROSEN, D., C. J. HEINRICH, L. CHEEVER, H. KHANER & P. C. SIMPSON. 1990. A protein kinase C isoenzyme is translocated to cytoskeletal elements on activation. Cell Regul. **1:** 693–706.
57. WEINBRENNER, C. E., G. SIMONIS, R. MARQUETANT & R. H. STRASSER. 1993. Selective regulation of calcium-dependent and calcium-independent subtypes of protein kinase C in acute and prolonged myocardial ischemia. Circulation **88**(Suppl. 1): I-101.
58. BOGOYEVITCH, M. A., P. J. PARKER & P. H. SUGDEN. 1993. Characterization of protein kinase C isotype expression in adult rat heart. Circ. Res. **72:** 757–767.
59. VOGT, A., M. BARANCIK, D. WEIHRAUCH, M. ARRAS, T. PODZUWEIT & W. SCHAPER. 1994. Protein kinase C inhibitors reduce infarct size in pig hearts *in vivo*. Circulation **90**(Suppl. I): I-647.
60. SCHAAP, D. & P. J. PARKER. 1990. Expression, purification, and characterization of protein kinase C-ε. J. Biol. Chem. **265:** 7301–7307.
61. CLERK, A., M. A. BOGOYEVITSCH, M. B. ANDERSON & P. SUGDEN. 1994. Differential activation of protein kinase C isoforms by endothelin-1, and phenylephrine and subsequent stimulation of p42 and p44 mitogen-activated protein kinases in ventricular myocytes cultured from neonatal rat hearts. J. Biol. Chem. **269:** 32848–32857.
62. LINDMAR, R., K. LÖFFELHOLZ & J. SANDMANN. 1988. On the mechanism of muscarinic hydrolysis of choline phospholipids. Biochem. Pharmacol. **37:** 4689–4695.
63. PANAGIA, V., C. OU, Y. TAIRA, J. DAI & N. S. DHALLA. 1991. Phospholipase D activity in subcellular membranes of rat ventricular myocardium. Biochim. Biophys. Acta **1064**(2): 242–250.
64. TAKI, T. & J. N. KANFER. 1981. Phospholipase D from rat brain. Methods Enzymol. **71:** 746–750.
65. SADOSHIMA, J. & S. IZUMO. 1993. Signal transduction pathways of angiotensin II-induced c-fos gene expression in cardiac myocytes *in vitro*. Circ. Res. **73:** 424–438.
66. HONGPING, Y., R. A. WOLF, T. KURZ & P. B. CORR. 1994. Phosphatidic acid increases

in response to noradrenaline and endothelin-1 in adult rabbit ventricular myocytes. Cardiovasc. Res. **28:** 18128–18134.

67. KURZ, T., R. A. WOLF & P. B. CORR. 1993. Phosphatidic acid stimulates inositol 1,4,5-triphosphate production in adult cardiac myocytes. Circ. Res. **72:** 701–706.

68. BERRIDGE, M. J. 1987. Inositol trisphosphate and diacylglycerol: two interacting second messengers. Annu. Rev. Biochem. **56:** 159–193.

69. THOMPSON, N. T., R. W. BONSER & L. G. GARLAND. 1991. Receptor-coupled phospholipase D and its inhibition. Trends Pharmacol. Sci. **12:** 404–408.

70. DE JONGE, H. W., H. A. A. VAN HEUGTEN, K. BEZSTAROSTI & J. M. J. LAMERS. 1994. Distinct α_1-adrenergic agonist- and ET-1 evoked phosphoinositide cycle responses in cultured neonatal rat cardiomyocytes. Biochem. Biophys. Res. Commun. **203:** 422–429.

71. PESSIN, M. S. & D. M. RABEN. 1989. Molecular species analysis of 1,2-diglycerides stimulated by α-thrombin in cultured fibroblasts. J. Biol. Chem. **264:** 8729–8738.

72. LEE, M. W. & D. L. SEVERSON. 1994. Signal transduction in vascular smooth muscle: diacylglycerol messengers and PKC action. Am. J. Physiol. **267:** C659–C678.

73. VAN HEUGTEN, H. A. A., H. W. DE JONGE, K. BEZSTAROSTI, H. S. SHARMA, P. D. VERDOUW & J. M. J. LAMERS. 1995. Intracellular signalling and genetic reprogramming during agonist-induced hypertrophy of cardiomyocytes. Ann. N. Y. Acad. Sci. **752:** 343–352.

74. VAN HEUGTEN, H. A. A., H. W. DE JONGE, K. BEZSTAROSTI & J. M. J. LAMERS. 1994. Calcium and endothelin-1 and the α_1-adrenergic stimulated phosphatidylinositol cycle in cultured rat cardiomyocytes. J. Mol. Cell. Cardiol. **26:** 1081–1093.

75. VAN HEUGTEN, H. A. A., K. BEZSTAROSTI, D. H. W. DEKKERS & J. M. J. LAMERS. 1993. Homologous desensitization of the endothelin-1 receptor mediated phosphoinositide response in cultured neonatal rat cardiomyocytes. J. Mol. Cell. Cardiol. **25:** 41–52.

76. THOMPSON, N. T., K. G. GARLAND & R. W. BONSER. 1993. Phospholipase D: regulation and functional significance. Adv. Pharmacol. **24:** 199–238.

77. CLERK, A., M. A. BOGOYEVITCH, M. B. ANDERSSON & P. SUGDEN. 1994. Differential activation of protein kinase C isoforms by endothelin-1 and phenylephrine and subsequent stimulation of p42 and p44 mitogen-activated protein kinases in ventricular myocytes cultured from neonatal rat hearts. J. Biol. Chem. **269:** 32848–32857.

78. BRUNNER, F. 1995. Tissue endothelin-1 levels in perfused rat heart following stimulation with agonists and in ischaemia and reperfusion. J. Mol. Cell. Cardiol. **27:** 1953–1963.

79. LISCOVITCH, M., P. BEN-AV, M. DANIN, G. FAIMAN, H. ELDAR & E. LIVNEH. 1993. Phosphatidylcholine: a role in cell signalling. J. Lipid Mediators **8:** 177–182.

Stress-Induced Cardioadaptation Reveals a Code Linking Hormone Receptors and Spatial Redistribution of PKC Isoforms

ANIRBAN BANERJEE,[a] FABIA GAMBONI-ROBERTSON,
MAX B. MITCHELL, THOMAS F. REHRING,
KARYN BUTLER, JOSEPH CLEVELAND,
DANIEL R. MELDRUM, JOSEPH I. SHAPIRO, AND
XIA-ZHONG MENG

*University of Colorado
Health Sciences Center
Denver, Colorado, 80262*

INTRODUCTION

Ischemic injury to the heart is a common problem, both as a disease and as an iatrogenic component of cardiac by-pass surgery. The enormous complexity inherent in simultaneous deprivation of oxygen and substrates from the myocardium as well as accumulation of metabolic wastes, is the focus of active investigation. Moreover, in the whole organ, myocytes experience a dynamic milieu (including neuroendocrine, vascular, and leucocytic factors) that changes during both ischemia and resumption of perfusion. A most promising therapeutic avenue may lie in the cardioadaptive "preconditioning" against sustained ischemia provided by transient episode(s) of ischemic stress preceding the insult.[2,10,20] This naturally protective mechanism is induced within 10 minutes of the stimulus and involves a variety of neuroendocrine agonists produced within the ischemic myocardium. The dominant receptor subtypes have been identified for several species, and appear linked to PKC.[10,16,18,22] However what actual protective mechanisms are engaged by PKC phosphorylation are not known.

The challenge is to find the proteins targeted by PKC so that these can eventually lead to an understanding of the rapid cardioprotective effect. At present, the consensus sequence is still that based on the initially discovered Ca^{++}-dependent isoforms (cPKC), which simply specifies phosphorylation of Ser/Thr residues that are surrounded by basic aminoacids.[8] This description is quite general, and could include a prohibitively large number of enzymes conducting diverse aspects of biochemistry including metabolic transformations, ion homeostasis, or contractility. Recently, sequene homology techniques revealed that PKC is actually a family of related isoforms. These PKC isoforms are distinct[8,14] in that they appear to i) have different structures, ii) be regulated by unique combinations of factors (cPKC,

[a] Address correspondence to: Dr. Anirban Banerjee, Assoc. Professor, Dept. of Surgery, University of Colorado, Health Sciences Center, Denver, CO 80262. Tel.: (303) 270-4545; Fax: (303) 270-4545; E-mail: banerjee_a@uchsc.edu.

nPKC etc.), iii) have distinct locations iv) have distinct translocations, and v) prefer distinct protein sequences specifically for phosphotransfer (targets). Lastly a very large number of hormone receptors appear to affect PKC and may direct isoform translocation to specific compartments. Thus regulation of target proteins (and hence entire pathways) by combinations of extracellular stimuli is likely to be intricate (and also the norm), because several serine and threonine residues in a target protein, could be phosphorylated by several isoforms with synergistic or conflicting results.

We hypothesized that extracellular stimuli may affect PKC translocation in characteristic combinations thereby altering distinct aspects of cellular regulation. For PKC-linked preconditioning stimuli, a few of the isoforms localizing in key compartments may lead to the induction of distinct cardioprotective mechanisms. A comparison of translocation profiles with physiological endpoints, could suggest a common code for inducing cardioadaptation. With the availability of new antibodies (*e.g.* against PKC η) and our growing awareness that translocation is not restricted to the sarcolemma alone, we proceeded to: i) delineate the distribution of PKC isoforms in isolated rat heart; ii) correlate each PKC activator to the translocation of individual PKC isoforms into specific intracellular locations; and iii) contrast the mosaic of PKC isoform translocation by all stimuli, to each other and to the improvement of postischemic functional recovery.

METHODS

Animals and Materials

Male Sprague-Dawley rats (325–350 gm; Sasco Inc., Omaha, NE) were fed a standard diet and acclimated in a quiet quarantine room for two weeks before experimentation. The animal protocol was reviewed and approved by the Animal Care and Research Committee, University of Colorado Health Sciences Center. All animals received humane care in compliance with the "Guide for the Care and Use of Laboratory Animals" (NIH publication No. 85-23, revised 1985). Sheep FITC-conjugated anti-mouse-IgG antibody was from Amersham (Arlington Heights, IL). Phenylephrine was obtained from American Regent Laboratories, Inc. (Shirley, NY). Bradykinin (BK) was obtained from Bachem California (Torrance, CA). 25% albumin (Plasbumin-25) and OCT compound were from Miles (Elkhart, IN). 2-Methylbutane was from Fisher (Pittsburg, PA). Rabbit polyclonal isoform-specific anti-PKC antibodies were from Santa Cruz Biotechnology (Santa Cruz, CA). These antibodies were raised (in rabbits) using isoform-unique peptide sequences (α:651–672, β1: 656–671, β2:657–673, γ:679–697, δ:657–673, ε:722–736, η:699–683, and ζ:573–592), and specificity has been verified by both the supplier and by ourselves with Western blotting. Cy-3 conjugated anti-rabbit-IgG antibody was from Jackwon Immunoresearch (West Grove, PA).

Perfusion of Isolated Rat Heart

The isolated crystalloid-perfused rat heart used in our laboratory was previously described.[2,6] Rats were anesthetized (sodium pentobarbital, 60 mg/kg, ip) and heparinized (500 units, ip). Hearts were excised, immediately arrested in iced oxygenated perfusate, mounted and perfused on a modified Langendorff apparatus at a constant pressure of 70 mmHg with Krebs-Henseleit solution (5 mM glucose, 1.2 mM Ca^{++}, 4.7 mM KCl, 25.0 mM $NaHCO_3$) in the nonrecirculating retrograde mode. The time from excision to perfusion was approximately 60–80 sec. The perfusate was saturated with a gas mixture of 92.5% O_2, 7.5% CO_2 achieving a pO_2 of 440–460 mmHg, pCO_2 of 39–41 mmHg, and pH 7.39–7.41 (ABL-4 blood gas analyzer, Radiometer; Copenhagen, Denmark). A water-filled latex balloon was inserted into the left ventricle through a left atriotomy, and the volume was adjusted to achieve a stable left ventricular end diastolic pressure of 5–6 mmHg during initial equilibration. Thereafter the balloon volume was not changed. Pacing wires were fixed to the right atrium, and hearts were paced at 350 bpm except during transient and sustained ischemia. Pacing was re-initiated only after three min of reperfusion in all groups. The index of myocardial function was left ventricular developed pressure (LVDP, in mmHg), which was continuously recorded with a direct pressure amplifier (RS-3200; Gould Electronics, Houston, TX) and later with a computerized bridge amplifier/digitizer (Maclab 8, AD Instruments, Milford, MA) and a Macintosh Quadra 800 minicomputer (Apple Computer, Cupertino, CA). Hearts that could not initially produce 90–120 mmHg LVDP when paced at 350 bpm were discarded. A three-way stopcock above the aortic root was turned to create global ischemia, during which time the heart was placed in a degassed perfusate-filled organ bath maintained at 37.5°C.

Stimulation Protocols

All hearts were equilibrated for 8 min prior to any stimulation. Preconditioning with single transient ischemia was for 2 min (TI), followed by 20 min of global ischemia and 40 min of reperfusion. Pharmacological agents were delivered for 2 min through an infusion port directly above the aortic canula (not circulated) at 0.068 ml/min (except when noted) using a Harvard infusion pump followed by 10 min of normal perfusion, 20 min of global ischemia, and 40 min of reperfusion. Phenylephrine (PE) was dissolved in PBS and infused at 1 μmole/min. Bradykinin was dissolved in buffer and infused at 20 nmoles/min.

Experimental Design of Preconditioning Experiments

Preconditioning experiments were conducted as previously described.[2] All hearts were perfused a total of 80 min, consisting of a 20-min preischemic period followed by a standardized IR challenge: 20 min global 37.5°C ischemia, 40 min reperfusion that allows substantial (50%) functional recovery (Ctrl). Three groups of hearts were pretreated with the different stimuli for exactly two min, 10 min prior to the onset of sustained global ischemia. These agonists included: transient ischemia (TI),[5,18] phenylephrine (PE),[2,18] and bradykinin (B2).[5] Hearts were not paced during transient and sustained ischemia. In all experiments, pacing following sustained ischemia was re-initiated only after three min of reperfusion. TABLE 1 shows the final, stable recovery after 40 min reperfusion (% of initial prestimulated baseline).

Immunofluorescence Microscopy

Subcellular localization and translocation studies of PKC isoforms after TI and PE stimulation were performed using immunofluorescence staining and

TABLE 1. Functional Recovery after Global Ischemia and Reperfusion in Isolated Rat Heart Is Expressed as the Final Developed Pressure Normalized to the Baseline Equilibration Developed Pressure for Each Heart: PKC Isoform Distributions in Control Hearts, after Various Preconditioning Stimuli[a]

	Cntl	TI	PE	B2
% DP recovered after 20 minutes ischemia	53.5 ± 3.7	79.9 ± 1.5	73.8 ± 1.6	80.3 ± 4.3
PKC α	C-ID	C-ID	**S**-C-ID	C-ID
β	P-N-C	P-N-C	P-N-C	P-N-C
δ	C-P	**S**-C-ID-P	**S**-C-ID-P	**S**-C-P
ε	ID-N-P-C	ID-**S**-N-P-C	ID-N-P-C	**S**-ID-N-P
η	C-P	C-**ID-N**-P	C-**ID-N**-P	C-**ID-N**-P
ζ	P	N-P	N-P	N-P

[a] C: cytoplasm, S: sarcolemma, P: perinuclear, N: nuclear, ID: intercalated discs. Bold letters denote prominent and consistent difference from control, while the first letter represents the most occupied compartment.

compared to control heart sections. In these experiments hearts were harvested and perfused as described above. Five hearts from each group (Ctrl, TI, PE, B2) were examined (10–15 sections per heart). Specimens were obtained at the end of drug infusion (2 min of PE, B2) and at the end of the ischemic preconditioning protocols (TI). Control specimens were harvested after 10 min equilibration. Ventricular tissue was excised from beating isolated hearts, blotted, embedded in OCT compound, rapidly frozen in dry ice-cooled 2-methylbutane, and stored at −70°C until used. Transverse 5-μm cryosections were prepared with a cryostate (2800 Frigocut E, Reichert-Jung, Germany) and collected on poly-l-lysine-coated slides. All sections were fixed for 10 min in a 70% acetone–30% methanol mixture at −20°C. Normal goat serum (10% in PBS) was applied as a blocking agent and briefly rinsed with PBS. Sections from each experimental group were then incubated for 1 hr with diluted primary antibodies (*i.e.*, rabbit polyclonal antibody against PKC isoenzymes) at room temperature with or without mouse antisarcomeric-α-actin antibody. For all groups individual PKC isoform staining was performed on adjacent sections. After washing the sections with PBS 3 times (3 min each), they were incubated with Cy-3 conjugated goat anti-rabbit-IgG for 1 hr. During this step sections also exposed to antisarcomeric-α-actin antibody were coincubated with FITC-conjugated sheep anti-mouse-IgG. Sections were then washed 3 times (3 min each) with PBS followed once for 3 min with 0.1% Triton X-100 in PBS. Nuclei were then stained with bis-benzamidine (10 mg/ml in PBS) for 30 sec and washed with PBS 3 times (2 min each). Slides were mounted with a glycerol-based anti-quenching media (O-phenylene diamine.HCl) and stored at 4°C.

To test for nonspecific fluorescence, adjacent sections of each experimental group were incubated with nonimmune purified rabbit IgG instead of primary antibodies. Specificity of the staining by the PKC antibodies was determined by preabsorption of the antibodies (1 : 100) with the immunizing peptides (0.1 mg.) for 2 hr at 4°C. Sections were viewed and photographed with a microscope equipped with fluorescence optics (Axioskop with MC-100 camera, Zeiss, Germany).

Statistical Analysis

All reported values are means ± SEM. Differences in % LVDP were considered significant at the 95% confidence level using analysis of variance (StatView 4.0, Abacus Concepts, Berkeley, CA). Post hoc testing was performed with the Bonferroni/Dunn procedure. Immunohistofluorescent slides were viewed by 2 blinded experts and reported translocations represent consensus.

RESULTS

Distribution of PKC Isoforms in Isolated Rat Heart

Here, the critical component for detecting the isoforms is the quality of the antigen-directed antibodies. We replaced our previous source[5,18] with improved antibodies from Santa Cruz Biochemicals. These newer antibodies are directed toward somewhat longer sequences than before and are more specific as assessed by the fewer number of bands on Western blots, regardless of ECL exposure time. With these improved antibodies we successfully detected PKC α, β_I, δ, ε, η and ζ isoforms in whole rat heart tissue but not PKC γ, or θ. PKC β_{II} is found in only nonmyocytic cells. All antibody binding on immunofluorescence section and stains and Western blots (SDS solubilized whole heart homogenate) could be completely blocked by prior incubation of the primary with excess isoform specific antigen peptide. Nonimmune normal rabbit serum did not detect any protein in either assay. These results reported here supersede our previous observations.[5,18]

TABLE 1 lists the six PKC isoforms identified in unique intracellular zones and related to activating stimuli. We have conservatively focused our attention on five defined compartments C: cytoplasm, S: sarcolemma, P: perinuclear, N: nuclear, ID: intercalated discs. Bold letters denote prominent and consistent difference from control, while the first letter represents the most occupied compartment. Other subtleties such as more defined staining in the endocardium, staining of nonmyocytic structures, and the statistical prevalence of staining exist but are not noted formally, in favor of the 'clear cut' nonparametric changes (TABLE 1). None of the PKC isoforms locations were different in isolated buffer-perfused hearts (15 min) compared to freshly excised and rapidly frozen rat hearts (data not shown).

In control hearts we find PKC α distributed throughout in the cytosol. Filamentous structures running the length of the myocyte and at the intercalated discs appear to be associated with brighter immunofluorescence. PKC β_I fluorescence was concentrated tightly around the perinuclear membranes in myocytes and faint cytosolic distributions. However, in about 30% of control cells also showed intranuclear presence. (PKC β_{II} was prominently detected on nonmyocellular structures such as interstitial cells and coronary endothelium and are therefore not discussed further). PKC δ is distributed evenly in the cytosol and clearly demarcates the perinuclear membranes in control hearts. PKC δ is also strongly apparent in endothelial cells, coronary smooth muscle cells and interstitial cells. Immunohistochemical localization of PKC ε in control rat heart indicates it is associated with multiple cell structures including perinuclear membranes, intercalated discs and the nucleus. Cytosolic presence, especially concentrated in 'clumps' can be discerned, but all these features are eliminated by the antigenic peptide. PKC η is present in the cytosol and perikarya in control hearts. In rat hearts we find PKC ζ in perinuclear membranes and more faintly in sarcolemmal membranes. Coronary vessels are strongly stained but the exact cell types have not been resolved. In longitudinal sections staining of interstitial cells running lengthwise between myocardial layers appears stronger.

Protection of Functional Recovery by PKC-Linked Stimuli

We focused on a few putative components of the simplest preconditioning stimulus that we could detect: a single transient ischemic (TI) episode of 2 min.[2,5,18] This minimal stimulus is best detected by modest ischemia-reperfusion challenge (20 min, global, 37°C) (TABLE 1). Detecting preconditioning against this reversible injury (about 50% lost developed pressure) requires a sensitive index. We exploited functional recovery (TABLE 1) as end-point,[2,5,18] because it is the composite of several vital myocardial processes (stunning, metabolic dysregulation and viability). These studies[2,18] and work from other laboratories[3,13,25] have established that TI stress stimulates noradrenergic termini to release neurotransmitter and that the α_1 adrenoreceptor is a necessary mediator of protection in the rat. This naturally encouraged the examination of protein kinase C (PKC) as the effector of cardioadaptation. We found that both TI and α_1 adrenoreceptor-induced protection (TABLE 1) was abolished by the PKC blockers chelerythrine and staurosporine.[18] Extrapolating from the α_1 adrenoreceptor, we investigated and found that bradykinin[11] (formed by the postischemic endothelium) induced preconditioning within 10 min of treatment[5] (TABLE 1). Acute cardioadaptation after the TI stress stimulus could be partially inhibited by bradykinin B_2 antagonist ($\sim$50%), while bradykinin-induced protection was inhibited by a PKC antagonist.[5]

Stimulated Translocation of PKC Isoforms in Isolated Rat Heart

We then proceeded to characterize the locations of PKC isoforms immediately following the PKC-linked stimuli. The hearts were taken down and frozen to preserve the translocation and later were examined with fluorescent-tagged antibodies to each PKC isoform (FIG. 1). The observations include translocation to the five compartments specified above (C, P, N, ID, S) and go beyond the two or three compartments described before.[5,18] Although translocation to cytoplasmic substructures could be seen, these are at present difficult to describe semiquantitatively.

For PKC α only PE induced significant translocation (about 75% of all fields) in the isolated perfused heart. For the examined stimuli, PCK β_1 appeared similar to untreated controls (mostly perinuclear, faint cytoplasmic staining and $\sim$30 intranuclear). PKC δ translocation to sarcolemmal membranes is unequivocal (FIG. 1) (accompanied by conspicuous decrease in diffuse cytosol staining) and observed for all stimuli examined here. The translocation is most apparent in endocardial layers. (However, in the present report we do not formally include quantitation of the degree of translocation in TABLE 1). Translocation of PKC ε to the sarcolemma is very prominent after bradykinin treatment and to a lesser extent after a single transient ischemic stress episode. All examined preconditioning stimuli (*i.e.*, protective) elicit dramatic translocation of PKC η to the intercalated discs and into the nucleus (FIG. 1). Staining could be abolished by coincubation with excess antigen peptide. In the cytosol, staining along cross-striations[9] is very prominent (but translocation to discrete cytoplasmic structures is not formally categorized in TABLE 1). PKC ζ which lacks the regulatory site for Ca^{++}

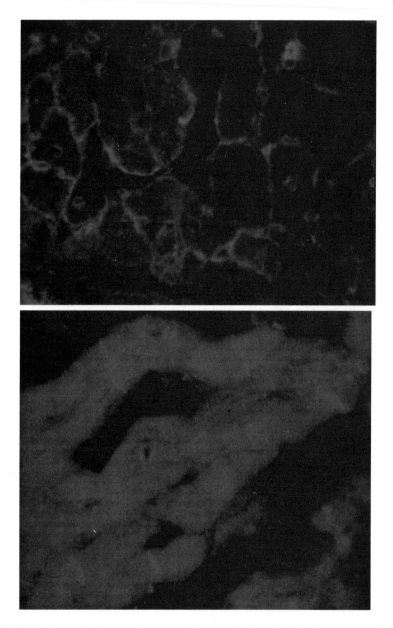

FIGURE 1. Illustrative immunofluorescent images showing the typical compartments utilized by PKC isoforms. The *top panel* shows a cross section of a TI-treated heart stained with primary antibodies against PKC δ. Sarcolemma (S), perinuclear membranes (P) and remnant of cytoplasmic staining are clearly visible. (Unstimulated controls contain PKC δ diffusely in the cytosol and perinuclear membranes,[18] not shown). The *lower panel* shows a longitudinal section in a PE-treated heart stained with primary antibodies against PKC η. Perinuclear membranes (P), and brighter intercalated discs (ID) where two cells meet can be seen. Also visible are the cross-striations along myofibrils.

and only one zinc finger, is prominently translocated into the nucleus by all PKC-linked preconditioning stimuli.

DISCUSSION

These results show the distribution of all known isoforms in the adult rat heart and that these isoforms are linked to various extracellular stimuli in characteristic patterns. While some isoform translocations such as δ_S and η_{ID} occur often (3/3), others such as ε_S (2/3), α_S (1/3), and β_I (0/3), occur infrequently and indeed constitute the difference in profile between the receptor stimuli considered here (*e.g.*, PE and B2). Although the functional recovery after the modest ischemic injury (20 min) appears similar, the different PKC isoform translocations suggest that the mechanisms of protection may not be exactly identical. Thus, additional endpoints such as infarction, arrhythmias or functional recovery after longer ischemic challenges could help distinguish the efficacies of these preconditioning stimuli.

Our results provide the first glimpses of distribution and translocation in *intact* heart. Cross-checking the literature shows that the isoforms detected in rat heart is rather dependent on the method for isolating myocytes, and differs from the isoforms found in ventricular protein extracts.[4,12,21] Certainly, developmental age[19,21] and presence of growth factors during myocyte culture[9] cause drastic changes from the phenotype in toto.[21] The predominance of studies using centrifugal fractionation to document translocation also obscures the characteristic location of each isoform within the numerous biochemical distinct membranous compartments of the myocyte. The anomalous translocation of certain isoforms during cell lysis in the presence of Ca^{++} adds another convoluting factor in destructive separation techniques.

Similarities and Dissimilarities of PKC Isoforms Reported in Heart

PKC α appears to be abundant in neonatal myocytes.[9,15,19,21] Some investigators have presented evidence for its presence in adult tissue by RT-PCR[15] and by immunoblot.[12,19] Others have been unable to detect PKC α in isolated adult myocytes,[4,21] perhaps because the isoform apparently decreases with neonatal age.[19,21] Of course, the uncertain quality of their noncommercial antibodies remains the critical determinant of successful detection. In adult myocytes, membrane translocation could be observed after phorbol esters (but not phenylephrine or endothelin).[19] Similarly, in neonatal myocyte culture, translocation of PKC α immunofluorescence from the cytosol to the perikarya was clearer after phorbol esters than after adrenergic agonist.[9]

The paucity of PKC β[15] and its easy precipitation with nuclear pellets may explain conflicting results in adult heart.[4,12,19,21] Using similar commercial antibodies Gu and Bishop[12] as well as Rybin and Steinberg[21] both detected PKC β in adult ventricles. However, the latter workers[21] were unable to detect it in cultured myocytes that had also been irradiated (to decrease fibroblasts). Under different culture conditions, Disatnik *et al.*[9] found both PKC β_I and β_{II} by immunocytofluorescence in neonatal hearts. The perinuclear predominance of the β_I isoform and its translocation into the nucleus[9] has parallels with our observations in adult heart (TABLE 1). The presence of fetal calf serum appeared to strongly translocate PKC β_I into the sarcolemma.[9]

Although an earlier study using noncommercial antibodies failed to detect the isoform in adult tissue,[4] both RT-PCR[15] and immunoblots have detected PKC δ in neonatal and adult myocytes.[12,19,21] There is nearly complete discrepancy between reports on the intracellular location of PKC δ and also its posttranslocation compartment. Puceat *et al.*[19] found 45% of the isoform in 'membrane' fractions (37,000-g pellet) in neonatal myocytes which decreased to 25% in adult myocytes. On the other hand, Rybin and Steinberg[21] found 80–90% of the isoform in a 100,000-g 'particulate' fraction for both adult and neonatal myocytes. However, their polyclonal antibody appears to recognize several proteins, especially at higher loads. Again using PKC δ antibody from the same commercial source, Gu and Bishop[12] found the isoform restricted to a nuclear-cytoskeletal' fraction (mild detergent resistant 800-g pellet). In contrast, immunocytofluorescence[9] depicts a predominant intranuclear location for PKC δ in cultured neonatal myocytes. Our results are consistent with reports that PMA[9,19,21] and adrenergic agonists[9,19] translocate the isoform (to the 37,000-g 'membrane pellet and to the perinuclear membrane in adult and neonatal myocytes, respectively).

PKC ε has been detected by all studies in heart tissue.[9,12,15,19,21] Differences in fractionation procedures find differences in membrane to the cytosolic distribution ratio but membrane translocation after PMA or adrenergic agonists have been observed. Curiously, in cultured neonatal myocytes immunofluorescence shows intranuclear locations as well as fascinating 'cross-striations' that are thought to be associated with myofibrils.[9]

Comparatively fewer studies have examined PKC η in heart. Remarkably, Bogoyevitch *et al.*,[4] who found it in immunoblots of adult ventricular extracts, lost the band after myocyte isolation procedures. In rat hearts the translocation of this Ca^{++}-independent isoform to significant cardiac compartments (in the context of acute cardioadaptation) is seen frequently. Taken together with its tissue-specific distribution suggests that PKC η may play a significant role differentiating cardiac physiology from that of other muscle cells.

PKC ζ content of adult hearts appears to be smaller than in neonatal tissue. In partial agreement with our results, immunofluorescence staining of neonatal cells showed the isoform was translocated into the nucleus by adrenergic agonists.[9]

Similarities and Dissimilarities between Stimuli

Examination of TABLE 1 shows that the different stimuli alter about 4 isoform-location profiles from the control state. Preconditioning stimuli appear to be more similar to each other than not. Bradykinin and TI show the highest degree of similarity, along with the fewest differences. The latter similarity to TI is not altogether convincing, because bradykinin receptor blockade was only partially successful.[5] PE, TI and B2 share four similar translocations (δ_S, η_{ID}, η_N, ζ_N) and two differences (either α_S or ε_S).

In control hearts PKC Isoforms are mostly cytosolic (α, δ, η) while PKC ε occupies positions at the intercalated discs, and PKC β_I and ζ occupy perinuclear membranes prominently. Remarkably, in intact rat heart, sarcolemma staining is not prominent in the control state for any isoform. All stimuli force translocation of PKC δ consistently to the sarcolemma. Other isoforms that reach the sarcolemmal compartment include ε (by both TI and B2) and α (by PE). Translocation to the intercalated discs is very striking for PKC η (all stimuli) and less so for δ. All stimuli translocate PKC isoforms η and ζ into the nucleus. Noticeably, both these isoforms are poised at perinuclear membranes in the control state, but this feature

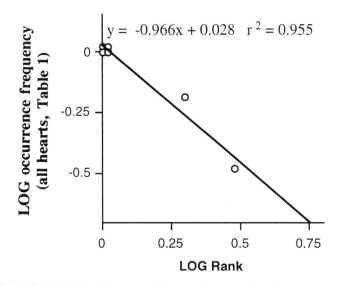

FIGURE 2. Zipf plot of log frequency of a prominent translocation against its log rank ($\delta_S = \eta_{ID} = \eta_N = \zeta_N > \varepsilon_S > \alpha_S$). The log-log plot shows the slope of -0.966 (close to -1) expected for languages which contain an implicit order (grammar).

is preserved even after stimulation. PKC α and δ which also show basal perinuclear staining do not show intranuclear translocation, at least with the stimuli described here. Overall, the nPKC isoforms δ, and η (and ε less so) are translocated more frequently, versus the lone case of cPKC α translocated by PE.

The appearance of distinct isoform translocations, depending on the particulars of the stimulus and its signal transduction, suggests that there may be an intracellular language where each isoform in a compartment constitutes a 'word.' The overall message ('sentence') may then be represented by the combinations of isoforms activated by the stimuli (or even by combinations of stimuli, such as TI). Recently, Zipf's law (which shows that log frequency of appearance of common words in any human language plotted against log rank has a slope of -1) was applied to assert that sequences of 'junk' intronic DNA has long-range order (*i.e.*, grammar).[17] We therefore listed the prominent translocations (that are different from the control state) and created a histogram of the frequency of appearance. After assigning ranks the log-log plot shows a slope of -0.966 (close to -1) which supports the notion that the stimulated PKC isoform translocations may constitute a syntactically constrained language (FIG. 2).

PKC in Preconditioning/Cardioadaptation

In this study we investigate the effect of stimuli of increasing complexity on the pattern of isoform redistribution in adult heart. The large number of isoform-distribution combinations are either all physiologically equivalent or else represent mechanistically distinct strategies available to realize ischemic cardioprotection. The signal syntax (or depth) could range in complexity from i) all receptors redistribute a single isoform, to ii) different stimuli redistribute different isoforms but result in identical physiological effects, to iii) different stimuli redistribute PKC isoforms in characteristic profiles that include algebraic sums of positive and negative effects. Higher order messages can be conveyed by time-dependent PKC redistribution and by the imposition of biphasic conditional thresholds at one or more isoforms before the final effects are achieved. However, FIGURE 2 suggests that interpretation iii, with undiscovered grammatical rules governing the interactions of isoforms, may be correct. Comparable protection against ischemia-reperfusion injury by diverse stimuli (interpretation ii) could imply that the receptor to PKC coupling is massively redundant. Alternatively, this could be a misperception reflecting inadequate discrimination in the indexes of protection (usually mechanical function, infarction, ATP catabolism or arrhythmogenesis).

It is not clear how the different PKC isoform translocation profiles are achieved by the signal transduction apparatus in heart. For example, PE and B2 should engage PLC to make DAG and IP_3 but their patterns are nonidentical (different α_S and ε_S). This may indicate the utilization of slightly different phospholipase isoforms by the receptors. Similarly α_1 noradrenergic blockade completely abolished protection induced by TI preconditioning, but the isoform profiles translocated by PE and TI are again nonidentical (different α_S and ε_S). One possibility is that elimination of the α_1 noradrenergic component eliminates (or attenuates) the translocation of PKC δ_S, $\eta_{N,ID}$ and ζ_N but still leaves the ε_S component intact (also stimulated by bradykinin). If so, PKC ε_S by itself may not be very protective toward postischemic functional recovery.

We have explored a very limited set of PKC-linked receptors and other stimuli that may induce cardioprotection in rat (TABLE 1). Another component of the poststress neuroendocrine environment in heart is adenosine, which plays a more prominent role in preconditioning rabbit heart.[10] In this species, protection against cell necrosis induced by adenosine A_1 or (A_3) receptors is also blocked by PKC inhibitors. Another DAG (oleyl acetyl glycerol), and PMA were both cardioprotective. This same DAG promotes cardioprotection in intact rats when myocardial survival is challenged by surgical vessel occlusion *in vivo*.[22] Again ischemic stress-induced cardioadaptation could be inhibited by PKC blockade with chelerythrine.[22] In this same vein, Downey and colleagues have induced preconditioning in rabbit heart by angiotensin II and acetycholine, and have suggested that cardioprotective signaling is potentially redundant.[10] Therefore, how DAG and adenosine append the PKC isoform translocation scheme proposed here remains to be seen.

Correlation of Stimulated Isoform Profiles with Functional Preconditioning

We first examined TABLE 1 to see if a common isoform was stimulated by all functionally protective agents. Three isoforms, PKC δ_S, $\eta_{N,ID}$ and ζ_N were translocated reproducibly and distinguishably from control, untreated hearts. PKC α_S was translocated only by PE but not by the others. Nevertheless, all three stimuli protected postischemic recovery. Therefore, PKC α_S may not be critical for recovery. Similarly, PKC ε_S was not observed consistently and may also not be essential for inducing cardioadaptation. However, it is entirely possible that PKC α_S and PKC ε_S act in lieu of each other (interchangeable) to complete the mechanistic regulation initiated by the other three consistently translocated isoforms (δ_S, $\eta_{N,ID}$ and ζ_N).

One set of cardioprotective mechanisms could involve modification of ion channels and exchangers that are located densely at these membranous sites.

Ischemic preconditioning attenuates lethal ionic disbalances (often initiated by acidosis) during ischemia.[23,26] Since all protective stimuli translocate PKC δ to the sarcolemma and η to the ID, these isoforms could be prime candidates for adaptive mechanisms involving colocalization and regulation of these ion transporter targets by phosphorylation. Translocation of the other common isoform PKC ζ to the nucleus cannot be understood easily since the complete zinc finger site is lacking in this isomer. Nuclear translocation in general (such as η_{ID} and ζ_N) may not be as important in the rapid preconditioning which occurs within minutes. It may be more important in the longer-term protection that takes several hours to develop. There is evidence that rapid preconditioning after single ischemic stress does not involve protein transcription or translation.[24] The preconditioning stimuli shown in TABLE 1 are completed within 2 min and the cardioprotection is induced rapidly (usually 5–10 min.[1,5,18]

Although the hypothesis of a common mediator is attractive, there is the distinct possibility of the fallacy of syllogism. In effect, PKC δ, η and ζ could be simply permissive. There could also be isoforms in the heart that are presently unknown but which are the true common mediators of protection. However, this latter possibility has been contested by RT-PCR studies.[15] Currently, nonselective PKD blockade makes it clear that some isoform(s) can mediate cardioprotection; but further tests of this hypothesis await translocation studies on a larger range of 'PKD linked' stimuli and the advent of isoform selective inhibitors.

Nevertheless, PKC η and ζ could be suitable candidates for transient expression experiments provided the activities could be directed to the appropriate myocellular compartments.

SUMMARY

Extracellular agents, including growth factors, cytokines and hormones, transmit their information into cells utilizing a balanced mosaic of intracellular phosphatases and kinases.[7] How do these agonists select the correct substrates and modify them in order to produce defined physiological responses? Our studies have centered on the mechanisms of stress-induced cardioprotection (preconditioning) against postischemic dysfunction. In several species, the ischemia-reperfusion resistant phenotype appears to be induced by metabotropic-receptor pathways linked to PKC. Our results on the isolated rat heart show that each protective stimulus involves a characteristic mosaic of PKC isoforms, translocating into distinct cellular compartments. The distinct receptor-stimulated PKC isoform profile engaged by each extracellular metabotropic agent could allow the heart several overlapping modes of phenotypic adaptation to ischemia.

REFERENCES

1. BANERJEE, A., M. A. GROSSO, J. M. BROWN, K. ROGERS & G. J. R. WHITMAN. 1991. Oxygen metabolite effects on creatine kinase and cardiac energetics after reperfusion. Am. J. Physiol. **261:** H590–H597.
2. BANERJEE, A., C. LOCKE-WINTER, K. B. ROGERS, M. B. MITCHELL, D. D. BENSARD, E. C. BREW, C. B. CAIRNS & A. H. HARKEN. 1993. Transient ischemia preconditions against subsequent cardiac ischemia reperfusion injury by an alpha-1 adrenergic mechanism. Circ. Res. **73:** 656–670.
3. BANKWALA, Z., S. L. HALE & R. A. KLONER. 1994. α-Adrenoceptor stimulation with

exogenous norepinephrine or release of endogenous catecholamines mimics ischemic preconditioning. Circulation **90**(2): 1023–1028.

4. BOGOYEVITCH, M. A., P. J. PARKER & P. H. SUGDEN. 1993. Characterization of protein kinase C isotype expression in adult rat heart. Circ. Res. **72**(4): 757–767.

5. BREW, E. B., M. B. MITCHELL, T. F. REHRING, F. GAMBONI-ROBERTSON, R. C. MCINTYRE, A. H. HARKEN & A. BANERJEE. 1995. The role of bradykinin in cardiac functional protection after global ischemia-reperfusion in the rat heart. Am. J. Physiol. In press.

6. BROWN, J. M., M. A. GROSSO, L. S. TERADA, G. J. WHITMAN, A. BANERJEE, L. W. WHITE, A. H. HARKEN & J. E. REPINE. 1989. Endotoxin pretreatment increases endogenous myocardial catalase activity and decrease ischemia-reperfusion injury of isolated rat hearts. Proc. Natl. Acad. Sci. USA **86**: 2516–2520.

7. COHEN, P. 1992. Signal integration at the level of protein kinases, protein phosphatases and their substrates. *In* Trends in Biochemical Sciences. H. G. M. Purton, Ed. 408–413. Elsevier Trends Journals/David Bousfield. Cambridge.

8. DEKKER, L. V. & P. J. PARKER. 1994. Protein kinase C—a question of specificity. Trends Biochem. Sci. **19**(2): 73–77.

9. DISATNIK, M-H., G. BURAGGI & D. MOCHLY-ROSEN. 1994. Localization of protein kinase C isozymes in cardiac myocytes. Exp. Cell Res. **210**: 287–297.

10. DOWNEY, J. M., M. V. COHEN, K. YTREHUS & Y. LIU. 1994. Cellular mechanisms in ischemic preconditioning: the role of adenosine and PKC. Ann. N.Y. Acad. Sci. **723**: 82–98.

11. GOTO, M., Y. LIU, X-M. YANG, J. L. ARDELL, M. V. COHEN & J. M. DOWNEY. 1995. Role of bradykinin in protection of ischemic preconditioning in rabbit hearts. Circ. Res. **77**: 611–621.

12. GU, X. & P. BISHOP. 1994. Increased protein kinase C and isozyme redistribution in pressure-overload cardiac hypertrophy in the rat. Circ. Res. **75**: 926–931.

13. HU, K. & S. NATTEL. 1995. Mechanisms of ischemic preconditioning in rat hearts. Involvement of α_{1b} adrenoreceptors, pertussis sensitive G proteins, and protein kinase C. Circulation **92**: 2259–2265.

14. INAGAKI, N., M. ITO, T. NAKANO & M. INAGAKI. 1994. Spatiotemporal distribution of protein kinase and phosphatase activities. Trends Biochem. Sci. **19**: 439–518.

15. KOHOUT, T. A. & T. B. ROGERS. 1993. Use of a PCR-based method to characterize protein kinase C isoform expression in cardiac cells. Am. J. Physiol. **264**: C1350–C1359.

16. LI, Y. & R. A. KLONER. 1995. Does protein kinase C play a role in ischemic preconditioning in rat hearts? Am. J. Physiol. **268**: H426–H431.

17. MANTEGNA, R. N., S. V. BULDYREV & H. E. STANLEY. 1994. Linguistic features of noncoding DNA sequences. Physiol. Rev. Lett. **73**: 3169.

18. MITCHELL, M. B., X. MENG, J. BROWN, A. H. HARKEN & A. BANERJEE. 1995. Preconditioning of isolated rat heart is mediated by protein kinase C. Circ. Res. **76**: 73–81.

19. PUCEAT, M., R. HILAL-DANDAN, B. STRULOVICI, L. L. BRUNTON & J. H. BROWN. 1994. Differential regulation of protein kinase C isoforms in isolated neonatal and adult rat cardiomyocytes. J. Biol. Chem. **269**: 16938–16944.

20. REIMER, K. A. & R. B. JENNINGS. 1992. Preconditioning. Definitions, proposed mechanisms, and implications for myocardial protection in ischemia and reperfusion. *In* Myocardial Protection: the Pathophysiology of Reperfusion and Reperfusion Injury. D. M. Yellon & R. B. Jennings, Eds. 165–183. Raven Press, Ltd. New York.

21. RYBIN, V. O. & S. F. STEINBERG. 1994. Protein kinase C isoform expression and regulation in the developing rat heart. Circ. Res. **74**: 299–309.

22. SPEECHLY-DICK, M. E., M. M. MOCANU & D. M. YELLON. 1994. Protein kinase C. Its role in ischemic preconditioning in the rat. Circ. Res. **75**: 586–590.

23. STEENBERGEN, C., M. E. PERLMAN, R. E. LONDON & E. MURPHY. 1993. Mechanism of preconditioning: ionic alterations. Circ. Res. **72**(1): 112–125.

24. THORNTON, J., S. STRIPLIN, G. S. LIU, A. SWAFFORD, A. W. H. STANLEY, D. M. VAN WINKLE & J. M. DOWNEY. 1990. Inhibition of protein synthesis does not block

myocardial protection afforded by preconditioning. Am. J. Physiol. **259:** H1822–H1825.

25. TOSAKI, A., N. S. BEHJET, D. T. ENGELMAN, R. M. ENGELMAN & D. K. DAS. 1995. Alpha-1 adrenergic receptor agonist-induced preconditioning in isolated working rat hearts. J. Pharmacol. Exp. Ther. **273:** 689–694.

26. TOSAKI, A., G. A. CORDIS, P. SZERDAHELYI, R. M. ENGELMAN & D. K. DAS. 1994. Effects of preconditioning on reperfusion arrhythmias, myocardial functions, formation of free radicals, and ion shifts in isolated ischemic/reperfused rat hearts. J. Cardiovasc. Pharmacol. **23:** 365–373.

Hunting for Differentially Expressed mRNA Species in Preconditioned Myocardium[a]

NILANJANA MAULIK,[b] RICHARD M. ENGELMAN,
AND DIPAK K. DAS

Cardiovascular Division
Department of Surgery
University of Connecticut School of Medicine
Farmington, Connecticut

INTRODUCTION

A growing body of evidence indicates that ischemic preconditioning/myocardial adaptation rapidly induces the expression of a wide variety of the mRNAs of the stress-related proteins in mammalian hearts. These include mRNAs of heat shock proteins,[1-8] antioxidants,[1,8] Ca^{2+}-regulated proteins,[9] and growth hormones.[10] Most of these stress genes are also induced when hearts are subjected to heat shock or oxidative stress.[11-20] It seems reasonable, therefore, to postulate that there may be a common inducible pathway for the stress-mediated induction of gene expression.

It has long been known that cells exhibit specific responses when confronted with sudden changes in their environmental conditions. The ability of the cells to acclimate to their new environment is the integral driving force for the new environment's adaptive modification of the cells. Such adaptation involves a number of cellular and biochemical alterations including metabolic homeostasis and reprogramming of gene expression. The changes in the metabolic pathways are generally short-lived and reversible, while the consequences of gene expression are a long-term process and may lead to the permanent alteration in the pattern of gene expression.

Why gene expression? It is believed that constitutive cellular protection against acute stress such as ischemia is provided by a variety of intracellular components including antioxidants and perhaps heat shock proteins. These components are the integral part of the defense system of the heart. When myocardial cells sense stress, they readily react by increasing the elements of the defense system. Antioxidants/antioxidant enzymes are likely to comprise the first line of defense, because they undergo rapid changes as a consequence of the development of oxidative stress associated with a large number of cardiovascular diseases including ischemia and reperfusion.[21] Hearts are also protected by a second line of defense consisting of lipolytic and proteolytic enzymes, proteases, and phospholipases, which is

[a] This study was supported by NIH Grants HL 22559 and HL 34360, and by a Grant-in-Aid from the American Heart Association.

[b] Correspondence: Nilanjana Maulik, Ph.D, Molecular Cardiology Laboratory, Cardiovascular Div., Dept. of Surgery, University of Connecticut School of Medicine, Farmington, CT 06030-1110. Tel.: (203) 679-2857; Fax: (203) 679-2451.

involved in the systematic recognition and removal of the injured cell components. Recent evidence suggests that myocardial cells possess an inducible pathway for cellular defense presumably translated by the signal transduction pathway. The intracellular signaling now believed to be mediated by the action of multiple kinases[22] is likely to be instrumental for the induction of the expression of the mRNAs of a variety of stress proteins including heat shock and oxidative stress-inducible proteins. This may lead to the systhesis of the related proteins involved in cellular protection or repair of injury. This phenomenon related to specific gene expression has been viewed as the third line of defense, and may reflect the ultimate adaptive stress responses.

Most of the gene expression is regulated at the level of transcription. Therefore, the evaluation of gene transcripts has become an important tool in the study of control and adaptive processes. Measurement of mRNA transcript levels is usually confined to selected genes of interest and often requires information about the gene sequence. By contrast, polymerase chain reaction-based differential display techniques (PCR-DDR) used in this study allowed us to detect, characterize, and differentiate between normal and precondition-mediated altered gene expression.

One of the principal advantages of the PCR-DDR technique is that it permits simultaneous identification of genes that are upregulated as well as genes that are downregulated. Therefore, we used this technique to evaluate gene expression directly in the isolated rat hearts that were preconditioned (PC) by subjecting them to 5 min ischemia followed by 10 min of reperfusion (1 × PC). Another group of hearts was preconditioned by repeating this process four times (4 × PC). The third group of hearts was subjected to 5 min of ischemia, while a fourth group was not subjected to any experimental protocol. Total RNA was extracted from the hearts followed by reverse transcription with the use of one-base anchored oligo-deoxythymidine (dT) primers, which bind to the 5′ boundary of a poly A tail, followed by PCR amplification with the rationally designed arbitrary 13 mers. Amplified cDNA fragments of 3′termini of mRNA were thus separated by size on a denaturing polyacrylamide gel. The DNA fragments of interest were reamplified using the same primer set. Amplified DNAs were separated by agarose gel electrophoresis, verified by Northern blot analysis prior to cloning and sequencing. DNA sequence revealed homology of several clones to known gene sequences and many others for unknown genes. Several clones revealed differential gene expression by Northern blot analysis in both 1 × PC and 4 × PC hearts.

MATERIALS AND METHODS

Male Sprague Dawley rats weighing about 300–350 gm were anesthetized with 100 mg/kg intraperitoneal sodium pentobarbital. Hearts were quickly removed, and perfused using a Langendorff setup with Krebs-Henseleit bicarbonate buffer (KHB), pH 7.4 as described elsewhere.[1] The rats were divided into four different groups. In the first group, control experiments were performed by perfusing the hearts with KHB buffer only for 60 min. The second group of rat hearts were equilibrated for 5 min with KHB buffer, and then subjected to 5 min of global ischemia by terminating the aortic flow. The third group of hearts were subjected to ischemic preconditioning by inducing 5 min of ischemia followed by 10 min of reperfusion (1 × PC). In the fourth group of hearts, this process of 1 × PC was repeated four times (4 × PC). The hearts were then removed from the perfusion setup, and left ventricular biopsies were quickly frozen in liquid nitrogen.

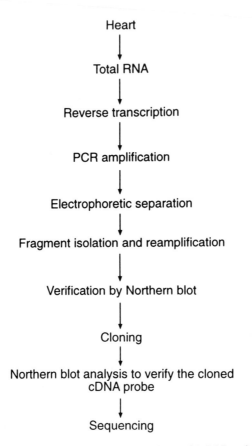

FIGURE 1. Schematic representation of the PCR-DDR technique.

Total cellular RNA was extracted from the hearts according to the modified acid guanidinium-thiocyanate-phenol-chloroform method[23] using Promega's total RNA isolation kit (Promega, Madison, WI).

PCR-DDR analysis was carried out as described by Liang *et al.*[24] Total RNA was used in our study to obtain clear background signal, easy purification, and integrity verification as compared to poly (A^+) RNA. The flow diagram of the procedure is depicted in FIGURE 1. We used three one-base anchored oligo-dT primers[25] to subdivide the mRNA population. The reverse transcription of mRNA and PCR reactions were done as follows. Total RNA (0.2 μg) was reverse transcribed in a 20-μl reaction mixture containing Superscript reverse transcriptase (Gibco/BRL, Grand Island, NY), deoxynucleoside triphosphate (dNTP) mix (250 μM), 5 $\times$ reverse transcriptase (RT) buffer and oligo-(dT) primer, H-T_{11}M (2 μM) (where M may be G, A or C). Three reverse transcription reactions for each RNA sample were prepared in PCR tubes (0.5-ml size), each containing one of the three different one-base anchored H-T_{11}M primers in duplicate. Control reactions were performed in the absence of reverse transcriptase. The thermo-

A

H-T$_{11}$G	5'-AAGCTTTTTTTTTTTTG-3'
H-T$_{11}$A	5'-AAGCTTTTTTTTTTTTA-3'
H-T$_{11}$C	5'-AAGCTTTTTTTTTTTTC-3'

B

H-AP1	5'-AAGCTTGATTGCC-3'
H-AP2	5'-AAGCTTCGACTGT-3'
H-AP3	5'-AAGCTTTGGTCAG-3'
H-AP4	5'-AAGCTTCTCAACG-3'
H-AP5	5'-AAGCTTAGTAGGC-3'
H-AP6	5'-AAGCTTGCACCAT-3'
H-AP7	5'-AAGCTTAACGAGG-3'
H-AP8	5'-AAGCTTTTACCGC-3'

FIGURE 2. (A) The sequence of the three one-base anchored oligo-dT primers. **(B)** The sequence of the arbitrary, 13 mer primers used in combination with the three one-base anchored oligo-dT primers shown in (A). Note the Hind III restriction site (5'-AAGCTT-3') at the 5' ends of both the arbitrary and the anchored primers for the easier manipulation of the amplified cDNAs after cloning into the PCR trap cloning vector.

cycler was then programmed to operate as follows: 65°C for 5 min, 37°C for 60 min, 75°C for 5 min. The tubes were then cooled down to 4°C. The cDNAs were amplified by PCR in the presence of α[^{33}P]2'-deoxy-adenosine-5'-triphosphate (dATP) (2,000 Ci/mmol) using a Perkin Elmer 9600 thermal cycler (Foster City, CA). Control experiments were performed by substituting water for cDNA. The reaction mixtures (20 μl) included arbitrary primers, H-AP$_1$ to H-AP$_8$. We used eight different arbitrary primers in combination with three anchored primers in different reactions (FIG. 2). The reaction mixture also contained 10 × PCR buffer (2 μM), dNTP mixture (25 μM), H-T$_{11}$M (2 μM), RT mixture from the reverse transcription reaction, which contained the same H-T$_{11}$M used for PCR as well as Ampli Taq DNA polymerase (Perkin Elmer). The PCR was programmed for 40 cycles as follows: denaturation at 94°C for 15 sec (for the Perkin Elmer 9600 thermocycler), annealing at 40°C for 2 min, and extension at 72°C for 30 sec for 40 cycles, at 72°C for 5 min for one cycle. The tubes were then cooled down to 4°C. Radiolabeled PCR amplification products were analyzed by electrophoresis in denaturing 6% polyacrylamide gels. M$_{13}$ cycle DNA sequencer (Genomyx Corporation, Foster City, CA) was used to obtain DNA standard ladder on differential display gels. A variability of 5–15% was observed in the number and intensity of bands among given samples on repeated PCR analysis. To confirm the reproducibility of amplification for selected bands, the reactions were repeated at least three times using different cDNA preparations. PCR bands of interest were recovered from the sequencing gels and reamplified in a 40-cycle PCR (40 μl mixture) in the absence of isotope. For differential display gel band reamplification, expand PCR (Taq + Pwo) High Fidelity Ampli Taq (Boehringer Mannheim, Indianapolis, IN) was used consisting of a unique enzyme mixture containing thermostable Taq DNA and Pwo DNA polymerase.[26]

Thirty μl of the reamplified cDNA was run on a 1.5% agarose gel using xylene cyanole as loading dye. The gel was stained with ethidium bromide. The remaining PCR samples were saved at $-20°C$ for cloning. About 90% of the probes were found after the first round of PCR. The size of the reamplified PCR products were the same as those on the DNA sequencing gel (not shown). The reamplified cDNA probes were cut out from the agarose gel and extracted by means of a Qiaex kit (Qiagen, Chatsworth, CA). The extracted cDNA probes were eluted in 20 μl H_2O, and saved for Northern blot analysis.

Northern blot analysis was used to verify the differential expression of the genes. For this, reamplified cDNA probes were used directly.

Reamplified cDNA probes were cloned into the PCR-TRAP cloning vector. The cloned PCR inserts were isolated, radiolabeled and used as probes for RNA blot analysis. cDNA fragments that generated a specific hybridization pattern on RNA blots were sequenced from both directions using the Sequence kit 2.0 (USB, Cleveland, Ohio). The nucleotide sequences obtained were compared with known sequences by searching the GenBank and EMBL data bases using the FASTA program software (Genetics Computer Group, Madison, WI).

RESULTS

Differential mRNA Display

To identify transcriptionally regulated genes potentially involved in ischemic preconditioning, differential mRNA display patterns from control and precondi- tioned hearts were compared. As mentioned in the Methods section, PCR amplifi- cations were performed with eight arbitrary (H-AP$_1$, H-AP$_2$, H-AP$_3$, H-AP$_4$, H-AP$_5$, H-AP$_6$, H-AP$_7$, and H-AP$_8$) and three anchored primers (H-T$_{11}$G, H-T$_{11}$C, and H-T$_{11}$A) in combinations (FIG. 2). The results of our study are shown in FIGURES 3–8 and are summarized in TABLE 1. The differentially displayed bands are identified by size and rank of the fragments from the top to the bottom of the gels obtained from four different groups of RNA samples (A: control, B: 5-min ischemia, C: 1 × PC, D: 4 × PC). FIGURE 3A and FIGURES 4–8 show representative autoradiographs of the differential display comparing RNAs from control, ischemic and preconditioned hearts. In the autoradiograph shown in FIGURE 3A, four differ- entially expressed bands were obtained using H-T$_{11}$G anchored primer in combina- tion with H-AP$_1$, H-AP$_2$, and H-AP$_3$ arbitrary primers (see the sequence in FIG. 2). These results are summarized in TABLE 1 where the first, second, and third bands are from the control (A) sample, while the fourth band is from the 1 × PC sample. With H-AP$_4$ arbitrary primer, the autoradiograph showed no difference between the bands. Using a different anchored primer, H-T$_{11}$C, but the same arbitrary primers, five differentially expressed bands were obtained (FIG. 4; summarized in TABLE 1 for numbers 5–9). Using H-AP$_2$ arbitrary primer in combination with H-T$_{11}$C anchored primer failed to show any such bands (FIG. 4). As shown in this figure, band number 5 corresponds to the 5′I sample and band number 6 to the 1 × PC sample, while band number 7 is present in both the 5′I and 1 × PC RNA samples, and the 8th and 9th bands are present in both the 1 × PC and 4 × PC hearts. Using another anchored primer, H-T$_{11}$A, in combination with the same arbitrary primers, H-AP$_1$ to H-AP$_4$, six differentially expressed bands represented by numbers 10–15 were found (FIG. 5). In TABLE 1, these bands represent control RNA samples and are designated as A.

Using different arbitrary primers, H-AP$_5$–H-AP$_8$, with H-T$_{11}$G anchored primer, 4 bands were recovered (numbers 16–19) (FIG. 6) which were differentially

TABLE 1. The Display of the Results Obtained after Polyacrylamide Gel Electrophoresis

Band I.D.[a]	RNA Sample	Fragment Size	Signal Strength	H-AP Primer	Anchored Primer
1. G3-1A	A	725	+++	H-AP$_3$	HT$_{11}$G
2. G3-2A	A	710	+++	H-AP$_3$	HT$_{11}$G
3. G2-3A	A	660	+++	H-AP$_2$	HT$_{11}$G
4. G1-4C	C	575	+++	H-AP$_1$	HT$_{11}$G
5. C1-5B	B	775	+++	H-AP$_1$	HT$_{11}$C
6. C4-6C	C	725	+++	H-AP$_4$	HT$_{11}$C
7. C3-7B, C	B, C	525	+++	H-AP$_3$	HT$_{11}$C
8. C1-8C, D	C, D	460	+++	H-AP$_1$	HT$_{11}$C
9. C1-9C, D	C, D	450	+++	H-AP$_1$	HT$_{11}$C
10. A2-10A	A	560	++	H-AP$_2$	HT$_{11}$A
11. A2-11A	A	550	++	H-AP$_2$	HT$_{11}$A
12. A3-12A	A	425	+++	H-AP$_3$	HT$_{11}$A
13. A3-13A	A	420	++	H-AP$_3$	HT$_{11}$A
14. A3-14A	A	410	++	H-AP$_3$	HT$_{11}$A
15. A3-15A	A	405	++	H-AP$_3$	HT$_{11}$A
16. G5-16D	D	550	+++	H-AP$_5$	HT$_{11}$G
17. G5-17C	C	540	+++	H-AP$_5$	HT$_{11}$G
18. G7-18B, D	B, D	390	+++	H-AP$_7$	HT$_{11}$G
19. G7-19C, D	C, D	340	++	H-AP$_7$	HT$_{11}$G
20. C5-20C	C	925	+++	H-AP$_5$	HT$_{11}$C
21. C5-21C	C	850	+++	H-AP$_5$	HT$_{11}$C
22. C7-22C, D	C, D	800	++	H-AP$_7$	HT$_{11}$C
23. C7-23C	C	590	++	H-AP$_7$	HT$_{11}$C
24. C7-24C	C	580	+++	H-AP$_7$	HT$_{11}$C
25. C5-25C	C	520	++	H-AP$_5$	HT$_{11}$C
26. C5-26C	C	510	++	H-AP$_5$	HT$_{11}$C
27. C7-27C, D	C, D	530	+++	H-AP$_7$	HT$_{11}$C
28. C7-28C, D	C, D	525	+++	H-AP$_7$	HT$_{11}$C
29. C6-29B	B	470	++	H-AP$_7$	HT$_{11}$C
30. C7-30B, C, D	B, C, D	425	+++	H-AP$_7$	HT$_{11}$C
31. C7-31C	C	415	+++	H-AP$_7$	HT$_{11}$C
32. A5-32A	A	760	++	H-AP$_5$	HT$_{11}$A
33. A5-33A	A	710	++	H-AP$_5$	HT$_{11}$A
34. A7-34A, B	A, B	515	+++	H-AP$_7$	HT$_{11}$A
35. A5-35A	A	420	++	H-AP$_5$	HT$_{11}$A
36. A5-36A	A	410	++	H-AP$_5$	HT$_{11}$A

[a] Bands are identified by code: anchored primer (G, C or A); arbitrary primers 1 to 8; (hyphen); size rank of band from top of the gel to bottom of the gel; RNA sample (A: control; B: 5′I; C: 1 × PC; D: 4 × PC).

expressed in the 4 × PC (band 16), 1 × PC (band 17), 5′I and 4 × PC (band 18), and 1 × PC and 4 × PC (band 19) samples as described in TABLE 1. The maximum number of differentially expressed bands were obtained using H-T$_{11}$C anchored primer and H-AP$_5$–H-AP$_8$ arbitrary primer combinations. These results are shown in FIGURE 7. Band number 20 was differentially expressed in 1 × PC, band 21 in 1 × PC, but band number 22 was present in both 1 × PC and 4 × PC hearts. Bands 23 to 26 were differentially expressed only in the 1 × PC sample, while bands 27 and 28 were expressed in both the 1 × PC and 4 × PC groups. Band number 29 was present only in the 5′ ischemic sample (see TABLE 1). Band number

30 was present in the 5'I, 1 × PC, and 4 × PC samples, but not in the control group. Band 31 was differentially expressed only in the 1 × PC RNA sample. With H-T$_{11}$A anchored primer and four arbitrary primers H-AP$_5$–H-AP$_8$, five differentially expressed bands were obtained (shown in FIG. 8), numbered 32–36 in TABLE 1. Bands 32–33 and 35–36 were differentially expressed only in the control A sample, but are absent in other samples, whereas band 34 was present in both the control and 5'I RNA samples.

In order to confirm that the bands had indeed been removed from the differential display autoradiographs, we re-exposed the films after removing the fragments. FIGURE 3B is one of the representative postexcision autoradiographs for FIGURE 3A. Comparison between FIGURE 3A and FIGURE 3B clearly demonstrates the disappearance of the bands from the box of FIGURE 3A after excision of the desired fragment, which was differentially expressed for further studies.

RNA Blot Analysis with PCR-Amplified Fragments

To confirm the gene regulation patterns observed in the differential display study, we recovered 36 selected bands, reamplified 20 of them, and used them to probe RNA blots prepared with total RNAs from the control, 5'I, 1 × PC, and 4 × PC rat hearts. When used as probes, 4 out of 20 PCR-amplified fragments (numbers 8, 27, 28, 30) generated hybridization patterns that reproduced ischemia-induced preconditioning specific expression of genes. Eight out of 20 reamplified PCR fragments hybridized nonspecifically to all 4 lanes, and were not studied further (TABLE 2). The remaining 8 fragments did not detect any transcripts (TABLE 2). Such transcripts may not have been detected possibly because their levels were below the sensitivity of the RNA blot analyses. Glycerol 3-phosphate dehydrogenase (GAPDH) was used as house keeping gene in our experiments.

RNA Blot Analysis with Cloned Fragments

The PCR products that generated hybridization patterns were cloned into the PCR-TRAP cloning vector and used as hybridization probes in RNA blot analysis to identify single clones corresponding to specific mRNA transcripts. Analyses were performed in hearts from the control, 5'I, 1 × PC, and 4 × PC groups with the fragments obtained from the bands numbered 8, 27, 28 and 30. A faint hybridization signal was obtained in control (lane A) as compared to 5'I (3-fold and 2.5-fold, respectively) and 1 × PC (4.4-fold and 2.9-fold, respectively) and 4 × PC (5.8-fold and 3.5-fold, respectively) with band number 8 (fragment size 460 bp, message length 0.7 kb) (TABLE 3) and with band number 27 and 28 (fragment size 530 bp and 525 bp, respectively). The transcript (1.1 kb) levels were enhanced after 5' ischemia, 1 × PC and 4 × PC hearts compared to that for the control group. Band number 30 also showed enhanced expression in the preconditioned and ischemic groups compared to control.

Sequence Homology

The results of partial sequence and preliminary homology searches are summarized in TABLE 2. The cDNA fragment from band number 8 was found to be highly homologous to one of the mitochondrial gene, ATPase 6. Fragments 27 (530 bp)

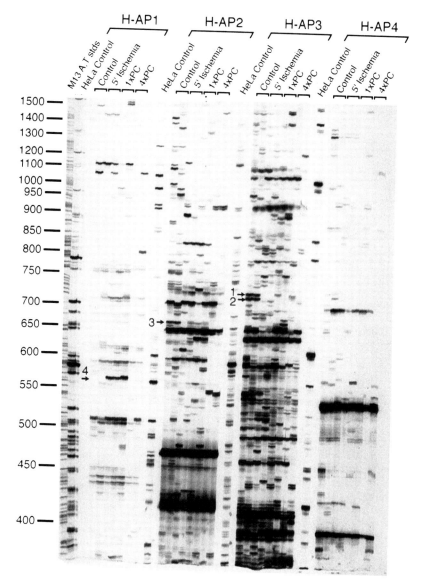

FIGURE 3A. Differential display gene expression using $H\text{-}T_{11}G$ anchored primer in combination with four arbitrary primers ($H\text{-}AP_1$, $H\text{-}AP_2$, $H\text{-}AP_3$, and $H\text{-}AP_4$). Note the upregulation and/or downregulation of four differentially expressed bands denoted by 1, 2, 3, and 4.

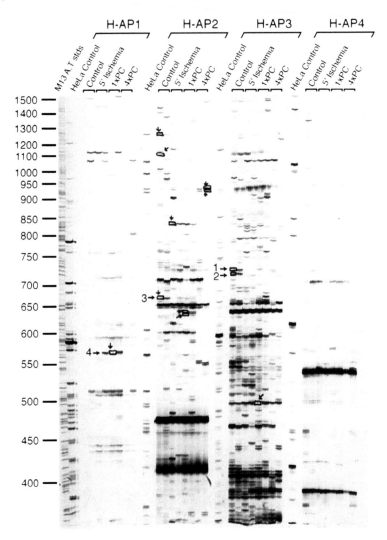

FIGURE 3B. Post-excision autoradiograph of the Figure shown in 3A. Please note the disappearance of the bands 1, 2, 3 and 4 (shown in Figure 3A) from the boxes.

and 28 (525 bp) were homologous with the mitochondrial gene, cyt b. Fragment 30 revealed 100% homology with the rat ribosomal protein L23a sequence.

DISCUSSION

PCR-DDR is a powerful technique for analyzing differences in gene expression that can be used to identify novel genes and their functions during preconditioning.

Differential gene expression can result from a number of factors including mutations, viral infections, and cellular differentiation, as well as in response to stress and environmental agents, such as hormones, drugs, and metals. These influencing factors make differential display especially beneficial in analyzing disease states, characterizing pharmacologically active compounds, discovering novel drug targets, and determining the functions of oligonucleotides or gene therapy agents. Differential display functions by selectively amplifying large numbers of expressed sequences (cDNAs) in individual analysis and then displaying these sequences

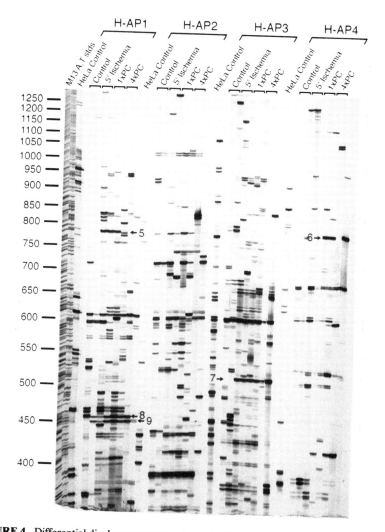

FIGURE 4. Differential display gene expression using H-T$_{11}$C anchored primer in combination with four arbitrary primers (H-AP$_1$, H-AP$_2$, H-AP$_3$, and H-AP$_4$). Note the upregulation and/or downregulation of five differentially expressed bands denoted by 5, 6, 7, 8, and 9.

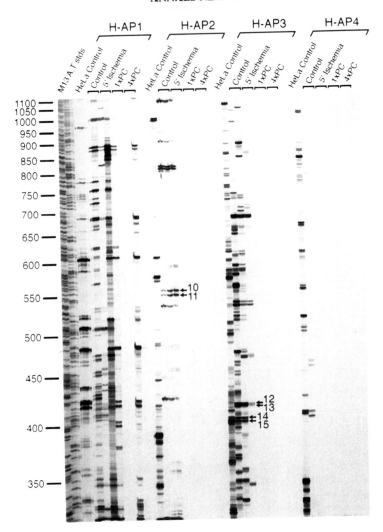

FIGURE 5. Differential display gene expression using H-T$_{11}$A anchored primer in combination with four arbitrary primers (H-AP$_1$, H-AP$_2$, H-AP$_3$, and H-AP$_4$). Note the upregulation and/or downregulation of five differentially expressed bands denoted by 10, 11, 12, 13, 14, and 15.

(cDNA fragments) by gel electrophoresis. PCR-differential display technology used in our study was developed by Drs. Arthur B. Pardee and Peng Liang.[24] This method involves reverse transcription of the mRNAs with oligo-dT primers anchored to the beginning of the poly (A) tail followed by the PCR reaction in the presence of a second 13 mer arbitrary in sequence. The amplified cDNA subpopulations of 3'-termini of mRNAs as defined by this pair of primers are

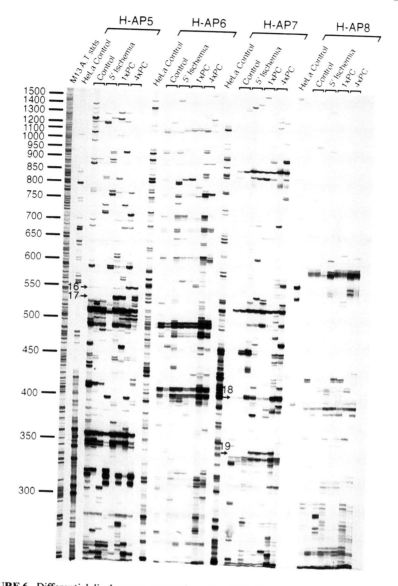

FIGURE 6. Differential display gene expression using H-T$_{11}$G anchored primer in combination with four arbitrary primers (H-AP$_5$, H-AP$_6$, H-AP$_7$, and H-AP$_8$). Note the upregulation and/or downregulation of four differentially expressed bands denoted by 16, 17, 18, and 19.

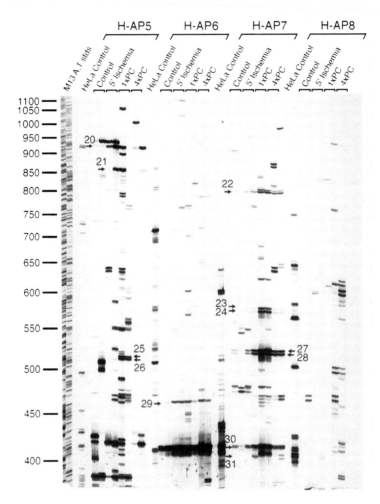

FIGURE 7. Differential display gene expression using H-T$_{11}$C anchored primer in combination with four arbitrary primers (H-AP$_5$, H-AP$_6$, H-AP$_7$, and H-AP$_8$). Note the upregulation and/or downregulation of four differentially expressed bands denoted by numbers 20 to 31.

distributed on a sequencing gel. By changing primer combination, it is possible to sequence approximately 95% of all mRNA species from the total RNA preparation of a given tissue or cell type.

In this study, we adapted the PCR-DDR technique[25] to examine the induction of gene expression that occurs during ischemic preconditioning. Two different preconditioning protocols were used, 1 × PC and 4 × PC, because our previous studies indicated that a number of stress-related genes and oncogenes are only induced in 4 × PC hearts.[1,8] Moreover, since our recent studies using the subtractive hybridization technique indicated rapid expression of several mitochondrial genes after short-term ischemia,[27,28] attempts were also made to examine the gene

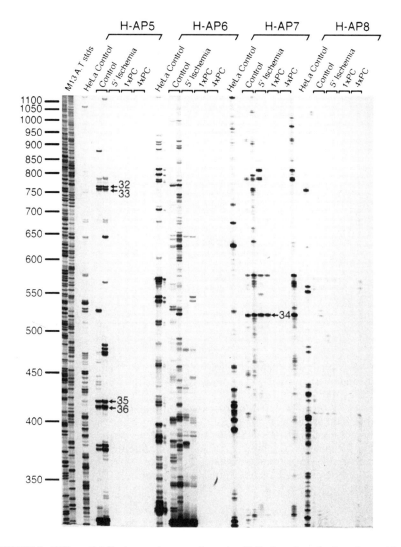

FIGURE 8. Differential display gene expression using H-T_{11}A anchored primer in combination with four arbitrary primers (H-AP_5, H-AP_6, H-AP_7, and H-AP_8). Note the upregulation and/or downregulation of five differentially expressed bands denoted by 32, 33, 34, 35 and 36.

regulation in 5-min ischemic heart. In essence, we compared both upregulation and downregulation of the gene expression between four groups of hearts, control, 5′I, 1 × PC, and 4 × PC. Each differential display analysis was repeated at least three times to confirm reproducibility of our results. Using 24 primer combinations, we identified 36 differential display cDNA bands. Out of 36 bands, 20 were reamplified. Four of these 20 bands were reproduced on RNA blot analysis. After sequencing (partial) and homology searches, 4 bands were matched with three different

TABLE 2. Analysis of cDNA Fragments Identified by Differential mRNA Display

Band #	Differential Display	Northern Analysis	Transcript Size (kb)	Sequence Homology
1	control	no hybridization	—	not sequenced
2	control	no hybridization	—	not sequenced
4	1 × PC	no hybridization	—	not sequenced
6	1 × PC	no hybridization	—	not sequenced
8	1 × PC, 4 × PC	preconditioned	0.7	ATPase 6
18	5′I, 4 × PC	no hybridization	—	not sequenced
19	1 × PC, 4 × PC	nonspecific	5.0	not sequenced
20	1 × PC	nonspecific	2.0	not sequenced
22	1 × PC, 4 × PC	nonspecific	2.5	not sequenced
27	1 × PC, 4 × PC	preconditioned	1.1	cyt b
28	1 × PC, 4 × PC	preconditioned	1.2	cyt b
29	5′I	nonspecific	3.0	not sequenced
30	5′I, 1 × PC, 4 × PC	preconditioned	2.3	r-protein L23a
31	1 × PC	nonspecific	1.0	not sequenced
32	1 × PC	nonspecific	0.9	not sequenced
32	control	no hybridization	—	not sequenced
33	control	no hybridization	—	not sequenced
34	control, 5′I	no hybridization	—	not sequenced
35	control	nonspecific	0.7	not sequenced
36	control	nonspecific	1.8	not sequenced

genes: the first band was identical with ATPase 6 (>95% homology), the second and third bands with cyt b (>98% homology), while the fourth one matched with protein L23a (100% homology).

Since we first reported that ischemic preconditioning could lead to the induction of the expression of oncogenes such as c-fos and c-myc and the mRNAs for major heat shock proteins, HSP 27, HSP 70, and HSP 89 as well as antioxidant genes for SOD and catalase,[1] a number of studies from different laboratories also observed gene expression in preconditioned hearts. In our study, we identified the differences in the pattern of gene expression between 1 × PC and 4 × PC hearts. For example, only repeatedly ischemic preconditioned hearts 4 × PC, and not

TABLE 3. Expression of Mitochondrial Genes (ATPase 6 and Cyt b) and Gene for a Ribosomal Protein L-23a

Fragment #	Genes	Control	5′I (Arbitrary Units)[a]	1 × PC	4 × PC
8	ATPase 6	0.5	1.5	2.2	2.9
27, 28	cyt b	1.1	2.8	3.2	3.9
30	ribosomal protein L-23a	0.3	1.8	2.1	2.6

[a] Total RNA (10 μg in each case) was isolated from hearts and used for Northern blot analysis. The blots were probed with ATPase 6, cyt b, and ribosomal protein L-23a cDNAs, separately. The blots were then stripped and re-probed with [^{32}P] GAPDH. The filters were exposed at −80°C using an intensifying screen. The results of densitometric scanning are shown in the table.

1 × PC, caused the induction of the expression of mRNAs for HSPs and antioxidants.[1,8] On the other hand, a short duration of ischemia triggered the induction of the expression of several mitochondrial genes.[28] This study was performed using the subtractive hybridization technique. One of the interesting findings of this study was that subtractive hybridization revealed the identity of many genes both unknown and known including mitochondrial[28] and other[29] genes, but none of them matched with the most commonly identified genes such as HSPs and antioxidants. Most of the studies on gene expression have been performed based on our knowledge of stress-induced proteins, such as HSPs and antioxidants. Traditionally, these studies are performed to identify these genes with their respective cDNA probes using Northern hybridization. Our approach using subtractive hybridization revealed for the first time the identity of many other genes which had not been identified previously in the ischemic myocardium.

The subtractive hybridization technique, however, can only identify upregulated genes. There is no doubt that many genes are also downregulated in response to ischemia and reperfusion. It is for this reason that we have now adapted the PCR-DDR technique to identify the pattern of gene expression in the preconditioned myocardium. Indeed, the results of our study clearly demonstrate that genes are both upregulated and downregulated during preconditioning. For example, as shown in TABLE 1 and FIGURES 3–8, band number 30 (C7-30 B, C, D) was not present in the control heart, but induced in 5'I, 1 × PC and 4 × PC hearts. On the other hand, bands 32–33 (A5-32A; A5-33A) and 35–36 (A5-35A; A5-36A) were differentially expressed only in the control sample, but were found to be absent in the ischemically preconditioned hearts. The mitochondrial genes, ATPase 6 and cyt b were present in the normal hearts, upregulated in 1 × PC hearts, and further upregulated in 4 × PC hearts.

The results of this study support our previous findings of subtractive hybridization that mitochondrial genes are expressed after a short period of ischemia and further demonstrates that expression of these genes is additionally stimulated after preconditioning. For example, ATPase 6 and cyt b genes were induced after 5 min of ischemia (3-fold and 2.5-fold, respectively) and further stimulated in 1 × PC (4.4-fold and 2.9-fold, respectively) and 4 × PC (5.8-fold and 3.5-fold, respectively) hearts. Very little is known regarding mitochondrial transcription although the initiation is known to be under the control of nuclear derived transcription factor TF-1.[30] A recent report showed elevated mRNA expression in mitochondrial as well as nuclear oxidative phosphorylation genes in the myocardium of patients with chronic ischemic heart disease.[31] Both ATPase 6 and cytochrome b genes are involved in oxidative ATP synthesis at the inner mitochondrial membrane and are located on the mitochondrial DNA. Upregulation of these genes during ischemic preconditioning is likely to be the adaptive response, because synthesis of these mitochondrial protein is essential for the heart to maintain cellular function during ischemia. However, mitochondrial gene expression is not self-sufficient, since some of the components that are essential for transcription and translation for these mitochondrial genes are encoded in the nucleus. It should be noted that overexpression of ATPase 6 and cyt b genes in the ischemic myocardium were previously reported by our laboratory.[28]

Another gene that was found to be upregulated after preconditioning is ribosomal protein L23a. This gene is related to *Saccharomyces cerevisiae* L25 and to *Eschericia coli* L23 ribosomal proteins that bind to a specific site in domain III of 26S and of 23S rRNAs.[32] Ribosomal protein L23a (molecular weight of 17.7 kd) contains 156 amino acids, and participates in the initiation of the assembly of the large ribosomal subunits for the synthesis of proteins. Very little is known about the functions of this ribosomal protein. It presumably plays a role in the development and differentiation of the cells. Transcription of a ribosomal protein encoding gene in the nucleoplasm is first transported to the cytoplasm where it is translated into ribosomal proteins followed by translocation to the nuclei, where it becomes associated with nacent rRNA, processed and assembled into small and large ribosomal subunits, and finally re-translocation into cytoplasm. It is known that ribosomal biogenesis fluctuates in response to cellular demand and under both transcriptional and translational control.[33] It is tempting to speculate that induction of L23a mRNA during ischemic preconditioning is the result of adaptive response of the heart to ischemia and reperfusion.

One of our goals in undertaking this study was to identify mediators that might be selective for a specific (ischemic preconditioning) or a small duration of ischemia. More bands (fragments) have to be sequenced to further identify known as well as unknown genes that are expressed during ischemic preconditioning. For this, it is necessary to use more primer combinations in order to screen additional mRNA species. So far we have used three anchored and only eight arbitrary primers. Our goal is to use 72 additional arbitrary primers in combination with three anchored primers, *i.e.*, 216 primer combinations. It is our hope that our PCR-DDR approach will allow us to hunt for as yet unknown genes in an attempt to identify important candidate factors or mediators (both known and unknown) from the jungle of 15,000 mRNA species.

REFERENCES

1. DAS, D. K., R. M. ENGELMAN & Y. KIMURA. 1993. Molecular adaptation of cellular defences following preconditioning of the heart by repeated ischemia. Cardiovasc. Res. **27:** 578–584.
2. CURRIE, R. W. 1987. Effects of ischemia and reperfusion on the synthesis of stress-induced (heat shock) proteins in isolated and perfused rat hearts. J. Mol. Cell. Cardiol. **19:** 795–808.
3. ANDRES, J., H. S. SHARMA, R. KNOLL, J. STAHL, L. M. A. SASSEN, P. D. VERDOUW & W. SCHAPER. 1993. Expression of heat shock proteins in the normal and stunned myocardium. Cardiovasc. Res. **27:** 1421–1429.
4. DONNELLY, T. J. R. E. SIEVERS, F. L. J. VISSERN, W. J. WELCH & C. L. WOLFE. 1992. Heat shock protein induction in rat hearts: a role for improved salvage after ischemia and reperfusion? Circulation **85:** 769–778.
5. KNOWLTON, A. A., P. BRECHER & C. S. APSTEIN. 1991. Rapid expression of heat shock protein in the rabbit after brief cardiac ischemia. J. Clin. Invest. **87:** 139–147.
6. HUTTER, M. M., R. E. SIEVERS, V. BARBOSA & C. L. WOLFE. 1994. Heat-shock protein induction in rat hearts. A direct correlation between the amount of heat-shock protein induced and the degree of myocardial protection. Circulation **89:** 355–360.
7. MEHTA, H. B., B. K. POPOVICH & W. H. DILLMAN. 1988. Ischemia induces changes in the level of mRNAs coding for stress protein 71 and certain kinase M. Circ. Res. **63:** 512–517.
8. DAS, D. K. & N. MAULIK. 1995. Cross talk between heat shock and oxidative stress inducible genes during myocardial adaptation to ischemia. *In*: Cell Biology of Trauma. J. J. Lemasters & C. Oliver, Eds. 193–212. CRC Press. Boca Raton, FL.
9. FRASS, O., H. S. SHARMA, R. KNOLL, D. J. DUNCKER, E. O. McFALLS, P. D. VERDOUW & W. SCHAPER. 1993. Enhanced gene expression of calcium regulatory proteins in stunned porcine myocardium. Cardiovasc. Res. **27:** 2037–2043.
10. SHARMA, H. S., M. WUNCH, R. KANDOLF & W. SCHAPER. 1989. Angiogenesis by slow coronary artery occlusion in the pig heart: expression of different growth factors mRNAs. J. Mol. Cell. Cardiol. **21**(Suppl. III): 69.
11. MAULIK, N., M. WATANABE, D. ENGELMAN, R. M. ENGELMAN & D. K. DAS. 1995.

Oxidative stress adaptation improves postischemic ventricular recovery. Mol. Cell. Biochem. **144:** 67–74.

12. MAULIK, N., M. WATANABE, D. ENGELMAN, R. M. ENGELMAN, V. E. KAGAN, E. KISIN, V. TYURIN, G. A. CORDIS & D. K. DAS. 1995. Myocardial adaptation to ischemia by oxidative stress induced by endotoxin. Am. J. Physiol. **269:** C907–C916.

13. MAULIK, N., R. M. ENGELMAN, Z. WEI, D. LU, J. A. ROUSOU & D. K. DAS. 1993. Interleukin-1α preconditioning reduces myocardial ischemia reperfusion injury. Circulation **88**(Suppl. II): 387–394.

14. MAULIK, N., Z. WEI, X. LIU, R. M. ENGELMAN, J. A. ROUSOU & D. K. DAS. 1994. Improved postischemic ventricular recovery by amphetamine is linked with its ability to induce heat shock. Mol. Cell. Biochem. **137:** 17–24.

15. LIU, X., R. M. ENGELMAN, I. I. MORARU, J. A. ROUSOU, J. E. FLACK, D. W. DEATON, N. MAULIK & D. K. DAS. 1992. Heat shock: a new approach for myocardial preservation in cardiac surgery. Circulation **86**(Suppl. II): 358–363.

16. LU, D., & D. K. DAS. 1993. Induction of differential heat shock gene expression in heart, lung liver, brain and kidney by a sympathomimetic drug, amphetamine. Biochem. Biophys. Res. Commun. **192:** 808–812.

17. MAULIK, N., R. M. ENGELMAN, Z. WEI, D. LU, J. A. ROUSOU & D. K. DAS. 1993. Interleukin-1α preconditioning reduced myocardial ischemia reperfusion injury. Circulation **88**(Part II): 387–394.

18. MAULIK, N., Z. WEI, X. LIU, R. M. ENGELMAN, J. A. ROUSOU & D. K. DAS. 1994. Improved postischemic ventricular functional recovery by amphetamine is linked with its ability to induce heat shock. Cell. Mol. Biol. **137:** 17–24.

19. MAULIK, N., H. S. SHARMA & D. K. DAS. Induction of haem oxygenase gene expression during the reperfusion of ischemic myocardium. J. Mol. Cell. Cardiol. In press.

20. MAULIK, N., R. M. ENGELMAN, Z. WEI, X. LIU, J. A. ROUSOU, J. FLACK, D. DEATON & D. K. DAS. 1995. Drug-induced heat shock improves post-ischemic ventricular recovery after cardiopulmonary bypass. Circulation **92**(Suppl. II): 381–388.

21. DAS, D. K., N. MAULIK & I. I. MORARU. 1995. Gene expression in acute myocardial stress. Induction by hypoxia, ischemia, reperfusion, hyperthermia and oxidative stress. J. Mol. Cell. Cardiol. **27:** 181–193.

22. DAS, D. K., N. MAULIK, T. YOSHIDA, R. M. ENGELMAN & Y-L. ZU. 1996. Preconditioning potentiates molecular signaling for myocardial adaptation to ischemia. Ann. N. Y. Acad. Sci. This volume.

23. CHOMCZYNSKI, P. & N. SACCHI. 1987. Single step method of RNA isolation by acid guanidinium thiocyanate-phenol-chloroform extraction. Anal. Biochem. **162:** 156–159.

24. LIANG, P. & A. B. PARDEE. 1992. Differential display of eukaryotic messenger RNA by means of the polymerase chain reaction. Science **257:** 967–971.

25. LIANG, P., W. ZHU, X. ZHANG, Z. GUO, P. O. O'CONNELL, L. AVERBOUKH, F. WANG & A. B. PARDEE. 1994. Differential display using one-base anchored oligo-dT primers. Nucleic Acid Res. **22:** 5763–5764.

26. BARNES, W. M. 1994. PCR amplification of up to 35 kb DNA with high fidelity and high yield from λ bacteriophage templates. Proc. Natl. Acad. Sci. USA **91:** 2216–2220.

27. DAS, D. K., I. I. MORARU, N. MAULIK & R. M. ENGELMAN. 1994. Gene expression during myocardial adaptation to ischemia and reperfusion. Ann. N. Y. Acad. Sci. **723:** 292–307.

28. MORARU, I. I., D. T. ENGELMAN, R. M. ENGELMAN, J. A. ROUSOU, J. E. FLACK, D. W. DEATON & D. K. DAS. 1994. Myocardial ischemia triggers rapid expression of mitochondrial genes. Surg. Forum **40:** 315–317.

29. MAULIK, N. & D. K. DAS. Molecular cloning, sequencing and expression analysis of a fatty acid transport gene in rat heart induced by ischemic preconditioning and oxidative stress. Mol. Cell. Biochem. In press.

30. SHADE, G. S. & D. A. CLAYTON. 1993. Mitochondrial transcription initiation. J. Biol. Chem. **268:** 16083–16086.

31. CORRAL-DEBRINSKI, M., G. STEPIEN, J. M. SHOFFNER, M. T. LOTT, K. KANTER & D C. WALLACE. 1991. Hypoxemia is associated with mitochondrial DNA damage and gene induction. JAMA **266:** 1812–1816.

32. SUZUKI, K., & I. G. WOOL. 1993. The primary structure of rat ribosomal protein L-23a. The application of homology search to the identification of genes for mammalian and yeast ribosomal proteins and a correlation of rat and yeast ribosomal proteins. J. Biol. Chem. **268:** 2755–27861.
33. MAGER, W. H. 1988. Control of ribosomal gene expression. Biochim. Biophys. Acta **949:** 1–15.

Molecular Basis of Cardiocyte Cell Specification

SHYAMAL K. GOSWAMI AND M. A. Q. SIDDIQUI[a]

Center for Cardiovascular and Muscle Research
Department of Anatomy and Cell Biology
State University of New York Health Science Center
at Brooklyn
Brooklyn, New York 11203

Despite significant progress in our understanding of the molecular basis of skeletal muscle development,[1] relatively little is known about the regulatory events that initiate and propagate the myocardial lineage to terminally differentiated cardiocytes. The lack of progress in this regard can in part be attributed to the nonavailability of a cardiac muscle cell line amenable to differentiation *in vitro*. This limitation has, however, been compensated for to some extent by the volume of information that has accumulated over the past decade on the development of cardiovasculature,[2-4] on the biochemical and genetic analysis of the role of peptide growth factors in heart development,[5] and on the molecular mechanism underlying heart muscle differentiation.[6] The experimental approaches currently being taken to understand cardiac muscle lineage specification is directed toward the mapping analysis of the myocardial cell lineage, and toward identification of regulatory factors that trigger the transcriptional events that ultimately lead the progenitor cells to differentiated cardiocytes.[2-4] This review is mainly concerned with recent progress on identification and characterization of key transcription factors that are potentially involved in cardiomyocyte specification and cell differentiation.

Regulation of Sarcomeric Gene Expression: a Paradigm of Myocardial Development

Although differentiating cardiac muscle cells do not form multinucleated myotubes like skeletal muscle, cardiac myocytes contain sarcomeric arrays with their structural organization and function similar to skeletal muscle. Many contractile protein genes are members of multigene families expressing differentially in cardiac chambers and in different skeletal muscles types,[7] while other muscle genes, such as muscle creatine kinase (MCK), are single gene products expressing in both cardiac and skeletal muscle. As a consequence, it was expected that the molecular mechanism that drives the expression of cardiac genes must share features similar to skeletal muscle genes.[8] Indeed, several muscle-specific genes share common regulatory elements for their expression in both cardiac and skeletal muscles. This notion was further enforced by observations that following hypertrophic stimuli cardiac myocytes undergo a genetic reprogramming that causes expression of

[a] Address for correspondence: M. A. Q. Siddiqui, Department of Anatomy and Cell Biology, State University of New York Health Science Center at Brooklyn, Brooklyn, NY 11203. Tel.: (718) 270-1014; Fax: (718) 270-3732.

certain skeletal genes.[9] But it is now becoming clear that cardiac muscle cells have a distinct transcriptional strategy for a programmed pattern of gene expression specific for the cardiac phenotype, which depends upon the availability of specific regulatory factors.[10]

Muscle genes that have been subject to regulatory analysis can be divided into four categories: (i) genes that are tissue restricted, such as cardiac myosin light chain 2 (MLC2); (ii) genes that are expressed in both cardiac and skeletal muscle cells, such as MCK; (iii) genes that are expressed in both cardiac and skeletal muscle cells during early embryonic development, but are subsequently turned off in one or the other muscle, such as cardiac α-actin and cardiac troponin T; and (iv) genes that are normally expressed in skeletal muscle but are activated in cardiac muscle following hypertrophic stimuli, such as skeletal α-actin. Since the majority of these genes are expressed in both cardiac and skeletal muscle cells at some stage of development, it was hypothesized that the cardiac and skeletal muscle-specific genes have a common molecular ancestor among the determinant factors.

Following the discovery of the myogenic basic-helix-loop-helix (bHLH) family of transcription factors as the determinant of skeletal muscle development, a significant effort was made to find the cardiac homologue of these proteins. However, no bHLH family of factors, other than the ubiquitously expressed E2 gene products, has yet been detected in cardiac muscle cells.[11] For human cardiac α-actin gene expression in neonatal rat cardiomyocytes, however, a regulatory domain containing the MyoD binding site (E-box) has been found to be necessary,[12] even though, the regulatory protein that occupies the E-box sequence in cardiac myocytes is not known. On the other hand, the tissue-specific cardiac MLC2 promoter, which lacks a functional E-box can be transactivated by ectopic expression of MyoD,[13] suggesting that a common regulatory factor that can mediate activation of both skeletal and cardiac genes (see below) might be the target of MyoD. Neonatal rat cardiac myocytes, upon treatment with norepinephrine, develop hypertrophy, which is associated with the induction of skeletal α-actin gene. However, the 700-bp-long regulatory region, which is required for its upregulation in cardiac myocytes, is nonessential for expression in skeletal muscle cells.[14] Similarly, the regulatory elements involved in the cardiac tissue restricted expression of cardiac troponin T (cTnT) gene has also been dissociated from those required for its expression in skeletal muscle. During early chicken embryonic development, the cTnT gene is expressed at a low level in both skeletal and cardiac muscles, but after 12 days, its expression goes up dramatically in cardiac muscle and is repressed concomitantly in skeletal muscle. While the proximal region up to -129 bp in the cTnT promoter is sufficient for its expression in skeletal muscle, the cardiac tissue-specific expression requires an additional sequence located at -247 to -201. This region contains two distinct *cis*-acting elements, an A/T rich sequence that is indistinguishable from the MEF-2 (myocyte enhancer factor-2) and a unique sequence that recognizes a novel factor, CEBF. These two elements work in conjunction with the two M-CAT sequences located in the proximal cTnT promoter region.[15,16] Similar studies with mouse cardiac troponin C (cTnC) gene also identified divergent regulatory pathways for its expression in cardiac and slow skeletal muscle.[17,18]

Mammalian cardiac muscle cells contain two isozymes of myosin heavy chain (MHC), namely α and β, of which the β-isoform is expressed in slow skeletal muscle as well. α-MHC, on the other hand, is expressed exclusively in cardiac muscle. In small mammals, such as rat and mouse, the expression of both isoforms are developmentally and hormonally (thyroid hormone) regulated. During fetal development, the β-isoform is predominant and its expression is downregulated after birth, while that of α-MHC goes up. A common muscle-specific enhancer is sufficient for expression of β-MHC in both cardiac and skeletal muscle cells.[19] The tissue-specific expression of cardiac MLC2, on the other hand, is regulated by a distinct negative regulatory element that accounts for its repression in skeletal muscle.[20] A cardiac specific sequence (CSS) has been described[20] that is responsible for the repression of cardiac MLC2 in skeletal muscle. It was recently discovered in our laboratory (Dhar, Ph. D. thesis) that the functional domains of CSS consists of three distinct protein binding sites with a common motif (GAAG) essential for repression of transcription and that CSS-mediated transcriptional inhibition is contingent upon the presence of a downstream modulatory sequence which also contains the GAAG motif.

In the MCK gene, which is expressed in both cardiac and skeletal muscle cells, a distal enhancer element, located at 1.1 kb upstream, contains multiple functional DNA binding domains, including a CArG box, an A/T rich sequence targeted by muscle-specific homeo box factor M-Hox, an AP-2 site, two E-boxes (CANNTG, target site for MyoD and myogenin) and an MEF-2 binding site (TATTTTTA). Interestingly, the contribution of these elements in MCK gene expression is different in cardiac and skeletal muscle tissues. In skeletal muscle, the order of the relative importance of these elements is E-box>A/T rich sequence>MEF-2>CArG; while that in cardiac muscle it is A/T rich sequence>CArG>MEF-2>E-boxes. Furthermore, in cardiac muscle, the enhancer activity is orientation dependent.[21] Studies with rabbit MCK promoter-enhancer, on the other hand, showed that the enhancer elements, comprising a CArG box, an A/T rich sequence, two E-boxes and one MEF-2 site were required for expression in skeletal muscle. But the cardiac muscle-specific expression was determined by the CArG element alone present in the proximal promoter region.[22] Thus, taken together, it appears that although a number of muscle-specific genes contain common regulatory elements involved in their expression in both cardiac and skeletal muscle cells, the regulatory mechanisms responsible for their expression in two distinct muscle types are divergent.

Role of the MEF-2 Family of Transcription Factors in Cardiac Muscle Differentiation

MEF-2 was originally identified as a DNA binding protein that recognizes the A/T rich sequence TTATTTTTA in the MCK enhancer.[23] Subsequently, the MEF-2 sequence was identified in the promoter/enhancer regions of several cardiac and skeletal muscle-specific genes, including the gene for cardiac MLC2.[24,25] MEF-2 from both cardiac and skeletal muscles belongs to the MADS-box (MCM1, Agamous and Deficiens and Serum Response Factor) family of transcription factors and is characterized by (i) the sequence specific binding to the MEF-2 sequence (TTATTTTTA), (ii) the presence of conserved MADS domain at the amino terminus (see Ref. 24 and reference therein), (iii) the presence of an additional domain, MEF-2 domain, which is located at the carboxyl terminal side of the MADS box and is conserved only among the members of the MEF-2 family, and (iv) the existence of multiple isoforms generated either from different genes or/and by the alternative splicing of the primary transcripts. To date, four *mef*-2 genes have been identified in vertebrates.[24] Recent data also implicated MEF-2 in cell lineage determination.[26] It appears that MEF-2 activity is caused by a group of MEF-2 proteins, rather than by a single polypeptide.[24] Some members of MEF-2 proteins are tissue restricted, while others are ubiquitous.[26] The fact that multiple isoforms of MEF-2 proteins, generated by alternatively spliced genes, exist which bind to functional DNA sites as dimmers considerably raises their potential in executing diverse regulatory functions. Taken together, these observations strongly suggest that the MEF-2 proteins play a pivotal role in the control of myogenesis and point to their potential as regulator of cell commitment.[24,26] Interestingly, a number of other transcription factors, which lack the above features but exhibit the binding to the MEF-2 sequence, have also been reported.[25,28,29] These include the paired-like homeodomain protein, Mhox and POU domain protein, oct-1,[24,28] and the zinc finger protein, HF-1b.[29] The physiological relevance of these transcription factors in muscle specific gene expression has yet to be demonstrated.

The Cardiac-Specific Transcription Factor BBF-1 Is a Novel Protein and Is an Early Marker for Cardiogenesis

The MyoD family proteins, which are considered to be the hallmark of skeletal myogenesis, are absent in cardiac muscle and therefore, there is no known marker for identifying the onset of cardiac muscle differentiation during early embryonic development and the mechanism for activation of cardiac muscle genes expression remains enigmatic. It would appear that tissue-specific regulatory factors divergent from the myogenic HLH proteins are involved in activation of cardiogenic program. We recently identified and characterized a new transcription factor, BBF-1, in chicken embryonic cardiac muscle, which recognizes the MEF-2 binding site. BBF-1 is distinguishable from MEF-2, since it is not immunoprecipitated by the MEF-2 specific antibodies (Ref. 25, unpublished data). Also, unlike MEF-2, which is present in both cardiac and skeletal muscles cells and possibly in other tissues, expression of BBF-1 is restricted to cardiac tissue only.[24,25] Since MEF-2 has already been implicated in myogenic lineage determination and BBF-1 appears to be a cardiac-specific transcription factor that binds to the MEF-2 sequence, we examined the potential of BBF-1 as the marker for cardiac muscle differentiation. In avian embryo, the mesodermal precursors of the cardiac muscle have been mapped, and the location, morphogenetic movement and the differentiative transition of these cells have been delineated, beginning with the assignment of cardiogenic fate at stage 4 ($\simeq$ 20 hr)[30] in gastrulating embryo.[31,32] The molecular aspects of these early embryonic changes, especially during the period beginning from the assignment of the cardiogenic fate to the onset of morphogenetic differentiation, have not been studied, and it is not clear what developmental and spatial signals responsible for cardiac tissue specification emanate during early embryogenesis. The genes appearing during this critical period, especially those appearing at or immediately before the cardiac fate assignment at stage 4,[30] are candidates for cardiac lineage-specific regulatory factors. Therefore, we analyzed the onset of cardiac myogenesis by monitoring the appearance of cardiac muscle-specific MLC2 and cardiac α-actin mRNAs in single embryos followed by that of BBF-1 and MEF-2 binding activities at defined stages of early blastodermal development. We also examined the same single embryos for the appearance of MyoD mRNAs. We observed that the first discernible signals for cardiac and skeletal MLC2 mRNAs appear at stages 5 and 8, respectively. Consistent with the onset of MLC2, cardiac α-actin mRNA was also detected at stage 5 and skeletal α-actin at stage 7, respectively (see FIG. 1 and Ref. 33 for details). It is well established that the first heart-forming precursor cells can be located in the bilateral regions around Henson's node at the full primitive streak stage, stage 4, of chicken development,[30,32] while the first progenitors of somite cells can be located in stage 7

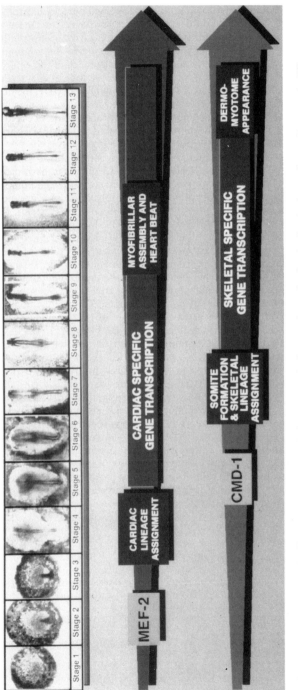

FIGURE 1. Expression of different marker genes during myogenic lineage determination in developing embryo. *Top panel*: different stages (Hamburger & Hamilton[30]) of chicken embryonic development is shown. *Bottom panel*: temporal expression of different marker genes are identified. The myogenic regulatory factor MEF-2 appears at stage 2. The cardiac myocyte specific factor BBF-1 appears at stage 4, when the transcripts for cardiac MLC2 and cardiac α-actin appear. The skeletal muscle specification factor CMD1 appears at stage 5, prior to the appearance of the first somite and the skeletal MLC2 transcript at stage 7. The appearances of specific transcripts were identified by sensitive RT-PCR analysis using gene-specific primers.[33]

blasotderms. Therefore, it appears that cardiac and skeletal muscle differentiation begins at or immediately after the assignment of the respective cell lineage at stages 4 and 7 in developing embryo, which is well before the onset of morphological differentiation at stages 10 and 13, respectively. This temporal separation of the two transcriptional events (stage 5 and stage 7) is consistent with the established separation in appearance of the two tissue-specific morphological characteristics (stage 10 and stage 13). We also observed that the first signal of CMD1, the chicken skeletal muscle homologue of MyoD, can be detected as early as stage 5, *i.e.*, prior to the appearance of first somite and the onset of transcription of the skeletal MLC2 gene at stage 8. This is consistent with the expected role of HLH proteins in programming only the skeletal, but not the cardiac, myogenesis.

To examine the possibility whether the functional expression of BBF-1 and MEF-2 DNA-binding activities are developmentally regulated in harmony with the appearance of MLC2 mRNAs, we isolated protein extracts from embryos of defined stages and tested for DNA-protein complex formation in a gel mobility shift assay. We observed that a defined BBF-1/DNA complex appears first at stage 5, with a barely detectable signal at stage 4. The MEF-2-like activity, on the other hand, begins to appear only at stage 8 and becomes defined at stage 12.[33] Subsequent analysis of protein extracts from isolated heart tubes of embryos at stage 12 of development and those from the remaining embryos, further confirmed that the origin of BBF-1 and MEF-2 activities were predominantly located in the heart tube.[33] Since the functional appearance of BBF-1 is temporally linked to the appearance of cardiac muscle-specific transcripts, we propose that BBF-1 is the earliest marker for the identification of the onset of cardiogenic differentiation. In order to delineate the precise regulatory role BBF-1 plays in the development of cardiac muscle lineage, we recently isolated the BBF-1 cDNA from a cDNA library constructed from the RNA isolated from the heart-forming region of stage 6 chick embryo. Characterization of this cDNA following its expression in *E. coli* shows its binding to the MEF-2 sequence (data not shown). *In situ* hybridization analysis demonstrated its expression in the precardiac mesodermal region during an early stage of development (data not shown). The nucleotide sequence analysis of the cDNA clone and DNA binding properties of the bacterially expressed recombinant protein revealed BBF-1 is a novel transcription factor, with no homology to known MEF-2 proteins. Taken together, these data suggest that BBF-1 is an important regulator of the cardiogenic lineage in avian development. Further confirmation of the role of this putative cardiac lineage associated protein will depend upon its successful expression in noncardiogenic cells and the capacity to transform them to the cardiogenic lineage.

REFERENCES

1. BUCKINGHAM, M. 1994. Molecular biology of muscle development. Cell **78:** 15–21.
2. YUTZEY, K. E. & D. BADER. 1995. Diversification of cardiomyogenic cell lineages during early heart development. Circ. Res. **77:** 216–219.
3. KIRBY, M. L. & K. L. WALDO. 1995. Neural crest and cardiovascular patterning. Circ. Res. **77:** 211–215.
4. FISHMAN, M. C. & D. Y. STAINIE. 1994. Cardiovascular development. Prospects for a genetic approach. Circ. Res. **74:** 757–763.
5. ENGELMANN, G. L., C. A. DIONNE & M. C. JAYE. 1993. Acidic fibroblast growth factor and heart development. Role in myocyte proliferation and capillary angiogenesis. Circ. Res. **72:** 7–19.

6. CHIEN, K. R., H. ZHU, K. U. KNOWLTON, W. MILLER-HANCE, M. VAN-BILSEN, T. X. O'BRIEN & S. M. EVANS. 1993. Transcriptional regulation during cardiac growth and development. Annu. Rev. Physiol. **55:** 77–95.

7. WADE, R. & L. KEDES. 1989. Developmental regulation of contractile protein genes. Annu. Rev. Physiol. **51:** 179–188.

8. SARTORELLI, V., M. KURABAYASHI & L. KEDES. 1993. Muscle-specific gene expression. A comparison of cardiac and skeletal muscle transcription strategies. Circ. Res. **72:** 925–931.

9. CHIEN, K. R., K. U. KNOWLTON, H. ZHU & S. CHIEN. 1991. Regulation of cardiac gene expression during myocardial growth and hypertrophy: molecular studies of an adaptive physiologic response. FASEB J. **5:** 3037–3046.

10. E. N. OLSON. 1993. Regulation of muscle transcription by the MyoD family. The heart of the matter. Circ. Res. **72:** 1–6.

11. EDMONDSON, D. G. & E. N. OLSON. 1993. Helix-loop-helix proteins as regulators of muscle-specific transcription. J. Biol. Chem. **268:** 755–758.

12. SARTORELLI, V., N. A. HONG, N. H. BISHOPRIC & L. KEDES. 1990. Myocardial activation of the human cardiac alpha actin promoter by helix-loop-helix proteins. Proc. Natl. Acad. Sci. USA **89:** 4047–4051.

13. GOSWAMI, S. & M. A. Q. SIDDIQUI. 1995. Transactivation of cardiac MLC-2 promoter by MyoD in 10T1/2 fibroblast cells is independent of E-box requirement but depends upon new proteins that recognize MEF-2 site. Cell. Mol. Biol. Res. **41:** 199–205.

14. BISHOPRIC, N. H. & L. KEDES. 1991. Adrenergic regulation of the skeletal alpha-actin gene promoter during myocardial cell hypertrophy. Proc. Natl. Acad. Sci. USA **88:** 2132–2136.

15. IANNELLO, R. C., J. H. MAR & C. P. ORDAHL. 1991. Characterization of a promoter element required for transcription in myocardial cells. J. Biol. Chem. **266:** 3309–3316.

16. MAR, J. H. & C. P. ORDAHL. 1990. M-CAT binding factor, a novel trans-acting factor governing muscle-specific transcription. Mol. Cell. Biol. **10:** 4271–4283.

17. SCHREIER, T., L. KEDES & R. GAHLMANN. 1990. Cloning, structural analysis, and expression of the human slow twitch skeletal muscle/cardiac troponin C gene. J. Biol. Chem. **265:** 21247–21253.

18. PARMACEK, M. S., A. J. VORA, T. SHEN, E. BRAR, F. JUNG & J. M. LEIDEN. 1994. A novel myogenic regulatory circuit controls slow/cardiac troponin C gene transcription in skeletal muscle. Mol. Cell. Biol. **14:** 1870–1885.

19. THOMPSON, W. R., B. NADAL-GINARD & V. MAHDAVI. 1991. A MyoD1-independent muscle-specific enhancer controls the expression of the beta-myosin heavy chain gene in skeletal and cardiac muscle cells. J. Biol. Chem. **266:** 22678–22688.

20. SHEN, R. A., S. K. GOSWAMI, E. MASCARENO, A. KUMAR & M. A. SIDDIQUI. 1991. Tissue-specific transcription of the cardiac myosin light-chain 2 gene is regulated by an upstream repressor element. Mol. Cell. Biol. **11:** 1676–1685.

21. AMACHER, S. L., J. N. BUSKIN & S. D. HAUSCHKA. 1993. Multiple regulatory elements contribute differentially to muscle creatine kinase enhancer activity in skeletal and cardiac muscle. Mol. Cell. Biol. **13:** 2753–2764.

22. VINCENT, C. K., A. GUALBERTO, C. V. PATEL & K. WALSH. 1993. Different regulatory sequences control creatine kinase-M gene expression in directly injected skeletal and cardiac muscle. Mol. Cell. Biol. **13:** 1264–1272.

23. GOSSETT, L. A., D. KELVIN, E. STERNBERG & E. N. OLSON. 1989. A new myocyte specific enhancer binding factor that recognizes a conserved element associated with multiple muscle specific genes. Mol. Cell. Biol. **9:** 5022–5033.

24. OLSON, E. N., M. PERRY & R. A. SCHULZ. 1995. Regulation of muscle differentiation by the MEF-2 family of MADS box transcription factors. Dev. Biol. **172:** 2–14.

25. ZHOU, M. D., S. K. GOSWAMI, M. E. MARTIN & M. A. SIDDIQUI. 1993. A new serum-responsive, cardiac tissue-specific transcription factor that recognizes the MEF-2 site in the myosin light chain-2 promoter. Mol. Cell. Biol. **13:** 1222–1231.

26. EDMONDSON, D. G., G. E. LYONS, J. F. MARTIN & E. N. OLSON. 1994. MEF2 gene expression marks the cardiac and skeletal muscle lineages during mouse embryogenesis. Development **120:** 1251–1263.

27. HAN, T. H. & R. PRYWES. 1995. Regulatory role of MEF-2D in serum induction of the c-jun promoter. Mol. Cell. Biol. **15:** 2907–2915.

28. CSERJESI, P., P. LILLY, C. HINCLEY, M. PERRY & E. N. OLSON. 1994. Homeodomain protein MHox and MADS protein myocyte enhancer-binding factor-2 converge on a common element in the muscle creatine kinase enhancer. J. Biol. Chem. **269:** 16740–16745.

29. ZHU, H., V. T. NGUYEN, A. B. BROWN, A. POURHOSSEINI, A. V. GARCIA, M. VAN BILSON & K. R. CHIEN. 1993. A novel, tissue restricted zinc finger protein (HF-1b) binds to the cardiac regulatory element (HF-1b/MEF-2) in the rat myosin light chain-2 gene. Mol. Cell. Biol. **13:** 4432–4444.

30. HAMBURGER, V. & H. L. HAMILTON. 1951. A series of normal stages in the development of the chick embryo. J. Morphol. **88:** 49–92.

31. MANASEK, F. J. & R. G. MONROE. 1972. Early cardiac morphogenesis is independent of function. Dev. Biol. **27:** 584–588.

32. GONZALEZ-SANCHEZ, A. & D. BADER. 1990. *In vitro* analysis of cardiac progenitor cell differentiation. Dev. Biol. **139:** 197–209.

33. GOSWAMI, S., P. QASBA, S. GHATPANDE, S. CARLETON, A. K. DESHPANDE, M. BAIG & M. A. SIDDIQUI. 1994. Differential expression of the myocyte enhancer factor 2 family of transcription factors in development: the cardiac factor BBF-1 is an early marker for cardiogenesis. Mol. Cell. Biol. **14:** 5130–5138.

Tumor Necrosis Factor-α-Induced Cytoprotective Mechanisms in Cardiomyocytes

Analysis by mRNA Phenotyping

HARI S. SHARMA,[a,c] DIRK WEISENSEE,[b] AND
IRIS LÖW-FRIEDRICH[b]

aCardiovascular and Molecular Biology Laboratory
Institute of Pharmacology
Erasmus University
Rotterdam, The Netherlands
and
bCenter for Internal Medicine
J. W. Goethe University Hospital
Frankfurt am Main, Germany

INTRODUCTION

Tumor necrosis factor-α (TNF-α) belongs to a class of hormone-like molecules termed cytokines, a group of soluble factors that includes interferons, interleukins and hematopoietic growth factors.[1,2] These polypeptide mediators form a complex network of interactive signals that regulate their own production and thereby the growth, differentiation and function of virtually every cell.[1] TNF-α, a polypeptide of 17 kDa, is one of the principle endogenous mediators of endotoxic shock, and it has been implicated in inflammation, immunoregulation, cytotoxicity, cytoprotection and angiogenesis.[3–5] TNF-α, predominantly produced and secreted by monocytes and macrophages stimulates extracellular matrix degradation and prostaglandin E_2 expression, and hence plays a role in both degenerative and inflammatory diseases.[2,6,7] Biological effects of TNF-α in the target cell are initiated by binding of TNF-α to high affinity cell surface receptors expressed on the membranes of almost all somatic cell types.[8–10] TNF receptors channel signals to the cytoplasm and nucleus, and thereby initiate profound alterations in the cellular metabolic pathway as well as in transcriptional machinery. Two immunologically distinct TNF receptors of 55 kDa (TNF-R55) and 75 kDa (TNF-R75) apparent molecular mass have been identified and characterized.[9–11]

A number of studies in different cell types including cardiomyocytes have shown that TNF-α induces phosphorylation of a stress protein belonging to the heat shock protein family with an apparent molecular weight of about 28 kDa.[12–16] TNF-α stimulates a rapid and transient expression of *c-myc* and *c-fos* mRNAs in quiescent human FS-4 fibroblasts indicating its growth promoting action on these

---

c Address for correspondence and requests for reprints: Hari S. Sharma, Ph.D., Institute of Pharmacology, Erasmus University, Faculty of Medicine & Health Sciences, P.O. Box 1738, 3000 DR Rotterdam, The Netherlands. E-mail: SHARMA@FARMA.FGG.EUR.NL.

cells.[17] Furthermore, TNF-α is a potent noncytotoxic growth inhibitor for endothelial cells *in vitro*, but enhances neovascularization *in vivo*.[5,18] TNF-α-induced signaling pathway downstream to the ligand receptor binding in cardiomyocytes has been characterized to be mediated via $G_{i\alpha}$ and G_β proteins coupled to adenylyl cyclase.[19] However, the intracellular mediators of TNF-α action involved in endogenous nuclear events leading to cytoprotective mechanisms are not known.

In the heart, myocardial ischemia causes injury that is characterized by several parameters including an increase in local expression as well as in circulating cytokines such as TNF-α.[20–22] Expression of TNF-α has been shown to be enhanced and localized to microvascular endothelium in the postischemic heart.[22] In a recent report, it was shown that pretreatment of rat hearts with TNF-α protects them from ischemia and reperfusion injury.[24] It is believed that TNF-α induces manganous superoxide dismutase (MnSOD) gene expression conferring resistance to TNF-α cytotoxicity.[23–24] In the normal heart, TNF-α may exert negative inotropic effects by directly altering intracellular calcium homeostasis in a concentration- and time-dependent manner.[25] Perfusion of spontaneously contracting cultures of cardiomyocytes with a high concentration of TNF-α (10,000 Units/ml) induced arrhythmias with time resulting in a complete cessation of spontaneous contractions and severe loss of myocyte inotropy.[46] In a test model of monitoring cardiotoxicity, we have shown that TNF-α as well as interleukins (IL-2, IL-3, IL-6) induce the formation of stress proteins in cultured cardiomyocytes.[14] We hypothesized that TNF-α stimulates cytoprotective mechanisms in cardiomyocytes, and such mechanisms can be examined by investigating the expression pattern of various heat shock/stress protein genes.

Heat shock and other environmental as well as pathophysiological stresses stimulate cellular synthesis of a highly conserved group of proteins called heat shock proteins (HSPs).[26–37] HSPs are members of stress proteins, which also include the glucose regulated proteins (GRPs), ubiquitin, $\alpha\beta$-crystalline and heme oxygenase.[28–32,35] These proteins enable cells to survive and recover from stressful conditions.[26,29,38] It is proposed that the heart has its own systems of protection against ischemia-reperfusion injury, probably by production of a number of HSPs that may act as chaperones in protecting vital cellular proteins from degradation.[28,32,34,36–42] Relatively well characterized, the HSP 70 family of proteins bind to ATP and help in posttranslational import of proteins into endoplasmic reticulum and mitochondria.[26,29,42] HSP 27, found in normal as well as cancer cells migrates to the nucleus upon stress, and it acts as a molecular chaperone, and plays an important role in signal transduction and drug resistance.[30,43] Ubiquitin (HSP 8) is a polypeptide of 8 kDa involved in ATP-dependent proteolysis.[31,44]

Therefore, with the background knowledge of interaction between TNF-α and heat shock protein genes, we conducted the present study. Our objectives were to get an insight into TNF-α-induced endogenous cytoprotective mechanisms. We developed an *in vitro* model based on cultured cardiomyocytes treated with an adequate amount of TNF-α and examined the expression pattern of mRNAs encoding heat shock proteins (HSP 27 and HSP 70) and ubiquitin.

MATERIALS

Alpha medium, Dulbecco's minimum essential medium (DMEM), fetal calf serum (FCS), trypsin, phosphate buffered saline (PBS), HEPES, L-glutamine, penicillin and streptomycin were supplied by Biochrom KG (Berlin, FRG). Minimum essential medium (MEM) and dialyzed FCS were purchased from Gibco-BRL (St. Louis, MO). TNF-α was obtained from British Bio-technology Limited (via H. Biermann GmbH, Bad Nauheim, FRG). DNase I Type IV (150 KU/mg) was provided from Sigma (Deisenhofen, FRG). Anti-titin and anti-mouse IgG antibodies were from Boehringer Mannheim GmbH (Mannheim, FRG). Deionized formamide was purchased from Life Technologies B.V., Breda, The Netherlands. [α-^{32}P]-dCTP (3000 Ci/mmol) and a random prime labeling system were procured from Amersham Nederland B.V., Den Bosch. All other chemicals were of the highest purity available and/or molecular biological grade.

METHODS

Isolation and Culture of Fetal Mouse Cardiomyocytes

Cardiomyocytes were isolated and maintained in culture as described previously.[14,45,46] Briefly, hearts from approximately 18-day-old fetal mice (NMRI strain) were dissected in calcium- and magnesium-free phosphate buffered saline (PBS). Tissue digestion was started by addition of trypsin (final concentration 0.1%) for 15 min at room temperature. The first supernatant was discarded, the following were collected in equal volumes of ice cold alpha medium including 20% fetal calf serum (FCS). The yield of intact cells was increased by the permanent presence of 0.05 mg/ml DNase I Type IV to the trypsin solution, which prevented the accumulation of sticky DNA released from damaged cells. The pooled cell suspension was centrifuged for 10 min in a Sorvall SS 34 rotor (1500 rpm; 4°C). After washing the pellet twice, the cells were resuspended in alpha medium and plated in culture dishes with a density of 5×10^4 cells/cm^2. Thereafter the cells were incubated at 37°C in a humidified atmosphere with 5% CO$_2$, which allowed them to attach tightly to the substrate. Adhered cells to culture dishes were characterized as beating cardiomyocytes and further verified by immunocytochemical staining technique to be more than 90% pure in cultures. The culture medium was alpha medium supplemented with 20% FCS for the first two days and was replaced by Dulbecco's modified Eagle's medium (DMEM) with 10% FCS for further two days. Fibroblast growth was prevented by using L-valine deficient minimum essential medium (MEM) and dialyzed FCS afterwards. Before the experiments started cells were cultured for 5–10 days forming a synchronously and rhythmically contracting monolayer. PBS and all media contained 25 U/ml penicillin and 25 μg/ml streptomycin; the culture media were additionally supplemented with 10 mM HEPES and 0.5 mM L-glutamine.

Characterization of Cells by Immunofluorescence Staining

In order to check the purity of cardiomyocytes, culture dishes were fixed in ice cold methanol/acetone 1 : 1 for 10 min and washed in PBS. Incubation followed with anti-titin antibody (1 : 50) diluted in PBS with 0.5% BSA for 60 min at room temperature. After washing twice with PBS slides were incubated with TRITC-conjugated secondary antibody against mouse IgG (1 : 10) for a further 60 min at room temperature. The preparations were washed again, covered with "mounting medium" (Bios GmbH) and photographed under a fluorescence microscope (Axioskop, Zeiss, Oberkochen, FRG) using a Kodak Tri-X film (400 ASA). Additionally, we also stained cardiomyocytes grown for 5 days in culture with anti-titin or anti-actin antibodies using rhodamine phalloidin, and these were photographed using a fluorescence microscope equipped with epi-illumination.

Incubation of Cardiomyocytes with TNF-α

A synchronously and rhythmically contracting confluent monolayer of cardiomyocytes in culture was serum deprived for 24 hrs and incubated with the recombinant TNF-α (1000 units/ml culture medium) for 1, 2, 4, 6, 8, 12 and 24 hrs. TNF-α was directly added to the culture dishes without exchanging the medium to avoid any culture shock. We used 3×10^6 cardiomyocytes for each incubation time point and repeated the experiments at least three times. Cells were harvested after each incubation in guanidinium isothiocynate buffer and processed for the isolation of total cellular RNA.

Determination of Contractility in Cardiomyocytes

The contractility of cardiomyocytes was followed in a microscope perfusion system according to Schlage and Bereiter-Hahn[47] consisting of an operating perfusion pump with constant volume output, a modified Dvorak-Stotler perfusion chamber, gas light connections of stainless steel tubings with dead volume free fittings, and a temperature control unit providing a constant temperature of 37°C. The perfusion chamber was mounted to the stage of a light microscope (e.g., Axiovert, Zeiss, Oberkochen, FRG.) attached to a video camera for the continuous recording of cardiomyocyte contractions under perfusion with DMEM or DMEM containing TNF-α. The image of the cells was analyzed using an image analysis unit (Leica, Bensheim, FRG) and contractility was determined.[46]

Isolation of Total Cellular RNA and Northern Blot Analysis

Total cellular RNA was isolated from the cardiomyocytes, treated or untreated with TNF-α for different time periods by the guanidinium isothiocynate-phenol-chloroform method described earlier and processed further for Northern hybridization.[48–50] The RNA concentration was measured by optical density, and the quality of RNA was tested on a denatured formaldehyde agarose gel. For Northern hybridization, 15 μg of total RNA was denatured at 65°C in buffer containing formamide and ethidium bromide and electrophoresed on a 1% agarose gel containing 2.2 M formaldehyde. RNA was transferred to Hybond-N membrane by vacuum blotting. Thereafter, filters were air dried and UV cross linked in a gene linker (Bio-Rad Laboratories B.V., The Netherlands), and ribosomal RNA bands were marked under UV light. Blots were kept in a rotating glass tube in an air oven for hybridization at 42°C in buffer containing 50% deionized formamide, 1.0 M sodium chloride, 1% sodium dodecylsulfate (SDS), 0.2% polyvinyl pyrrolidone, 0.2% ficoll, 0.2% bovine serum albumin, 50 mM Tris-HCl (pH 7.5), 0.1% sodium pyrophosphate, 10% dextran sulfate and denatured salmon sperm DNA (100 μg/ml). Blots were hybridized with radiolabeled cDNA probes encoding HSP 27, HSP 70 and ubiquitin.[44,51,52] cDNA inserts were labeled employing a multiprime labeling system (Amersham Nederland B.V., Den Bosch), to a specific activity of 10^9 cpm/μg DNA using [^{32}P]-dCTP (3000 Ci/mmol). After the labeling reaction, probes were purified using nuctrap push columns (Stratagene Inc., USA) to remove unincorporated radioactive dCTP. Filters were washed at room temperature for 5 min in 2 × SSC (1 × SSC = 150 mM NaCl, 15 mM trisodium citrate) and 0.1% SDS and at 55°C in 0.1 × SSC containing 0.1% SDS for 20 min. Subsequently, filters were wrapped in household plastic wrap and exposed to Kodak X-OMAT AR films (Kodak Nederland B.V., Odijk) at −80°C for 1–3 days. A glyceraldehyde-3-phosphate dehydrogenase (GAPDH) cDNA probe[53] (a 1.2-kb PstI fragment of human cDNA, procured from ATCC, USA) was used to rehybridize membranes for reference purposes. Furthermore, filters were rehybridized with a cDNA insert of 770 bp encoding 28S rRNA in order to calculate the fold induction of HSPs expression after correcting the RNA loading differences.[50] Hybridization signals on autoradiographs were quantified by video scanning in optical density mode using a Bioprofil version 4.6 computer program (Vilber Lourmat, France). Several exposures of the Northern blots were taken to ensure that quantitation of hybridization signals was in linear range. For normalization, optical density (OD) of hybridization signal for each gene was divided by the OD of the corresponding GAPDH or 28S rRNA signal. Induction of each gene was calculated and expressed as % relative mRNA values (mean ± SEM) in TNF-α-treated cardiomyocytes relative to control. Expression was statistically analyzed using Student's *t* test, and significance was accepted at $p < 0.05$.

RESULTS AND DISCUSSION

Effect of TNF-α on Structure and Contractility of Cardiomyocytes

Mouse fetal cardiomyocytes under normal culture conditions depict a monolayer of spontaneously contractile cells. These cells display rhythmic and synchronous contractions for several days with an average frequency of 97 ± 29 cycles/min. FIGURE 1 shows a microphotograph of spontaneously contractile fetal cardiomyocytes cultured on a coverslip for 5 days and photographed in phase contrast. Even when serum is reduced to 2% or absolutely absent, these cells are able to contract for more than 24 hours without any sign of cellular damage.[45,46] On a routine basis, we checked the purity of cardiomyocytes in culture by plating them on glass coverslips and growing them for 72 hours prior to staining them with anti-titin as well as anti-actin antibodies. The contractile cardiomyocytes display regular cross striation due to titin staining, which represents a major consituent protein in intact myofibrils.[54] Actin was localized in isolated cardiomyocytes in cross striation in a very specific and regular manner with interspacing.[54]

When serum-deprived cardiomyocytes were treated with recombinant TNF-α (1000 units/ml), they showed disruption in spontaneous contractions in a time-dependent manner, and eventually arrhythmias were observed after 4 hours of incubation. TNF-α resulted in complete cessation of spontaneous contractions after 8 hours of incubation of serum-depleted cells. In another study, we found that a higher dose of TNF-α (10,000 Units/ml) caused complete cessation of spontaneous contractions already in the 11th minute of perfusion.[46] This effect lasted for some more additional minutes and changed to arrhythmias of variable extent as long as the TNF-α was present in the perfusion medium. This inhibitory effect of TNF-α on contractility of cardiomyocytes was reversible upon the incubation of cells in the growth medium containing 10% of FCS. In this study, 24 hrs of TNF-α incubation resulted in cellular necrosis leaving

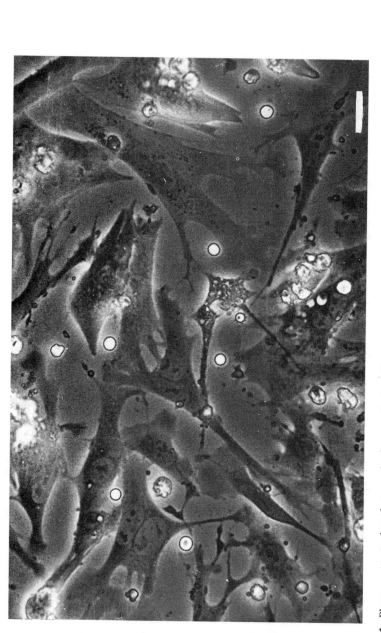

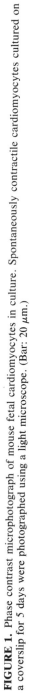

FIGURE 1. Phase contrast microphotograph of mouse fetal cardiomyocytes in culture. Spontaneously contractile cardiomyocytes cultured on a coverslip for 5 days were photographed using a light microscope. (Bar: 20 μm.)

a high number of floating dead cells in the culture medium. Our results indicate a direct impact of TNF-α on contractility of cultured cardiomyocytes in a time- and concentration-dependent manner. These effects of TNF-α in experimental animals have already been evaluated, *e.g.*, in the adult cat heart TNF-α exerted

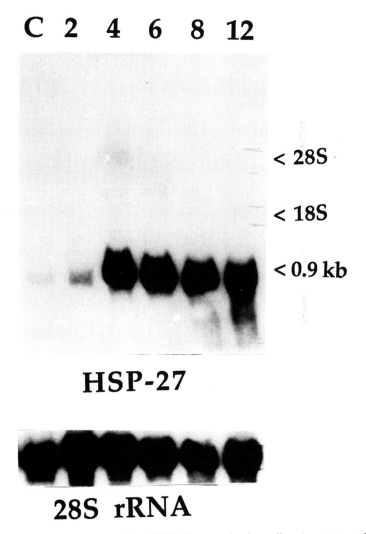

FIGURE 2a. Northern blot analysis of HSP 27 expression in cardiomyocytes treated with TNF-α. A representative Northern blot showing a major 0.9-kb mRNA band encoding HSP 27. 15 μg of total RNA extracted from untreated (C) and TNF-α-treated cardiomyocytes was hybridized with a cDNA insert encoding human HSP 27. Cardiomyocytes were incubated with TNF-α (1000 units/ml) in serum free growth medium for the times indicated on the *top*. Filters were rehybridized with a radiolabeled cDNA probe for 28S rRNA (*lower panel*) for reference purposes.

a concentration- and time-dependent negative inotropic effect that was fully reversible upon removal of this cytokine.[25] Under pathophysiological conditions like myocardial infarction or ischemia, increased concentration of circulating TNF-α in humans has been reported that may mimic the tissue injury.[20-22] In our experiments, decreased cellular inotropy accompanied by arrhythmias in TNF-α-treated cardiomyocytes was observed with time. The tendency of cardiomyocytes to develop arrhythmias may be attributed to the decreased resting membrane potential due to TNF-α treatment.[45] The intracellular signaling cascade involves the adenylyl cyclase system coupled to G proteins, which has been shown to be activated by the treatment of TNF-α. This results in the hypersensitivity of this system, which may account for the depressed contractile state of cardiomyocytes.[19] However, the intracellular mediators of TNF-α-induced cytoprotective events are not yet characterized. Therefore, it is important to understand the intricacy of cellular mechanisms responsible for the pleiotropic effects of TNF-α on the cardiomyocytes and to determine whether this cytokine exerts its effect(s) directly or indirectly by stimulating and releasing other autocrine factors.

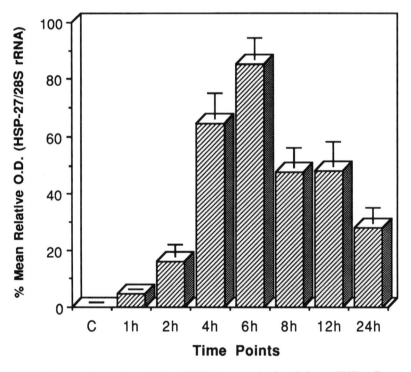

FIGURE 2b. Densitometric analysis of HSP 27 expression in relation to TNF-α. Bar graph showing quantitative analysis of the TNF-α-induced HSP 27 mRNA expression in cardiomyocytes. Hybridization signals (mRNA bands) of HSP 27 as well as from 28S rRNA blots were quantified by video densitometry as described in the text. Data are means of the normalized signal $\pm$ SEM (n = 4) and expressed as % mean relative O.D. of HSP 27 and 28S rRNA hybridization signals.

Expression of Heat Shock Proteins in Relation to TNF-α

In order to examine whether TNF-α exerts its effect(s) on cardiomyocytes by altering the nuclear transcriptional machinery, we investigated the expression pattern of a number of genes involved in cellular defense. TNF-α-treated cells as well as untreated cells were processed for the extraction of total RNA and the gene expression was assessed by Northern blot analysis. We detected an mRNA species of 0.9 kb encoding HSP 27 in untreated (control, C) as well as TNF-α-treated cardiomyocytes (FIG. 2a). The expression of HSP 27 was drastically induced in cells treated with TNF-α already at 2 hr and the expression remained elevated until 12 hr of incubation (FIGS. 2a and b). HSP 27 expression was maximum (more than 80 times vs control) at 6 hr of TNF-α incubation (FIG. 2b). In the case of HSP 70, there was no detectable mRNA expression in control cardiomyocytes, whereas the treatment of cells with TNF-α induced the expression of the HSP 70 gene. The mRNA signal of about 2.7 kb hybridizing to the HSP 70 cDNA probe was detectable at 2 hr of incubation, and the intensity of signal

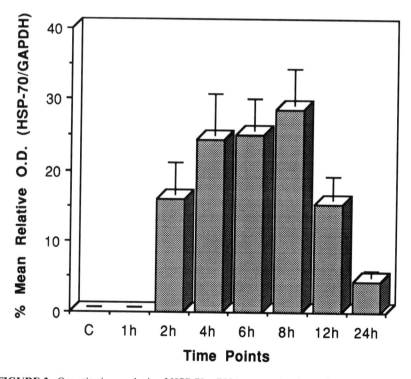

FIGURE 3. Quantitative analysis of HSP 70 mRNA expression in cardiomyocytes treated with TNF-α. Bar graph showing quantitative analysis of the TNF-α-induced HSP 70 mRNA expression. Hybridization signals from HSP 70 as well as from GAPDH blots were quantified by video densitometry as described in Methods. Data are means of the normalized signal $\pm$ SEM (n = 4) and expressed as % mean relative O.D. of HSP 70 and GAPDH hybridization signals.

C   1   2   4   6   8   12   24

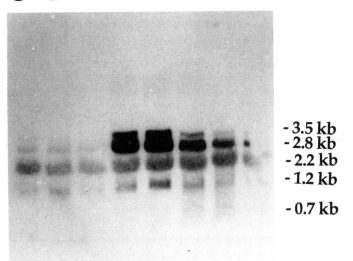

- 3.5 kb
- 2.8 kb
- 2.2 kb
- 1.2 kb
- 0.7 kb

Ubiquitin

28S rRNA

FIGURE 4a. Northern blot analysis of ubiquitin expression in cardiomyocytes treated with TNF-α. A representative Northern blot showing multiple mRNA bands encoding ubiquitin. 15 μg of total RNA extracted from control (untreated) and TNF-α-treated cardiomyocytes was hybridized with a cDNA insert encoding porcine ubiquitin. Fetal cardiomyocytes were incubated with TNF-α (1000 units/ml) in serum free growth medium for the times indicated on the *top*. Filters were rehybridized with a radiolabled cDNA probe for 28S rRNA (*lower panel*) for reference purposes.

increased dramatically after 2 hr of TNF-α incubation and remained increased until 12 hr, with maximal expression at 8 hr (FIG. 3). 24 hr of TNF-α incubation of cardiomyocytes resulted in decreased mRNA expression of HSP 70. We and others have shown that myocardial ischemia and reperfusion induce the expression of HSPs that may be involved in the myocardial adaptation to ischemic stress.[28,34,36–39,55–57] Myocardial ischemia is known to produce a number of intra-cellular changes within cardiomyocytes including increased cellular calcium levels, free radical production, decreased intracellular pH, decreased ATP and glucose levels, etc. These cellular alterations leading to a metabolic or hypoxic stress result in cellular injury that may be characterized by denaturation and/or disturbance in

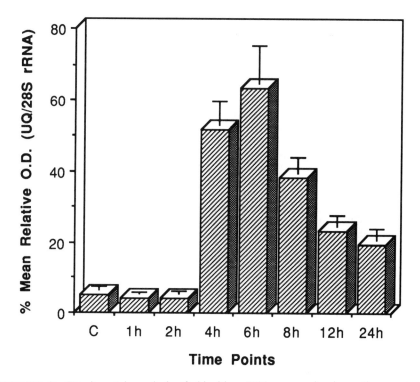

FIGURE 4b. Densitometric analysis of ubiquitin mRNAs expression in cardiomyocytes treated with TNF-α. Bar graph showing quantitative analysis of the TNF-α-induced expression of ubiquitin (UQ). Multiple mRNA signals from hybridization blots of UQ as well as a single mRNA band from 28S rRNA blots were quantified by video densitometry as described in Methods. Data are means of the normalized signal ± SEM (n = 4) and expressed as % mean relative O.D. of UQ and 28S rRNA hybridization signals.

the three dimensional structure of many proteins. TNF-α has been shown to be produced in the postischemic and/or infarcted myocardium which probably accounts for the enhanced circulating levels of this cytokine.[20-22] It is believed that HSPs play an important role in transient rearrangements in cellular activities, thereby coping with the stress period by protecting essential components of the cell and allowing the cell to recover from the stress.[26-30] Our results on HSPs expression in cardiomyocytes indicate for TNF-α-induced heat shock response for transient cellular adaptation. It may be noted that TNF-α pretreatment for 24 hr in rats has been beneficial for the heart against ischemia-reperfusion injury,[24] and this beneficial effect could be mediated via increased levels of MnSOD.[23,24] Though we did not test the expression of MnSOD, an enzyme involved in detoxification of superoxide anions in the mitochondria in our cardiomyocytes model, it is plausible that TNF-α may also induce the expression of this enzyme, which may play a role in cytoprotection. Furthermore, the phosphorylation and intracellular organization of HSP 27[12-16] in cardiomyocytes treated with TNF-α may be related to the cytoprotective activity of this protein against the deleterious effects of this cytokine.

Ubiquitin is a highly conserved protein found in all cell types, and it participates in ATP-dependent cytosolic proteolysis. We examined TNF-α-treated cultured cardiomyocytes for the expression of ubiquitin in order to evaluate the extent of cellular protein damage by this cytokine. As depicted in FIGURE 4a, multiple mRNA bands encoding monomer as well as polymers of ubiquitin were detected in cardiomyocytes. Steady state mRNA levels of ubiquitin were drastically induced (>10 fold vs untreated cells) by TNF-α, being maximal at 6 hr of stimulation, and thereafter expression of this stress gene declined but remained elevated as compared to control (FIG. 4b). In a porcine model of myocardial ischemia and reperfusion, we reported earlier that ubiquitin mRNAs as well as monomer and conjugated ubiquitin proteins levels were enhanced in the postischemic heart.[28] Enhanced expression of ubiquitin in cardiomyocytes treated with TNF-α is an indication of cellular protein damage. Recently, it was shown that an acute intravenous administration of TNF-α (100 μg/kg body weight) in rats resulted in a time-dependent increase in the levels of both free and conjugated ubiquitin in skeletal muscle.[58] Our results on ubiquitin expression indicate that TNF-α induces the nonlysosomal protein degradation pathway for the clearance of damaged/denatured proteins in cardiomyocytes.

Taken together, our results demonstrate that an adequate dose of TNF-α rapidly and transiently induces the mRNA expression of cytoprotective molecules such as HSP 27, HSP 70 and ubiquitin in cardiomyocytes. Furthermore, the ubiquitin system could play an important role in the cytosolic degradation of damaged proteins in TNF-α-treated cardiomyocytes where HSPs may counteract the proteolytic events and preserve many vital proteins. We conclude that the enhanced transcription of HSPs in response to TNF-α in cardiomyocytes suggests the activation of protective/defense mechanisms that may contribute, for example, during cardiac protection against ischemia.

REFERENCES

1. KRONKE, M., S. SCHUTZE, P. SCHEURICH et al. 1990. Tumour necrosis factor signal transduction. [Review]. Cell. Signalling **2:** 1–8.
2. WRIDE, M. A. & E. J. SANDERS. 1995. Potential roles for tumor necrosis factor α during embryonic development. Anat. Embryol. **191:** 1–10.
3. TRACEY, K. J. & A. CERAMI. 1994. Tumor necrosis factor: a pleiotropic cytokine and therapeutic target. [Review]. Annu. Rev. Med. **45:** 491–503.
4. BEYAERT, R. & W. FIERS. 1994. Molecular mechanisms of tumor necrosis factor-induced cytotoxicity. What we do understand and what we do not. [Review]. FEBS Lett. **340:** 9–12.
5. FRATER-SCHRÖDER, M., W. RISAU, R. HALLMANN, P. GAUTSCHI & P. BÖHLEN. 1987. Tumor necrosis factortype a, a potent inhibitor of endothelial cell growth in vitro, is angiogenic in vivo. Proc. Natl. Acad. Sci. USA **84:** 5277–5281.
6. DAYER, J. M., B. BEUTLER & A. CERAMI. 1985. Cachectin/tumor necrosis factor stimulates collagenase and prostaglandin E_2 production by human synovial cells and dermal fibroblasts. J. Exp. Med. **162:** 2163–2168.
7. STRIETER, R. M., S. L. KUNKEL & R. C. BONE. 1993. Role of tumor necrosis factor-alpha in disease states and inflammation. [Review]. Crit. Care Med. **21:** S447–S463.
8. LOETSCHER, H., Y. C. PAN, H. W. LAHM et al. 1990. Molecular cloning and expression of the human 55 kd tumor necrosis factor receptor. Cell **61:** 351–359.
9. TARTAGLIA, L. A., R. F. WEBER, I. S. FIGARI, C. REYNOLDS, M. J. PALLADINO & D. V. GOEDDEL. 1991. The two different receptors for tumor necrosis factor mediate distinct cellular responses. Proc. Natl. Acad. Sci. USA **88:** 9292–9296.
10. HELLER, R. A. & M. KRONKE. 1994. Tumor necrosis factor receptor-mediated signaling pathways. [Review]. J. Cell Biol. **126:** 5–12.

11. ROTHE, J., G. GEHR, H. LOETSCHER & W. LESSLAUER. 1992. Tumor necrosis factor receptors—structure and function. [Review]. Immunol. Res. **11:** 81–90.
12. ARRIGO, A. P. 1990. Tumor necrosis factor induces the rapid phosphorylation of the mammalian heat shock protein hsp28. Mol. Cell. Biol. **10:** 1276–1280.
13. KAUR, P., W. J. WELCH & J. SAKLATVALA. 1989. Interleukin 1 and tumour necrosis factor increase phosphorylation of the small heat shock protein. Effects in fibroblasts, Hep G2 and U937 cells. FEBS Lett. **258:** 269–273.
14. LÖW, F. I., D. WEISENSEE, P. MITROU & W. SCHOEPPE. 1992. Cytokines induce stress protein formation in cultured cardiac myocytes. Basic Res. Cardiol. **87:** 12–18.
15. SATOH, J. & S. U. KIM. 1995. Cytokines and growth factors induce hsp27 phosphorylation in human astrocytes. J. Neuropathol. Exp. Neurol. **54,** 504–512.
16. MEHLEN, P., A. MEHLEN, D. GUILLET, X. PREVILLE & A-P. ARRIGO. 1995. Tumor necrosis factor-α induces changes in the phosphorylation, cellular localization, and oligomerization of human hsp27, a stress protein that confers cellular resistance to this cytokine. J. Cell. Biochem. **58:** 248–259.
17. LIN, J. X. & J. VILCEK. 1987. Tumor necrosis factor and interleukin-1 cause a rapid and transient stimulation of c-fos and c-myc mRNA levels in human fibroblasts. J. Biol. Chem. **262:** 11908–11911.
18. JÄÄTTELA, M., M. PINOLA & E. SAKSELA. 1991. Heat shock inhibits the cytotoxic action of TNF-alpha in tumor cells but does not alter its noncytotoxic actions in endothelial and adrenal cells. Lymphokine Cytokine Res. **10:** 119–125.
19. REITHMANN, C., P. GIERSCHIK, K. WERDAN & K. H. JAKOBS. 1991. Tumor necrosis factor alpha up-regulates Gi alpha and G beta proteins and adenylyl cyclase responsiveness in rat cardiomyocytes. Eur. J. Pharmacol. **206:** 53–60.
20. MAURY, C. P. & A. M. TEMPO. 1989. Circulating tumor necrosis factor-α (cachectin) in myocardial infarction. Am. J. Pathol. **139:** 709–715.
21. LEFER, A. M., P. TSAO, N. AOKI & M. J. PALLADINO. 1990. Mediation of cardioprotection by transforming growth factor-beta. Science **249:** 61–64.
22. HERSKOWITZ, A., S. CHOI, A. A. ANSARI & S. WESSELINGH. 1995. Cytokine mRNA expression in postischemic/reperfused myocardium. Am. J. Pathol. **146:** 419–428.
23. WONG, G. H., J. H. ELWELL, L. W. OBERLEY & D. V. GOEDDEL. 1989. Manganous superoxide dismutase is essential for cellular resistance to cytotoxicity of tumor necrosis factor. Cell **58:** 923–931.
24. EDDY, L. J., D. V. GOEDDEL & G. H. WONG. 1992. Tumor necrosis factor-α pretreatment is protective in a rat model of myocardial ischemia-reperfusion injury. Biochem. Biophys. Res. Commun. **184:** 1056–1059.
25. YOKOYAMA, T., L. VACA, R. D. ROSSEN, W. DURANTE, P. HAZARIKA & D. L. MANN. 1993. Cellular basis for the negative inotropic effects of tumor necrosis factor-alpha in the adult mammalian heart. J. Clin. Invest. **92:** 2303–2312.
26. WELCH, W. J. 1992. Mammalian stress response: cell physiology, structure, function, of stress proteins, and implications for medicine and disease. Physiol. Rev. **72:** 1063–1081.
27. MESTRIL, R. & W. H. DILLMANN. 1995. Heat shock proteins and protection against myocardial ischemia. [Review]. J. Mol. Cell. Cardiol. **27:** 45–52.
28. ANDRES, J., H. S. SHARMA, R. KNÖLL, J. STAHL, L. M. A. SASSEN, P. D. VERDOUW & W. SCHAPER. 1993. Expression of heat shock proteins in the normal and stunned porcine myocardium. Cardiovasc. Res. **27:** 1421–1429.
29. SCHLESINGER, M. 1990. Heat shock proteins. J. Biol. Chem. **265:** 12111–12114.
30. CIOCCA, D. R., S. OESTERREICH, G. C. CHAMNESS, W. L. MCGUIRE & S. A. FUQUA. 1993. Biological and clinical implications of heat shock protein 27,000 (HSP27): a review. J. Natl. Cancer Inst. **85:** 1558–1570.
31. JENTSCH, S. 1992. Ubiquitin-dependent protein degradation: a cellular perspective. Trends Cell Biol. **2:** 98–103.
32. HAYASHI, T., J. TANAKA, T. KAMIKUBO, K. TAKADA & M. MATSUDA. 1993. Increase in ubiquitin conjugates dependent on ischemic damage. Brain Res. **620:** 171–173.
33. JANSSEN, Y. M., H. B. VAN, P. J. BORM & B. T. MOSSMAN. 1993. Cell and tissue responses to oxidative damage. [Review]. Lab. Invest. **69:** 261–274.

34. IWAKI, K., S. H. CHI, W. H. DILLMANN & R. MESTRIL. 1993. Induction of HSP70 in cultured rat neonatal cardiomyocytes by hypoxia and metabolic stress. Circulation **87:** 2023–2032.

35. TACCHINI, L., L. SCHIAFFONATI, C. PAPPALARDO, S. GATTI & Z. A. BERNELLI. 1993. Expression of HSP 70, immediate-early response and heme oxygenase genes in ischemic-reperfused rat liver. Lab. Invest. **68:** 465–471.

36. SHARMA, H. S., L. H. SNOECKX, L. M. A. SASSEN, R. KNOEL, J. ANDRES, P. D. VERDOUW & W. SCHAPER. 1993. Expression and immunohistochemical localization of heat shock protein-70 in preconditioned porcine myocardium. Ann. N. Y. Acad. Sci. **723:** 491–494.

37. KNOWLTON, A., P. BRECHER, C. APSTEIN, S. NGOY & G. ROMO. 1991. Rapid expression of heat shock protein in the rabbit after brief cardiac ischemia. J. Clin. Invest. **87:** 139–147.

38. YELLON, D. & D. S. LATCHMAN. 1992. Stress proteins and myocardial protection. J. Mol. Cell. Cardiol. **24:** 113–124.

39. DAS, D. K., R. M. ENGELMAN & Y. KIMURA. 1993. Molecular adaptation of cellular defences following preconditioning of the heart by repeated ischaemia. Cardiovasc. Res. **27:** 578– .

40. PLUMIER, J. C., B. M. ROSS, R. W. CURRIE *et al.* 1995. Transgenic mice expressing the human heat shock protein 70 have improved post-ischemic myocardial recovery. J. Clin. Invest. **95:** 1854–1860.

41. MARBER, M. S., R. MESTRIL, S. H. CHI, M. R. SAYEN, D. M. YELLON & W. H. DILLMANN. 1995. Overexpression of the rat inducible 70-kD heat stress protein in a transgenic mouse increases the resistance of the heat to ischemic injury. J. Clin. Invest. **95:** 1446–1456.

42. KNOWLTON, A. A. 1995. The role of heat shock proteins in the heart. J. Mol. Cell. Cardiol. **27:** 121–131.

43. ARRIGO, A. P. & W. J. WELCH. 1987. Characterization and purification of the small 28,000-dalton mammalian heat shock protein. J. Biol. Chem. **262:** 15359–15369.

44. EINSPANIER, R., H. S. SHARMA & K. H. SCHEIT. 1987. An mRNA encoding poly-ubiquitin in porcine corpus luteum: identification by cDNA cloning and sequencing. DNA **6:** 395–400.

45. WEISENSEE, D., T. SEEGER, A. BITTNER, H. J. BEREITER, W. SCHOEPPE & F. I. LOW. 1995. Cocultures of fetal and adult cardiomyocytes yield rhythmically eating rod shaped heart cells from adult rats. In Vitro Cell. Dev. Biol. Anim. **31:** 190–195.

46. WEISENSEE, D., H. J. BEREITER, W. SCHOEPPE & F. I. LOW. 1993. Effects of cytokines on the contractility of cultured cardiac myocytes. Int. J. Immunopharmacol. **15:** 581–587.

47. SCHLAGE, W. K. & H. J. BEREITER. 1983. A microscope perfusion respirometer for continuous respiration measurement of cultured cells during microscopic observation. Microsc. Acta **87:** 19–34.

48. CHOMCZYNSKI, P. & N. SACCHI. 1987. Single step method of RNA isolation by acid guanidinium thiocyanate-phenol-chloroform extraction. Anal. Biochem. **162:** 156–159.

49. BRAND, T., H. S. SHARMA, K. FLEISCHMANN *et al.* 1992. Proto-oncogene expression in porcine myocardium subjected to ischemia and reperfusion. Circ. Res. **71:** 1351–1360.

50. SHARMA, H. S., H. A. A. VAN HEUGTEN, M. A. GOEDBLOED, P. D. VERDOUW *et al.* 1994. Angiotensin II induced expression of transcription factors precedes increase in transforming growth factor-$\beta 1$ mRNA in neonatal cardiac fibroblasts. Biochem. Biophys. Res. Commun. **205:** 105–112.

51. WU, B., C. HUNT & R. MORIMOTO. 1985. Structure and expression of the human gene encoding major heat shock protein HSP70. Mol. Cell. Biol. **5:** 330–341.

52. HICKEY, E., S. E. BRANDON, R. POTTER, G. STEIN, J. STEIN & L. A. WEBER. 1986. Sequence and organization of genes encoding the human 27 kDa heat shock protein. Nucleic Acids Res. **14:** 4127–4145.

53. TSO, J., X-H. SUN, T. KAO, K. REECE & R. WU. 1985. Isolation and characterization of rat and human glyceraldehyde-3-phosphate dehydrogenase cDNAs: genomic complexity and molecular evolution. Nucleic Acids Res. **13:** 2485–2502.

54. SCHAPER, J., S. HEIN, T. BRAND & W. SCHAPER. 1989. Contractile proteins and the cytoskeleton is isolated rat myocytes. J. Appl. Cardiol. **4:** 423–429.
55. DELCAYRE, C., J. L. SAMUEL, F. MAROTTE, B. M. BEST, J. J. MERCADIER & L. RAPPAPORT. 1988. Synthesis of stress proteins in rat cardiac myocytes 2–4 days after imposition of hemodynamic overload. J. Clin. Invest. **82:** 460–468.
56. DONNELLY, T. J., R. E. SIEVERS, F. L. VISSERN, W. J. WELCH & C. L. WOLFE. 1992. Heat shock protein induction in rat hearts: a role for improved myocardial salvage after ischemia and reperfusion? Circulation **85:** 769–778.
57. HEADS, R. J., D. M. YELLON & D. S. LATCHMAN. 1995. Differential cytoprotection against heat stress or hypoxia following expression of specific stress protein genes in myogenic cells. J. Mol. Cell. Cardiol. **27:** 1669–1678.
58. GARCIA, M. C., N. AGELL, M. LLOVERA, S. F. LOPEZ & J. M. ARGILES. 1993. Tumour necrosis factor-alpha increases the ubiquitinization of rat skeletal muscle proteins. FEBS Lett. **323:** 211–214.

Myocardial Adaptive Changes and Damage in Ischemic Heart Disease

NOBUAKIRA TAKEDA,[a] YUKO OTA,
YASUYUKI TANAKA, CHIHIRO SHIKATA,
YUUSAKU HAYASHI, SATOKO NEMOTO,
AKIRA TANAMURA, TAKAAKI IWAI, AND
IZURU NAKAMURA

Department of Internal Medicine
Aoto Hospital
Jikei University School of Medicine
Tokyo, Japan

INTRODUCTION

Long-term myocardial ischemia induces various changes in myocardial subcellular organelles as an adaptation to ischemic conditions. If the duration and/or severity of myocardial ischemia exceeds a certain level, these myocardial adaptations become insufficient to sustain normal functioning and myocardial failure occurs. In this study, changes in two of the elements of myocardial subcellular organelles relating to cardiac energetics were investigated using autopsy materials from patients with ischemic heart disease. These were ventricular myosin isozymes, investigated by pyrophosphate gel electrophoresis, and myocardial mitochondrial DNA mutations, detected by the polymerase chain reaction (PCR).

MATERIALS AND METHODS

Small pieces of left ventricular free walls, weighing approximately 0.5 g, were obtained at autopsy and were used in these experiments. Post-mortem times were all within 3 h of death. From each patient, a small piece of tissue was dissected from an area of the left ventricle which appeared macroscopically to be unaffected by ischemia. Myosin was extracted from the ventricular samples according to the method of Martin *et al.*[1] The following procedure was then carried out at a temperature of 0–4°C. The ventricular myocardial sample was minced and homogenized in 40 mM NaCl, 5 μg/ml leupeptin and 3 mM Na-phosphate buffer (pH 7.0) with a glass homogenizer. The homogenate was centrifuged at 1,000 × g for 15 min; then the pellet was resuspended in the same solution and centrifuged again. The resulting pellet was suspended in 5 mM dithiothreitol, 5 mM EGTA, 5 μg/ml leupeptin and 0.1 M Na-pyrophosphate buffer (pH 8.6) and left for 1 h. The

[a] Corresponding author: Nobuakira Takeda, M.D., Ph.D., Department of Internal Medicine, Aoto Hospital, Jikei University School of Medicine, Aoto 6-41-2, Katsushika-ku, Tokyo 125, Japan. Fax: 81-3-3602-2839.

suspension was then centrifuged at $100,000 \times g$ for 1 h. An equivalent volume of glycerol was added to the supernatant and the solution, containing myosin, was stored at $-20°C$. Myosin isozymes were separated by polyacrylamide gel electrophoresis in the presence of pyrophosphate (pyrophosphate gel electrophoresis) according to the method of Hoh *et al.*[3] The gel contained 3.88% acrylamide and 0.12% N,N'-methylene-bis-acrylamide. The running buffer consisted of 20 mM $Na_4P_2O_7$ (pH 8.8) in the presence of 10% glycerol. Electrophoresis was carried out over 30 h at 2°C and a constant voltage of 13.3 V/cm. The gels were stained with Coomassie brilliant blue R-250, G-250 and destained with 7.5% acetic acid and 5% methanol. The bands revealed on the gels were recorded by densitometry. Sodium dodecyl sulfate (SDS) polyacrylamide gel electrophoresis was then performed according to the method of Weber and Osborn[4] in order to examine whether the components revealed by pyrophosphate gel electrophoresis contained all the subunits of myosin, *i.e.*, the heavy chain (HC) and light chains (LC) 1 and 2.

DNA was extracted from human left ventricular myocardial samples weighing approximately 20 g, obtained at autopsy.[5] Each sample was homogenized then digested over 12 h at 37°C in 10 mM Tris-HCl and 0.1 M EDTA (pH 7.4) containing 0.1 mg/ml proteinase K and 0.5% SDS. DNA was extracted with phenol, chloroform, and isoamylalcohol, after which it was precipitated with 3 M sodium acetate (pH 7.4) and ethanol at $-80°C$ over 30 min. A template DNA solution was obtained by dissolving the centrifuged pellet, rinsed with 70% ethanol, in 30 μl 10 mM Tris-HCl and 0.1 M EDTA (pH 8.0). Oligonucleotide primers for PCR were synthesized and purified on cartridges. PCR amplification was performed using a reaction mixture of template DNA, two primers, dNTPs, PCR buffer, and Taq DNA polymerase. Amplification was carried out for 30 cycles under the following conditions: denaturation at 94°C for 15 s, annealing at 50°C for 15 s, and primer extension at 72°C for 80 s. Amplified DNA fragments were separated by agarose gel electrophoresis, stained with ethidium bromide, and detected by photofluorography.

Statistical comparisons were made by Student *t* test.

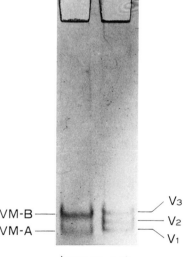

FIGURE 1. Pyrophosphate gel electrophoresis of human and rat left ventricular myocardium.[6] Human VM-A corresponds to rat V_1, and human VM-B to rat V_3 ventricular myosin isozyme, respectively.

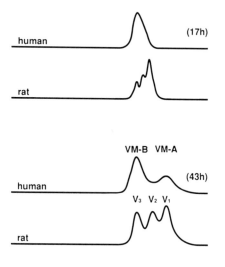

FIGURE 2. Ventricular myosin isozyme pattern revealed by densitometry.[6] VM-A has faster and VM-B slower electrophoretical mobility.

RESULTS

Myosin from human left ventricles was separated into two bands by pyrophosphate gel electrophoresis. These contained VM-A, which exhibited faster electrophoretic mobility and was present at a lower concentration, and VM-B, which had slower mobility and a higher concentration (FIGS. 1, 2), as described in our previous report.[6] SDS polyacrylamide gel electrophoresis revealed that these two components contained all the subunits of myosin, *i.e.*, the heavy chain and light chains 1 and 2[2] (FIG. 3). VM-A tended to occur in higher concentrations in patients with ischemic heart disease than in control patients who had no heart disease (FIG. 4).

A 7.4-kb deletion was detected between the D-loop and the ATPase 6 genes of mitochondrial DNA from the myocardium of 6 out of 10 patients with myocardial infarction.

DISCUSSION

The ventricular myosin isozyme pattern in rats alters under certain physiological and pathological conditions.[7-15] In pressure-overload cardiac hypertrophy, the pattern shifts towards V_3, which exhibits the lowest ATPase activity. This change is thought to be an adaptation which occurs in order to enable myocardial contractility to be maintained with low energy and oxygen consumption.[16-19] The human left ventricular myosin isozyme patterns in this study revealed that VM-B or V_3 is the predominant isozyme and that its concentration can change only within a small range. This means that adaptive changes in human ventricular myosin isozymes are limited. This may be one explanation of the fact that humans develop heart failure more easily than rats.

Mitochondrial DNA mutations are thought to play some causal role in mitochondrial myopathy, cardiomyopathy and diabetes mellitus.[20-23] These mutations can be hereditary or acquired. The mitochondrial DNA deletions detected in this study were thought to be induced by free radicals which are produced during myocardial ischemia. These deletions might lead to disturbed energy production in myocardial mitochondria.

In this study, all patients died from heart failure due to myocardial infarction. While changes in other subcellular organelles such as the sarcolemma or sarcoplasmic reticulum must play an important role in inducing heart failure, disordered energy production due to mitochondrial DNA deletions and the limited ability to

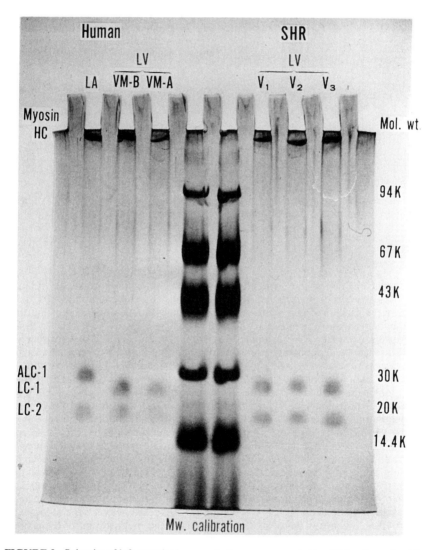

FIGURE 3. Subunits of left ventricular myosin isozyme separated by SDS polyacrylamide gel electrophoresis.[2] Both VM-A and VM-B contain all the subunits of ventricular myosin.

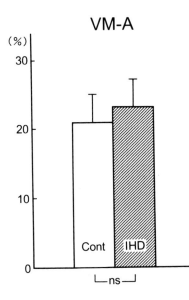

FIGURE 4. Comparison of VM-A concentrations in the ventricular myocardium of patients with and without ischemia. The concentration of VM-A tended to be higher in the myocardium of patients with ischemia. Cont: controls, IHD: ischemic heart disease, ns: not significant. *Vertical lines* indicate SD.

alter the relative proportions of ventricular myosin isozymes might also have been involved in the mechanism of heart failure in these patients.

SUMMARY

Changes in two of the elements of myocardial subcellular organelles relating to cardiac energetics, ventricular myosin isozymes and mitochondrial DNA mutations, were examined using left ventricular tissue samples obtained at autopsy from patients with ischemic heart disease.

Myosin isozymes were examined in tissues from nine patients with ischemic heart disease and 12 control patients with cancer but no heart disease. Extracted myosin was separated by pyrophosphate gel electrophoresis. The relative concentration of each component was determined by densitometry. Mitochondrial DNA mutations were evaluated in tissues from ten patients with myocardial infarction and 11 control patients with cancer but no heart disease. DNA was extracted and mitochondrial DNA mutations were detected by the polymerase chain reaction.

Two bands were revealed by pyrophosphate gel electrophoresis. These contained VM-A, which exhibited faster electrophoretic mobility and was present in lower concentrations, and VM-B, which had a lower mobility and a higher concentration, respectively. SDS polyacrylamide gel electrophoresis showed that these two components contained the heavy chain and light chains 1 and 2 of myosin. VM-A concentrations tended to be higher in patients with ischemic heart disease than in controls. A 7.4-kb deletion was detected between the D-loop and the ATPase 6 genes of mitochondrial DNA from the myocardium of 6 out of 10 patients with myocardial infarction.

The relative amounts of the two myosin isozymes could be altered by ischemic heart disease, although the functional significance of these components is unclear.

The changes in the two myosin isozymes might be an adaptive change to disordered energy metabolism, but this change was small. The myocardial mitochondrial DNA deletions in patients with myocardial infarction were thought to result from ischemic damage.

REFERENCES

1. MARTIN, A. F., E. D. PAGANI & R. J. SOLARO. 1982. Thyroxine-induced redistribution of isoenzymes of rabbit ventricular myosin. Circ. Res. **50:** 117–124.
2. NAKAMURA, I. 1988. Myosin isoenzymes of human ventricular myocardium obtained by pyrophosphate gel electrophoresis. Jikeikai Med. J. **35:** 351–360.
3. HOH, J. F. Y., P. A. MCGRATH & P. T. HALE. 1978. Electrophoretic analysis of multiple forms of rat cardiac myosin: effects of hypophysectomy and thyroxine replacement. J. Mol. Cell. Cardiol. **10:** 1053–1076.
4. WEBER, K. & N. OSBORN. 1969. The reliability of molecular weight determinations by dodecyl sulfate polyacrylamide gel electrophoresis. **244:** 4406–4412.
5. TAKEDA, N., A. TANAMURA, T. IWAI, I. NAKAMURA, M. KATO, T. OHKUBO & K. NOMA. 1993. Mitochondrial DNA deletion in human myocardium. Mol. Cell. Biochem. **119:** 105–108.
6. TAKEDA, N., H. RUPP, G. FENCHEL, H-E. HOFFMEISTER & R. JACOB. 1985. Relationship between the myofibrillar ATPase activity of human biopsy material and hemodynamic parameters. Jpn. Heart J. **26:** 909–922.
7. LOMPRE, A. M., K. SCHWARTZ, A. D'ALBIS, G. LACOMBE, N. V. THIEM & B. SWYNGHEDAUW. 1979. Myosin isoenzyme redistribution in chronic heart overload. Nature **282:** 105–107.
8. DILMANN, W. H. 1980. Diabetes mellitus induces changes in cardiac myosin of the rat. Diabetes **29:** 579–582.
9. MERCADIER, J. J., A. M. LOMPRE, C. WISNEWSKY, J. L. SAMUEL, J. BERCOVICI, B. SWYNGHEDAUW & K. SCHWARTZ. 1981. Myosin isoenzymic changes in several models of rat cardiac hypertrophy. Circ. Res. **49:** 525–532.
10. RUPP, H. 1981. The adaptive changes in the isoenzyme pattern of myosin from hypertrophied rat myocardium as a result of pressure overload and physical training. Basic Res. Cardiol. **76:** 79–88.
11. RUPP, H. & R. JACOB. 1982. Response of blood pressure and cardiac myosin polymorphism to swimming training in the spontaneously hypertensive rat. Can. J. Physiol. Pharmacol. **60:** 1098–1103.
12. TAKEDA, N., P. DOMINIAK, D. TURCH, H. RUPP & R. JACOB. 1985. The influence of endurance training on mechanical catecholamine responsiveness, beta-adrenoceptor density and myosin isoenzyme pattern of rat ventricular myocardium. Basic Res. Cardiol. **80:** 88–99.
13. TAKEDA, N., T. OHKUBO, T. HATANAKA, A. TAKEDA, I. NAKAMURA & M. NAGANO. 1987. Myocardial contractility and left ventricular myosin isoenzyme pattern in cardiac hypertrophy due to chronic volume overload. Basic Res. Cardiol. **82**(Suppl. 2): 215–221.
14. TAKEDA, N., I. NAKAMURA, T. HATANAKA, T. OHKUBO & M. NAGANO. 1988. Myocardial mechanical and myosin isoenzyme alterations in streptozotocin-diabetic rats. Jpn. Heart J. **29:** 455–463.
15. TAKEDA, N. 1990. Effects of thyroid hormones on myocardial contractility and ventricular myosin isoenzymes. Jikeikai Med. J. **37**(Suppl.): 45–52.
16. ALPERT, N. R. & L. A. MULIERI. 1982. Increased myothermal economy of isometric force generation in compensated cardiac hypertrophy induced by pulmonary artery constriction in the rabbit. Circ. Res. **50:** 491–500.
17. KISSLING, G., H. RUPP, L. MALLOY & R. JACOB. 1982. Alteration in cardiac oxygen consumption under chronic pressure overload. Significance of the isoenzyme pattern of myosin. Basic Res. Cardiol. **77:** 255–269.
18. JACOB, R., G. KISSLING, G. EBRECHT, C. HOLUBARSCH, I. MEDUGORAC & H. RUPP.

1983. Adaptive and pathological alterations in experimental cardiac hypertrophy. *In* Advances in Myocardiology. E. Chazov, V. Saks & G. Rona, Eds. 55–77. Plenum Press. New York, NY.

19. HOLUBARSCH, C., R. Z. LITTEN, L. A. MULIERI & N. R. ALPERT. 1985. Energetic changes of myocardium as an adaptation to chronic hemodynamic overload and thyroid gland activity. Basic Res. Cardiol. **80:** 582–593.

20. GOTO, Y., I. NONAKA & S. HORAI. 1990. A mutation in the tRNA[Leu(UUR)] gene associated with MELAS subgroup of mitochondrial encephalomyopathies. Nature **348:** 651–653.

21. OZAWA, T., M. TANAKA, S. SUGIYAMA, K. HATTORI, T. ITO, K. OHNO, A. TAKAHASHI, W. SATO, G. TAKADA, B. MAYUMI, K. YAMAMOTO, K. ADACHI, Y. KOGA & H. TOSHIMA. 1990. Multiple mitochondrial DNA deletions exist in cardiomyocytes of patients with hypertrophic or dilated cardiomyopathy. Biochem. Biophys. Res. Commun. **170:** 830–836.

22. OBAYASHI, T., K. HATTORI, S. SUGIYAMA, M. TANAKA, T. TANAKA, S. ITOYAMA, H. DEGUCHI, K. KAWAMURA, Y. KOGA, H. TOSHIMA, N. TAKEDA, M. NAGANO, T. ITO & T. OZAWA. 1992. Point mutations in mitochondrial DNA in patients with hypertrophic cardiomyopathy. Am. Heart J. **124:** 1263–1269.

23. VAN DEN OUWELAND, J. M. W., H. H. P. J. LEMKES, W. RUITENBEEK, L. A. SAND-KUIJL, M. E. VIJLDER, P. A. A. STRUYVENBERG, J. J. P. KAMP & J. A. MASSEN. 1992. Mutation in mitochondrial tRNA[Leu(UUR)] gene in a large pedigree with maternally transmitted type II diabetes mellitus and deafness. Nature Genet. **1:** 368–371.

Redox Potential Regulation and Ascorbate Oxidase/Gene Expression in Humans

PARINAM S. RAO, SRINIVASA K. RAO,
ROBERT S. PALAZZO, HELENE N. METZ,
DAVID W. WILSON, G. CHEN, L. MICHAEL GRAVER,
AND JON R. COHEN

Department of Surgery
Long Island Jewish Medical Center
Long Island Campus of Albert Einstein College of Medicine
New Hyde Park, New York 11042

INTRODUCTION

Oxidative damage has now been implicated in the pathogenesis of a number of diseases including atherosclerosis, rheumatoid arthritis, diabetes mellitus, neoplasia and ischemia-reperfusion injuries associated with revascularization.[1-4] Aerobic metabolism in biological systems results in the production of reactive free radicals that are oxidants. Mitochondria respiration, enzymatic oxidases, dehydrogenases and phagocytosis are the main sources of endogenous oxidants while diet, environmental pollution, cigarette smoke and products of ionizing radiation are the sources of exogenous oxidants. A variety of oxidants are produced but the most important ones are free radicals (FR) derived from oxygen. FR are highly reactive species capable of taking electrons (oxidizing) from surrounding molecules in the intracellular and extracellular fluids and in biological fluids such as plasma. The reactive species damage the molecules they attack such as proteins, lipids and DNA, and alter the redox potential of the biological fluids disrupting the cellular function. There about sixty enzymes that are shown to be involved in the antioxidant activity in vertebrate animals including humans.[5] Super oxide dismutase (SOD), CAT, glutathione peroxidase (GSH/GPx) are the important intercellular antioxidants. Extracellular, including membrane associated, antioxidant activity in plasma is carried out by the proteins such as transferrin, lactoferrin, ceruloplasmin, haptoglobin, hemopexin, carotenoids and albumin that sequester the free transition metal ions which produce FR. Small molecules like vitamin C (ascorbate, Asc), vitamin E (α-tocopherol) and urate are well-known antioxidants (TABLE 1).

In addition, several other substances present in much lower concentrations such as bilirubin and glutathione also carry out the antioxidant activity. These compounds that break the pro-oxidant chain reactions are consumed in the process. A method to measure the antioxidant capacity of biological fluids by chemiluminescence was developed,[6] but it cannot give the net redox potential (RP). In the past we reported a method we developed to estimate the scavenging capacity of the plasma oxygen radical scavengers.[7] The net result of the individual reactions between the oxidants and the corresponding antioxidants is an important parameter as it directly relates to the capacity of the system to contain the oxidative damage

289

TABLE 1. Important Antioxidants (Human)

Intracellular	Extracellular	Membranes
SOD	Asc	vit E
CAT	urate	carotenoids
GSH/GPx	SH	ceruloplasmin
	bilirubin	haptoglobin
	albumin	hemopexin
	lactoferrin	transferrin

or stress. Therefore it is important to have a measurable single parameter of plasma that acts as a marker of the antioxidant capacity of the sample. Ascorbate radical correlations with age, as measured by electron spin resonance (ESR) intensity, are found to be weak.[8]

Redox Potential

The oxidation reduction activity of the plasma constituents is always in a kinetic flux. The net activity can be represented by the RP which can be determined by the standard Nernst equation.

$$E_h = E_0 + \frac{RT}{nF} \ln \frac{[\text{Oxidant}]}{[\text{Reductant}]}$$

Where E_h and E_0 are the measured and standard RP, n is the number of electrons taking part in the process, F is the Faraday's constant, R is the gas contant and T is absolute temperature. The following is the simplified representation of the effects of oxidation reduction in biological systems (TABLE 2).

Antioxidant therapy associated with the reversal of oxidative stress delays the pathogenesis of heart failure.[9] Measurement of plasma RP of rabbits subjected to shock showed a marked change, and it returned to normal by infusion of albumin,[10] indicating its utility as a marker of some importance in the treatment of even acute conditions. Our previous work on the kinetics of free radical reactions in aqueous solutions shows that RP can be considered as a parameter for the net antioxidant status.[11] We report here a method used to measure plasma RP of 100 volunteers of normal (different age and ethnic groups) and patients.

Though the consumption of saturated fats in France is greater than in UK, the mortality rate from coronary artery disease in France is only one third of the UK

TABLE 2. Reduction Oxidation States in Biological Systems

Oxid.	Prooxid.	Vasconstr.	Stress
Red	Antioxid.	Vasodil.	Relax

If $\frac{\text{Reduction}}{\text{Oxidation}} = 1$ normal

< 1 ischemia/reperfusion, disease

positive E_0^1 (kinetic RP)

TABLE 3. Biochemical Parameters Measured Listed by Method Employed

RIA	ELISA	HPLC, EPR Spin Trap	Fluorometry	Spectrophotometry
	FPA	$\cdot O_2^-$	GSH	
C_3a	b-TG	$\cdot OH$		NO (GRIESS)
C_5a		Fe^{2+}		Hb, HPT
TxB_2		MDA		oxy/
6Keto-PGF1a				methemoglobin
$ET_{1,2}$				PMN-elastase
PAF				Ascorbic acid

rate.[12] It has been postulated that the high consumption of red wine is responsible for this "French Paradox" of coronary artery disease, attributing the positive effects to the high flavonoid content and other antioxidant polyphenols of the wine that act as antioxidants.[13] However, red wine contains pro-oxidant Fe^{2+}. Therefore we have investigated the French Paradox with the method we developed to measure the RP, as this can give a net antioxidant indicator of the plasma.

Plasma antioxidant enzymes that act as sensitive markers of the oxidative stress are also important to monitor the RP changes. Therefore measuring the antioxidant enzymes through their gene expression may be a powerful and reliable method to monitor the RP regulation. Initial studies on redox regulation in human myocardial antioxidant gene expression through GSHpx-1[14] indicate that the monitoring of gene expression is another important step in the direction of analyzing the antioxidant role and its utility as a marker of clinical significance. Ascorbate oxidase (AO), an important antioxidant enzyme activity in human plasma, is probably associated with the ceruloplasmin complex.[15] However, the measurements of plasma ascorbate oxidase with the existing method, developed for aqueous systems, did not give reliable results, as the plasma constituents interfere with the assay. Therefore we looked for the gene expression of AO in human tissues. We report the presence of detectable gene expression of plant ascorbate oxidase homologue in human tissues.

MATERIALS AND METHODS

Several biochemical parameters that play a role or reflect the oxidative reductive states of the plasma were measured. A list of all the biochemical methods used in this study is shown in TABLE 3. Methods are carried out as described in our previous work and that of others with appropriate modifications.[16–18]

TABLE 4. Protocols

Normal volunteers: n = 100, ages 5–90
Elective CABG patients: n = 30, control: n = 60
In-house patients: n = 100
Volunteers on red wine (250 mL): n = 20, placebos: n = 10
Heat stress preconditioning
  Pigs: n = 40, wt = 15–20 kg
  Control: n = 30, 30 min CC, 45 min CPB
  Heat stress: n = 10, 5 min 42.5°C, 30 min CC, 45 min CPB

TABLE 5. Precision and Validity of the Redox Potential Measurements

Precision: n = 100, CV = 7.4%	
Validity	
EPR spectrometry (Cu*)	$r = 0.416$
Luminol chemiluminescence	$r = 0.810$
Oxidized protein, carbonyl content	$r = 0.486$
Ascorbate	$r = 0.008$
Glutathione	$r = 0.116$

Redox Potential Measurements

Apparent RP (E_m) of known oxidant and reductant in the plasma sample was measured using a micro Pt/AgCl combination electrode (MI-800, ME Inc., CA). Kinetic RP (E_0^1) of the sample was obtained from a plot of E_0^1 (known kinetic redox potential of compounds in aqueous solutions) plotted against the E_m (RP measured in the presence of plasma). For this purpose 10 μL of each agent, various chemical and cardiovascular drugs at 20 mM concentration, was added to 100 μL plasma and the voltage potential in mV was measured.

The Precision and Validity of the Method

The RP measurements are verified with standard electron paramagnetic resonance (EPR) spectroscopy[17] and luminol chemiluminescence.[19] In addition, other parameters such as oxidized protein, carbonyl content,[20] ascorbate[16] and glutathione[18] of the samples from patients and normal pigs preconditioned with heat stress[21] and control plasma samples were measured. The protocols followed are shown in TABLE 4.

Plasma was prepared from the blood samples drawn into non-coagulant vacutainer tubes from normal human volunteers, elective coronary artery bypass graft (CABG) patients, controls, in-house patients, and RP (E_m) of the plasma was measured. Plasma samples were prepared before and one hour after 250 ml of

TABLE 6. Apparent Redox Potential of Chemicals of Biological Importance in Plasma (pH 7.4, 25°Celsius)

Antioxidants	mV	Pro/Antioxidants	mV	Pro-Oxidants	mV
POBN	−26	NEM	−3	Potassium permanganate	120
PBN	−28	Vit E	−5	Copper (2) chloride	56
Luminol	−28	Ubiquinone	−5	Potassium dichromate	25
p-Nitrophenol	−29	Thiodiglycolic acid	−9	TEMPOL	45
Imidazole	−33	Menaquinone	−10	MB	39
Dimethyl thiovera	−38	Vit C	−15	FAD	18
BHT	−34			Ferricyanide	14
NAC	−74			Rose Bengal	6
GSH	−80			L-Histidine	5
L-Cysteine	−90			Glucose	3
DTT	−129			N,N, Dimethyl p-nitro alanine	1.5

TABLE 7. Apparent Redox Potential of Cardiovascular Drugs in Plasma (pH 7.4, 25°Celsius)

Antioxidants	mV	Pro/Antioxidants	mV	Pro-Oxidants	mV
Indomethacin	−7	Quinidine sulfate	2	Nitroglycerine	39
Theophylline	−16	Propranolol	1.9	Procardia	27
Lidocaine	−16	Procainamide	−3.7	Metaprolol	25
L-Dopa	−19			Enalapril maleate	18
Hydrochlorothiazide	−20			Cardizem	16
Diltiazem	−21			Isosorbide	15
Verapamil	−23			Codeine	15
Nifedipine	−24			Altace	10
Methyl prednisolone	−28			Norvasc	8
Dobutrex	−44			Tenormin	6
Zocor	−53				
Hydralazine	−59				

French red wine was given to volunteers and placebos. RP (E_m) of these samples was also measured. Plasma samples of pigs preconditioned by heat shock and controls for undergoing cardiopulmonary bypass (CPB) were collected to measure RP. As there are no good methods for measuring AO in plasma, we measured AO enzymatic activity in plasma by differential oxidation of ascorbate in plasma by heat and also by controlled reduction of cytochrome C by ascorbate in native and AO-depleted plasma.

Putative Ascorbate Oxidase Gene Expression

In order to probe the AO-like gene expression in oligonucleotide primers of DNA sequence (Primer 1. 5′TCCAYTTRATARTG3′, Primer 2. 5′AA-CATRTAYTCNACRTCCCA3′, Primer 3. 5′CACCCTTGGCATTTGCAT3′, Primer 4. 5′TCCCATTCCCATATGCAA 3′; (N = A, G, T or C:R = G or A:Y = C or T) from plant ascorbate oxidase gene[22] were synthesized. Multiple

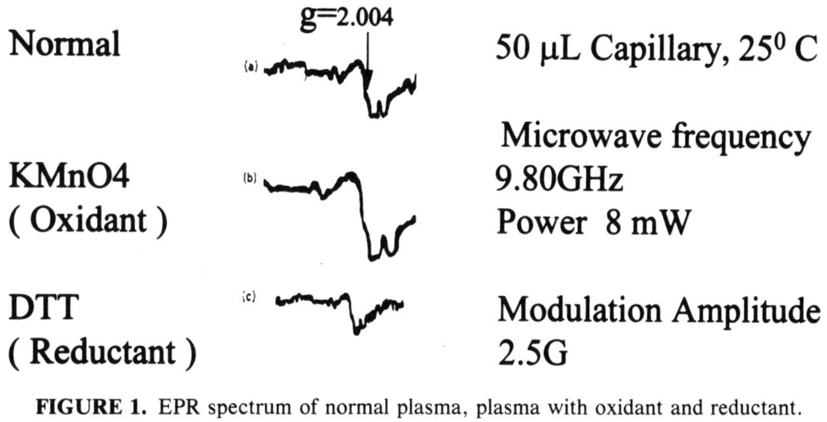

FIGURE 1. EPR spectrum of normal plasma, plasma with oxidant and reductant.

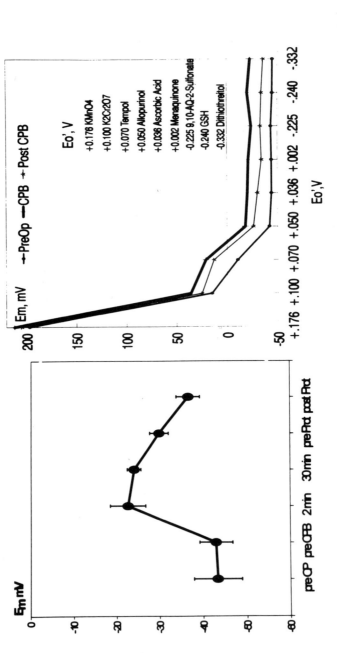

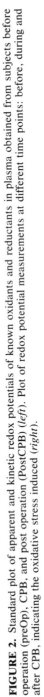

FIGURE 2. Standard plot of apparent and kinetic redox potentials of known oxidants and reductants in plasma obtained from subjects before operation (preOp), CPB, and post operation (PostCPB) (*left*). Plot of redox potential measurements at different time points: before, during and after CPB, indicating the oxidative stress induced (*right*).

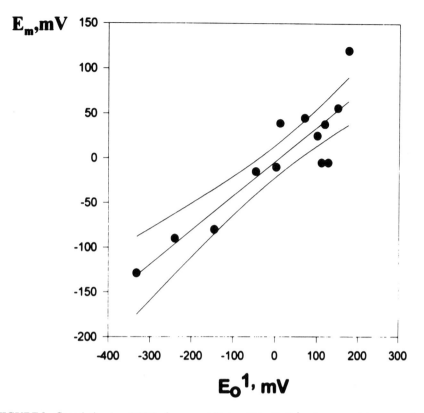

FIGURE 3. Correlation ($r = 0.901$) of apparent (E_m) and kinetic E_0^1 redox potential measured in plasma.

human tissue Northern blot (MTN-HumanII) was obtained from Clontech, Palo Alto, CA. The oligonucleotide primers were end labeled with a nonradioactive, enhanced chemiluminescence (ECL) kit from Amersham Life Science Inc., Arlington Heights, IL. Northern hybridization of the blot was carried out according to the standard methods.[23] The hybridized blot was exposed to x-ray film to obtain the signal.

RESULTS AND DISCUSSION

The data obtained from different experiments conducted to analyze the role and importance of RP are presented here. The relation between RP and other parameters that play a role in the redox balance in the human plasma under normal, disease and experimental conditions (such as CPB, wine and heat stress) tested in this study is also presented. The data obtained from the measurements of various biochemical parameters (Asc, GSH, etc.,) was used to establish the influence of these parameters on RP.

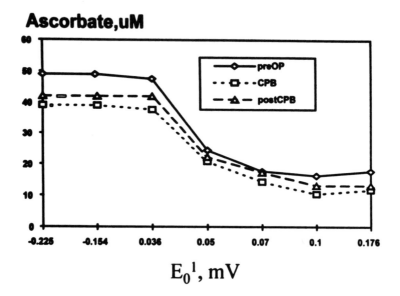

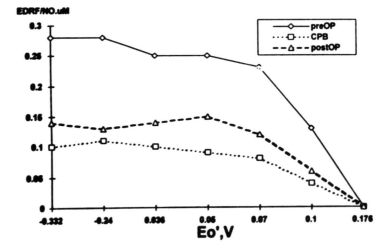

FIGURE 4. Plot showing the relation between antioxidant concentration and RP values in plasma before, during and post CPB (for ascorbate, GSH and EDRF/NO) and CPB (for CPK). The positive relation between the reduction in the antioxidant concentration and shift of kinetic redox potential towards more oxidative state is observed.

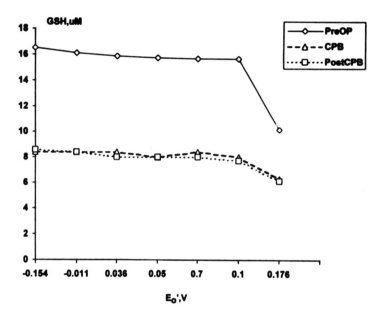

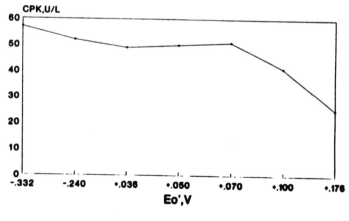

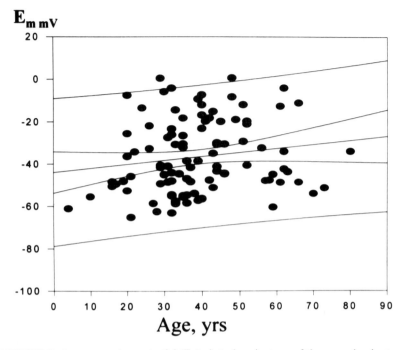

FIGURE 5. Apparent redox potential (E_m) plotted against age of the normal volunteers.

Redox Potential Measurements

Precision of the method is calculated and found to be 7.4% (n = 100). The validity of the method is tested by various other standard methods. The correlation coefficients of the results between the obtained values are presented in TABLE 5. RP correlated much better than ascorbate than other values, indicating the major role of ascorbate in maintaining the RP of the plasma. The apparent RPs of several chemicals of biological importance in the presence of plasma are presented in TABLE 6. In addition, the RPs of various cardiovascular drugs in the presence of plasma are presented in TABLE 7. Based on the values obtained they are classified as antioxidants, pro/antioxidants and oxidants. These data are valuable in estimating the effect of these compounds on the RP of the samples in plasma. Representative EPR spectra of normal plasma, and plasma with oxidant ($KMnO_4$) and reductant (DTT) are shown (FIG. 1). As described in the Methods section, we obtained the kinetic RP of the plasma samples from a standard plot of E_0^1 (known redox compounds in aqueous solutions) plotted against the E_m, RP measured in the presence of plasma (FIG. 2). Correlation of E_m versus E_0^1 with a regression coefficient of 0.901 is shown in FIGURE 3. CPB induces oxidative stress and as a result the concentration of antioxidants decreases. The concentrations of four different antioxidants—Asc, GSH, endothelium-derived relaxing factor/nitric oxide (EDRF/NO), and creatine phosphokinase (CPK)—were measured and plotted against kinetic RP (E_0^1) of the CPB samples (FIG. 4). The decrease in the concentration of these antioxidants clearly showed a shift in the kinetic RP.

Redox Potential, Antioxidant Concentration and Age

RP data from the plasma of healthy normal volunteers are presented as a plot; age against apparent RP (E_m) (FIG. 5) and log E_m (FIG. 6). The E_0^1 increased progressively with age. In patients E_0^1 is significantly lower ($p < 0.001$) and oxidative than normals. Plasma kinetic RP and antioxidant (Asc and GSH) concentrations of plasma were correlated (TABLE 8). It appears that kinetic RP correlates better with Asc concentration than with GSH in all groups compared. In general, the correlation between kinetic RP and Asc is much better in females compared to males (0.65 vs 0.449) and in the subset of Asians, this is even better in the case of females compared to males (0.892 vs 0.501).

Effect of Red Wine on Plasma Redox Potential

Plasma RP of volunteers given red wine and placebos was measured before and one hour after giving wine to normal volunteers and controls. The iron content of the plasma was also measured as red wine contains the oxidant iron Fe^{2+}. The data were plotted and are presented in FIGURE 7. Though the iron content did not increase, the RP values increased towards the reduced state of the plasma reflecting the positive effects observed.

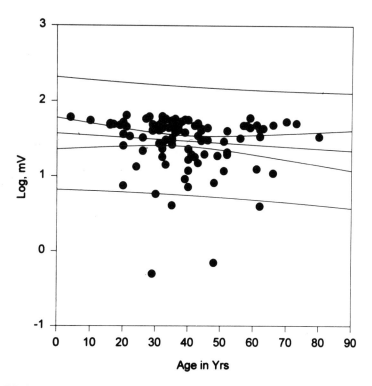

FIGURE 6. Apparent redox potential (Log, mV) plotted against age of the normal volunteers.

TABLE 8. Correlation between Redox Potential and Antioxidants (Asc, GSH) in Normal Volunteers

	Volunteers			White		Asian	
	All	Male	Female	Male	Female	Male	Female
E_0^1 vs Asc	0.563	0.449	0.65	0.448	0.669	0.501	0.892
E_0^1 vs GSH	0.236	0.167	0.31	0.169	0.344	0.164	0.360
Asc vs GSH	0.166	0.241	0.125	0.241	0.096	0.364	0.485

Heat Stress Preconditioning and Effect on Redox Potential

We measured the RP of the preconditioned (heat stress) pigs undergoing CPB. It is known that CPB induces oxidative stress, and heat preconditioning gives protection against oxidative stress. Ratios of RP from preOp, CPB and postOp samples of heat stress animals and controls were calculated and are presented in FIGURE 8. The protection given by the preconditioning reflected very well as seen in the RP values. Plasma E_m values of pigs treated and untreated, before and after CPB, were significantly different ($p < 0.001$).

Putative Human Ascorbate Oxidase (AO) Gene Expression

Biochemical measurement of AO did not give reliable results; therefore we focused on measuring the AO gene expression via its Northern analysis. Multiple tissue mRNA blot of human tissues shows a reasonable level of signal corresponding to the homologous AO expression in different tissues (FIG. 9). The AO expression in blood probably relates to the ascorbate oxidase-like activity of the plasma

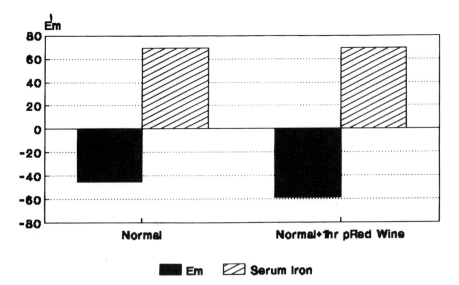

FIGURE 7. Effect of red wine on apparent redox potential of plasma.

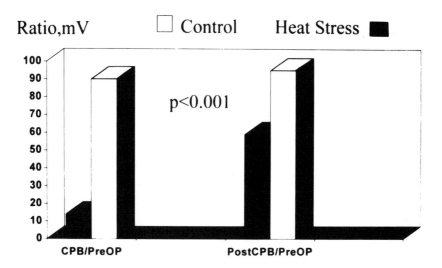

FIGURE 8. Plot showing the protective effect of heat stress on CPB as measured by redox potential of plasma.

in the ceruloplasmin complex. However, the signal is diffuse, indicating the presence of either several homologous species or a non-specific signal with limited homology to the plant AO. In any case, the presence of a signal is a positive indication towards the identification and analysis of AO gene expression. Further work with more specific regions of AO cDNA is necessary. Recently we obtained such a cDNA from Pioneer Corporation.

CONCLUSIONS

We present a novel, sensitive method to determine the apparent and kinetic RP of plasma that has a potential to conduct *in vivo* studies. We measured this parameter in various conditions and several volunteers. Also our data and the method used to measure the kinetic RP of pro- and antioxidants of biological importance and cardiovascular drugs will lead us to predict their efficacy and clinical significance. The measured RP of plasma correlates better with ascorbate than GSH. The kinetic RP values towards the oxidative state increased progressively with age, indicating its usefulness as a putative marker of aging. Our results demonstrating the positive influence of red wine on human plasma is another good example of the usefulness of this method and lends strong support in understanding the French Paradox, showing that the antioxidant capacity increases significantly in the wine-administered individuals compared to normals.

The simplicity of the method presented allows one to distinguish between the pro- and antioxidant activity of the plasma leading to ascertain their total antioxidant capacity in healthy, sick and aged individuals. Not only can this be measured in the collected samples but it is also possible to have a continuous monitoring of *in vivo* RP to measure the antioxidant capacity/oxidative damage. This is an important step towards the antioxidant therapy.

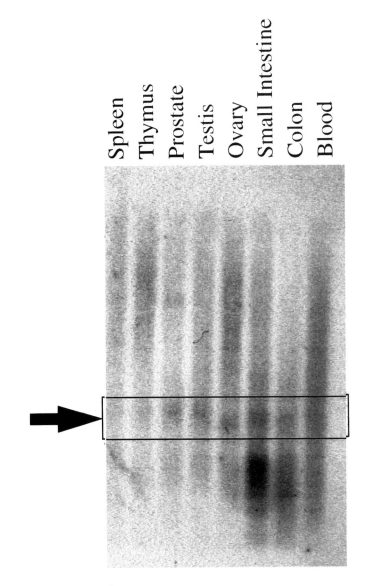

FIGURE 9. Northern blot of multiple human tissue mRNA probed with the primers specific to ascorbate oxidase (plant). The *arrow* indicates the expected plant ascorbate oxidase mRNA. Intense signal *lower* than the plant mRNA expected size may represent smaller ascorbate oxidase homologue in humans.

REFERENCES

1. HOLLAN, S. 1995. Free radicals in health and disease. Haematologia **26**(4): 117–189.
2. HAWLWELL, B. & J. M. C. GUTTERIDGE. 1989. Free Radicals in Biology and Medicine, 2nd edit. 416–494. Clarendon Press. Oxford.
3. STEINBERG, D. S., PARTHASARATHY, T. E. CAREW, J. C. KHOO & J. L. WITZTUM. 1989. Beyond cholesterol: modification of low density lipoproteins that increases atherogenicity. N. Eng. J. Med. **320**: 915–923.
4. WEDENBERG, K., G. RONQUIST, U. ULMSTEN, & A. WALDENSTROM. 1995. Energy economy of human uterine muscle strips under different *in vitro* conditions and its dependence on tissue redox potential. Eur. J. Obs. Reprod. Biol. **62**(1): 115–119.
5. VANDERKOOI, J. M., M. ERCINSKA, & I. A. SILVER. 1991. Oxygen in mammalian tissue: methods of measurement and affinities of various reactions. Am. J. Physiol. **260**(Cell Physiol. 29): C1131–C1150.
6. WHITEHEAD, T. P., G. H. G. THROPE & S. R. J. MAXWELL. 1992. Enhanced chemiluminescence assays for antioxidant capacity in biological fluid. Anal. Chim. Acta **266**: 265–277.
7. RAO, P. S. *et al.* 1988. Specificity of oxygen radical scavengers and assessment of free radical scavenging efficiency using luminol enhanced chemiluminescence. Biochem. Biophys. Res. Commun. **150**(1): 39–44.
8. SASAKI, R., T. KUROKAWA & S. TERO-KUBOTA. 1983. Ascorbate radical and ascorbic acid levels in human serum and age. J. Gerontol. **38**(1): 26–30.
9. DHALLA, A. K., N. SINGH & P. K. SINGAL. 1994. Antioxidant therapy associated with the reversal of oxidative stress delays the pathogenesis of heart failure. Circulation **90**(4): I-491.
10. JELINEK, M. *et al.* 1992. The effect of shock on blood oxidation and reduction potential. Experientia **48**: 980–985.
11. RAO, P. S. & E. HAYON. 1975. Redox potential of free radicals. III. Reevaluation of method. J. Am. Chem. Soc. **97**: 2986–2989.
12. RENAUD, F. & M. DE LOGERIL. 1992. Wine, alcohol, platelets and French paradox for coronary artery diseases. Lancet **341**: 1523–1526.
13. WHITEHEAD, P. T., D. ROBINSON, S. ALLAWAY, J. SYMS & A. HALE. 1995. Clin. Chem. **41**(1): 32–35.
14. MICKLE, D. A. & R. D. WEISEL. 1994. Redox regulation of human myocardial antioxidant gene expression. Circulation **90**(4): I-250.
15. OSAKI, S., J. A. MCDEERMOTT & E. FRIEDEN. 1964. Proof for the ascorbate oxidase activity of ceruloplasmin. J. Biol. Chem. **239**(10): 3570–3575.
16. ZANNIONI, V., M. LYNCH, S. GOLDSTEIN & P. SATO. 1974. A rapid micro method for determination of ascorbic acid in plasma and tissues. Biochem. Med. **11**: 41–44.
17. RAO, P. S., G. S. WEINSTEIN, N. RUJIKARA, J. M. LUBER & D. H. TYRAS. 1990. An HPLC method for *in vivo* quantitation of oxygen free radicals using spin and chemical traps. Chromatographia **30**: 19–23.
18. COHN, V. A. & J. LYLE. 1966. A fluorimetric method for determination of oxidized GSH. Anal. Biochem. **14**: 434–437.
19. RAO, P. S., J. M. LUBER, J. MILINOWICZ, P. LALEZAR & H. S. MULLER. 1988. Specificity of oxygen radical scavengers and assessment of free radical scavenger efficiency using luminol enhanced chemiluminescence. Biochem. Biophys. Res. Commun. **150**: 39–44.
20. LENZ, A-G. U. COSTABLE, S. SHALTIEL & R. L. LEVINE. 1989. Determination of carbonyl groups in oxidatively modified proteins by reduction with titrated sodium borohydride. Anal. Biochem. **177**: 419–425.
21. ROBINSON, B. L., T. MORITA, O. TOFT & J. J. MORRIS. 1985. Accelerated recovery of postischemic stunned myocardium after induced expression of myocardial heat-shock protein (Hsp 70). J. Thorac. Cardiovasc. Surg. **109**(4): 23–28.

22. OHKAWA, J., N. OKADA, A. SHINMYO & M. TAKANO. 1989. Primary structure of cucumber (*cuminis sativus*) ascorbate oxidase deduced from cDNA sequence: homology with blue copper proteins and tissue specific expression. Proc. Natl. Acad. Sci. USA **86:** 1239–1243.

23. SAMBROOK, J., E. F. FRITSCH & T. MANIATIS. 1989. Molecular Cloning: a Laboratory Manual. 2nd edit. Cold Spring Harbor Press. Cold Spring Harbor, NY.

Myocardial Protection in the Elderly

Biology of the Senescent Heart[a]

JAMES D. McCULLY AND SIDNEY LEVITSKY[b]

Division of Cardiothoracic Surgery
New England Deaconess Hospital
and
Harvard Medical School
Boston, Massachusetts

Studies examining the effects of aging on the myocardium have indicated that with advancing age there are anatomical, mechanical, ultrastructural, and biochemical alterations which compromise the adaptive response of the heart.[1–2] These alterations cause the senescent myocardium to be less tolerant to surgically induced ischemia than the mature myocardium and aggravate surgical complications in the elderly. With the increased incidence of elderly patients as candidates for complex cardiac surgery, the investigation into methods which will increase survivability and enhance cardiac protection are of paramount importance.

The susceptibility of the aged myocardium to ischemia-induced injury is evident at many levels. Morphologically, left ventricular mass is increased with age, as is a reduction in the size of the left ventricular cavity, although this predominately is found to occur in the elderly female.[3] There is also evidence of increased calcification of the valve annulus and epicardial coronary arteries as well as temporal alteration in the myocardial conduction system.[4,5] Ultrastructurally, the effect of aging is evidenced in a decreased mitochondria-to-myofibril ratio, cardiac myocyte enlargement and loss of mitochondrial organization,[6] as well as alteration in myocardial contractile properties.[2]

The mechanistic delineation of the aging process on myocardial function has often been obscured by intervening disease processes and epidemiological evaluation of myocardial complications associated with the elderly; while essential, this has not allowed for delineation between the effects of the temporal alteration of the myocardium and concurrent and/or preceding disease states. Recent experimental models, however, offer new insights into this dilemma through the use of experimental protocols, utilizing aging sheep. In this model, sheep provide a paradigm of pure senescence, free of cardiac disease, and the complicating variables of hypertrophy, dilatation, and coronary stenosis.[7]

In a recent report, it was shown using this model that the senescent myocardium is less tolerant of ischemia than the mature heart.[7,8] Investigations in which sexually mature (0.75 ± 0.11 years) and senescent (7.1 ± 0.45 years) sheep were used to contrast myocardial recovery following surgically induced global ischemia indi-

[a] Supported by the National Institutes of Health (HL 29077), and the American Heart Association (AHA 95006300).

[b] Address correspondence and reprint requests to: Sidney Levitsky, M.D., Division of Cardiothoracic Surgery, New England Deaconess Hospital, 110 Francis Street, Suite 2C, Boston, MA 02215. Tel.: 617-632-8383; Fax: 617-734-1656.

cated that postischemic, global, normothermic, systolic, and functional injury at 30 min normothermic reperfusion was significantly greater ($p < 0.05$) in the senescent as compared to the mature sheep heart.[7] These results indicate that in a pure senescent model the effect of aging alone, without intervening complications, detrimentally modulated functional recovery following surgically induced global ischemia.

In a separate series of experiments, mature and senescent sheep were subjected to 55 min of hypothermic blood cardioplegia arrest followed by 5 min of warm blood cardioplegia and 30 min of vented reperfusion.[8] Results from these experiments indicated that in the mature heart myocardial contractility was preserved with an insignificant 9% decrease in the slope of the preload recruitable stroke work relationship. In contrast, postarrest contractility in the senescent heart was returned to only 38% of the control value ($p < 0.05$). No significant change in passive compliance was identified in either group and MVO_2 was unchanged. These results suggest that even with current optimum myoprotective strategies the senescent myocardium exhibits a greater decrement in systolic function following surgically induced ischemia compared to the mature myocardium, suggesting that specific intraoperative myocardial management strategies may be required to preserve myocardial function in the aged patient.

Towards Development of Alternative Myoprotective Strategies for the Elderly Patient

Contingent upon the development of alternative myoprotective strategies is the determination of the intrinsic mechanisms of temporally modulated myocardial functional injury. The mechanism leading to myocardial ischemic injury remains controversial, but it has been generally accepted that the cessation of coronary blood flow and, thus, oxygen delivery is the initial step in the process leading to myocardial ischemic injury.[9] One mechanism postulated to play a central role leading to the eventual impairment of myocyte cellular function following surgically induced ischemia, in the senescent myocardium, involves the regulation of cellular calcium transport.[10]

Free cytosolic calcium is required for the proper function of the myocardial cellular contractile apparatus. In cardiac myocytes the cytosolic free calcium concentration is regulated by a variety of energy-dependent processes that maintain a concentration gradient greater than 10,000-fold across the plasma membrane with resting cytosolic calcium concentration being maintained at less than 10^{-7} mol/l.[10] The imposition of surgically induced global ischemia and the resultant cessation of myocardial coronary blood flow increases cytosolic calcium accumulation through a cascade of cellular events, which include the induction of metabolic acidosis and the activation of the sodium-proton exchanger.[11] These events result in the transport of hydrogen ions to the extracellular space, and the movement of sodium into the cytosol, increasing cytosolic sodium ion concentration and activating the sodium-calcium exchanger. Sodium is transported to extracellular space and calcium is taken up into the cytosol, increasing cytosolic calcium ($[Ca^{2+}]_i$) concentration. Increased $[Ca^{2+}]_i$ accumulation during ischemia is also augmented by ischemia-induced depolarization of the membrane potential, which allows for the opening of the l-type calcium channels and further calcium entry into the myocyte.[11] the increased $[Ca^{2+}]_i$ accumulation is then believed to activate cellular and cytosolic calcium-dependent phospholipases and proteases, which induce membrane injury and the further entry of calcium into the cell. These

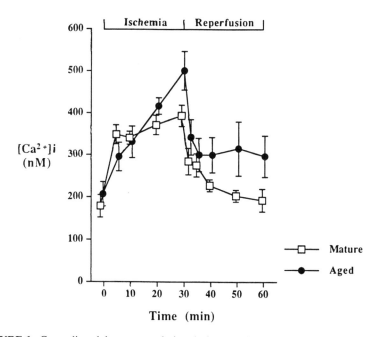

FIGURE 1. Cytosolic calcium accumulation during 30 min of normothermic ischemia and reperfusion. Cytosolic calcium accumulation in mature (15–20 weeks) and aged hearts (>130 weeks) was measured, quantitatively, using Fura-2. Results indicate a significant increase ($p < 0.05$) in cytosolic calcium accumulation during 30 min normothermic global ischemia, which rapidly returned to preischemic levels during reperfusion. In aged hearts, cytosolic calcium accumulation was increased approximately 30% greater at 30 min of normothermic ischemia as compared to mature hearts. This increase was correlated with decreased functional recovery in the aged heart during reperfusion.

processes act to rapidly alter myocardial cellular homeostasis leading to cellular dysfunction, or if of sufficient duration or intensity, cell injury of death.[11]

The etiological importance of intracellular calcium overload in the senescent myocardium has been illustrated in a series of experiments utilizing the calcium sensitive, second generation fluorescent calcium indicator fura-2 to quantitatively measure $[Ca^{2+}]_i$ accumulation in the isolated perfused rabbit heart.[12,13] In these experiments, $[Ca^{2+}]_i$ accumulation during 30 min of normothermic global ischemia and reperfusion was serially quantitated in sexually mature (15–20 weeks) and aged rabbit (135 weeks) hearts.[12,13] These results (FIG. 1) indicated that the aged heart accumulated 30% more $[Ca^{2+}]_i$ during ischemia than the mature heart.[12,13] Upon reperfusion $[Ca^{2+}]_i$ immediately returned to preischemic levels in both mature and aged hearts; however, comparison of left ventricular (LV) pressure and LV dP/dT max (change in pressure/change in time) after 30 min of reperfusion indicated that increased $[Ca^{2+}]_i$ during ischemia was correlated with reduced myocardial functional recovery and that these functional decrements were amplified in the aged heart as compared to the mature heart, despite the fact that $[Ca^{2+}]_i$ accumulation rapidly returned to preischemic levels at the onset of reperfusion.[13]

Amelioration of Cytosolic Calcium Accumulation

The intrinsic importance of calcium homeostasis has led to the development of cardioplegic protocols that attempt to limit the deleterious effects of ischemia-reperfusion injury. Cardioplegia is used as a myoprotective agent for the alleviation of surgically induced ischemic injury, incurred during cardiac operative procedures, to allow for the functional preservation of the myocardium. These solutions allow for the rapid electromechanical arrest of the myocardium through alteration of cellular electrochemical gradients. Partial control of $[Ca^{2+}]_i$ accumulation from surgically induced myocardial ischemia during open heart surgery is achieved through the use of cardioplegic solutions.[14–16] Most cardioplegia solutions use high potassium to arrest the heart.[14] The use of hypothermic potassium cardioplegia in adult open heart surgery increases the available intraoperative time and has been correlated with improved postischemic myocardial functional recovery, and reduced postoperative mortality.[14] Potassium-induced arrest maintains the heart in a depolarized state, significantly decreasing the energy demand of the myocardium.[2] Basal metabolic energy requirements are sustained under potassium-induced arrest and thus still constitute a significant energy expenditure.[9] In addition, depolarization leads to the alteration of the ion flux across the sarcolemmal membrane and is associated with both increased $[Ca^{2+}]_i$ accumulation and the significant depletion of cellular ATP reserves.[9]

Alternatives to potassium cardioplegia have been suggested to allow for enhanced functional recovery of the myocardium following ischemia/reperfusion. Hearse et al.[16] have reported that magnesium, when included in potassium cardioplegia (St. Thomas' Hospital), was beneficial to coronary flow and aided in the reduction of myocardial enzymatic leakage in the ischemic and reperfused heart. Recently, Steenbergen et al.[10] examined the relationship between ATP depletion, $[Ca^{2+}]_i$ concentration, and lethal myocardial ischemic injury in the perfused rat heart using nuclear magnetic resonance (NMR) and reported that high magnesium (16 mM) arrest delayed $[Ca^{2+}]_i$ accumulation and ATP depletion longer than high potassium (30 mM) arrest during normothermic ischemia in the mature rat heart.

The mechanism of action of magnesium supplemented cardioplegia as compared to potassium cardioplegia is less well known. In the myocardium, magnesium has been shown to act as a physiological calcium blocker as well as being required as an essential cofactor complexed to ATP and other adenine nucleotides for energy transfer reactions.[17–18] It has also been shown that high magnesium concentrations in the extracellular space inhibit calcium entry into the cell by displacing calcium from its binding sites in the sarcolemmal membrane.[19]

We compared the efficacy of potassium and/or magnesium cardioplegia in controlling $[Ca^{2+}]_i$ accumulation during ischemia/reperfusion in mature (15–20 weeks) and aged (>130 weeks) isolated perfused rabbit hearts.[12,13] Our results (FIG. 2) indicated that while potassium cardioplegia moderately ameliorated $[Ca^{2+}]_i$ accumulation during the 30 minutes of normothermic global ischemia, the use of magnesium-supplemented potassium cardioplegia obviated $[Ca^{2+}]_i$ accumulation during the 30 min of normothermic global ischemia in the mature and aged myocardium.[12,13]

As stated earlier, the effect of increased $[Ca^{2+}]_i$ accumulation during normothermic global ischemia in mature hearts had only nominal effects on myocardial functional recovery but, in the aged myocardium, increased $[Ca^{2+}]_i$ accumulation was correlated with reduced functional recovery. This detrimental effect was ameliorated with the use of potassium and magnesium-supplemented potassium cardioplegia in the aged heart. While potassium cardioplegia was less efficient

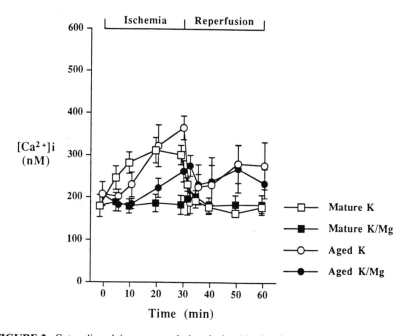

FIGURE 2. Cytosolic calcium accumulation during 30 min of normothermic ischemia and reperfusion in mature and aged hearts. Comparison of cytosolic calcium accumulation following potassium cardioplegia (20 mM KCl, K), and magnesium-supplemented potassium cardioplegia (20 mM KCl and 20 mM $MgSO_4$, K/Mg). Results indicate a significant decrease in cytosolic calcium accumulation with magnesium-supplemented potassium cardioplegia in both the mature and aged myocardium as compared to potassium cardioplegia alone. The use of magnesium-supplemented potassium cardioplegia maintained cytosolic calcium concentrations within normal physiological parameters throughout 30 min normothermic global ischemia in both mature and aged hearts. Enhanced functional recovery during reperfusion was correlated with the use of magnesium-supplemented potassium cardioplegia.

than magnesium-supplemented potassium cardioplegia in ameliorating $[Ca^{2+}]_i$ accumulation during normothermic global ischemia, both cardioplegias were correlated with enhanced left ventricular functional recovery, but the effects were more pronounced with magnesium-supplemented potassium cardioplegia than potassium cardioplegia alone.[12,13]

The mechanisms of $[Ca^{2+}]_i$ accumulation in the myocardium during normothermic global ischemia were recently investigated using the specific calcium channel inhibitors of the sarcolemmal voltage-gated l-type calcium channel (nifedipine), the sodium-calcium exchanger (dimethyltiourea), and the calcium release channel of the sarcoplasmic reticulum (ryanodine).[20] These experiments indicated that in the myocardium, $[Ca^{2+}]_i$ accumulation during normothermic global ischemia occurs mainly via the sarcolemmal l-type Ca^{2+} channel and the sarcoplasmic reticulum release channel in agreement with previous observations.[21] The modulating action of magnesium-supplemented potassium cardioplegia on $[Ca^{2+}]_i$ accumulation during normothermic global ischemia would appear to act through the inhibition of both the l-type Ca^{2+} channel and the sarcoplasmic reticulum release channel.[20]

Intracellular Calcium Overload and Intracellular Function: Role of the Mitochondria

Our investigations and the investigations of others suggest that the maintenance of mitochondrial calcium homeostasis plays a central role in the attenuation of myocardial injury in the aged myocardium following normothermic global ischemia. Several lines of evidence indicate that mitochondrial efficiency decreases with age and with ischemia. Investigation of myocardial energy metabolism with aging, in intact hearts and isolated mitochondria, has shown that maximal myocardial substrate oxidation rates decline approximately 20% from the mature heart to the aged heart in the rat.[22] In addition, studies in isolated mitochondria have shown that aging is associated with reduced oxidation rates.[23] In the isolated perfused rat heart, the effect of anoxia followed by reoxygenation, in isolation mitochondria, has been shown to induce mitochondrial enzyme release, and that the magnitude of the release was dependent upon the duration of the anoxic period and the concentration of cytosolic ATP.[24] It has also been shown that in isolated heart mitochondria treated with ischemia and reperfusion, there was incomplete collapse of the transmembrane proton gradient, and the impairment of respiration linked ATP generation.[25]

Myocardial tissue is primarily aerobic and its metabolism is closely dependent upon oxygen, as confirmed by the abundance of mitochondria (30% of the total volume). The high energy requirement of the myocardium is almost exclusively met by mitochondrial oxidative phosphorylation.[26] This leads to a high sensitivity of the myocardial cell to oxygen deficiency.[27] Under normal (nonischemia) conditions, calcium transport from the myocyte during diastole occurs against an electrochemical gradient requiring the use of adenosine triphosphate (ATP)-dependent calcium transport mechanisms.[28] The induction of normothermic global ischemia has been shown to rapidly reduce cellular high energy phosphates. This reduction occurs in the ischemic myocardium through the continuance of a number of reactions that persist during ischemia and include the energy dependent cellular transport mechanisms and enzymatic reactions.[28]

Early investigation has shown that rabbit hearts subjected to normothermic global ischemia are rapidly depleted of ATP tissue stores, and that the accumulation of $[Ca^{2+}]_i$ is associated with or precedes the changes in cellular high energy phosphates.[29] Experiments using newborn (3–5 day) and adult (4–5 month) rabbit hearts indicate an age-related susceptibility to ischemia/reperfusion injury.[10–12] When challenged with 30 min of warm global ischemia followed by 30 min of normothermic reperfusion, newborn hearts were found to be able to return rapidly to preischemic cardiac function and restore myocardial high energy phosphate stores. In the adult hearts subjected to the same protocol, functional recovery was significantly delayed and the recovery high energy phosphate stores were much slower in returning to preischemic levels.[11] These age-related differences in functional recovery were correlated with lower $[Ca^{2+}]_i$ accumulation during ischemia in the newborn as compared to the adult myocardium.[11]

The inability of the senescent myocardium to respond to ischemic stress has been associated with alterations in myocardial high energy phosphate restoration following surgically induced global ischemia. High energy phosphates are required for the proper maintenance of the heart as an aerobic organ. Under homeostatic conditions the mitochondrial inner membrane (cristae) which contains the electron transport chain, expels protons to the cytosol, creating a charge gradient that provides the passive energy for Ca^{2+} influx by the Ca^{2+} uniporter. Increased $[Ca^{2+}]_{mt}$ accumulation destabilizes the inner mitochondrial membrane and causes the inner membrane pore to open and permit further cation movement ("futile calcium cycling").[30] It has been speculated that this "futile calcium cycling" in the mitochondrion, an energy-dependent process requiring ATP to transport calcium against the electrochemical gradient out of the mitochondrion, utilizes needed ATP required for the maintenance of cell viability.[30] With subsequent depletion of ATP during ischemia, mitochondrial function may play a central role in the molecular events leading to tissue injury, especially in the aged myocardium.

One enzyme that may be an indicator of impaired mitochondrial function is cytochrome oxidase. Cytochrome oxidase is the terminal enzyme complex of the inner mitochondrial electron transport chain and has been shown to be vital in the production of high energy phosphate.[26] The activity of cytochrome oxidase has been shown to sharply decline in the latter part of the life and may compromise high energy phosphate preservation in the aged.[31] Recently, we showed that following 30 min of normothermic global ischemia $[Ca^{2+}]_{mt}$ accumulation was significantly increased ($p < 0.05$) in aged but not mature hearts.[32] When aged hearts were treated with magnesium-supplemented potassium cardioplegia, $[Ca^{2+}]_{mt}$ accumulation was ameliorated and these effects were correlated with enhanced functional recovery in the aged myocardium. Northern hybridization and run-on transcriptional analysis indicated that cytochrome oxidase (COX I) mRNA expression was decreased in the aged as compared to the mature heart.[32] The use of magnesium-supplemented potassium cardioplegia was found to increase COX I mRNA levels to a level not significantly different from that found in mature hearts and to significantly increase cytochrome oxidase activity.

Recently, the etiological significance of these biochemical alterations was substantiated using ^{31}P-NMR (nuclear magnetic resonance) spectroscopy. In a series of experiments using aged rabbit hearts, we have been able to show that amelioration of cytosolic and mitochondrial calcium accumulation with magnesium-supplemented potassium cardioplegia preserves high energy phosphates during ischemia and enhances high energy phosphate recovery during reperfusion in the senescent myocardium.

Role of the Nucleus

The interrelationship between nuclear and mitochondrial function has been well established, and it has been postulated that since the majority of mitochondrial proteins are encoded by nuclear genes and then imported into the appropriate mitochondrial compartment following completion of their synthesis in the cytoplasm that alteration in cytoplasmic homeostasis would detrimentally affect both intracellular organelles.[33,34] Previous reports suggested that the modulation of $[Ca^{2+}]_i$ accumulation may be involved in the regulation of nuclear function through the alteration of the cytosolic : nuclear calcium gradient.[33] The modulation of nuclear calcium ($[Ca^{2+}]_n$) has been proposed to be regulated by an ATP-dependent and a calmodulin-dependent mechanism which allows for the selective accumulation of calcium in the nucleus.[34] Recently, Brini et al.[35] reported that in HeLa cells, $[Ca^{2+}]_n$ is rapidly equilibrated with $[Ca^{2+}]_i$, suggesting that the nuclear membrane does not represent a major barrier to the diffusion of Ca^{2+} ions and that $[Ca^{2+}]_n$ is not regulated by a nuclear transport mechanism.

Our investigations have shown that in highly purified myocardial nuclei, myocardial nuclear calcium $[Ca^{2+}]_n$ accumulation (expressed as $[Ca^{2+}]_n$ nmol/μg DNA) is not significantly different between mature and aged hearts prior to the onset of ischemia, indicating that initial $[Ca^{2+}]_n$ concentration does not influence $[Ca^{2+}]_n$

accumulation during normothermic global ischemia.[13] $[Ca^{2+}]_n$ in mature hearts subjected to ischemia with or without cardioplegia was found to be unchanged. However, in aged hearts, the level of $[Ca^{2+}]_n$ was significantly increased during normothermic global ischemia without cardioplegia, and in hearts subjected to 30 min of normothermic global ischemia with potassium cardioplegia ($p < 0.05$ vs control). The use of magnesium or magnesium-supplemented potassium cardioplegia was found to significantly ($p < 0.05$) attenuate $[Ca^{2+}]_n$ accumulation in aged hearts.[13] These results indicate that the mechanism of $[Ca^{2+}]_n$ accumulation in the mature and aged heart may be different. In the mature heart $[Ca^{2+}]_n$ accumulation would appear to be unaffected by alteration of $[Ca^{2+}]_i$ accumulation, whereas in the aged heart $[Ca^{2+}]_n$ and $[Ca^{2+}]_i$ accumulation would appear to be associated.

The role of $[Ca^{2+}]_n$ is not clearly defined, but has been proposed as a possible mechanism involved in the regulation of key nuclear processes, such as gene expression, degradation of the nuclear envelope and apoptosis.[33,34] Previous authors have suggested that $[Ca^{2+}]_i$ may be involved in the regulation of nuclear function through the alteration of the cytosolic : nuclear calcium gradient.[34] Recently, we showed that increased $[Ca^{2+}]_n$ accumulation during normothermic global ischemia in aged hearts is correlated with increased nuclear DNA fragmentation.[13] The use of magnesium or magnesium-supplemented potassium cardioplegia was found to significantly attenuate nuclear DNA fragmentation in the aged myocardium. In the mature heart, wherein no increase in $[Ca^{2+}]_n$ accumulation was found to occur during 30 min of normothermic global ischemia, there was no DNA fragmentation evident.[13]

The mechanism of action of magnesium-supplemented potassium cardioplegia in ameliorating nuclear DNA fragmentation in the aged myocardium would appear to involve, at least at one level, the modulation of mitochondrial calcium homeostasis.[36] Earlier work by Benzi and Lerch[37] showed that postischemic perfusion with ruthenium red, a hexavalent dye that inhibits mitochondrial calcium uptake, significantly decreased oxygen consumption in the ischemic heart, and enhanced contractile function. (To date ruthenium red and magnesium are the only two reported agents to block calcium influx via the mitochondrial uniporter.[38]) The authors provided no mechanism of action but speculated that the protective mechanism of ruthenium red could possibly involve the maintenance of essential processes required for cell viability or act by the direct inhibition of calcium entry into the cell.[37] In a series of experiments using mature and aged rabbit hearts, we have been able to show that ruthenium red significantly ameliorates $[Ca^{2+}]_{mt}$ accumulation and is associated with both decreased DNA fragmentation and decreased $[Ca^{2+}]_n$ accumulation even though $[Ca^{2+}]_i$ accumulation is increased.[36] These results mimic those found when magnesium-supplemented potassium cardioplegia is used and suggest that modulation of the mitochondrion and, in particular, "futile calcium cycling" may be of significance in the modulation of ischemic myocardial injury.

Aging would appear to limit the capacity of the myocardium to regulate $[Ca^{2+}]_n$ accumulation and DNA fragmentation. The mechanism leading to increased nuclear DNA fragmentation remains speculative, but may involve the activation of calcium-dependent endonucleases. These endonucleases have been shown to generate specific DNA breaks that would impair the proper transcription of that segment of the DNA.[34] Al-Mohnna et al.[39] have shown that the nuclear envelope is not a barrier to calcium, and that small increases in $[Ca^{2+}]_i$ are rapidly transmitted to the nucleus, but that the nucleus appears to have an insulation mechanism that protects the nucleus from calcium transients of greater than 300 nmol. These authors propose that this mechanism would allow for the activation of cytosolic calcium-dependent enzymes while maintaining the nuclear enzymes largely inactive. Nuclear calcium-dependent enzymes would become active only with a long-lived $[Ca^{2+}]_i$ change, such as that found in our normothermic global ischemia model. This mechanism would only partially explain the differences observed in mature and aged DNA fragmentation, but does not address the differences observed in $[Ca^{2+}]_n$ accumulation.[39] In the mature heart $[Ca^{2+}]_n$ accumulation would not appear to be regulated by a calcium concentration-dependent mechanism, whereas in the aged myocardium both ATP and calcium-dependent mechanisms may be of importance in the eventual increase in $[Ca^{2+}]_n$ accumulation during normothermic ischemia.

Since DNA fragmentation has been shown to be a key feature in the events leading to cell death, the increased DNA fragmentation observed in the aged heart following 30 min of normothermic global ischemia may be of importance in the understanding of the factors modulating the impaired functional recovery of the aged heart.

Role of Nuclear DNA Fragmentation

Eukaryotic DNA has been regarded as a relatively static structure in which variation in content is brought about by mutation, although structural rearrangements are occasionally observed at the chromosomal level.[40] During cellular differentiation, selective regions of conformationally relaxed DNA are activated and inactivated (repressed) according to developmental mechanism(s) regulating gene expression.

Gene expression in the myocardium, as in all other cells, flows from the DNA via transcription to the RNA transcript and thence via translation to the protein product. This flow of genetic information is complex, consisting of a coordinated series of processes which include RNA transcription, processing, transport and translation and which act in a sequentially ordered fashion to regulate gene expression. In the aged myocardium, in which DNA synthesis and RNA transcription and translation are reduced in comparison to the neonatal myocardium, increased DNA fragmentation may act to limit significantly the heart's ability to respond to altered physiological stress.[41,42] It could be speculated that the modulation of increased $[Ca^{2+}]_n$ accumulation in the aged myocardium during normothermic global ischemia would allow for the maintenance of essential synergistic intracellular homeostatic processes and DNA integrity. The maintenance of DNA integrity would in turn provide for transcriptional fidelity of genomic sequences required for the proper functional recovery of the myocardium.

Our data indicate that the use of magnesium-supplemented potassium cardioplegia ameliorates cytosolic and nuclear calcium accumulation, modulates DNA fragmentation, and is associated with enhanced functional recovery.[13,36] The correlation between DNA fragmentation and functional recovery has led us to speculate that the mechanism of magnesium-supplemented potassium cardioplegia may involve either an RNA or a protein-dependent mechanism. Recently, we tested this hypothesis using magnesium-supplemented potassium cardioplegia with the addition of specific blockers of RNA (α-amanitin, a specific RNA polymerase II inhibitor) and protein synthesis (cycloheximide) to evaluate their hemodynamic and biochemical effects on cardioplegic protection in the aged rabbit heart.[43] The mechanism of action of these two inhibitors allowed us to differentiate between the putative RNA and protein-dependent mechanism of magnesium-supplemented potassium cardioplegia. Our results indicate that inhibition of protein synthesis did not affect the cardioprotection afforded by magnesium-supplemented potassium cardioplegia in the aged myocardium. Inhibition of RNA synthesis, however, was found to significantly ($p < 0.05$) decrease the preservation of myocardial functional recovery afforded by magnesium-supplemented potassium cardioplegia in the aged myocardium following 30 min of normothermic, to levels not significantly different from that seen in unprotected global ischemia without cardioplegia.[43] Of significance to our hypothesis was the finding that the decreased functional recovery found to occur in hearts treated with magnesium-supplemented potassium cardioplegia in which RNA synthesis was inhibited was the finding of increased DNA fragmentation ($p < 0.05$) compared to hearts treated with magnesium-supplemented potassium cardioplegia alone and magnesium-supplemented potassium cardioplegia with addition of cycloheximide, the protein synthesis inhibitor.[43] These results indicate that when RNA synthesis is inhibited the protection afforded by magnesium-supplemented potassium cardioplegia is abolished, such that there is no difference from global ischemia without cardioplegia.

The relative contribution of RNA and protein synthesis in the acquisition of cardioprotection is not yet fully elucidated. Previous investigations have indicated that following ischemia and reperfusion there are altered mRNA transcript levels. However, little data is available to indicate if these mRNA's ultimately result in the synthesis of myocardial proteins essential for enhanced myocardial functional recovery.[32,44–47] Our results suggest that the synthesis of de novo proteins may not be involved in the myocardial protection afforded in the aged myocardium by magnesium-supplemented potassium cardioplegia.[43] This would agree with the findings of Thornton et al.,[47] who showed that inhibition of protein synthesis with actinomycin D and cycloheximide had no effect on the myocardial protection from infarct afforded by preconditioning. In their rabbit model, preconditioned groups had a greatly reduced infarct size in either the presence or the absence of the protein synthesis inhibitors, actinomycin D and cycloheximide. From these data the authors concluded that protein synthesis had no relation with the mechanism of cardioprotection.

These data do not exclude the role of proteins in providing for cardioprotection. In fact, there is sufficient data to suggest that protein phosphorylation, changes in protein conformation and protein translocation may all play an essential role in conferring cardioprotection. The relative synthesis rates and the related mechanisms required for de novo protein intervention, however, make it unlikely that direct transcription-translation linkage is involved in cardioprotection.

Our investigations have led us to speculate that the mechanism leading to reduced functional recovery following surgically induced ischemia, in the aged as compared to the mature myocardium, is the result of the progressive accumulation of genetic damage which exceeds the capacity of the mechanisms for repair, renewal and removal of damaged genomic molecules. Support for this hypothesis are studies showing that following phenotypic development of the myocardium, myocyte DNA synthesis ceases, and DNA α and β polymerase activity in the cardiac myocyte is decreased such that only maintenance DNA repair is maintained.[41] The age-related reduction of DNA α and β polymerase activity compromises the efficient repair of myocyte nuclear DNA, leading to increased nuclear DNA fragmentation.[41,42] Sufficient evidence is currently available to indicate that increased DNA fragmentation leads to cell death. Protection from cellular necrosis is in part afforded by DNA nucleotide excision repair mechanisms, which function to remove and correct injurious DNA damage.[48–50] Of primary importance in this mechanism is the recognition of DNA damage sites. Recently, it was shown that DNA damage is repaired more efficiently

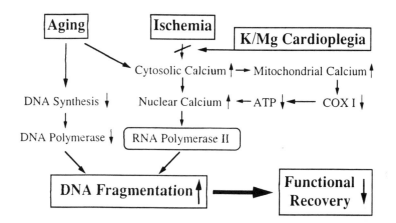

FIGURE 3. Hypothetical mechanism for loss of ischemic tolerance in the aged myocardium, and the role of magnesium supplemented potassium (K/Mg) cardioplegia. Aging is associated with decreased DNA synthesis and DNA α and β polymerase activity. This leads to an increased DNA fragility in the aged myocardium. The imposition of surgically induced global ischemia increases cytosolic calcium accumulation in the aged myocardium, resulting in increased mitochondrial calcium accumulation and decreased high energy phosphate preservation/resynthesis. Increased cytosolic calcium accumulation and decreased high energy phosphates increase nuclear calcium accumulation leading to increased DNA fragmentation. These phenomena are associated with decreased functional recovery following surgically induced global ischemia. The use of magnesium-supplemented potassium cardioplegia ameliorates these phenomena and enhances functional recovery in the aged myocardium. The mechanism of action of magnesium-supplemented potassium cardioplegia is regulated through an RNA-dependent mechanism which modulates DNA fragmentation and ultimately functional recovery in the aged myocardium.

in actively transcribed genes and that this repair is directly involved with the transcriptional apparatus.[51] The mechanism of transcription-dependent DNA excision-repair has been proposed to involve the stalling of the RNA polymerase II on the DNA template, thus signalling the location of DNA damage and facilitating DNA repair.[50] Our data, indicating increased DNA fragmentation in hearts treated with magnesium-supplemented potassium cardioplegia with the addition α-amanitin, would appear to support the mechanism of transcription-dependent DNA excision-repair.[43] Etiologically, such a system would be of benefit to the aging myocardium with its reduced DNA polymerase activities, by allowing for the more efficient usage of polymerase activity and the maintenance of cellular viability (FIG. 3).

The inability of the senescent myocardium to respond to ischemic stress has been suggested to involve many mechanisms. Herein, we have attempted to show that unmodulated calcium accumulation is directly involved in the mechanisms leading to reduced functional recovery in the aged myocardium following surgically induced global ischemia. While many of these mechanisms remain at present, controversial and speculative, further research will allow for their incorporation into the development of a unified hypothesis elaborating procedures for myocardial protection in the elderly.

REFERENCES

1. ROBERTS, W. C. 1988. The aging heart. Mayo Clin. Proc. **63:** 205–206.
2. LAKATTA, E. G., J. H. MITCHELL, A. POMERANCE & G. G. ROWE. 1987. Human aging: changes in structure and function. JACC **10:** 42–47.
3. RICE, D. P. & J. J. FELDMANN. 1983. Living longer in the United States. demographic changes and health needs. Milbank Mem. Fund Quart. **61:** 362–396.
4. LIE, J. T. & P. I. HAMMOND. 1988. Pathology of the senescent heart: anatomic observations on 237 autopsy studies of patients 90 to 105 years old. Mayo Clinc. Proc. **63:** 552–564.
5. LAKATTA, E. G. 1993. Cardiovascular regulatory mechanisms in advanced age. Physiol. Rev. **73:** 413–467.
6. FRENZEL, H. & J. FEINMAN. 1984. Age-dependent structural changes in the myocardium of rats. A quantitative light- and electron-microscopic study on the right and left chamber wall. Mech. Ageing Dev. **27:** 29–41.
7. MISARE, B. D., I. B. KRUKENKAMP & S. LEVITSKY. 1992. Age-dependent sensitivity to unprotected cardiac ischemia: the senescent myocardium. J. Thorac. Cardiovasc. Surg. **103:** 60–65.
8. CALDERONE, C. A., I. B. KRUKENKAMP, P. G. BURNS, G. R. GAUDETTE, J. SCHULMAN & S. LEVITSKY. 1995. Blood cardioplegia in the senescent heart. J. Thorac. Cardiovasc. Surg. **109:** 269–274.
9. STERNBERGH, W. C., L. A. BRUNSTING, A. S. ABD-ELFATTAH & A. S. WECHSLER. 1989. Basal metabolic energy requirements of polarized and depolarized arrest in rat heart. Am. J. Physiol. **256:** H846–H851.
10. STEENBERGEN, C., E. MURPHY, J. WATTS & R. LONDON. 1990. Correlation between cytocolic free calcium, contracture, ATP, and irreversible ischemic injury in perfused rat heart. Circ. Res. **66:** 135–146.
11. JIMENEZ, E., P. DEL NIDO, H. FEINBERG & S. LEVITSKY. 1993. Redistribution of myocardial calcium during ischemia. Relationship to onset of contracture. J. Thorac. Cardiovasc. Surg. **105:** 988–994.
12. ATAKA, K., D. CHEN, J. D. MCCULLY, S. LEVITSKY & H. FEINBERG. 1993. Magnesium cardioplegia prevents accumulation of cytosolic calcium in the ischemic myocardium. J. Mol. Cell. Cardiol. **25:** 1387–1390.
13. TSUKUBE, T., J. D. MCCULLY, E. A. FAULK, M. FEDERMAN, J. LOCICERO, I. B. KRUKENKAMP & S. LEVITSKY. 1994. Magnesium cardioplegia reduces cytosolic and nuclear calcium and DNA fragmentation in the senescent myocardium. Ann. Thorac. Surg. **58:** 1005–1011.
14. WRIGHT, R., S. LEVITSKY, K. RAO, C. HOLLAND & H. FEINBERG. 1978. Potassium cardioplegia. Arch. Surg. **113:** 976–980.
15. BURKHOFF, D., R. KALIL-FILHO & G. GERSTENBLITH. 1990. Oxygen consumption is less in rat hearts arrested by low calcium than by high potassium at fixed flow. Am. J. Physiol. **259:** H1142–H1147.
16. HEARSE, D. J., P. B. GARLICK & S. M. HUMPHREY. 1977. Ischemic contracture of the myocardium. Mechanism and prevention. Am. J. Cardiol. **39:** 986–993.
17. SHINE, K. I. & A. M. DOUGLAS. 1975. Magnesium effects in rabbit ventricle. Am. J. Physiol. **288:** 1545–1554.
18. SHINE, K. I. 1979. Myocardial effects of magnesium. Am. J. Physiol. **237:** H413–H423.
19. LANSMAN, J. B., P. HESS & R. W. TSIEN. 1986. Blockade of current through single calcium channels by Cd^{2+}, Mg^{2+}, and Ca^{2+}. Voltage and concentration dependence of calcium entry into the pore. J. Gen. Physiol. **88:** 321–347.
20. TSUKUBE, T., J. D. MCCULLY, M. FEDERMAN, I. B. KRUKENKAMP & S. LEVITSKY. 1996. Developmental differences in cytosolic calcium accumulation associated with surgically induced global ischemia: optimization of cardioplegic protection and mechanism of action. J. Thorac. Cardiovasc. Surg. In press.
21. POWELL, T., P. TATHAM & V. TWIST. 1984. Cytoplasmic free calcium measured by Quin2 fluorescence in isolated ventricular myocytes at rest and during potassium-depolarization. Biochem. Biophys. Res. Commun. **122:** 1012–1020.

22. ABU-ERREISH, G., J. NEELY, J. WHITMER, V. WHITMAN & D. SANADI. 1977. Fatty acid oxidation by isolated perfused working hearts of aged rats. Am. J. Physiol. **232:** E258–E262.

23. CHEN, J., J. WARSHAW & D. SANADI. 1972. Regulation of mitochondrial respiration in senescence. J. Cell Physiol. **80:** 141–148.

24. NISHIMURA, M., H. TAKAMI, M. KANEKO et al. 1993. Mechanism of mitochondrial enzyme leakage during reoxygenation of the rat heart. Cardiovasc. Res. **27:** 1116–1122.

25. NOHL, H., V. KOLTOVER & K. STOLZE. 1993. Ischemia/reperfusion impairs mitochondrial energy conservation and triggers O_2 release as a byproduct of respiration. Free Radical. Res. Commun. **18:** 127–137.

26. FROLKIS, V. V., R. A. FROLKIS, L. S. MKHITARIAN, V. G. SHERCHUK, V. E. FRAIFELD, L. G. VAKULENKO & I. SYROUY. 1988. Contractile function and Ca^{2+} transport system of myocardium in ageing. Gerontology **34:** 64–74.

27. FERRARI, R., P. PEDERSINI, M. BONGRAZIO, G. GAIA, P. BERNOCCHI, F. DiLISA & O. VISIOLI. 1993. Mitochondrial energy production and cation control in myocardial ischaemia and reperfusion. Basic Res. Cardiol. **88:** 495–512.

28. JENNINGS, R. B. & C. STEENBERGEN. 1985. Nucleotide metabolism and cellular damage in myocardial ischemia. Annu. Rev. Physiol. **47:** 727–749.

29. NAYLER, W., S. PANAGIOTOPOULOS & J. ELZ. 1988. Calcium mediated damage during post-ischemic reperfusion. J. Mol. Cell. Cardiol. **20:** 41S11.

30. PENG, C. F., J. J. KANE, M. L. MURPHY & K. D. STRAUB. 1977. Abnormal mitochondrial oxidative phosphorylation of ischemic myocardium by calcium chelating agents. J. Mol. Cell. Cardiol. **9:** 897–908.

31. PIERI, C., R. RECCHIONI & F. MORONI. 1993. Age-dependent modifications of mitochondrial trans-membrane potential and mass in rat splenic lymphocytes during proliferation. Mech. Age. Dev. **70:** 201–212.

32. FAULK, E. A., J. D. McCULLY, N. C. HADLOW, T. TSUKUBE, I. B. KRUKENKAMP, M. FEDERMAN & S. LEVITSKY. 1995. Magnesium cardioplegia enhances mRNA levels and the maximal velocity of cytochrome oxidase I in the senescent myocardium during global ischemia. Circulation **92**(Suppl. II): II-405–II-412.

33. MAZZANTI, M., L. J. DeFELICE, J. COHEN & H. MALTER. 1990. Ion channels in the nuclear envelope. Nature **343:** 764–767.

34. NICOTERA, P., D. J. McCONKEY, D. P. JONES & S. ORRENIUS. 1989. ATP stimulates Ca^{2+} uptake and increases the free Ca^{2+} concentration in isolated rat liver nuclei. Proc. Natl. Acad. Sci. USA **86:** 453–457.

35. BRINI, M., M. MURGIA, L. PASTI, D. PICARD, T. POZZEN & R. RIZZUTO. 1993. Nuclear Ca^{2+} concentration measured with specifically targeted recombinant aequorin. EMBO J. **12:** 4813–4819.

36. FAULK, E. A., J. D. McCULLY, T. TSUKUBE, N. C. HADLOW, I. B. KRUKENKAMP & S. LEVITSKY. 1995. Myocardial mitochondrial calcium accumulation modulates nuclear calcium accumulation and DNA fragmentation. Ann. Thorac. Surg. **60:** 338–344.

37. BENZI, R. H. & R. LERCH. 1992. Dissociation between contractile function and oxidative metabolism in post-ischemic myocardium. Circ. Res. **71:** 567–576.

38. DENTON, R. M. & J. G. McCORMACK. 1990. Ca^{2+} as a second messenger within mitochondria of the heart and other tissues. Annu. Rev. Physiol. **52:** 451–466.

39. AL-MOHNNA, F. A., K. W. T. CADDY & S. R. BOLSOVER. 1994. The nucleus is insulated from large cytosolic calcium ion changes. Nature **367:** 745–749.

40. SHMOOKLER-REIS, R. J. & S. GOLDSTEIN. 1980. Loss of reiterated DNA sequences during serial passage of human diploid fibroblasts. Cell **21:** 739–746.

41. CLAYCOMB, W. C. 1979. DNA synthesis and DNA enzymes in terminally differentiating cardiac muscle cells. Exp. Cell Res. **118:** 111–114.

42. McCULLY, J. D., J. D. MALBY, M. J. SOLE & C. C. LIEW. 1991. RNA transcription and translation in the normal and cardiomyopathic Syrian hamster during the temporal development of the myocardium. Biochem. Cell Biol. **69:** 88–92.

43. MATSUDA, H., J. D. McCULLY, N. C. HADLOW, I. B. KRUKENKAMP & S. LEVITSKY.

1995. Evidence that cardioplegia enhances functional recovery in the senescent myocardium through an RNA dependent mechanism. Surg. Forum **46:** 211–213.

44. MYRMEL, T., J. D. MCCULLY, I. B. KRUKENKAMP & S. LEVITSKY. 1994. Warm ischemia triggers cardioprotective heat shock protein mRNA by anaerobic metabolism. Circulation **90**(Part II): II-299–II-305.

45. MCCULLY, J. D., T. MYRMEL, M. M. LOTZ, I. B. KRUKENKAMP & S. LEVITSKY. 1995. The rapid expression of myocardial Hsp 70 mRNA and the heat shock 70 kDa protein can be achieved after only a brief period of retrograde hyperthermic perfusion. J. Mol. Cell. Cardiol. **27:** 873–882.

46. ENTWISTLE, J. W. C., L. J. GRAHAM, E. R. JAKOI & A. S. WECHLER. 1995. Myocardial stunning: changes in cardiac gene expression after global ischemia and reperfusion. Surg. Forum **46:** 209–211.

47. THORNTON, J., S. STRIPLIN, G. S. LIU, A. SWAFFORD, A. W. H. STANLEY, D. M. VAN WINKLE & J. M. DOWNEY. 1990. Inhibition of protein synthesis does not block myocardial protection afforded by preconditioning. Am. J. Physiol. **259:** H1822–H1825.

48. FRIEDBERG, E. C. 1985. DNA Repair. Freeman and Co. San Francisco, CA.

49. HANAWALT, P. C., P. K. COOPER, A. K. GANESAN & C. A. SMITH. 1979. DNA repair in bacterial and mammalian cells. Annu. Rev. Biochem. **48:** 783–836.

50. MELLON, I., G. SPIVAK & P. C. HANAWALT. 1987. Selective removal of transcriptional blocking DNA damage from the transcribed strand of the mammalian DHFR gene. Cell **51:** 241–249.

51. LEADON, S. A. & D. A. LAWRENCE. 1991. Preferential repair of DNA damage on the transcribed strand of the human metallothionein genes requires RNA polymerase II. Mutat. Res. **255:** 67–78.

The Influence of Myocardial Temperature on Stunning following Coronary Revascularization[a]

RICHARD M. ENGELMAN, DANIEL T. ENGELMAN,
JOHN A. ROUSOU, JOSEPH E. FLACK, III,
DAVID W. DEATON, DENNIS A. TIGHE,
ROBERT D. RIFKIN, AND CHERYL A. GREGORY

Departments of Surgery and Medicine
Baystate Medical Center
759 Chestnut Street
Springfield, Massachusetts 01107
and
The University of Connecticut School of Medicine
263 Farmington Avenue
Farmington, Connecticut 06032

Myocardial stunning is best defined as reversible postischemic contractile dysfunction which is not associated with myocardial infarction.[1] One of the primary factors thought to be responsible is cytosolic calcium overload during reperfusion due to increased calcium entry into the cell and decreased uptake by the sarcoplasmic reticulum.[1,2] In the nonsurgical patient, transient ischemia occurs in the catheterization laboratory during angioplasty, at normothermia, followed by reperfusion. During cardiac surgery, however, a range of myocardial temperatures is available during ischemia and reperfusion. The subject of this report is a randomized prospective trial carried out in 33 patients undergoing coronary revascularization at three temperatures comparing preoperative and postoperative sophisticated parameters of ventricular systolic and diastolic function. The goal was to determine whether temperature is a factor in recovery of myocardial function following a period of cardioplegia in patients undergoing coronary revascularization.

METHODS

An NIH-funded clinical trial has been ongoing at the Baystate Medical Center for two years. This randomized prospective clinical study involves patients undergoing coronary revascularization who have a preoperative left ventricular ejection fraction greater than 30%, age less than or equal to 75 years and anatomy requiring three or more coronary bypass grafts. Patients were approached preoperatively with the intent of evaluating myocardial preservation and cardiopulmonary bypass at three different temperatures, cold (myocardial temperature less than 15°C and systemic perfusion temperature at 20°C), tepid (myocardial and perfusion tempera-

[a] Supported by NIH Grants #HL22559-14 and #HL48631-02.

ture at 32°C), and warm (myocardial and perfusion temperature at 37°C). Myocardial contractility was studied prior to cardiopulmonary bypass and one-half hour after completing coronary revascularization and weaning from cardiopulmonary bypass.

Measurements of Myocardial Contractility

A commercially available echocardiographic system (Hewlett Packard Transesophageal Echocardiography, Andover, MA) was equipped with circuitry (Acoustic Quantification Package) which provides real time two-dimensional ultrasonic integrated backscatter imaging. Unique software was utilized to permit on-line and real time delineation and tracking of the sharply demarcated borders between endocardium and blood based on integrated backscatter imaging (FIG. 1). Quantification and display of cardiac chamber cavity areas were implemented on-line, permitting serial derivation and display of indices of ventricular function in real time. This methodology has been published by Perez et al.[3] and is commercially available.

Prior to introduction of systemic heparinization, the patients were anesthetized, and a transesophageal echocardiograph probe was placed. A Sonos 1500 echocardiographic machine (Hewlett Packard, Andover, MA) was utilized.

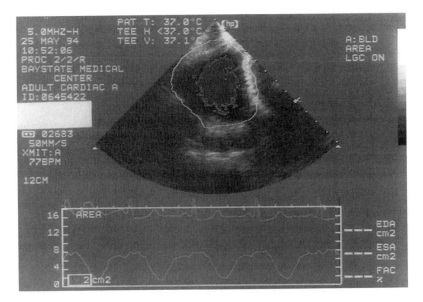

FIGURE 1. This is an end-diastolic frame of a four-chamber automatic boundary-detected image obtained by a transgastric view utilizing transesophageal echocardiography. The region of interest, which is the left ventricular chamber, is documented by a *solid white line* drawn around the LV cavity. The endocardial border is fully defined. The graphics below the echo show the cavity area computed and displayed instantaneously with calibration marks in square centimeters and with the electrocardiograph displayed for timing purposes.

Following introduction of general endotracheal anesthesia, a mid-sternotomy incision was carried out and heparin administered. After appropriate preparation for cardiopulmonary bypass with dissection of an internal mammary artery, a mikro-tip transducer catheter (Millar Model TCB-500, Millar Instruments, Inc., Houston, TX) was placed through the right superior pulmonary vein, into the left ventricular chamber. A right atrial pacing catheter was placed for uniformity of measurement and atrial pacing initiated at 90 beats/minute. A snare was placed around the inferior vena cava for subsequent preload reduction during data acquisition.

Hemodynamic variables continuously recorded were heart rate, left ventricular pressure, and left ventricular dimensions. The data were digitized and recorded in real time with a 12-bit A-D convertor sampling at 200 Hz using the Cordat II data acquisition, analysis and presentation system (Data Integrated Scientific Systems, Pinckney, MI and Triton Technologies, Inc., San Diego, CA). Utilizing the Cordat II system, the data can be analyzed in real time or subsequently interpreted utilizing the CV Autoreport Cardiovascular Analysis Program (Scitelligence, Inc., Brighton, MI). This approach substitutes the single-plane area-length method for quantification of left ventricular volume.[4] This methodology has been validated as a reliable approach for estimating left ventricular volume.[5]

Obtaining adequate pressure-volume relationships requires reduction and expansion of ventricular preload. This is accomplished by transient occlusion of the inferior vena cava to produce a 30-mmHg reduction in maximal left ventricular pressure. At each sampling time, data are recorded over a ten-second period with the respirator off at end-expiration. The patient is allowed to equilibrate and caval occlusion data are obtained. Three sets of occlusion data are obtained at each time point. Global functional data are analyzed during each preload reduction, which is accomplished both prior to the introduction of cardiopulmonary bypass and 30 minutes after completing the operation and discontinuing cardiopulmonary bypass.

The relationship between end-systolic pressure (P_{es}) and/or volume (V_{es}) is described in the equation $P_{es} = E_{max}(V_{es} - V_0)$, where E_{max} is the slope and V_0 is the X-intercept of the linear regression.[6] Maximal elastance or E_{max} is defined as the point along the pressure-volume loop where the ratio of instantaneous LV pressure to LV volume is maximized during the cardiac cycle. The "stiffness" coefficient (β) is derived from exponential modeling of the end diastolic pressure (EDP)-volume (EDV) relationship by the equation $EDP = \alpha \times e^{(\beta \times EDV)}$.[7] The stiffness coefficient is the inverse of compliance. The first derivative of left ventricular pressure ($LV_{dP/dt}$) is calculated as a polynomial approximation from the digital LV pressure signal. End diastolic volume (EDV) is defined as the LV volume at the first positive $LV_{dP/dt}$. LV stroke work is defined as the integral of LV pressure (P) and volume (V) by the equation $SW = \int PdV$ (pressure times the derivative of the volume). A linear regression analysis is performed on the stroke work-end diastolic volume relationship, which is called the preload recruitable stroke work (PRSW) with slope (Mw) and × intercept (V_0). FIGURE 2 illustrates a representative pressure volume loop and FIGURE 3, a representative global PRSW relationship. FIGURE 4 is a schematic of the pressure-volume relationship. External work is the area within the pressure-volume loop (FIG. 4), while potential energy is the area below the end-systolic P-V slope but outside the loop. The summation of potential energy and external work is the total mechanical energy generated by ventricular contractions.[8] The analysis of these functions was performed after recording data using the Cordat II system.

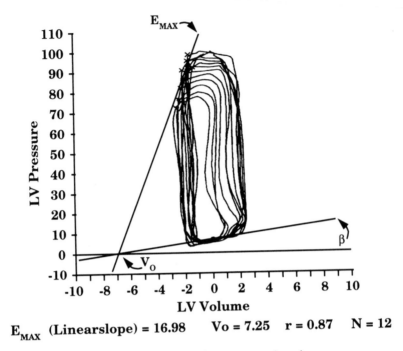

E_{MAX} (Linearslope) = 16.98   Vo = 7.25   r = 0.87   N = 12

FIGURE 2. A representative pressure-volume loop.

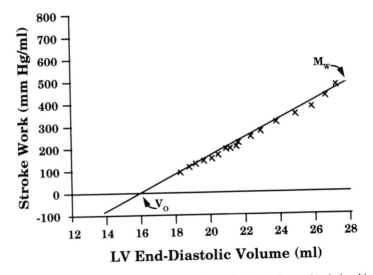

FIGURE 3. A representative global preload recruitable stroke work relationship.

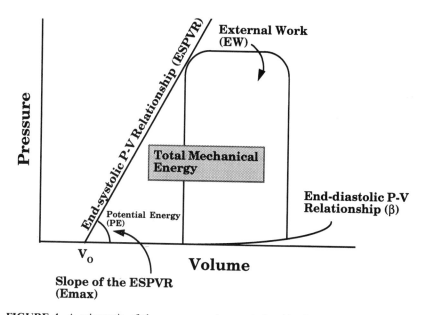

FIGURE 4. A schematic of the pressure-volume relationship. External work is the area within the pressure-volume loop, while potential energy is the area below the end systolic pressure-volume slope outside the pressure-volume loop. The summation of potential energy and external work is the total mechanical energy generated by ventricular contractions.

Patient Population

Thirty-three patients were randomly divided into the three study groups, 9 cold patients, 11 tepid and 13 warm. Preoperative parameters in each of these groups were not significantly different. The patient groups are illustrated in TABLE I. Ejection fraction was near 54%, the number of grafts per patient near four. Cardiopulmonary bypass time was 130 to 140 minutes and the cardioplegic arrest time was 82–86 minutes. All 33 patients had an uncomplicated recuperation. No patient had a perioperative myocardial infarct.

Statistical Analysis

Data were analyzed using the BMDP dynamic, release 7.0 and BMDP New System Version 1.0 (BMDP Statistical Software, Inc., Los Angeles, CA). All comparisons are done for each patient between the preoperative value, which is taken as the control level and the individual patient's postoperative determination. All measurements are expressed as a per cent difference from the preoperative to the postoperative value, and accordingly, are expressed as either a minus or a plus depending upon whether the postoperative determination was increased or decreased relative to the preoperative value. Results were expressed as mean ± standard error of the mean. The comparison of variables among the groups was tested by analysis of variance, and when significant by F test; mean values were

TABLE 1. Patient Groups

	N	Preoperative Data						Operative Data		
		Age (Years)	Age Range (Years)	Male (%)	Diabetes (%)	HTN (%)	EF (%)	No. of Grafts	CPB	X-Clamp
Cold	9	67 ± 3	50–79	56	33	78	55 ± 2	4.1 ± 0.4	146.6 ± 16.9	85.8 ± 10.6
Tepid	1	60 ± 2	41–73	91	27	55	53 ± 2	3.9 ± 0.2	132 ± 11.0	82.5 ± 7.4
Warm	13	61 ± 2	49–71	77	23	62	55 ± 2	4.0 ± 0.2	139.2 ± 9.8	83.4 ± 6.6

compared by the least significant method. Probability less than 0.05 was considered significant.

RESULTS

By 30 minutes of weaning from cardiopulmonary bypass, all patients were independent of pump support and did not require inotropes or pressors. The data were recorded in a reproducible manner as illustrated in FIGURE 1. This figure documents an end-diastolic frame of a four-chamber automatic boundary-detected image with the region of interest documented by a solid white line drawn around the left ventricular cavity. The graphics below the echo show the cavity area computed and displayed instantaneously with calibration marks in centimeters and with the electrocardiogram displayed for timing purposes. This illustration can be reproducibly duplicated for each patient.

The results are presented in TABLE 2 for all studies. The most significant data surrounded the measurement of preload recruitable stroke work and external mechanical work. In the cold group, there was a decrease in stroke work of 40% from baseline on an average for all nine patients. In the tepid group, this decrease was only 2% and in the warm group, there was an actual increase in contractility of 4%. The difference between the cold and the warm groups is significant at a $p < 0.05$ level. Indeed, the difference between preoperative and postoperative PRSW was significantly decreased in the cold group. In the tepid and warm groups, the difference from preoperative to postoperative was not significant.

External work, a determination of the mechanical work of the heart, a reflection of PRSW, documents a similar change with the cold group having a significant decrease compared to warm preservation. There was also a significant decrease in the cold group from the preoperative to the postoperative level with a mean decrease of 23%. The warm group on the other hand had a mean increase of 17% in the two determinations. Comparable data was obtained for total mechanical energy and maximal elastance (E_{max}) with the cold group having the largest decrease from preoperative to postoperative. However, the difference was not significant due to patient variability.

The isovolumic relaxation constant (tau) was not significantly different between the three patient groups. However, the stiffness coefficient (β), derived from modeling of the end diastolic pressure-volume relationship (FIGS. 2 and 4), which is the inverse of compliance, showed an increase in the cold and tepid

TABLE 2. Results from All Studies[a]

	PRSW	EW	ME	E_{max}	tau	β
Cold	$-40 \pm 10^*$	$-23 \pm 12^*$	-14 ± 8	-32 ± 17	-5 ± 4	↑
Tepid	-2 ± 7	-5 ± 9	-13 ± 9	-4 ± 8	-14 ± 5	↑
Warm	$+4 \pm 6$	$+17 \pm 5$	$+7 \pm 10$	-15 ± 11	-7 ± 2	unchanged

[a] All data are presented as percentage change from preoperative to postoperative ± SEM. PRSW: preload recruitable stroke work; EW: external mechanical work; ME: total mechanical energy; E_{max}: maximal elastance; tau: isovolumic relaxation constant; β: stiffness coefficient, the inverse of compliance.
* Significant difference between cold and warm groups, $p < 0.05$.

groups with no change in the warm patients. This documents decreased diastolic compliance or increased stiffness in the cold and tepid patients.

DISCUSSION

Myocardial stunning is clearly associated with everyday cardiac surgery. The fact that there is postischemic contractile dysfunction, which is reversible and not associated with infarction, is well known to cardiac surgeons.[1] We feel that calcium overload during reperfusion may well be a feature of this phenomenon.[2] Studies in our laboratory have attempted to document the temperature relationship of postischemic ventricular dysfunction in the experimental model. Two studies have been carried out which have been reported in detail by our laboratory.[9,10] In the first, we documented depression of Ca^{2+}-ATPase activity in the pig heart model during reperfusion in the cold blood cardioplegia group compared to the warm cardioplegia group. A higher Ca^{2+}-ATPase activity corresponds to a higher rate of sarcoplasmic reticulum calcium uptake, which would be consistent with a reduction of intracellular Ca^{2+}. In a rat study, measuring intracellular calcium levels, cold cardioplegia at 4°C resulted in significantly increased intracellular calcium during both arrest and reperfusion, while at 20°C the intracellular calcium level increased only during reperfusion. At 28°C and 37°C, intracellular calcium was stable during both arrest and reperfusion.

Our present clinical study documents that a more rapid recovery of normal contractile function occurs with warm cardioplegia/preservation. This is associated with improved or unchanged postoperative compliance but a decrease in compliance associated with cold preservation. Particularly, there was a dramatic reduction in preload recruitable stroke work and external mechanical work associated with the cold group. However, the fact that the cold patients did not recover complete ventricular function by 30 minutes after discontinuance of cardiopulmonary bypass does not imply that the patients are going to develop any significant long-term deterioration of left ventricular function. In fact, this is not the case. What it implies is that for rapid recovery of optimal function following cardiopulmonary bypass, warm preservation may be preferred. This approach may not necessarily be optimal, however, and indeed has the potential for other adverse sequelae such as depressed neurologic function.[11]

The imperative of this study rests with the use of warm preservation in instances when myocardial function is preoperatively so depressed that any reduction in postoperative function is clearly detrimental to patient care. In these instances, warm preservation is recommended. The etiology of depressed function in the cold patient is supported by the basic research described in our laboratory which documents that increased intracellular calcium accumulation occurs in the reperfused cold myocardium, and is associated with a decrease in sarcoplasmic reticulum Ca^{2+}-ATPase function. This occurs in the experimental animal, and probably occurs in the human heart as well.

REFERENCES

1. BOLLI, R. 1990. Mechanism of "myocardial stunning." Circulation **82:** 723–738.
2. KRAUSE, S. M. & M. L. HESS. 1985. Characterization of cardiac sarcoplasmic reticulum dysfunction during short-term normothermic global ischemia. Circ. Res. **55:** 176–184.
3. PEREZ, J. E., A. D. WAGGONER, B. BARZILAI, H. E. MELTON, JR., J. G. MILLER &

B. E. SOBEL. 1992. On-line assessment of ventricular function by automatic boundary detection and ultrasonic backscatter imaging. J. Am. Coll. Cardiol. **19:** 313–320.

4. SHAH, P. M., M. CRAWFORD, A. DEMARIA *et al.* 1989. Recommendations for quantitation of the left ventricle by two-dimensional echocardiography. J. Am. Soc. Echo. **2:** 358–367.

5. QUINONES, M. A., A. D. WAGGONER, L. A. REDUTO *et al.* 1981. A new, simplified and accurate method for determining ejection fraction with two-dimensional echocardiography. Circulation **64:** 744–753.

6. OSAMU, K., J. S. SAPIRSTEIN, W. B. DAILY, W. E. PAE & W. S. PIERCE. 1994. Left ventricular mechanics during synchronous left atrial-aortic bypass. J. Thorac. Cardiovasc. Surg. **107:** 1503–1511.

7. MISARE, B. D., I. B. KRUKENKAMP, Z. P. LAAR & S. LEVITSKY. 1992. Retrograde is superior to antegrade continuous warm blood cardioplegia for acute cardiac ischemia. Circulation **86**(Suppl. 2): 393–397.

8. SUGA, H. 1990. Ventricular energetics. Physiol. Rev. **70:** 247–277.

9. LIU, X., R. M. ENGELMAN, Z. WEI, N. MAULIK, J. A. ROUSOU, J. E. FLACK, III, D. W. DEATON & D. K. DAS. 1993. Postischemic deterioration of sarcoplasmic reticulum; warm vs. cold blood cardioplegia. Ann. Thorac. Surg. **56:** 1154–1159.

10. ENGELMAN, R. M., Z. KIU, J. A. ROUSOU, J. E. FLACK, III, D. W. DEATON & D. K. DAS. 1994. Intracellular Ca^{2+} transients during open heart surgery: hypothermic versus normothermic cardioplegic arrest. Ann. N. Y. Acad. Sci. **723:** 229–238.

11. MARTIN, T. D., J. M. CRAVER, J. P. GOTT, W. S. WEINTRAUB, J. RAMSAY, C. T. MORA & R. A. GUYTON. 1994. Prospective randomized trial of retrograde warm blood cardioplegia: myocardial benefit and neurologic threat. Ann. Thorac. Surg. **57:** 298–304.

Normothermic Ischemia in Coronary Revascularization

SAMUEL V. LICHTENSTEIN,[a] JAMES G. ABEL, AND
STEPHEN E. FREMES

Division of Cardiovascular and Thoracic Surgery
St. Paul's Hospital Heart Centre
University of British Columbia
Vancouver, British Columbia, Canada
and
Sunnybrook Medical Centre
University of Toronto
Toronto, Ontario, Canada

INTRODUCTION

The goal of myocardial protection during cardiac surgery is to maintain myocardial energy supply at a level greater than demand and provide a surgical field that is dry, motionless, and well visualized.[1,2] Preservation with cardioplegia attempts to optimize the ratio of energy supply to consumption and facilitate myocardial utilization of oxygen and substrates.[1] The ability of the heart to optimally utilize oxygen and substrate will be ultimately determined by the composition, distribution, duration of infusion and temperature of the cardioplegia solution.

Warm heart surgery was recently introduced as an alternative to conventional methods of myocardial protection.[3,4] As initially proposed, warm heart surgery consisted of normothermic potassium arrest with attempted "continuous" perfusion of warm blood cardioplegia—warm aerobic arrest.[4] The technical constraints of coronary bypass surgery however, frequently necessitate the interruption of either global or regional coronary perfusion with resultant periods of warm ischemia. However, since myocardial oxygen consumption is reduced by 90% with electromechanical arrest alone with little further protection provided by even profound hypothermia,[5] one could reason on that basis alone, that with electromechanical arrest *limited* periods of ischemia should be equally well tolerated with normothermia as with hypothermia.[2,6]

As experience with warm heart surgery increased, surgeons who were at first reluctant to interrupt the flow of cardioplegia at normothermia slowly became more comfortable with the safety of stopping cardioplegia during the construction of distal anastomoses in coronary bypass surgery. What initially started with only judicious interruption of cardioplegia at normothermia has "degenerated" in our hands to a frankly intermittent method of warm blood cardioplegia for coronary revascularization.

This communication presents the historical precedence and possible physiologic rationale for the superior clinical results achieved with *intermittent* warm

[a] Address for correspondence and reprints: Dr. S. V. Lichtenstein, St. Paul's Hospital Heart Centre, 1081 Burrard St., Vancouver, B.C. V6Z 1Y6, Canada. Tel.: (604) 631-5501; Fax: (604) 631-5375.

blood cardioplegia in coronary bypass surgery despite the attendant periods of normothermic ischemia. The associated clinical results have been presented in great detail,[7] and will only be highlighted here to lend support to specific conclusions.

METHODS

Patient Selection

From November 5, 1990 to December 31, 1992, 1732 patients presenting for coronary bypass surgery were enrolled in a prospective randomized trial comparing myocardial protection with warm versus cold blood cardioplegia.[8] In the warm arm 720 patients received *intermittent* antegrade cardioplegia and form the clinical base for this report.[7]

Surgical Technique

The operative procedure was previously described.[7,8] Briefly, after sternotomy and heparinization cardiopulmonary bypass was initiated at 2.4 L/min/m². Systemic perfusion temperature was maintained at 37°C. After cross clamping the aorta high potassium blood cardioplegia at 37°C was introduced into the root of the aorta at a rate of 200–300 mls/min to induce arrest which uniformly occurred within 30 seconds of infusion. After approximately 1500 mls the infusion was switched to a low potassium warm blood cardioplegia solution delivered at about 50–150 ml/min. If the left ventricle distended, cardioplegia administration was transiently stopped and the aortic root temporarily vented (-20 cm H_2O suction) to actively decompress the left ventricle. Cardioplegia was then restarted with the vent off and increasing pressure in the aortic root confirming competence of the aortic valve.

With the intermittent technique warm blood cardioplegia was routinely interrupted after the coronary artery of choice was incised and the aortic root was actively vented to clear the operative field of blood and facilitate construction of the distal anastomosis. After completion of the distal anastomosis cardioplegia was restarted down the aortic root while the graft was sized for appropriate length. Adequate cardioplegia flow was simply determined by palpation of the aorta to ensure a satisfactory pressure in the root. Cardioplegia was kept running down the root ($\pm$ grafts) until the next coronary artery was opened. Proximal anastomoses were performed according to the surgeon's preference either prior to or after aortic declamping and using a partial occlusion clamp.

When the internal mammary artery was used as a conduit its anastomosis was the last distal fashioned and a gentle clamp was placed on the artery until removal of the aortic cross clamp.

Data Collection and Statistical Analysis

All data relating to cardioplegia volume administered and the length of interruptions was collected prospectively. Intermittency was operationalized as the longest time off cardioplegia per patient in minutes (LTOC) and also the total cumulative ischemic time as a proportion of the cross clamp time per patient (PTOC).

The primary outcome of this study was prespecified as the composite end point of mortality, myocardial infarction (MI) by enzyme criteria and low output syndrome (LOS).

Operative mortality included all cause 30 day mortality or in hospital death if not discharged. Perioperative MI was defined as the appearance of a new Q wave by computer analysis of the ECG.[8] Enzymatic MI was defined as an elevation in creatinine kinase isoenzyme obtained at 0, 4, 8, 12, 20, and 28 hours post operatively. Presence of LOS was determined by majority decision of three anesthetists reviewing critical care charts. Criteria for LOS was predefined as a need for inotropic agents or IABP or both for >60 min, to keep systolic blood pressure above 90 mmHg in the presence of a low cardiac output (cardiac index: <2.2 $L/min/m^2$) and optimized filling pressures (>18 mmHg).

RESULTS

The demographics of this intermittent warm group are similar with respect to age, sex, functional class, left ventricular grade and urgency of operation to those reported in the literature from our institution.[7]

In the intermittent warm group the cross clamp was applied an average of 61.8 ± 22.2 minutes. The total warm blood cardioplegia (4 parts blood : 1 part crystalloid) delivered averaged 4624 ± 1992 ml for a mean flow rate of 75 ml/min over the entire cross clamp period. During this time 3.2 ± 0.9 was the average number of grafts constructed requiring cardioplegia to be shut off for a total of 28 ± 12.4 min or 48.2 ± 18.6% of the cross clamp interval (PTOC). Cardioplegia was therefore interrupted for an average of approximately 9 minutes for each of the distal anastomoses. The number of interrupted periods of cardioplegia flow are equivalent to the number of distal anastomosis constructed (3.2 ± 0.9 grafts). The longest single period of cardioplegia interruption (LTOC) for each patient was 11.4 ± 4.0 minutes, with the maximum interruption in excess of 20 min.

The data pertaining to LTOC (FIG. 1) and PTOC (FIG. 2) were divided into quartiles with groups of similar size.[7] Demographic and angiographic characteristics did not differ significantly between LTOC and PTOC quartiles. By univariate statistics increased LTOC was harmful (>13 min, $p = 0.046$), whereas increased PTOC was beneficial ($p = 0.07$). Stepwise logistic regression was performed, controlling for demographic and angiographic predictors. In the multivariate models, LTOC remained detrimental ($p = 0.07$) and PTOC remained beneficial ($p = 0.053$). Additional modeling after entering surgeon identity into the risk equation, eliminated the PTOC effect, whereas longer LTOC remained marginally significant as a risk factor ($p = 0.053$).[7]

DISCUSSION

Conventional myocardial protection depends on chemical electromechanical arrest and *hypothermia* to compensate for the lack of capillary perfusion. Unfortunately, hypothermia is not without serious detrimental effects on membrane stability, myocardial O_2 delivery, myocardial O_2 utilization and energy generation.[10,11] Warm heart surgery as initially conceived,[3] depends similarly on chemical electro-

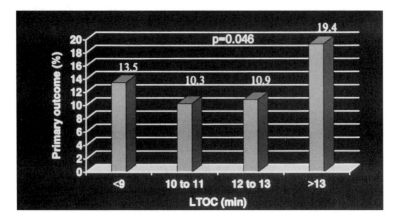

FIGURE 1. Primary outcome prespecified as the composite end point of mortality, myocardial infarction by enzyme criteria and low output syndrome versus single longest time off cardioplegia (LTOC).

mechanical arrest but with *continuous capillary perfusion* to compensate for normothermia.[4] This approach is sound physiologically and there are theoretical grounds for preferring continuous normothermic capillary perfusion.[9] However, the technical constraints of blood in the operating field, particularly in coronary bypass surgery may be exceedingly troublesome. A succesful surgical outcome demands a cardioplegic method which not only maximizes myocardial preservation but also permits a superior technical result. It is important to demonstrate there-

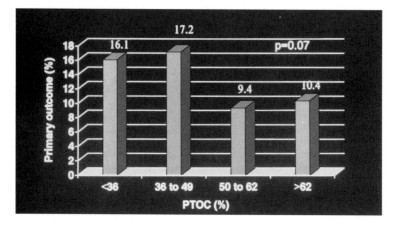

FIGURE 2. Primary outcome prespecified as the composite end point of mortality, myocardial infarction by enzyme criteria and low output syndrome versus percent time off cardioplegia (PTOC) as a proportion of the cross clamp time.

fore, that if attempts at local control fail to provide a bloodless field, warm blood cardioplegia can be safely interrupted for the period required to carefully construct a distal anastomosis under direct vision. Otherwise it might well remain a technically ineffective method despite its theoretical benefits.[9,12]

Of the two components of warm heart surgery—electromechanical arrest and continuous perfusion—the more important by far is the large decrease in myocardial O_2 consumption due to electromechanical arrest.[5] Without the order of magnitude reduction in myocardial O_2 consumption attending electromechanical arrest, continuous blood (Hct 20%) perfusion would have to be provided at an untenable rate of 500 mls/min to satisfy the energy demands of a normal heart of average weight. In contrast, electromechanical arrest reduces myocardial oxygen consumption to levels comparable to those found with profound hypothermia,[5] so short periods of normothermic ischemia should be equally well tolerated even in a hypertrophied heart.[6]

In this study the cardioplegia was interrupted for about 48% of the cross clamp time. It is important to note that this discontinuation of the cardioplegia did not occur over a single time period—the longest single ischemic interval in each patient extended from 6.8 ± 5.4 to 15.3 ± 5.0 min. Despite repeated episodes of normothermic ischemia with intermittent warm blood cardioplegia, the reported clinical outcomes are improved compared with those reported for intermittent hypothermic blood cardioplegia in a recent randomized trial.[8]

Although these outcomes may seem somewhat surprising, the data in the physiological[2,6] and often overlooked early clinical literature[13,14] would in fact predict that *brief* episodes (<13 min) of normothermic ischemia in the potassium-arrested heart are well tolerated. Melrose et al.[2] introduced elective cardiac arrest with potassium citrate (electromechanical arrest) at normothermia and showed that coronary flow could be safely interrupted for 15 min with return of normal cardiac activity and function. The safe period of nonperfused electromechanical arrest (normothermic ischemia) was extended to 30 min in subsequent experiments,[6] and it was suggested that even longer times could be tolerated if oxygenated blood was substituted for crystalloid. Some investigators found that even after 3 hours of normothermic nonperfused potassium-induced cardiac arrest in canine experiments the heart easily supported the circulation[13] without evidence of pathological changes in serial biopsies of the myocardium.

Effler et al.[13] at the Cleveland Clinic led in adopting normothermic elective cardiac arrest for clinical use. They were successful in 70 of their first 73 operations with a single bolus of blood and potassium citrate at normothermia followed by periods without coronary perfusion ranging from 6 to 58 minutes. Gerbode and Melrose described similar experiences with human hearts stopped at normothermia without perfusion for 50 to 65 minutes without ill effects.[14] For longer periods of arrest they felt a reasonable compromise was to perfuse the coronaries intermittently with a warm blood potassium solution—not unlike our present methodology.

The proposed myocardial tolerance to intermittent warm blood cardioplegia can be put in proper perspective if one considers the clinical experience[15,16] with normothermic *ischemic cardioplegia,* the antithesis of myocardial protection. In 1139 cases (636 valve procedures), at the Texas Heart Institute, the aorta was occluded at normal temperatures for 26 to 90 minutes and in many cases the hypertrophied heart allowed to beat until its energy stores were exhausted prior to standstill. Nevertheless, in this worst of all scenarios, the occurrence of stone heart was only 0.6% and only in the very hypertrophied hearts, or those with prior coronary artery disease and those with cross clamp times greater than 45 minutes.[15]

Accepting that truly continuous warm perfusion cannot be achieved in all cardiac procedures, it is interesting to speculate that compared to conventional hypothermic ischemia, normothermia may actually enhance the myocardial tolerance to short periods of ischemia. The advantages of cold ischemia are based on studies which have shown superior viability of the myocardium stored hypothermically for prolonged periods (4 hours).[17] The difference in O_2 debt between warm and cold arrest, if present, is relatively small over a 15–20-min period, but that difference is potentially magnified and its effects exaggerated with very long periods of ischemia. Since it is clinically rare (irrespective of the preservation method used) for the surgeon to simply stand by and record the ischemic time necessary for a heart to be irreversibly damaged, more relevant is the recently reported comparison of brief periods of normothermic versus hypothermic ischemia separated by intermittent periods of reperfusion.[8]

Several indirect pieces of evidence support the contention that maintaining the integrity of basal metabolism with normothermia as well as preserving the ability to quickly shift from aerobic to anaerobic metabolism and the capacity to deal with reperfusion may confer a benefit to short periods of ischemia at 37°C, which offsets the slightly higher oxygen consumption. Ischemic preconditioning of the myocardium may play an important role in this regard. It is known, for instance, that alternating intermittent periods of normothermic ischemia with periods of reperfusion in the working heart improves the myocardial tolerance to a subsequent episode of prolonged ischemia.[18–20] Preconditioning significantly reduces infarct size resulting from an extended period of coronary ligation and significantly improves systolic wall motion on subsequent reperfusion.[19] The mechanisms responsible for this curious response have not been well delineated but a slowed rate of ATP depletion[18] and release of adenosine during the period of ischemia have been implicated.[20] Since they were not surgically motivated, the preconditioning studies to date have been carried out in the working heart with high O_2 requirements, made ischemic at 37°C and allowed to beat until depletion of energy stores caused standstill. The potentially important effect of preconditioning with repetitive periods of normothermic ischemia and reperfusion in the context of surgical electromechanical arrest and an intrinsically diminished myocardial O_2 requirement,[7] is unfortunately not known at present and awaits evaluation.

There are several additional theoretical factors that may contribute to the safe outcome of intermittent normothermic ischemia as is surgically encountered (FIGS. 1 and 2). Interruption of cardioplegia flow renders the myocardium ischemic, but with O_2 needs at a minimum as a result of electromechanical arrest, the fully saturated reservoir of warm blood in the coronary vasculature may delay hypoxia and extend the time of aerobic metabolism despite the absence of coronary flow. Higher hematocrits, a real future possibility with warm blood cardioplegia would of course exaggerate this effect. Determination of the time when the myocardium shifts from aerobic to anaerobic metabolism will require technology such as probes capable of simultaneous measure of tissue pO_2 and tissue pCO_2 or pH. Noncoronary collateral flow, which may be substantial in normothermically perfused and systemically vasodilated patients, could maintain nutritive flow in hearts with minimal energy requirements. Short of resumption of electromechanical activity, noncoronary collateral flow would be beneficial in this regard. It has been calculated that cellular energy stores and anaerobic energy producing pathways should be able to maintain the viability of myocardial tissue, free of electromechanical activity, for many hours if metabolites are properly removed and substrate provided.[21] Repetitive prolonged infusions facilitate lactate and hydrogen ion washout, and the hyperglycemic cardioplegia solution used in this report[7,8] provides exogenous glucose substrate which may be protective during normothermic ischemia.[22] Supportive animal experiments have shown[14] that normothermic cardioplegia perfusion for 15 min alternating with 15 min of normothermic ischemia with sustained arrest may be carried on for as many as six hours and still obtain a normally active heart when the potassium citrate is washed away.

It should be appreciated that although warm blood cardioplegia delivery in this study was discontinuous, myocardial capillary perfusion was nevertheless occurring for better than 50% of the aortic cross clamp time during which activities not critical to the operation were carried out. It is not a return to the intermittent technique where a 500-ml bolus of 4°C solution is infused over 1–2 minutes perhaps 2–3 times during a one-hour cross clamp time for a total capillary perfusion time of 2–6 minutes. As one observer noted (W. M. Daggett, personal communication), in this current approach to myocardial protection the event is *cardioplegia off,* during which critical parts of the operation are performed, rather than the event being cardioplegia on with activity religiously suspended for the 2 min of cardioplegia infusion and then non-critical tasks performed with the cardioplegia flow turned off.

Since the myocardium takes up oxygen and substrate over time rather than by dose,[1] there may be an added benefit to an extended presentation of cardioplegia as opposed to the short vigorous bolus normally given after an ischemic episode. We believe that the reperfusion period after a normothermic ischemic episode is of paramount importance and should be ensured even if it means slowing of the operative pace. Ironically, those surgeons who are initially uncomfortable with warm cardioplegia, particularly when delivered intermittently, purposely increase the pace of the operation with compromise of the reperfusion periods and possibly surgical results. We would recommend based on conservative estimates of O_2 debt with potassium arrest and O_2 delivery with warm blood cardioplegia (Hct 20%), at least 5 min of reperfusion at 100–150 ml/min for every 15-min period of normothermic ischemia. Yau and associates[23] found that coronary patients who recieved intermittent warm blood cardioplegia following a similar protocol demonstrated improved diastolic compliance, reduction in CK-MB fraction, maintenance of mitochondrial function and adenine nucleotides and without a significant increase in lactate production when compared to intermittent cold blood cardioplegia. Their subgroup analysis suggested that the average flow rate of warm cardioplegia should equal or exceed 80 ml/min during the cross clamp period, which is similar to the average 75 ml/min infusion delivered in this study. More recently they randomized coronary bypass surgery patients to antegrade warm blood cardioplegia or retrograde warm blood cardioplegia or intermittent cold blood cardioplegia and found that antegrade warm blood cardioplegia delivered as described in this paper proved to be the best myocardial protection on the basis of metabolic parameters and clinical outcomes.[23] It is likely that at 37°C the myocardial cells having the abiliity to respond appropriately, through regulation of key enzyme systems and membrane functions, are able to protect themselves most effectively against the limited ischemic challenge.[18–21] Hence, repetitive short periods of normothermic ischemia followed by reperfusion may indeed be more adaptive than similar hypothermic ischemia,[8,18–20] in which the insult of ischemia is compounded by the added metabolic trauma of hypothermia.[3,10,11]

Continuous perfusion of warm blood cardioplegia has the potential to provide nearly ideal myocardial protection[4,12] and should be aimed for in all cardiac procedures. This is simply stating the obvious—blood flow is better than no blood flow—and needs no further comment. Equally obvious is that insistence on continuous perfusion cannot be allowed to compromise the technical standards of the operation. This perhaps is even more important with respect to graft patency and long-term survival than a potentially ideal method of intraoperative myocardial protection which jeopardizes surgical precision. The purpose of this communication is to demonstrate that when preferred methods at local control (irrigation, clamps, probes, snares, air jet) fail to provide satisfactory visibility, warm blood cardioplegia infusion may be safely interrupted for <13 min. It is a curious fact of our own preconditioning that hypothermic ischemia is well accepted and normothermic ischemia with electromechanical arrest causes grave concern, yet the negligible difference in O_2 requirements over a short period of time may well be overshadowed by the metabolic advantages of being warm. Any O_2 debt can very likely be repaid and utilized more effectively with appropriate reperfusion at normothermia.[11,8,23]

The safe time limit of elective cardiac arrest without coronary perfusion at normothermia has not been determined by this study.[7] Our own experience[7] and review of the literature[13,14,23] would suggest that repeated interruption of warm blood cardioplegia with generous intermittent reperfusion is safe, without attendant clinical or metabolic sequelae and provides superior myocardial protection to standard intermittent cold blood cardioplegia.[8]

Melrose *et al.*[2] originally introduced elective flaccid diastolic cardiac arrest with normothermic blood and potassium citrate to provide a surgical field that is dry, motionless and well visualized. Warm heart surgery is not meant to be a return to the "bloody, bold and resolute" surgery so necessary in the early days of poor operating conditions and time limitation.[24] Rather it is hopefully part of the evolution of cardiac surgery towards deliberate and precise techniques aimed at good long-term results as well as immediate operative survival.

SUMMARY

Warm heart surgery—continuous perfusion with normothermic blood cardioplegia—was introduced as an alternative to conventional intermittent hypothermic perfusion for myocardial protection. Interruption of global coronary flow, however, greatly facilitates the performance of distal coronary anastomoses and is the method that has evolved with many surgeons using warm blood cardioplegia for coronary revascularization. We present results (mean ± SD) in 720 patients undergoing coronary bypass surgery protected with intermittent warm blood cardioplegia and exposed to normothermic ischemia but with electromechanical arrest. An average of 3.2 ± 0.9 grafts were constructed per case with an average aortic cross clamp time of 61.8 ± 22.2 minutes. Cardioplegia was interrupted a total of 28.5 ± 12.4 min per operation. The percent time off cardioplegia (PTOC) expressed as a proportion of the cross clamp was 48.2 + 18.6%. The longest single time off cardioplegia (LTOC) was 11.4 ± 4.0 min per patient. Calculated mean cardioplegia delivery during the cross clamp period was 75 ml/min. PTOC and LTOC were divided into quartiles (PTOC: <36, 36–49, 50–62, >62%; LTOC: <10, 10–11, 12–13, >13 min) and related to prespecified composite outcome of mortality, enzymatic myocardial infarct and low output syndrome. PTOC was protective (event rate/quartile 16.1%, 17.2%, 9.4%, 10.6%, $p = 0.07$) and longer LTOC (event rate/quartile 13.5%, 10.3%, 10.9%, 19.0%, $p = 0.046$) borderline harmful. The data suggest that when necessary multiple periods of normothermic myocardial ischemia in the presence of electromechanical arrest are well tolerated and potentially protective provided that any single ischemic interval is <13 min.

REFERENCES

1. BUCKBERG, G. D. 1987. Strategies and logic of cardioplegic delivery to prevent, avoid, and reverse ischemic and reperfusion damage. J. Thorac. Cardiovasc. Surg. **93:** 127–139.
2. MELROSE, D. G., D. B. DIEGER, M. M. BENTALL & J. B. E. BAKER. 1955. Elective cardiac arrest; preliminary communication. Lancet **2:** 21–22.
3. LICHTENSTEIN, S. V., H. EL DALATI, A. PANOS & A. S. SLUTSKY. 1989. Long cross-clamp times with warm heart surgery. Lancet **1:** 1443.
4. LICHTENSTEIN, S. V., K. A. ASHE, H. EL DALATI, R. J. CUSIMANO, A. PANOS & A. S. SLUTSKY. 1991. Warm heart surgery. J. Thorac. Cadiovasc. Surg. **101:** 269–274.
5. BERNHARD, W. F., H. F. SCHWARTZ & N. P. MALICK. 1961. Selective hypothermic cardiac arrest in normothermic animals. Ann. Surg. **153:** 43–51.
6. BAKER, J. B. E., H. H. BENTALL, B. DREYER & D. G. MELROSE. 1957. Arrest of isolated heart with potassium citrate. Lancet **2:** 555–557.
7. LICHTENSTEIN, S. V., C. D. NAYLOR, C. M. FEINDEL et al. 1995. Intermittent warm blood cardioplegia. Circulation **92**(Suppl. II): II-341–II-346.
8. The Warm Heart Investigators. 1994. Randomized trial of normothermic verus hypothermic coronary bypass surgery. Lancet **343:** 559–563.
9. LICHTENSTEIN, S. V. & J. G. ABEL. 1992. Warm heart surgery; theory and current practice. In Advances in Cardiac Surgery. R. B. Karp, H. Laks & A. S. Wechsler, Eds. Vol. 3: 135–154. Mosby-Yearbook Inc. Chicago.
10. BALDERMAN, S. C., J. P. BINETTE, A. CHEN, J. N. BHAYANA & A. GAGE. 1983. The optimal temperature for preservation of the myocardium during global ischemia. Ann. Thorac. Surg. **35:** 605–614.
11. MAGOVERN, G. J., J. T. FLAHERTY, V. L. GOTT et al. 1982. Failure of blood cardioplegia to protect the myocardium at lower temperatures. Circulation **66**(Suppl. I): I-60–I-67.
12. LICHTENSTEIN, S. V., T. A. SALERNO & A. S. SLUTSKY. 1990. Warm continuous cardioplegia vs intermittent hypothermic protection during cardiopulmonary bypass; pro and con. J. Cardiothorac. Anesth. 4(2): 279–286.
13. EFFLER, D. B., H. F. KNIGHT, JR., L. K. GROVES & W. J. KOLFF. 1957. Elective cardiac arrest for open heart surgery. Surg. Gynecol. Obstet. **105:** 407–416.
14. GERBODE, F. & D. G. MELROSE. 1958. The use of potassium arrest in open cardiac surgery. Am. J. Surg. **96:** 221–227.
15. BLOODWELL, R. D., J. N. KIDD, G. L. HALLMAN, W. J. BURDETTE, M. J. McMURTREY & D. A. COOLEY. 1969. Cardiac valve replacement without coronary perfusion: clinical and laboratory observation. In Prosthetic Heart Valves. L. A. Brewer, Ed. 397–403. Charles C Thomas Inc. Springfield, IL.
16. MacGREGOR, D. C., V. S. MEHTA, F. N. METIS et al. 1972. Normothermic anoxic arrest of the heart. Is there a means of estimating the safe period? J. Thorac. Cardiovasc. Surg. **64**(6): 833–839.
17. FREMES, S. E., R. K. LI, R. D. WEISEL, D. A. G. MICKLE & L. C. TUMIATI. 1991. Prolonged hypothermic cardiac storage with University of Wisconsin solution; an assessment with human cell cultures. J. Thorac. Cardiovasc. Surg. **102:** 666–672.
18. MURRY, C. E., R. B. JENNINGS & K. A. REINER. 1986. Preconditioning with ischemia: a delay in lethal cell injury in ischemic myocardium. Circulation **74**(5): 1124–1126.
19. COHEN, M. V., G. S. LIN & J. M. DOWNEY. 1991. Preconditioning causes improved wall motion as well as smaller infarcts after transient coronary occlusion in rabbits. Circulation **84:** 341–349.
20. LIN, G. S., J. THORNTON, D. M. VAN WINKLE, A. W. H. STANLEY, R. A. OLSSON & J. M. DOWNEY. 1991. Protection against infarction afforded by preconditioning is mediated by A_1 adenosine receptors in rabbit hearts. Circulation **84:** 350–356.
21. SCHAPER, W., K. BINZ, S. SASS & B. WINKLER. 1987. Influence of collateral blood flow and of variations in MVO_2 on tissue-ATP content in ischemic and infarcted myocardium. J. Mol. Cell. Cardiol. **19:** 19–37.
22. EPSTEIN, C. S., F. N. GRAVINO & C. C. HAUDENSCHILD. 1983. Determinants of a

protective effect of glucose and insulin on the ischemic myocardium. Circ. Res. **52:** 515–526.

23. YAU, T. M., R. D. WEISEL, D. A. G. MICKLE, M. KOMEDA *et al.* 1991. Alternative techniques of cardioplegia. Circulation **84**(Suppl. II): II-686.

24. HEARSE, D. J., M. V. BRAIMBRIDGE & P. JYNGE. 1981. *In* Protection of the Ischemic Myocardium: Cardioplegia. 3–18. Raven Press. New York.

Preconditioning to Improve Myocardial Protection[a]

VIVEK RAO, JOHN S. IKONOMIDIS,
RICHARD D. WEISEL,[b] AND GIDEON COHEN

Centre for Cardiovascular Research
and
Division of Cardiovascular Surgery
The University of Toronto
Toronto, Ontario, Canada

INTRODUCTION

Coronary artery bypass surgery (CABG) has been shown to relieve angina and reduce mortality in patients with left main or proximal left anterior descending coronary artery disease,[1,2] triple vessel coronary artery disease,[3,4] and left ventricular dysfunction[5] and in patients with diabetes mellitus.[6]

Since Favaloro's original description,[7] the morbidity and mortality associated with CABG has steadily declined. The improved results of surgery are due in part to advances in surgical technique as well as improvements in perioperative myocardial protection. Despite the relatively low rates of morbidity and mortality currently associated with CABG,[8] patients with unstable angina, poor preoperative left ventricular function or a recent myocardial infarction still face an increased risk for surgery.[9] Further improvements in myocardial protection are required to reduce the risks of coronary bypass surgery for these patients.

This review summarizes the major developments in the composition and delivery of cardioplegia that have taken place at The Toronto Hospital. In addition, we highlight areas of current research aimed at unravelling the heart's endogenous ability to protect itself from ischemia (ischemic preconditioning). We discuss the relative advantages and disadvantages of various cardioplegic additives intended to improve myocardial protection during coronary bypass surgery.

The Introduction of Cardioplegia

The initial experience with coronary bypass grafting was associated with significant morbidity and mortality. The results of surgery were not only dependent on the technical success of the operation, but also on the ability of the surgeon

[a] Supported by the Heart and Stroke Foundation of Ontario (Grant B2267) and The Medical Research Council of Canada (Grant MT 9829). RDW is a career investigator of the Heart and Stroke Foundation of Canada. VR is a Research Fellow of the Heart and Stroke Foundation of Canada. JSI is a Research Fellow of the Heart and Stroke Foundation. GC is a Surgical Scientist at the Department of Surgery, University of Toronto.

[b] Address for correspondence: Richard D. Weisel, MD, Division of Cardiovascular Surgery, EN 14-215, The Toronto Hospital, 200 Elizabeth Street, Toronto, Ontario M5G 2C4, Canada.

to reduce intraoperative myocardial injury. The advent of elective cardiac arrest enabled surgeons to prolong the length of surgery and perform more complicated operations.

The benefits of hypothermia were first espoused by Dr. Wilfred G. Bigelow[10] at the University of Toronto. In a series of classical experiments, Bigelow and colleagues were able to show that moderate hypothermia (25–28°C) was able to protect the heart from ischemic injury. This technique, with or without intermittent aortic cross clamping was widely used in the 1970s.

Potassium arrest of the heart was first performed by Melrose and reported in 1955.[11] Unfortunately the high concentration of potassium (240 mmol) resulted in severe cardiac injury. The reintroduction of a crystalloid solution with a lower potassium concentration in the late 1970s enabled surgeons to electively arrest the heart with much less ischemic injury than with intermittent aortic cross clamping.[12]

Following Melrose's important discovery, several improvements were made in the composition and delivery of cardioplegia. The fundamental precepts of any cardioplegic technique involves protection against ischemic injury during the cross clamp period when normal antegrade coronary perfusion is lost. Optimizing the metabolic supply/demand ratio of the heart requires both a reduction in high energy phosphate utilization as well as an increase in the delivery of oxygen and metabolic substrates. The initial use of intermittent aortic cross clamping was abandoned by most surgeons with the realization that the ensuing ventricular fibrillation greatly increased the energy requirements of the heart. The introduction of hypothermic, hyperkalemic cardioplegic solutions was intended to induce asystolic arrest with minimal energy requirements. Intermittent doses of cardioplegia were then administered every 15–20 minutes in order to provide oxygen and metabolic substrates needed to satisfy the basal requirements of the arrested, hypothermic heart. In addition, multidose cardioplegic infusions were required to prevent the rise in myocardial temperatures and the replacement of cardioplegic solution caused by noncoronary collateral flow.

Cardioplegic Direction

Antegrade via the Aortic Root

At our institution, cardioplegia was traditionally delivered antegrade into the aortic root, a technique still employed by most surgeons. The initial arresting dose of between 500 and 1000 cc of cardioplegia is given immediately after aortic cross clamp application. Intermittent doses of cardioplegia can then be given through the aortic root at the completion of each distal anastomosis. In our institution, we attempt to provide the initial antegrade cardioplegia at a perfusion pressure of 70 mmHg. Although cardioplegia can be given continuously in an antegrade fashion, it usually results in flooding of the operative field and may compromise the technical success of the distal anastomosis. In patients with severe proximal disease, coronary stenoses may limit cardioplegic delivery and result in inhomogeneous myocardial perfusion.

Retrograde

Retrograde delivery of cardioplegia via the coronary sinus was described by Gott in 1957.[13] The advent of warm heart surgery has increased the interest in retrograde cardioplegia for coronary bypass surgery.[14] Retrograde cardioplegia has been employed to circumvent the inhomogeneous distribution of cardioplegia associated with antegrade delivery in the presence of severe proximal coronary artery stenoses. Unfortunately, evidence is mounting that retrograde perfusion does not adequately perfuse the right ventricle and does not provide as adequate capillary perfusion of the left ventricle as antegrade delivery.[15-19]

At our institution, we use a right atrial cannulation technique for retrograde delivery of cardioplegia. A purse-string suture is placed in the right atrium and the retrograde cannula is placed into the coronary sinus. The position of the cannula is confirmed by observing the distension of the posterior interventricular vein, monitoring the coronary sinus pressure (a sudden drop in pressure suggests that the cannula has slipped into the right atrium) and palpating the coronary sinus. Right atrial retrograde cardioplegia involves placing tapes on both cava and clamping the pulmonary artery. Cardioplegia is then delivered into the right atrium. Cardioplegia is delivered passively into the coronary sinus with the aortic root vented. However, valves in the orifice of the coronary sinus may prevent adequate retrograde delivery.[19,20]

Techniques have been proposed in an attempt to improve perfusion with retrograde delivery. A single prolene snare placed at the base of the coronary sinus just proximal to the posterior interventricular vein has been advocated to prevent dislocation of the cannula into the right atrium. There is a concern about injuring the coronary sinus and/or the posterolateral branch of the right coronary artery when placing this suture. Rudis et al.[21] found that coronary sinus occlusion during retrograde cardioplegia significantly improved perfusion to the right ventricle and posterior intraventricular septum while at the same time reducing the overall volume of cardioplegic solution administered. Menasche et al. proposed using a manually inflatable retrograde cannula in an attempt to secure its position.[22] The ideal positioning of the retrograde cannula is still unknown. Some surgeons insist on inserting the cannula as distal as possible into the coronary sinus while others feel that a more proximal position results in improved perfusion. At our institution, the cardioplegic cannula is placed as distally as possible into the coronary sinus and then withdrawn slowly until the posterior interventricular vein is seen to be distended.

When retrograde cardioplegia is given at normothermic temperatures, it is essential that it be given continuously to avoid normothermic ischemia. Proponents of continuous retrograde delivery claim that this technique does not flood the operative field to the same extent as continuous antegrade delivery. Nevertheless, most surgeons inevitably interrupt delivery of retrograde flow in order to optimize the completion of the distal anastomosis. Maatsura et al.[23] showed in a porcine model that three 7-minute interruptions during a 45-minute period of cardioplegic administration resulted in a larger infarct size, more myocardial acid production and a reduction in echocardiographic wall motion compared with intermittent cold antegrade/retrograde cardioplegia. Our clinical experience also indicates that warm cardioplegia interrupted for greater than 7 minutes results in ischemic myocardial metabolism.

Continuous retrograde cardioplegia is not truly continuous and the optimal rate that surgeons should attempt to deliver cardioplegia is not well defined. In a prospective, randomized trial[24] we found that retrograde flows of less than 100 mL/min were associated with myocardial lactate release and acid production following cross clamp removal. Flow rates of 200 mL/min minimized lactate production and maintained coronary venous pH within the physiologic range. Flow rates of 300 mL/min or higher did not confer any additional benefit, and thus we concluded that a minimum flow rate of 200 mL/min should be utilized during retrograde cardioplegia in an attempt to optimize distribution. In order to compensate for periods of interruption, "catch-up" infusions of cardioplegia are given following each interruption in order to maintain an average delivery of 200 mL/min.

Unfortunately, the major incumbrance to delivering high rates of retrograde flow is the developed coronary sinus pressure. Coronary sinus pressures above 40 mmHg may lead to perivascular hemorrhage and edema as well as direct coronary sinus injury.[25]

Combined Antegrade/Retrograde Delivery

The distribution of antegrade cardioplegia is potentially limited by proximal coronary artery stenoses. The distribution of retrograde cardioplegia may be unreliable, particularly to the right ventricle. A combination of both techniques may thus provide the optimal distribution of cardioplegia.[26-29]

One technique to provide combined antegrade and retrograde cardioplegia involves alternate infusions controlled by a stopcock on the cardioplegia line. Continuous retrograde delivery is attempted during the construction of the distal anastomosis. Distal and proximal anastomoses are completed in a sequential fashion. Following completion of each proximal anastomosis, the stopcock is turned to provide antegrade perfusion via the aortic root. Subsequent antegrade infusions then result in a combination of perfusion via the native coronary circulation as well as through all completed vein grafts. Care must be taken to carefully deair the aortic root prior to each antegrade infusion, and thus this technique is both time consuming and potentially dangerous should an air embolus travel down a vein graft or patent coronary artery. In a recent study of 75 patients undergoing isolated coronary artery bypass surgery,[30] we observed that the use of this technique using normothermic blood cardioplegia reduced lactate production, preserved high energy phosphate stores and provided greater perfusion of the heart during the cross clamp period than either antegrade or retrograde cardioplegic delivery alone.

A modification of this technique eliminated the requirement to repeatedly deair the aortic root. Following completion of each distal anastomosis, the proximal end of the vein graft is connected to a manifold system which runs in parallel to the retrograde delivery. This technique results in continuous cardioplegic delivery both retrograde via the coronary sinus and antegrade through each completed vein graft. In order to conserve saphenous vein, it is usually necessary to perform a proximal anastomosis following the second distal anastomosis. We usually perform the second distal anastomosis to the smallest vessel requiring a graft since this arterial territory will not be perfused by antegrade flow once the proximal anastomosis to the aortic root is completed. Simultaneous retrograde perfusion drains via Thebesian channels and the aortic root is vented to prevent venous congestion. We recently completed a clinical trial comparing these two techniques of combination cardioplegia and concluded that there were no clinically significant differences with respect to myocardial metabolism or recovery of left ventricular function.[31] However, the simultaneous technique was easier to perform and eliminated the risk of air embolism.

The optimal technique for delivering cardioplegia is still controversial. A combination of antegrade and retrograde delivery will likely provide the most uniform distribution of cardioplegia. New techniques of cardioplegic delivery will undoubtably result in improved perfusion to areas such as the right ventricle and posterior interventricular septum which are not adequately perfused with current cardioplegic techniques.

The Optimal Cardioplegic Temperature

Once homogeneous perfusion of the myocardium is established, the temperature and composition of the cardioplegia assume importance. The standard method of delivering either blood or crystalloid cardioplegia consisted of intermittent hypothermic (10°C) infusions. Hypothermia was often achieved with the supplemental use of a topical jacket or saline slush. We have found that the use of topical saline slush results in a phrenic nerve palsy with a risk of prolonged postoperative ventilation and respiratory complications. A similar observation was reported by Allen *et al.*, who found that topical hypothermia did not improve postoperative hemodynamics, did not reduce perioperative myocardial infarction or the need for inotropes, but did contribute to postoperative pulmonary morbidity.[32]

The aim of hypothermic arrest was to reduce myocardial oxygen requirements during the aortic cross clamp period. Buckberg *et al.*[33] found that hypothermia does not reduce myocardial oxygen requirements much beyond the reduction achieved with hyperkalemic arrest. In addition, hypothermic cardioplegia results in delayed recovery of both myocardial metabolism and ventricular function.[34-36] Rosenkranz *et al.* hypothesized that the metabolic dysfunction was due to the washout of Krebs cycle intermediates such as glutamate and aspartate and showed that a normothermic induction of glutamate and aspartate-enriched cardioplegia improved metabolic recovery in energy-depleted hearts.[37] Teoh *et al.*[38] demonstrated that a terminal infusion of warm blood cardioplegia (a "hot shot") immediately prior to cross clamp release resulted in a prolongation of electromechanical arrest, improvement in aerobic metabolism and increased diastolic compliance. The beneficial effect of the hot shot was thought to be due to early temperature-dependent mitochondrial respiration and ATP generation. Since this technique resulted in a prolongation of electromechanical arrest, the ATP produced was used for repair of intracellular ischemic injury and restoration of depleted energy stores.

It became evident that a normothermic induction combined with a normothermic terminal infusion permitted early recovery of myocardial metabolic function. Lichtenstein extrapolated these findings and proposed that normothermic (37°C) perfusion throughout the cross clamp period may be beneficial.[39] However, the modest increase in myocardial oxygen demand at normothermia necessitated continuous delivery of cardioplegia to avoid normothermic myocardial ischemia. Lichtenstein *et al.* employed normothermic antegrade blood cardioplegia in 121 consecutive patients and compared them to a historical cohort of 133 patients who recieved hypothermic (10°C) antegrade blood cardioplegia. Normothermic blood cardioplegia produced a significant reduction in perioperative myocardial infarction and the requirement for postoperative intraaortic balloon pump support. A subsequent prospective, randomized trial in 1732 patients revealed that normothermic blood cardioplegia led to a significant reduction in the incidence of postoperative low output syndrome.[40] This trial failed to show any differences in terms of perioperative myocardial infarction (by ECG criteria) or mortality. Another trial by the Emory group[41] confirmed the similarity of normothermia and hypothermia in terms of myocardial protection, but raised a concern regarding the increased incidence of postoperative neurologic events.

Another concern raised by opponents of normothermic surgery was the need to interrupt delivery of cardioplegia to permit adequate visualization of the distal anastamosis. We have found that interruptions greater than 7 minutes produce ischemic anaerobic metabolism detected by myocardial lactate release. Salerno et al.[14] introduced the concept of continuous, retrograde warm blood cardioplegia. Since retrograde delivery perfuses the heart via coronary veins, thereby avoiding proximal coronary artery stenoses, these authors hypothesized that perfusing an alternate capillary bed would allow for more continuous delivery of cardioplegia.

Our laboratory conducted a series of prospective, randomized clinical trials to determine the optimal composition and delivery of normothermic blood cardioplegia.[36,42-44] Fremes' original blood cardioplegic solution consisted of a 2:1 mixture of blood from the perfusion circuit to a crystalloid additive designed to achieve the same osmolarity and electrolyte composition of standard crystalloid cardioplegia.[45] We found that increasing the proportion of blood to 4:1 (achieving a hemoglobin concentration of 80 g/L) improved myocardial metabolic and functional recovery following cardioplegic arrest.[42] In addition, we found that an antegrade flow rate of 80 ml/min was required to ensure adequate perfusion with normothermic blood cardioplegia. In this study, "catch-up" infusions were given via the aortic root and each completed vein graft to compensate for periods of cardioplegic interruption necessary to complete the distal anastamosis. The volume of this infusion was calculated by the perfusionist to precisely compensate for the period of interruption and to maintain the average desired flow rate. We then proceeded to compare ventricular function following hypothermic and normothermic cardioplegia.[36] In this prospective trial involving 53 patients, we found that hypothermic cardioplegia resulted in a delay in recovery of postoperative left ventricular function. Normothermic cardioplegia resulted in increased systolic function and preload recruitable stroke work compared to hypothermic cardioplegia. In addition, patients in the normothermic group exhibited enhanced early diastolic relaxation (FIG. 1).

In a subsequent study comparing hypothermic and normothermic cardioplegia given either antegrade or retrograde, we found that warm blood cardioplegia resulted in greater lactate and acid washout with reperfusion.[43] In addition, this study examined the use of tepid (29°C) cardioplegia. We reasoned that tepid cardioplegia may provide the metabolic benefit of cold cardioplegia while permitting the immediate recovery of left ventricular function associated with normothermic cardioplegia. FIGURE 2 illustrates myocardial oxygen consumption, lactate release and acid release at 30 minutes of cardioplegic arrest in patients who received cold (8°C), tepid (29°C) or warm (37°C) cardioplegia. Tepid cardioplegia resulted in less lactate and acid washout compared to warm cardioplegia. In addition, at 12 hours following discontinuation of cardiopulmonary bypass, ventricular function remained depressed in patients who received cold blood cardioplegia. Both tepid and warm cardioplegia permitted recovery of left ventricular function at 12 hours following cardiopulmonary bypass. As a result of these prospective clinical studies, we now employ tepid blood cardioplegia for routine coronary bypass surgery.

Cardioplegic Additives

As the technique and temperature of cardioplegic perfusion becomes optimal, attention can then focus on various cardioplegic additives designed to mimic or enhance the heart's endogenous ability to protect itself against ischemia.

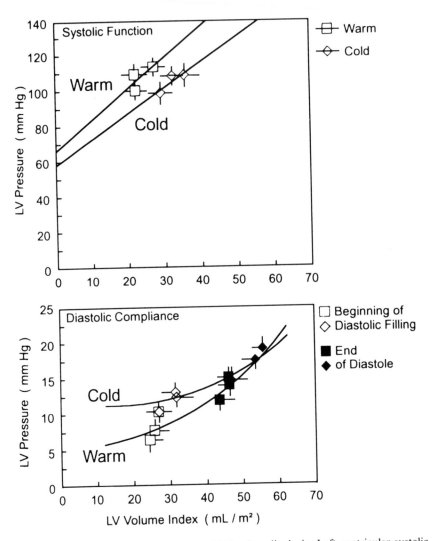

FIGURE 1. A comparison of warm and cold blood cardioplegia. Left ventricular systolic function and diastolic compliance are depicted as measured 3 hours following isolated coronary bypass surgery. Warm blood cardioplegia resulted in improved systolic function ($p = 0.001$ by ANOCOVA) and enhanced early diastolic relaxation ($p = 0.0002$ by ANOCOVA). (Adapted from Yau et al.[36])

Ischemic Preconditioning

In 1986, Murry, Jennings and Reimer reported that brief episodes of ischemia conferred protection against a subsequent prolonged ischemic insult.[46] They termed this phenomenon "ischemic preconditioning" and have since spawned an

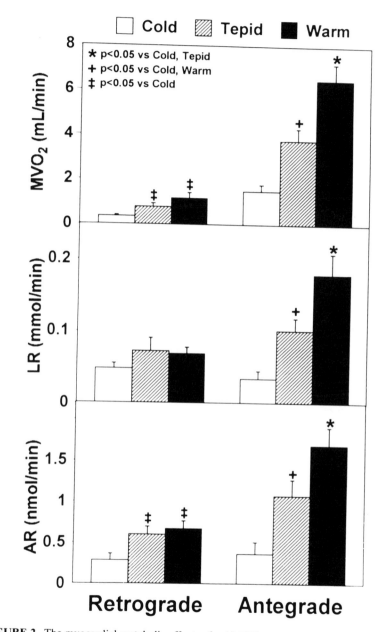

FIGURE 2. The myocardial metabolic effects of cold (8°C), tepid (29°C) and warm (37°C) blood cardioplegia. Regardless of direction, tepid cardioplegia reduced ischemic metabolism compared to warm. Cold cardioplegia was associated with the least ischemic myocardial metabolism, but resulted in a depression of early postoperative left ventricular function. MVO_2: myocardial oxygen consumption; LR: lactate release; AR: acid release.

extensive investigation into the characteristics, physiology and molecular mechanisms of this phenomenon. Ischemic preconditioning is perhaps the most powerful
endogenous protective mechanism discovered in the heart to date. In Murry's
experiments, preconditioning decreased infarct size from 20% to 5%. Similar
reductions in infarct size have been reproduced by a variety of investigators.

While preconditioning was initially described in a variety of animal models,
considerable evidence is now accumulating to suggest that a similar effect exists
in humans.[47–50] Yellon et al.[49] reported that brief periods of aortic cross clamping
prior to a sustained cross clamp period resulted in a preservation of high energy
phosphates. However, even brief periods of ischemia are undesirable and this
"mechanical preconditioning," albeit protective, is less attractive than a pharmacologic stimulation of the preconditioning effect.

In our laboratory, we have demonstrated that isolated monolayer cultures of
human ventricular cardiomyocytes were capable of producing a preconditioning
effect and we have subsequently shown that this effect is transferrable, suggesting
the presence of a humoral mediator[50] (FIG. 3).

Several pharmacological agents have been shown to mimic the preconditioning
effect including adrenergic agents, bradykinin, adenosine and amiloride. Unfortunately, most of these agents are either toxic or produce undesirable side-effects
when administered to humans. Adenosine is the agent most widely believed to

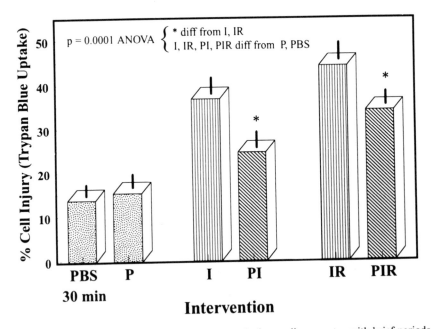

FIGURE 3. Preconditioning isolated human ventricular cardiomyocytes with brief periods
of ischemia. Preconditioning reduced injury as assessed by trypan blue uptake from 37 ±
2% to 15 ± 1% following a 90-minute exposure to simulated ischemia. PBS: phosphate
buffered saline (control); P: preconditioning stimulus (20 minutes of ischemia); I: 90 minutes
of prolonged ischemia; IR: ischemia followed by 30 minutes of normoxic reperfusion.
(Adapted from Ikonomidis et al.[50])

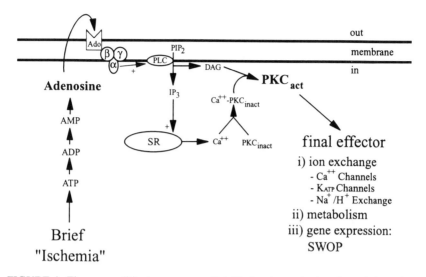

FIGURE 4. The preconditioning response. Brief ischemia results in a degradation of ATP into adenosine, the first diffusable metabolite. Adenosine permeates the cell membrane and then activates the adenosine receptor which stimulates the membrane bound G-protein. G-protein stimulation then precipitates the hydrolysis of membrane phospholipids such as PIP_3 (phosphatidyl inositol trisphosphate) to PIP_2, which in turn stimulates protein kinase C (PKC). PKC activation then stimulates an unknown effector protein which may be the K_{ATP} channel. The final mechanism by which the preconditioning response affords protection against ischemia remains unknown.

induce the preconditioning response.[51,52] However, its use in humans is limited by its potent vasodilatory effects.[53] As the molecular mechanisms of the preconditioning effect are clarified, new pharmacologic therapies will be developed which have the potential of having a significant myocardial protective effect (FIG. 4).

Glucose-Insulin-Potassium

Preconditioning is associated with a reduction in anaerobic metabolism. Pyruvate dehydrogenase (PDH) is an enzyme that regulates the metabolism of pyruvate by converting it into acetyl-CoA. When PDH is inhibited, pyruvate accumulates and is then converted into lactate with a corresponding production of acid protons. Insulin and dichloroacetate are two agents that can stimulate PDH activity and may therefore prove to be useful additives to cardioplegia.

In 1965, Sodi-Pollaris *et al.*[54] used a glucose-insulin-potassium solution to decrease electrocardiographic abnormalities in acutely infarcting myocardium. Since this initial report, several investigators have attempted to use glucose and insulin solutions either preoperatively, intraoperatively or postoperatively to improve the results of surgery.[55]

A direct inotropic effect of insulin has been suggested in animal models.[56] Gradinac *et al.*[57] administered insulin to patients who required intraaortic balloon pump (IABP) support following coronary bypass surgery and found an improvement in cardiac function. Svedjeholm *et al.*[58] used a glucose, insulin and glutamate solution for patients who could not be weaned from cardiopulmonary bypass. These authors identified sixteen patients who were unable to wean from bypass and administered the glutamate-GI solution prior to considering intraaortic balloon pump support. Only three of these patients subsequently required the IABP to be weaned from bypass and all three died of irreversible cardiac injury. The authors concluded that administration of glutamate-GI solution may potentially reverse transient myocardial dysfunction and avoid the use of mechanical support.

The role of exogenous glucose and insulin solutions in cardiac surgery remains unclear due to the lack of properly designed, prospective randomized trials. Basic science research combined with anectodal clinical evidence seems to suggest that insulin may be an important component in the cardioplegic formulations of the future. Reports from the diabetic literature indicate a relationship between insulin and protein kinase C activation.[59,60] In addition, insulin regulates the K_{ATP} channels in the β-cells of the pancreatic islet. Therefore, insulin-enhanced cardioplegia may represent a method of stimulating or augmenting the heart's preconditioning response.

Glutamate, Aspartate for Urgent Surgery

At our institution, Teoh *et al.*[61] used a glutamate and aspartate-enriched cardioplegic solution in patients undergoing isolated coronary bypass surgery. Although low risk elective patients did not benefit, there was a slight benefit of glutamate-aspartate to those patients undergoing urgent surgery for unstable angina. Similarly, Rosenkranz *et al.*[62] showed a benefit of glutamate-enriched blood cardioplegia in high risk patients with cardiogenic shock. These authors hypothesized that patients who present for surgery shortly after an ischemic event have a depletion of Krebs cycle intermediates such as glutamate and aspartate. Therefore, restoration of these metabolites should improve perioperative preservation of high energy phosphates. The preconditioning response is also associated with a preservation of high energy phosphates[50] and thus glutamate and aspartate may be able to act synergistically with a preconditioning-mimetic agent.

Calcium Channel Blockers

Calcium channel antagonists such as verapamil, nifedipine and diltiazem have been shown in experimental studies to preserve myocardial function and metabolism after normothermic ischemia,[63] crystalloid cardioplegia[64,65] and blood cardioplegia.[66] These agents prevent calcium influx and adenosine triphosphate hydrolysis during cardioplegic arrest. Calcium antagonists may also improve cardioplegic delivery by coronary vasodilation.

Unfortunately, calcium antagonists depress cardiac function and can induce heart block.[67,68] In a prospective randomized trial,[69] we found that diltiazem cardioplegia reduced perioperative ischemic injury, improved myocardial metabolic recovery and prevented postoperative tachycardia and hypertension. However, diltiazem cardioplegia was also associated with a depression of systolic function and atrioventricular block for a variable period after cross-clamp removal. As a result of this trial, we concluded that cardioplegia enhanced with calcium channel blockers may be beneficial for patients with normal preoperative left ventricular function who are at risk for postoperative hypertension, tachycardia, coronary spasm or ischemia, but may be detrimental for patients with poor ventricular function. In addition, we found a very narrow dose-response relation which limits the benefits of this cardioplegic additive.

Newer calcium channel antagonists such as amylodopine and felodopine may prove to have less of a myocardial depressant effect and thus may potentially have beneficial effects when added to cardioplegic solutions.

Antioxidants

Free radical-induced lipid peroxidation of the cell membrane has been shown to occur during cardiac surgery. Our laboratory showed a bimodal release of free radicals following cardioplegic arrest and reperfusion.[70]

Numerous laboratory and clinical studies have tried to assess the efficacy of a wide variety of antioxidant agents. Vitamin E and the cytosolic enzyme glutathione peroxidase are important endogenous protectors against free radical-induced injury. Unfortunately, a water soluble form of vitamin E is not currently available. In a prospective, randomized trial Yau *et al.*[71] were able to confer a protection against free radical injury by supplementing patients with a two week course of high dose vitamin E. Unfortunately, this protocol is impractical in high risk patients who require urgent or emergent surgery and do not have the luxury of time to increase vitamin E stores.

To date, there is very little evidence that the preconditioning response protects against oxyradical-induced injury. Therefore, antioxidant therapy may provide a useful adjunct to any myocardial protective strategy based upon the stimulation of myocardial preconditioning.

SUMMARY

Major advances in the composition and delivery of cardioplegia have helped to reduce the morbidity and mortality associated with coronary bypass surgery. The discovery of the preconditioning response should facilitate the development of more powerful myocardial protective agents. These new agents may act to directly stimulate the preconditioning response or may act in a supplementary fashion to either augment the response or provide protection from alternate pathways.

As new techniques of myocardial protection continue to be developed, the risk-to-benefit ratio of coronary bypass surgery will continue to improve. As a result of these improvements, surgeons will be able to offer surgery to an increasingly high risk patient population without increasing the morbidity or mortality currently associated with coronary bypass.

CONCLUSION

Coronary artery bypass surgery is currently associated with low morbidity and mortality; however, an increasing proportion of patients are presenting for surgery with increased risk due to unstable angina, poor preoperative left ventricular function or a recent myocardial infarct. Improved techniques of myocardial protection are required to lower the risks of surgery for these patients. The goal of any cardioplegic strategy is to resuscitate the ischemic have myocardium and maintain normal myocardial metabolism and function. We have reviewed the current strategy concerning both the composition and delivery of cardioplegia at The Toronto Hospital. In addition, we have highlighted the possible role of ischemic preconditioning in myocardial protection for patients undergoing coronary bypass surgery.

REFERENCES

1. TAKARO, T., P. PEDUZZI, D. M. DETRE, H. N. HULTGREN, M. L. MURPHY, J. VAN DER BEL-KAHN, J. THOMSEN & W. R. MEADOWS. 1982. Survival in subgroups of patients with left main coronary artery disease: Veterans Administration Cooperative Study of surgery for coronary arterial occlusive disease. Circulation **66:** 14–22.
2. VARNAUSKAS, E. and the European Coronary Surgery Study Group. 1989. Twelve-year follow-up of survival in the randomized European Coronary Surgery Study. N. Engl. J. Med. **319:** 332–337.
3. CALIFF, R. M., F. E. HARRELL, K. L. LEE, J. S. RANKIN, M. A. HLATKY, D. B. MARK, R. H. JONES, L. H. MUHLBAIER, H. N. OLDHAM & D. B. PRYOR. 1989. The evolution of medical and surgical therapy for coronary artery disease: a 15-year perspective. JAMA **261:** 2077–2086.
4. MYERS, W. O., B. J. GERSH, L. D. FISHER, M. B. MOCK, D. R. HOLMES, H. V. SCHAFF, S. GILLESPIE, T. J. RYAN, G. C. KAISER and other CASS investigators. 1987. Medical versus early surgical therapy in patients with triple vessel disease and mild angina pectoris: a CASS registry study of survival. Ann. Thorac. Surg. **44:** 471–486.
5. SCHAFF, H. V., B. J. GERSH, L. D. FISHER, R. L. FRYE, M. B. MOCK, T. B. RYAN, R. B. ELLS, B. R. CHAITMAN, E. L. ALDERMAN, G. C. KAISER, D. P. FAXON, M. G. BOURASSA and participants in the Coronary Artery Surgery Study. 1984. Detrimental effect of perioperative myocardial infarction on late survival after coronary artery bypass: report from the Coronary Artery Surgery Study. J. Thorac. Cardiovasc. Surg. **88:** 972–981.
6. POCOCK, S., R. HENDERSON, A. RICKARDS, J. HAMPTON, S. KING, C. HAMM, J. PUEL, W. HUEB, J-J GOY & A. RODRIGUEZ. 1995. Coronary angioplasty versus coronary artery bypass surgery: overview of the published randomized trials (abstract). Circulation **92:** I-476.
7. FAVALORO, R. G. 1968. Saphenous vein autograft replacement of severe segmental coronary artery occlusion: operative technique. Ann. Thorac. Surg. **5:** 334–339.
8. CHRISTAKIS, G. T., P. L. BIRNBAUM, R. D. WEISEL, J. IVANOV, T. E. DAVID, T. A. SALERNO and the Cardiovascular Surgeons at the University of Toronto. 1989. The changing pattern of coronary bypass surgery. Circulation **80**(Suppl. I): I51–I61.
9. RAO, V., J. IVANOV, R. D. WEISEL, J. S. IKONOMIDIS, G. T. CHRISTAKIS & T. E. DAVID. Predictors of low output syndrome following coronary bypass surgery. J. Thorac. Cardiovasc. Surg. In press.
10. BIGELOW, W. G., W. K. LINDSAY & W. F. GREENWOOD. 1950. Hypothermia: its possible role in cardiac surgery. Ann. Surg. **132:** 849–866.
11. MELROSE, D. G., B. DREYER, H. H. BENTALL & J. B. E. BAKER. 1955. Elective cardiac arrest. Lancet **2:** 21.
12. WEISEL, R. D., I. H. LIPTON, R. N. LYALL & R. J. BAIRD. 1978. Cardiac metabolism and performance following cold potassium cardioplegia. Circulation **58**(Suppl. I): I217–I226.
13. GOTT, V. L., J. L. GONZALEZ, M. N. ZUHDI et al. 1957. Retrograde perfusion of the coronary sinus for direct-vision aortic surgery. Surg. Gynecol. Obstet. **104:** 319.
14. SALERNO, T. A., J. P. HOUCK, C. A. M. BARROZO et al. 1992. Retrograde continuous warm blood cardioplegia: a new concept in myocardial protection. Ann. Thorac. Surg. **51:** 245–247.
15. PARTINGTON, M. T., C. ACAR, G. D. BUCKBERG, P. JULIA, E. R. KOFSKY & H. I. BUGYI. 1989. Studies of retrograde cardioplegia. I. Capillary blood flow distribution

to myocardium supplied by open and occluded arteries. J. Thorac. Cardiovasc. Surg. **97:** 605–612.

16. MENASCHE, P., J. B. SUBAYI, L. VEYSSIE, O. LE DREF, S. CHEVRET & A. PIWNICA. 1991. Efficacy of coronary sinus cardioplegia in patients with complete coronary artery occlusions. Ann. Thorac. Surg. **51:** 418–423.

17. CROOKE, G. A., L. H. HARRIS, E. A. GROSSI, F. G. BAUMANN, A. C. GALLOWAY & S. B. COLVIN. 1991. Biventricular distribution of cold blood cardioplegic solution administered by different retrograde techniques. J. Thorac. Cardiovasc. Surg. **102:** 631–637.

18. STIRLING, M. C., T. B. McCLANAHAN, R. J. SCHOTT, M. J. LYNCH, S. F. BOLLING, M. M. KIRSH & K. P. GALLAGHER. 1989. Distribution of cardioplegic solution infused antegradely and retrogradely in normal canine hearts. J. Thorac. Cardiovasc. Surg. **98:** 1066–1076.

19. QUINTILLO, C., P. VOCI, F. BILOTTA, G. LUZI, F. CHIAROTTI, M. C. ACCONCIA, C. MERCANTI & B. MARINO. 1995. Risk factors for incomplete distribution of cardioplegic solution during coronary artery grafting. J. Thorac. Cardiovasc. Surg. **109:** 439–447.

20. FABIANI, J. N., A. DELOCHE, J. SWANSON & A. CARPENTIER. 1988. Retrograde cardioplegia through the right atrium. Ann. Thorac. Surg. **45:** 595–602.

21. RUDIS, E., R. N. GATES, H. LAKS, D. C. DRINKWATER, A. ARDEHALI, A. AHARON & P. CHANG. 1995. Coronary sinus ostial occlusion during retrograde delivery of cardioplegic solution significantly improves cardioplegic distribution and efficacy. J. Thorac. Cardiovasc. Surg. **109:** 941–947.

22. MENASCHE, P. 1994. Experimental comparison between manually inflatable versus autoinflatable retrograde cardioplegia catheters. Ann. Thorac. Surg. **58:** 533–535.

23. MAATSURA, H., H. L. LAZAR, X. M. YANG *et al.* 1993. Detrimental effects of interrupting warm blood cardioplegia during coronary revascularization. J. Thorac. Cardiovasc. Surg. **106:** 357–361.

24. IKONOMIDIS, J. S., T. M. YAU, R. D. WEISEL, N. HAYASHIDA, X. P. FU, M. KOMEDA, J. IVANOV, S. M. CARSON, M. K. MOHABEER, L. C. TUMIATI & D. A. G. MICKLE. 1994. Optimal flow rates for retrograde warm cardioplegia. J. Thorac. Cardiovasc. Surg. **107:** 510–519.

25. PANOS, A. L., I. S. ALI, P. L. BIRNBAUM *et al.* 1992. Coronary sinus injuries during retrograde continuous, normothermic blood cardioplegia. Ann. Thorac. Surg. **54:** 1137–1138.

26. BHAYANA, J. N., T. KALMBACH, F. V. BOOTH, R. M. MENTZER & G. SCHIMERT. 1989. Combined antegrade/retrograde cardioplegia for myocardial protection: a clinical trial. J. Thorac. Cardiovasc. Surg. **98:** 956–960.

27. DRINKWATER, D. C., H. LAKS & G. D. BUCKBERG. 1990. A new simplified method of optimizing cardioplegic delivery without right heart isolation. Antegrade/retrograde blood cardioplegia. J. Thorac. Cardiovasc. Surg. **100:** 56–63.

28. KALMBACH, T. & J. N. BHAYANA. 1989. Cardioplegic delivery by combined aortic root and coronary sinus perfusion. Ann. Thorac. Surg. **47:** 316–317.

29. HAYASHIDA, N., R. D. WEISEL, T. SHIRAI, J. S. IKONOMIDIS, J. IVANOV, S. M. CARSON, M. K. MOHABEER, L. C. TUMIATI & D. A. G. MICKLE. 1995. Tepid antegrade and retrograde cardioplegia. Ann. Thorac. Surg. **59:** 723–729.

30. HAYASHIDA, N., J. S. IKONOMIDIS, R. D. WEISEL, T. SHIRAI, J. IVANOV, S. M. CARSON, M. K. MOHABEER, L. C. TUMIATI & D. A. G. MICKLE. 1995. Adequate distribution of cardioplegia. J. Thorac. Cardiovasc. Surg. **110:** 800–812.

31. SHIRAI, T., V. RAO, R. D. WEISEL, J. S. IKONOMIDIS, J. IVANOV & N. HAYASHIDA. Antegrade and retrograde cardioplegia: alternate or simultaneous? J. Thorac. Cardiovasc. Surg. In press.

32. ALLEN, B. S., G. D. BUCKBERG, E. R. ROSENKRANZ, W. PLESTED, J. SKOW, E. MAZZEI & R. SCANLAN. 1992. Topical cardiac hypothermia in patients with coronary disease. An unnecessary adjunct to cardioplegic protection and cause of pulmonary morbidity. J. Thorac. Cardiovasc. Surg. **104:** 626–631.

33. BUCKBERG, G. D., J. R. BRAZIER, R. L. NELSON *et al.* 1977. Studies of the effects of

hypothermia on reginal myocardial flow and metabolism during cardiopulmonary bypass. I. The adequately perfused beating, fibrillating and arrested heart. J. Thorac. Cardiovasc. Surg. **73:** 87–94.

34. FREMES, S. E., R. D. WEISEL, D. A. G. MICKLE, J. IVANOV, M. M. MADONIK, S. J. SEAWRIGHT, S. HOULE, P. R. MCLAUGHLIN & R. J. BAIRD. 1985. Myocardial metabolism and ventricular function following cold potassium cardioplegia. J. Thorac. Cardiovasc. Surg. **89:** 531–546.

35. WEISEL, R. D., D. A. G. MICKLE, C. D. FINKLE, L. C. TUMIATI, M. M. MADONIK & J. IVANOV. 1989. Delayed myocardial metabolic recovery after blood cardioplegia. Ann. Thorac. Surg. **48:** 503–507.

36. YAU, T. M., J. S. IKONOMIDIS, R. D. WEISEL, D. A. G. MICKLE, J. IVANOV, M. K. MOHABEER, L. C. TUMIATI, S. M. CARSON & P. LIU. 1993. Ventricular function after normothermic versus hypothermic cardioplegia. J. Thorac. Cardiovasc. Surg. **105:** 833–844.

37. ROSENKRANZ, E. R., G. D. BUCKBERG, H. LAKS & D. G. MULDER. 1983. Warm induction of cardioplegia with glutamate enriched blood in coronary patients with cardiogenic shock who are dependent on inotropic drugs and intra-aortic balloon support. J. Thorac. Cardiovasc. Surg. **86:** 507–518.

38. TEOH, K. H., G. T. CHRISTAKIS, R. D. WEISEL, S. E. FREMES, D. A. G. MICKLE, A. D. ROMASCHIN, R. S. HARDING, J. IVANOV, M. M. MADONIK, I. M. ROSS, P. R. MCLAUGHLIN & R. J. BAIRD. 1986. Accelerated myocardial metabolic recovery with terminal warm blood cardioplegia (hot shot). J. Thorac. Cardiovasc. Surg. **91:** 888–895.

39. LICHTENSTEIN, S. V., K. A. ASHE, H. EL DALATI et al. 1991. Warm heart surgery. J. Thorac. Cardiovasc. Surg. **101:** 269–274.

40. The Warm Heart Investigators. 1994. Randomised trial of normothermic versus hypothermic coronary bypass surgery. Lancet **343:** 559–563.

41. MARTIN, T. D., J. M. CRAVER, J. P. GOTT et al. 1994. Prospective, randomized trial of retrograde warm blood cardioplegia: myocardial benefit and neurologic threat. Ann. Thorac. Surg. **57:** 298–304.

42. YAU, T. M., R. D. WEISEL, D. A. G. MICKLE, J. IVANOV, M. K. MOHABEER, L. C. TUMIATI, S. M. CARSON & S. V. LICHTENSTEIN. 1991. Optimal delivery of blood cardioplegia. Circulation **84**(Suppl. III): III380–III388.

43. HAYASHIDA, N., J. S. IKONOMIDIS, R. D. WEISEL, T. SHIRAI, J. IVANOV, S. M. CARSON, M. K. MOHABEER, L. C. TUMIATI & D. A. G. MICKLE. 1994. The optimal cardioplegic temperature. Ann. Thorac. Surg. **58:** 961–971.

44. HAYASHIDA, N., R. D. WEISEL, T. SHIRAI, J. S. IKONOMIDIS, J. IVANOV, S. M. CARSON, M. K. MOHABEER, L. C. TUMIATI & D. A. G. MICKLE. 1995. Tepid antegrade and retrograde cardioplegia. Ann. Thorac. Surg. **59:** 723–729.

45. FREMES, S. E., G. T. CHRISTAKIS, R. D. WEISEL, D. A. G. MICKLE, M. M. MADONIK, J. IVANOV, R. HARDING, S. J. SEAWRIGHT, S. HOULE, P. R. MCLAUGHLIN & R. J. BAIRD. 1984. A clinical trial of blood and crystalloid cardioplegia. J. Thorac. Cardiovasc. Surg. **88:** 726–741.

46. MURRY, C. E., R. B. JENNINGS & K. A. REIMER. 1986. Preconditioning with ischemia: a delay of lethal cell injury in ischemic myocardium. Circulation **74**(5): 1124–1136.

47. LAWSON, C. S. 1994. Does ischemic preconditioning occur in the human heart? Cardiovasc. Res. **28:** 1461–1466.

48. KLONER, R. A. & D. M. YELLON. 1994. Does ischemic preconditioning occur in patients? J. Am. Coll. Cardiol. **24:** 1133–1142.

49. YELLON, D. M., A. M. ALKHULAIFI & W. B. PUGSLEY. 1993. Preconditioning the human myocardium. Lancet **342:** 276–277.

50. IKONOMIDIS, J. S., L. C. TUMIATI, R. D. WEISEL, D. A. G. MICKLE & R-K. LI. 1994. Preconditioning human ventricular cardiomyocytes with brief periods of simulated ischemia. Cardiovasc. Res. **28:** 1285–1291.

51. LIU, G. S., C. E. GANOTE & J. M. DOWNEY. 1994. Activation of adenosine receptors is required for protection from a direct opener of K_{ATP} channels in rabbit ventricular cardiomyocytes (abstract). Circulation **90**(Suppl. I): I478.

52. LIU, G. S., J. THORNTON, D. M. VAN WINKLE *et al.* 1991. Protection against infarction afforded by preconditioning is mediated by A_1 receptors in rabbit heart. Circulation **84:** 350–356.
53. BELARDINELLI, L., J. LINDEN & R. BERNE. 1989. The cardiac effects of adenosine. Prog. Cardiovasc. Dis. **32:** 73–97.
54. SODI-POLLARES, D., M. D. TESTELLI, B. L. FISLEDER *et al.* 1965. Effects of an intravenous infusion of a potassium-glucose-insulin solution on the electrocardiographic signs of myocardial infarction. Am. J. Cardiol. **5:** 166–181.
55. LAZAR, H. L. 1994. Enhanced preservation of acutely ischemic myocardium using glucose-insulin-potassium solutions. J. Cardiovasc. Surg. **9**(Suppl.): 474–478.
56. LUCCHESI, B. R., M. MEDIAN & F. J. KNIFFEN. 1972. The positive inotropic action of insulin in the canine heart. Eur. J. Pharmacol. **18:** 107–115.
57. GRADINAC, S., G. M. COLEMAN, H. TAEGTMEYER *et al.* 1989. Improved cardiac function with glucose-insulin-potassium after aortocoronary bypass grafting. Ann. Thorac. Surg. **48:** 484–489.
58. SVEDGEHOLM, R., I. HULJEBRANT, E. HAKANSON & I. VANHANEN. 1995. Glutamate and high-dose glucose-insulin-potassium (GIK) in the treatment of severe cardiac failure after cardiac operations. Ann. Thorac. Surg. **59:** S23–S30.
59. INCERPI, S., P. BALDINI, V. BELLUCCI, A. ZANNETTI & P. LULY. 1994. Modulation of the Na/H antiport by insulin: interplay between protein kinase C, tyrosine kinase and protein phosphatases. J. Cell Physiol. **159:** 205–212.
60. YU, B., M. STANDAERT, T. ARNOLD *et al.* 1992. Effects of insulin on diacylglycerol/ protein kinase C signalling and glucose transport in rat skeletal muscles in vivo and in vitro. Endocrinology **130:** 3345–3355.
61. TEOH, K. H., J. IVANOV, R. D. WEISEL, P. L. BIRNBAUM, M. M. MADONIK, D. A. G. MICKLE, T. E. DAVID, T. A. SALERNO and the Cardiovascular Surgeons at the University of Toronto. 1990. The surgical management of unstable angina: a clinical trial of warm induction glutamate aspartate blood cardioplegia for urgent revascularization. Abstracts of the American Association for Thoracic Surgery, Toronto, Ontario, May 1990.
62. ROSENKRANZ, E. R., G. D. BUCKBERG, H. LAKS & D. G. MULDER. 1983. Warm induction of cardioplegia with glutamate enriched blood in coronary patients with cardiogenic shock who are dependent on inotropic drugs and intra-aortic balloon pump support. J. Thorac. Cardiovasc. Surg. **86:** 507–518.
63. SMITH, S. J., B. N. SINGH, H. D. NISBET & R. M. NORRIS. 1975. Effects of verapamil on infarct size following experimental coronary occlusion. Cardiovasc. Res. **9:** 569–571.
64. LOWE, J. E., L. H. KLEINMAN, K. A. REIMER & A. R. WECHSLER. 1977. Effects of cardioplegia produced by calcium influx inhibition. Surg. Forum. **28:** 279–280.
65. MAGOVERN, G. J., C. M. DIXON & J. A. BURKHOLDER. 1981. Improved myocardial protection with nifedipine and potassium-based cardioplegia. J. Thorac. Cardiovasc. Surg. **82:** 239–244.
66. STANDEVEN, J. W., M. JELLINEK, L. J. MENZ *et al.* 1984. Cold blood potassium diltiazem cardioplegia. J. Thorac. Cardiovasc. Surg. **87:** 201–212.
67. MILLAR, R., D. A. LATHROP, G. GRUPP *et al.* 1981. Differential cardiovascular effects of calcium channel blocking agents. Potential mechanisms. Am. J. Cardiol. **49:** 499–506.
68. LATHROP, D. A., J. R. VALLE-AGUILERA, R. W. MILLARD *et al.* 1982. Comparative electrophysiologic and coronary hemodynamic effects of diltiazem, nisoldopine and verapamil on myocardial tissue. Am. J. Cardiol. **49:** 613–620.
69. CHRISTAKIS, G. T., S. E. FREMES, R. D. WEISEL, J. G. TITTLEY, D. A. G. MICKLE, J. IVANOV, M. M. MADONIK, A. M. BENAK, P. R. McLAUGHLIN & R. J. BAIRD. 1986. Diltiazem cardioplegia. A balance of risk and benefit. J. Thorac. Cardiovasc. Surg. **91:** 647–661.
70. WEISEL, R. D., D. A. G. MICKLE, C. D. FINKLE, L. C. TUMIATI, M. M. MADONIK, J. IVANOV, G. W. BURTON & K. U. INGOLD. 1989. Myocardial free-radical injury after cardioplegia. Circulation **80**(Suppl. III): III14–III18.
71. YAU, T. M., R. D. WEISEL, D. A. G. MICKLE, G. W. BURTON, K. U. INGOLD, J. IVANOV, M. K. MOHABEER, L. C. TUMIATI & S. M. CARSON. 1994. Vitamin E

for coronary bypass operations. A prospective, double-blind, randomized trial. J. Thorac. Cardiovasc. Surg. **108:** 302–310.

72. BUCKBERG, G. D., F. BEYERSDORF, B. S. ALLEN & J. M. ROBERTSON. 1995. Integrated myocardial management: background and initial application. J. Cardiovasc. Surg. **10:** 68–89.

Pediatric Myocardial Protection

From the Aspect of the Developmental Status of Myocardium

FUMIO YAMAMOTO,[a] SHIGEKO TAKAICHI,
TAKUMI ISHIKAWA, HIDEKAZU HIRAI, AND
TOSHIKATSU YAGIHARA

Department of Cardiovascular Surgery
National Cardiovascular Center
Fujishiro-dai
Suita 565, Osaka, Japan

INTRODUCTION

Since the chemical crystalloid cardioplegia was introduced into the clinical setting, clinical results of open heart surgery of adult patients have been improved significantly. However, pediatric cardiac surgeons are still in conflict over myocardial protection, because most techniques of myocardial protection available to pediatric cardiac surgery, at present, are based on myocardial protection conventionally obtained from clinical results of adult operation. And most techniques for pediatric myocardial protection used in the clinical setting require a theoretical rationale. On the other hand, there are a great number of papers[1-5] describing the difference between mature and immature cells in terms of anatomical, physiological, and pharmacological aspects. However, as most of these are from the animal experiments, the relevance of these experimental data to clinical application is not clear. Furthermore, the developing status of the neonatal heart depends on the life span of each animal species. Therefore, myocardial cells of some animals which have a relatively short life span such as rat and rabbit may show the relatively mature status of structure even at the age of one month. On the other hand, neonatal myocardial cells of relatively long life span animals such as human beings may show more immature status of structure. Furthermore, its maturity may also be influenced by underlying cardiac anomalies.

From this point of view, first of all, we have examined electronmicroscopically myocardial specimens obtained from human embryos and fetuses, and patients who received cardiac operation under cardioplegic arrest, to find out the relationship between the developing status of intracellular organelle and underlying anomalies. Secondly, rabbit myocardium at different ages was investigated in terms of cell maturity to ascertain which age of rabbit myocardium is equivalent to the human neonatal myocardium. Thirdly, using immature rabbit heart, the protective ability of several cardioplegic solutions was investigated in an isolated working preparation.

[a] Tel.: 06-833-5012; Fax: 06-872-7486.

TABLE 1. Materials for the Electronmicroscopic Study of Human Beings

No.	Age	Sex	Diagnosis	Operation
1	8 w	—	Embryo	—
2	9 w	—	Embryo	—
3	9 w	—	Embryo	—
4	9 w	—	Embryo	—
5	9 w	—	Embryo	—
6	24 w	—	Fetus	—
7	26 w	—	Fetus	—
8	0 m	M	TAPVC (IIa)	CPV-LA anastomosis
9	0 m	F	HLHS	Norwood procedure
10	0 m	F	TAPVC (Ib)	CPV-LA anastomosis
11	0 m	M	TAPVC (Ia)	CPV-LA anastomosis
12	0 m	M	HLHS	Norwood procedure
13	1 m	M	Cong. AS	OAC
14	1 m	M	Cong. AS	OAC
15	2 m	M	TGA (II)	arterial switch operation
16	2 m	F	Truncus Arteriosus (I)	Rastelli operation
17	2 m	M	VSD (II) PDA	closure and ligation
18	2 m	M	VSD (II)	closure
19	4 m	M	TAPVC (IIa)	cut back procedure
20	4 m	M	TGA (I)	Arterial switch operation
21	6 m	F	MR, P/o ECD repair	MVR
22	8 m	M	TGA (I)	arterial switch operation
23	9 m	M	TGA (I)	arterial switch operation
24	9 m	M	ASD (II)	closure
25	9 m	M	Cong. MR	MVR
26	10 m	M	TGA (I) PH	palliative Senning operation
27	10 m	M	cTGA TR	TVR
28	12 m	M	DORV PS	Rastelli operation
29	24 m	M	TAPVC (Ia)	CPV-LA anastomosis

MATERIALS AND METHODS

Electronmicroscopic Study with Human Specimens

Myocardial specimens were obtained from four embryos, two fetuses and 21 patients who underwent open heart surgery. The background of these specimens is shown in TABLE 1. In the case of the embryos, specimens were obtained from the ventricle under microscope, and in the case of the fetuses, myocardium of the left ventricle identified by microscope was obtained. In the case of the operated patient, myocardial specimens were obtained from the apex of the left ventricle before and after chemical cardioplegic arrest under extracorporeal circulation. All the specimens were stained with 2% osmic acid after fixation with 3% glutaraldehyde. After these treatments, about 30 to 50 electronmicrographs per specimen magnified 3500 times were taken to observe about 100 cells in terms of the developmental status of the intracellular organelle.

Criterion for Cell Maturity

The criterion for cell typing depending on cell maturity is described in TABLE 2A. Maturity of cell was classified according to conditions of the nucleus, myofibril, glycogen and mitochondria.

TABLE 2A. Criteria for Cell Typing

1) Nucleus-shape, condition of chromatin and nucleolus
2) Myofibril-localization and density
3) Glycogen-localization and compartment formation
4) Mitochondria-localization and density

Criterion for Cell Injury

After classification of cell type, severity of injury in each cell was determined according to the criterion of cell damage described in TABLE 2B such as conditions of the myofibril, mitochondria and nucleus. For example, when supercontraction of myofibrils was observed with normal mitochondrial cristae and perimembranous vacuole in the nucleus, it was classified as grade II injury.

RESULTS

Classification of Cell Maturity

All the cells that were examined in this study were classified into at least six types of cells.

Type A Cell

FIGURE 1A shows a typical electronmicrograph of this type of cell, which is the most immature cell. The nucleus is almost round, chromatin is uniformly distributed, and one or two nucleoluses are observed in the nucleus. Most of the cytosol is occupied by the glycogen compartment, although a few myofibrils are observed around the nucleus. A few mitochondrias are also observed in this type of cell.

Type B Cell

In FIGURE 1B, this type was identified with the irregular and oval shaped nucleus in which condensed chromatin was observed close to the inner membrane

TABLE 2B. Criteria for Cell Injury

	Myofibril		Mitochondria	
	Supercontraction	Disruption	Cristae	Nucleus
Grade I	(−)	(−)	normal	normal
Grade II	(+)	(−)	normal	perimembranous vacuole
Grade III	(+)	(+)	partially disappeared	perimembranous vacuole
Grade IV	(+)	(+)	partially disappeared	rupture

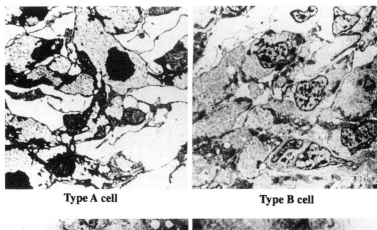

Type A cell   Type B cell

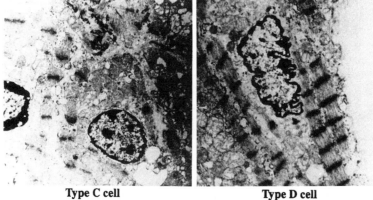

Type C cell   Type D cell

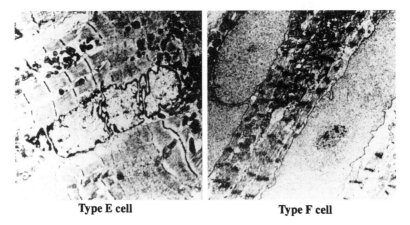

Type E cell   Type F cell

FIGURE 1. Electronmicroscopic finding of each type of cell.

of the nucleus. The developmental status of mitochondrias, myofibrils, Z-bands, as well as intercalated discs is more advanced in this type of cell.

Type C Cell

Type C cell is shown in FIGURE 1C with the difference in development and location of the mitochondria and myofibrils, although the nucleus is similar to the type B cell. Glycogen is distributed uniformly in the cytosol without making any compartment.

Type D Cell

Type D cell is shown in FIGURE 1D. The condition of the nucleus in this type of cell is very similar to that of type B or C cell. However, myofibrils are more developed to the whole cytosol and mitochondrias are also more developed between myofibrils.

Type E Cell

Type E cell is shown in FIGURE 1E, a typical mature cell which consists of oval shaped nucleus and mature intracellular organelles.

Type F Cell

In contrast with the similarity of the mitochondria, myofibrils, and other intracellular organelles except the nucleus to that of type E cell, a more advanced nucleus which possesses the oval shape and uniformly distributed chromatin is observed in this type of cell shown in FIGURE 1F. Therefore we classified this type of cell as an F type of cell, that is to say, supermatured cell.

The Relationship between Type of Cell and Age of Specimen

The relationship between cell types and age of specimen was analyzed and is shown in FIGURE 2. Type A cell was observed in specimens obtained from embryos, and type B cell was observed in specimens obtained from embryos and fetuses. Type C cell was observed in specimens obtained from fetuses as well as from patients operated on during the neonatal period. Type D cell was observed in specimens obtained from patients operated on during neonatal and early infancy. Type E cell was observed in the specimens obtained from the neonatal period to the age of two years. However, type F cell was observed just in the specimens obtained from 1-month-old patients of congenital aortic stenosis. Therefore neonatal myocardium consisted of at least three types of cells from the immature to the almost mature.

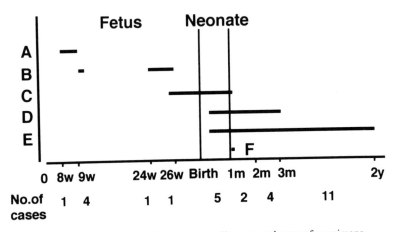

FIGURE 2. The relationship between cell types and ages of specimens.

Severity of Cell Damage

According to the criterion given in TABLE 2B, severity of cell injury before and after cardioplegic arrest was investigated. TABLE 3 shows the number of cells and its percent of all cells before and after cardioplegic arrest. The left hand column shows the severity of change of cell injury in specimens less than 3 months old. Eighty-seven percent of type C cells showed grade III injury after cardioplegic arrest, although 56% of type C cells showed grade II injury before cardioplegic arrest. In types D and E, there was no significant change before or after cardioplegic arrest. In type F cells observed in patients of congenital aortic stenosis, 54% of grade I and 46% of grade II injury were observed after cardioplegic arrest, because the specimen was not obtained before cardioplegic arrest due to deterioration of patient condition before the operation.

In the case of cells less than 1 month old, grade of injury in type C cells showed significant progress of injury after cardioplegic arrest although no significant change was observed in type D and E cells.

In the case of two patients with total anomalous of pulmonary venous drainage (TAPVC), type C cells again showed significant progress of cell injury after cardioplegic arrest. Type D and E cells again showed no significant change in the progress of cell injury before or after cardioplegic arrest (FIG. 3).

Electronmicroscopic Study of Rabbit Myocardium and Comparative Study of Several Cardioplegic Solutions in an Isolated Working Heart Preparation

Electronmicroscopic Study

Myocardial specimens obtained from rabbit heart at 1, 3, 7 and 30 days after birth were evaluated in terms of cell maturity according to the criterion described above (TABLE 2A). Electronmicrographs of 1 and 3 day rabbit hearts showed an immature status similar to type C cells of human beings and 7- and 30-day-old rabbit myocardial cells were similar to type E cells of human beings (FIG. 4).

TABLE 3. Grade of Cell Injury before and after Cardioplegic Arrest in Each Type of Cell of Operated Patients[a]

	Less than 3 Months Old					Less than 1 Month Old					2 Cases of TAPVC				
Grade	I	II	III	IV	Total	I	II	III	IV	Total	I	II	III	IV	Total
Type C															
pre-AC Number	0	72	7	50	129	0	72	7	50	129	0	72	7	0	79
%	0	56	5	39	100	0	56	5	39	100	0	91	9	0	100
post-AC Number	0	36	270	4	310	0	36	268	0	304	0	36	135	0	171
%	0	12	87	1	100	0	12	88	0	100	0	21	79	0	100
Type D															
pre-AC Number	25	124	0	6	155	0	122	0	6	128	0	122	0	0	122
%	16	80	0	4	100	0	95	0	5	100	0	100	0	0	100
post-AC Number	0	57	2	0	59	0	49	2	0	51	0	49	2	0	51
%	0	97	3	0	100	0	96	4	0	100	0	96	4	0	100
Type E															
pre-AC Number	463	554	29	7	1053	7	362	16	7	392	0	122	0	0	122
%	44	52	3	1	100	2	92	4	2	100	0	100	0	0	100
post-AC Number	0	115	20	0	135	0	65	8	0	73	0	65	8	0	73
%	0	85	15	0	100	0	89	11	0	100	0	89	11	0	100
Type F															
pre-AC Number	—	—	—	—	—										
%	—	—	—	—	—										
post-AC Number	75	65	0	0	140										
%	54	46	0	0	100										

[a] pre-AC: before aortic cross clamp on; post-AC: after aortic cross clamp off; Number: number of cells examined and classified according to the criteria of cell injury.

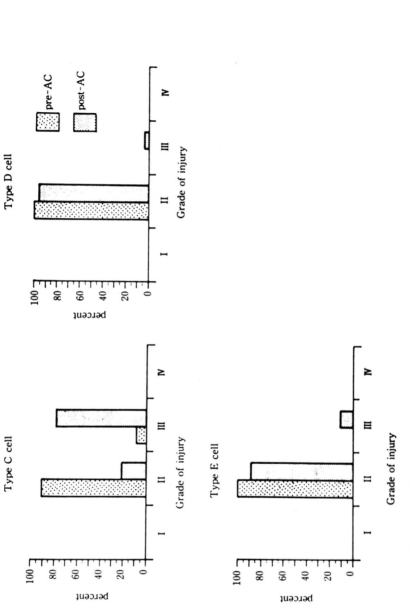

FIGURE 3. The change of degree in cell injury before and after cardioplegic arrest in two patients with total anomalous of pulmonary venous drainage (TAPVC).

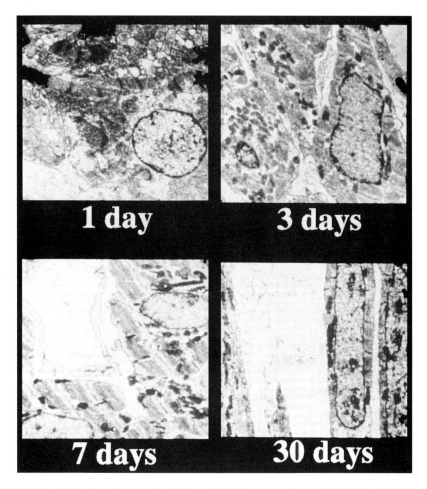

FIGURE 4. Electronmicroscopic finding of rabbit myocardium at 1, 3, 7 and 30 days after birth.

An Isolated Working Heart Study

Using an isolated working heart preparation of a three-day-old (perfusion medium was Krebs-Henseleit bicarbonate buffer containing 11 mM of glucose), several protective abilities of St. Thomas' solution and Bretschneiders' solution were investigated in terms of functional recovery and enzyme leakage. After 20 min of ischemia for the measurement of preischemic function such as aortic flow, coronary flow heart rate and aortic pressure, hearts were subjected to 3 min of cardioplegic infusion with St. Thomas' solution, Bretschneiders' solution, GIK solution and Krebs-Henseleit bicarbonate solution followed by 360 minutes ischemia at 20°C. Hearts were reperfused with the Langendorff mode at 37°C

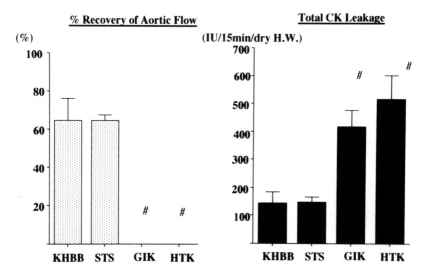

FIGURE 5. The effects of several cardioplegic solutions upon functional recovery and CK leakage in 3-day-old rabbit heart. *Left*: % recovery of aortic flow. Postischemic value of aortic flow was divided by preischemic control value and expressed by percent. *Right*: Total CK leakage. CK leakage during Langendorff reperfusion; IU/15 min/dry H. W. CK leakage was expressed by the international units per dry heart weight. #: $p < 0.05$ when compared to the KHBB group. Each group consisted of 6 hearts. KHBB: Krebs-Henseleit bicarbonate buffer; STS: St. Thomas' cardioplegic solution; GIK: glucose-insulin-potassium solution; HTK: Bretshneiders' solution.

followed by the working perfusion for the measurement of functional indices again. During Langendorff reperfusion, coronary effluent was collected and creatine kinase was measured as the tissue damage. Functional recovery was expressed by dividing the postischemic value of each function by the preischemic control value. FIGURE 5 shows the results of function and enzyme leakage and St. Thomas' solution improved postischemic recovery of function and enzyme leakage under hypothermic ischemia.

DISCUSSION

There is no established and standard method related to pediatric myocardial protection. There are many physiological differences between immature and mature hearts in anatomical, biochemical, and functional aspects,[1-5] and it is also unclear how these differences contribute to the extent of injury after ischemia. We have speculated about the reason for this obscurity and have arrived at the hypothesis that congenital heart anomalies possess the characteristic hemodynamics that may result in the different developmental status of the myocardium including the biochemical aspect. Therefore we investigated 1) how myocardial cells of human beings, especially operated patients, are different at different ages and different anomalies, and 2) how representative cardioplegic solutions protect immature cells against ischemia. In our electronmicroscopic study using specimens of human beings, these cells were classified into at least six types depending on the maturity of the intracellular organelle. It is particularly important to note that firstly, neonatal myocardium consisted of three types of cells and among these, type C cells showed less ischemic tolerance than D and E cells and, secondly, the developmental status of cells was influenced by the underlying anomalies. Of course, one needs to repeat the same study using patients who are accompanied with other anomalies not included in this study. However, this evidence can offer the beneficial viewpoint from which to choose the cardioplegic solution, especially in neonatal operation under cardioplegic arrest.

From the animal experiment using the three-day-old rabbit hearts whose cells were equivalent to type C cells of human beings, St. Thomas' solution offered the best protection in an isolated working preparation. These results may recommend the use of St. Thomas' solution among the several crystalloid cardioplegic solutions for neonatal cardioplegia, although we have to know the biochemical differences between six types of cells.

Therefore it is possible to conclude that, 1) neonatal myocardium consists of three different maturities of cells and their maturities are influenced by the underlying anomalies of the heart, and 2) St. Thomas' cardioplegic solution can offer, to some extent, beneficial effects upon myocardial protection of neonatal heart although room to modify the cardioplegic solution remains after elucidation of biochemical response of immature cells to the ischemia.

REFERENCES

1. JARMAKANI, J. M., M. NAKAZAWA & T. NAGATOMO. 1978. Effect of hypoxia on mechanical function in the neonatal mammalian heart. Am. J. Physiol. **224:** H469–H474.
2. WARSHAW, J. B. 1972. Cellular energy metabolism in the development. IV. Fatty acid activation, acyl transfer and fatty acid oxidation during development of the chicken and rat. Dev. Biol. **28:** 537–544.
3. BOLAND, R., A. MARTONOSI & T. W. TILLACK. 1983. Developmental change in the composition and function of sarcoplasmic reticulum. Am. J. Physiol. **245:** H998–H1006.
4. ROSS, B. A., C. L. SEIDAL & A. GARSON. 1984. Verapamil effect on vascular smooth muscle: variation in immature and mature animal. Pediatr. Cardiol. **252:** 5.
5. NAYLER, W. G. & E. FASSOLD. 1977. Calcium accumulating and ATPase activity of cardiac sarcoplasmic reticulum before and after birth. Cardiol. Res. **11:** 231–237.

Reactive Oxygen Species

Enzymatic and Nonenzymatic Antioxidants in Patients Undergoing Open Heart Surgery

R. K. SURI,[a,d] M. S. RATNA,[a] V. DHAWAN,[b] A. GUPTA,[b]
R. GUPTA,[a] K. SHARMA,[a] S. K. S. THINGNAM,[a]
G. D. PURI,[c] S. MADHULIKA,[b] AND N. K. GANGULY[b]

aDepartments of Cardiovascular and Thoracic Surgery,
bExperimental Medicine, and cAnesthesia
Postgraduate Institute of Medical Education and Research
Chandigarh, 160 012, India

INTRODUCTION

Open heart surgery during coronary artery bypass or surgery for valve replacement subjects the heart to the damaging effects of anoxic arrest and global ischemia resulting from cross clamping the ascending aorta. Reperfusion of the myocardium after removal of the aortic cross clamp paradoxically causes further damage (viz. reperfusion injury) to the myocardium.[1] Myocardial protection is an essential aspect of cardiac surgery, as the already ischemic and damaged myocardium is further vulnerable to such ischemic and reperfusion injuries.[2] The latter has been attributed to various mechanisms, of which reactive oxygen species (ROS) or oxygen free radical (OFR)-mediated injury is the most accepted.[3] Protective mechanisms against the ROS-induced damage are normally present in all cells. Antioxidants act by either preventing formation of ROS, or by converting them to less reactive substances, or by repairing the damage caused by them. These include enzymes like superoxide dismutase (SOD), catalase (CAT) and glutathione peroxidase (GP), which constitute the first line of defence against the ROS and other endogenous nonenzymatic antioxidants like reduced glutathione, vitamins A, E, and C and N-acetyl cysteine.[4]

The role of ROS in causing reperfusion injury has been proved[1] with evidence of reduced infarct size when scavengers of ROS (SOD and allopurinol) were exogenously administered after reperfusion.[5] No clinical study has been conducted so far that compares the generation of ROS with changes in antioxidant levels in patients of coronary artery disease and valvular heart disease.

The present study has therefore been undertaken i) to measure and find out the relative difference in levels of ROS activity and antioxidants in the two groups intraoperatively and postoperatively; ii) to localize the site of generation of ROS; and iii) to correlate these results with various clinical and hemodynamic parame-

---

[d] Address for reprints and correspondence: Dr. R. K. Suri, Prof. & Head, Department of Cardiovascular & Thoracic Surgery, Pgimer, Chandigarh (160 012), India. Tel.: (off.) 0091-0172-541031-39, Ext. 302; (res.) 0091-0172-545977; Fax: 0091-0172-540401.

ters, which would suggest the degree of oxidative damage caused by ROS and the possible role of antioxidants in myocardial protection against such damage.

MATERIALS AND METHODS

Between June 1994 and Jan 1995 20 patients undergoing open heart surgery were selected and divided into 2 groups of 10 each. Group I included 10 patients with coronary artery disease undergoing coronary artery bypass graft surgery, and 10 patients with chronic rheumatic heart disease requiring valve replacement surgery constituted group II. Patients with pulmonary and systemic infections, or hypersensitivity reactions were excluded from the study as these conditions are known to alter the levels of ROS and antioxidants. Drugs like xanthine oxidase inhibitors (allopurinol), captopril, nonsteroidal antiinflammatory drugs and steroids were stopped 72 hours before surgery. Preoperative clinical data and prebypass blood samples were used as control for the same patient.

Procedure

Similar myocardial protection methods were used in all the patients. Blood was sampled from three different sites: i) the radial artery; ii) from the right atrium, which is cannulated via the internal jugular vein with a Swan Ganz catheter; and (iii) from the coronary sinus using a 14 Fr retrograde perfusion cannula inserted immediately before bypass (and removed before the end of bypass).

Samples were taken just before going on CPB, at 30 min of global myocardial ischemia, *i.e.*, after application of the aortic cross clamp; at 10 min of myocardial reperfusion, *i.e.*, after unclamping the aorta; and 24 hr postoperatively. One sample of blood cardioplegia was also taken to exclude exogenous introduction of OFRs and enzymatic antioxidants. ROS generation assay and levels of antioxidants was conducted using standard methods described by earlier investigators.[6–11] Data analysis was done using Student t test (paired and unpaired) and coefficient of correlation, wherever applicable.

RESULTS

Generation of ROS (MDA & CL) and estimations of antioxidants (*i.e.*, SOD, GP, CAT, and vitamins A and E) were carried out from the three different sites. The results were compared between the groups, sites, and phases of surgery and were correlated with the various clinical (renal and pulmonary) and hemodynamic parameters.

There was a significant increase ($p < 0.01$) in ROS at 30 min of ischemia from baseline at all sites (TABLE 1). There was a further increase ($p < 0.01$) in ROS at 10 min after reperfusing the ischemic myocardium. There was a decrease in ROS at 24 hr after surgery as compared to their levels 10 min after reperfusion. This decrease was significant in the radial artery and coronary sinus samples. Of the three sampling sites, the CL was relatively high ($p < 0.01$) in the right atrium as compared to the other two sites. The oxidative damage caused by ROS was also detected by the increase in MDA levels, which followed a trend similar to that of the CL, at all the sites. The levels of vitamins A and E showed a maximum

TABLE 1. Pattern of OFRs, Enzymatic and Nonenzymatic Antioxidants during Various Phases of CPB between the 2 Groups and the 3 Different Sites[a]

		Group I			Group II		
		Rad	RA	CS	Rad	RA	CS
Baseline	CL	5.5	4.8	7.5	3.7	4.5	7.7
	MDA	5.0	5.2	4.9	5.9	4.8	5.8
	SOD	10.9	11.6	11.6	10.9	11.3	11.9
	CAT	38.7	40.1	43.3	38.1	35.9	36.3
	GP	58.1	65.6	68.6	63.5	65.6	64.8
	VIT A	19.2	49.6	25.4	4	14.0	13.2
	VIT E	14.6	31.5	21.8	3	23.8	22.9
30 min	CL	10.2	10.4	9.1	7.9	8.7	9.1
ischemia	MDA	10.7	10	9.4	10.5	10.8	9.9
	SOD	16.4	20.8	18	18.3	19.5	18.3
	CAT	56.4	56.5	52.8	61.4	56.4	49.5
	GP	72.7	81.5	76.5	78.5	81.5	77.8
	VIT A	0	2	0	0	0	13.2
	VIT E	3.2	0	0	6.9	13	22.9
10 min after	CL	11.1	13.4	9.8	9.4	13.6	10.4
reperfusion	MDA	12.0	13.0	10	12.7	13.1	10.4
	SOD	26.2	36.9	29.2	28.9	33.5	29.1
	CAT	77.7	71.8	69.6	80.7	22.5	63.1
	GP	84.8	98.5	104.8	97.7	98.5	99.3
	VIT A	0	10	1.9	0	3.6	0
	VIT E	0	0	5.3	27	19.3	20.8
24 hr postop	CL	8.3	8.2	—	7.1	7.7	—
	MDA	9.1	7.9	—	7.7	8.5	—
	SOD	36.1	47.2	—	38.6	46.2	—
	CAT	83.7	83.6	—	84.7	85.7	—
	GP	107.7	115.8	—	116.4	115.8	—
	VIT A	0	0.9	—	2.9	1.3	—
	VIT E	0	2.9	—	5.1	7	—

[a] CL: chemiluminescence (counts per minute/million cells $\times$ 10^4); MDA: malondialdehyde (nmole thiobarbituric acid reactive substances/mg protein); SOD: superoxide dismutase (U/mg protein); CAT: catalase (U/mg protein); GP: glutathione peroxidase (nmole/NADPH oxidized/min/mg protein); VIT A: vitamin A (μg/deciliter); VIT E: vitamin E (μg/deciliter); Rad: radial artery; RA: right atrium; CS: coronary sinus.

quantum of fall at 30 min ischemia from baseline. However, this fall correlated well with ROS levels, as maximum amount of increase in the ROS was also seen at 30 min after aortic cross clamping. There was a significant and continuous rise ($p < 0.01$) of all the three enzymes studied from the preoperative period, through 24 hr postoperatively (TABLE 1). Hemodynamic parameters improved remarkably in the postoperative period (TABLE 2). Other clinical parameters studied did not vary significantly in the postoperative period. There was no difference in the trends of ROS and enzymatic and nonenzymatic antioxidants between both the groups during various phases of surgery.

DISCUSSION

Various mechanisms have been proposed that could increase the ROS producing activity of phagocytes, especially polymorphonuclear leukocytes, in patients on cardiopulmonary bypass.[12] The increase in ROS seen at 30 min after aortic cross clamping and 10 min after reperfusion at the three sampling sites corroborated with earlier studies.[2] We did not find any difference in the trends of ROS between the two groups, which suggests that patients of valvular heart disease are equally prone to ROS generation as the patients of coronary artery disease. The higher levels of CL in the right atrium after reperfusion in comparison to the other two sites, with the lowest levels in the coronary sinus samples, indicates maximal contribution of ROS from the lungs and minimal contribution from the myocardium. Such findings were also reported by earlier investigators.[2,13] The levels of vitamins A and E showed a decreasing trend during cardiopulmonary bypass and did not reach baseline postoperatively, which was expected due to the increase in ROS level.

There was an improvement in cardiac index and pulmonary capillary wedge pressures postoperatively despite an increase in CL and MDA levels. This could be attributed to only minor and reversible alterations caused by the ROS, with the possible role of the antioxidants in myocardial recovery during and following surgery.

Thus, if the increased production of ROS and the simultaneous depletion of antioxidants can be further substantiated, the therapeutic role of antioxidants can be better defined. This understanding may go a long way towards reducing the incidence of myocardial dysfunctions related to reperfusion injury during cardiac surgery or cardiopulmonary bypass.

TABLE 2. Comparison of Hemodynamic Parameters during Surgery and Postoperative Periods in Group I (CABG) and Group II (Valve Replacement)[a]

	Group I				Group II		
	Baseline	Immediately Postop	24 Hr Postop	Baseline	Immediately Postop	24 Hr Postop	
HR	132	91	83	102	110	90	
BP	106/70(81)	125/73(91)	112/67(83)	156/70(91)	121/48(68)	116/60(75)	
PAP	15/7(10)	13/6(9)	20/10(15)	84/42(58)	37/27(31)	35/23(28)	
CVP	10	9	9	18	7	16	
PCWP	12.5	9.8	8.5	26	12.8	9.6	
COP	4.6	5	4.8	3.5	4.2	5.3	
CI	2.46	3.74	3.22	1.95	2.35	3.4	
SV	57	39	52	37	38	37	
TSR	853	850	852	1820	1432	882	
SVR	752	745	735	1460	1284	694	
PVR	108	98	105	688	484	329	
LCW	3.9	4.5	4.6	5	3.5	6.9	
LVSW	28.2	40.2	45.1	27.7	28.2	44.6	
RCW	1.5	1.5	1.4	3.1	1.6	1.42	
RVSW	10.3	10.2	9.8	30.9	14.6	12	

[a] HR: heart rate per minute; BP: arterial blood pressure in mmHg; PAP: pulmonary artery pressure in mmHg; CVP: central venous pressure in mmHg; PCWP: pulmonary capillary wedge pressure in mmHg; COP: cardiac output in liters/min; CI: cardiac index in liters/min/m^2; SV: stroke volume in ml/min; TSR: total systemic resistance in dyne-sec/cm^{-5}; SVR: systemic vascular resistance in dyne-sec/cm^{-5}; PVR: pulmonary vascular resistance in dyne-sec/cm^{-5}; LCW: left cardiac work in kg-m; RCW: right cardiac work in kg-m; LVSW: left ventricular stroke work in g-m; RVSW: right ventricular stroke work in g-m.

REFERENCES

1. FLAHERTY, J. T. 1991. Myocardial injury mediated by OFR. Am. J. Med. **91**(Suppl. 3C): 795–855.
2. DAVIES, S. W., S. M. UNDERWOOD, D. G. WICKENS, R. O. FENECK, T. L. DORMANDY & R. K. WALESBY. 1990. Systemic pattern of free radical generation during coronary bypass surgery. Br. Heart J. **64**: 236–240.
3. DAS, D. K. 1994. Introduction. *In* Cellular, Biochemical and Molecular Aspects of Reperfusion Injury. Ann. N. Y. Acad. Sci. **723**: xii–xvi.
4. HALLIWELL, B. 1994. Free radicals and anti-oxidants: a personal view. Nutr. Rev. **52**(8): 253–265.
5. GARDNER, T. J., J. R. STEWART, A. S. CASALE, J. M. DOWNEY & D. E. CHAMBERS. 1983. Reduction of myocardial ischemic injury with oxygen derived free radical scavengers. Surgery **94**: 423.
6. BOYUM, A. 1968. Isolation of mononuclear cells and granulocytes from human blood. Scand. J. Clin. Lab. Invest. **21**(S-97): 77–89.
7. CHEUNG, K., A. C. ARCHIBALD & M. F. ROBINSON. 1984. Luminol dependent chemi-luminescence produced by neutrophils stimulated by immune complexes. Aust. J. Biol. Med. Sci. **62**: 403–419.
8. SPITZ, G., N. J. LAWRIE, A. ZACCARIA, H. E. FERRARI, JR. & B. D. GOLDSTEIN. 1986. The reaction of 2-thiobarbituric acid with biologically active alpha, β-unsaturated aldehydes. Free Radic. Biol. Med. **2**: 33–39.
9. OBERLAY, L. W. & D. R. SPITZ. 1984. Assay of superoxide dismutase activity in tumor tissue. Methods Enzymol. **105**: 457–464.
10. BEERS, F. & I. W. SIZER. 1952. Spectrophotometric method for measuring the break of hydrogen peroxide by catalase. J. Biol. Chem. **195**: 133–140.
11. OHLORFF, C., G. LANGE & O. HOCKWIN. 1980. Post synthetic changes of glutathione peroxidase and glutathione reductase in the aging bovine. Mech. Ageing Dev. **14**: 153–158.
12. PRASAD, K., J. KALRA, B. BHARDWAJ & A. M. CHAUDHARY. 1992. Increased oxygen free radical activity in patients on cardiopulmonary bypass undergoing aorto-coronary bypass surgery. Am. Heart J. **123**: 7–45.
13. BANDO, K., R. PILLAI, D. E. CAMERON *et al.* 1992. Effect of oxygen tension and cardiovascular operation on myocardial anti-oxidant enzyme activities in patients with tetrology of fallot and aorto-coronary bypass. J. Thorac. Cardiovasc. Surg. **104**: 159–164.

Adaptive Defense of the Organism

Architecture of the Structural Trace and Cross Protective Effects of Adaptation

FELIX Z. MEERSON, MAYA G. PSHENNIKOVA, AND
IGOR YU. MALYSHEV

Institute of General Pathology and Pathophysiology
Academy of Medical Science
Baltijskaya 8
Moscow 125315, Russia

INTRODUCTION

Genotypic adaptation, as a result of which all animal and plant species have developed on the basis of heredity, mutations and natural selection, is a central phenomenon in biology as a whole and medicine in particular. For medicine it is essential that realization of genetic programs potentially embedded in the genetic apparatus predetermines to a great extent the resistance or, on the contrary, the vulnerability of an organism to specific factors of the environment. However, genotypic adaptation in itself neither concludes nor exhausts the content of the adaptation process. Ambient factors affecting the organism in the course of an individual life induce via control mechanisms a selective increase in expression of regulatory genes. As a result novel structural changes develop in the organism— the systemic structural "trace," which becomes the material base of stable long-term adaptation.[1,2] This individual phenotypic adaptation is, as it were, superimposed on genotypic adaptation; they are distinguishable only with difficult, but together they form the characteristic individual image of the organism and ensure enhanced resistance to environmental factors.

For biology and medicine it is important that adaptations, whose structural traces develop in vital organs or are very ramified, increase organismic resistance not only to a single influencing factor but also to many other factors. In other words, beside the direct protective effect, phenotypic adaptation possesses cross protective effects.[1,3]

The Role of the Architecture of the Adaptive Systemic Structural Trace and Selective Gene Expression in the Protective Effects of Adaptation

In adaptation to certain factors, the systemic structural trace proves spatially very limited, being localized in definite organs. For example, systematic administration of increasing doses of barbiturates, morphine, alcohol, and nicotine induced activation of nucleic acid and protein synthesis in the liver and not infrequently liver hypertrophy. Simultaneously, the potency of cytochrome P_{450} and the microsomal oxidation system was increased and the activity of cholesterol-7α-hydroxylase responsible for cholesterol oxidation was enhanced. As a result alimentary hypercholesterolemia appeared significantly reduced.[4,5] Thus under the action on the organism of poisons, this initial and rather simple in its construction systemic

371

SOME LINKS OF THE SYSTEMIC STRUCTURAL TRACE
OF ADAPTATION TO PHYSICAL LOADS

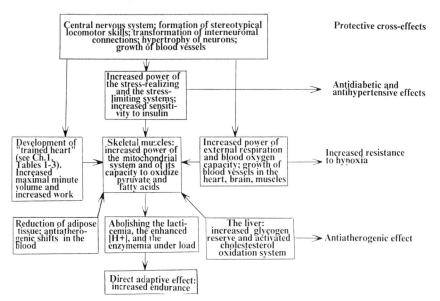

FIGURE 1. Some links of the systemic structural trace of adaptation to physical loads.

structural trace provides, in addition to the transition from urgent imperfect adaptation to stable protection against the poison (direct protection), an antiatherogenic effect (cross protection).

In adaptation to such factors as regular exercises or hypoxia, incomparably more ramified and complex structural traces form to provide the development of a much broader spectrum of protective cross effects. FIGURE 1 shows that, in adaptation to physical loads, the systemic structural trace occurs in nerve centers, endocrine gland, heart, skeletal muscles, etc. Consistently, adaptation to exercise possesses various protective cross effects: it limits atherogenic dyslipidemia,[6] reduces blood pressure at initial stages of hypertension,[7] beneficially affects diabetes,[8] and enhances the organism resistance to hypoxia and severe damaging stress exposures.[9] These diverse effects can explain the wide application of adaptation to exercise in prophylaxis and rehabilitation in diabetes, hypertension, and atherosclerosis.[6-8]

The mechanism of formation of many links of this ramified systemic structural trace is still far from being fully disclosed. Therefore, it is worthwhile to follow the relationship of cell structures determined by uneven gene expression in adaptation to high load by the example of such a vital organ as the heart. We shall try to systematize this by comparing the accumulation of definite myocardial structures in such disease-induced, *i.e.*, pathological reactions as cardiac compensatory hyperfunction under the conditions of heart defect, hypertension and intermittent physiological load in the training of a healthy organism.

The interrelations between structures in "trained" and "compensatory-hypertrophied" hearts presented in TABLES 1, 2 and 3 illustrate this regularity. The tables show that selective increases in mass and activity of strictly definite cardiomyocyte structures provide an increase in maximum performance, its economy and a high electric stability of trained hearts. The opposite complex of shifts being determined as seen from the tables by a reduced expression of respective genes, is associated with a decrease of all these parameters in compensatory-hypertrophied hearts. Apparently the adaptive shifts in trained hearts may be only due to increased expression of the same genes.

Of course, the pronouncement and the significance of each of these shifts are far from equivalent. For instance, the increase in mitochondrial mass induced by myocardial training is not large, while the increase in mass and potency of Ca-transport systems is considerable.

TABLE 4 reflects the results of our electronometric study.[21] It was shown that, first, with the adaptation regime used, the heart mass as a whole and the mitochondrial and myofibril volume per myocardium unit mass remained essentially unchanged. Only the size of each mitochondrion proved diminished and, naturally, the number of such smaller mitochondria per section unit area increased by 30% and the mitochondrial membrane surface per tissue unit volume increased by 28%, *i.e.*, moderately. Second, in animals adapted to physical load the surface of longitudinal channels of the SR was increased by 50%. At the same time, during adaptation to physical loads, an almost threefold increase was observed in the volume of the Golgi apparatus, where according to modern concepts cell-membrane forming processes take place, specifically those involving SR membranes. This may be indicative of the considerably activated formation of myocyte membrane structures during adaptation of the heart to physical loads.

According to current concepts, the membrane of the longitudinal channels of the SR and the sarcolemma are the sites where the Ca-activated Mg-dependent

TABLE 1. Differential Cation Transport and Electric Stability of the Trained Heart and of the Heart Subjected to Prominent Hypertrophy Due to Continuous Compensatory Hyperfunction[a]

Index	Trained Heart	Heart in Compensatory Hypertrophy
Ca-ATPase activity and volume of longitudinal SR channels per myocardium unit mass	Considerably increased (Penpargkul *et al.*, 1977; Guski *et al.*, 1981)	Reduced capacity to uptake Ca^{2+} (Harigaya & Schwartz, 1969; Chidsey, 1974)
Na,K-ATPase activity	Increased (Kyrge, 1976)	Decreased (Kaufman, 1972)
Relaxation velocity and relaxation index	Increased (Meerson & Kapelko, 1975)	Decreased (Meerson & Kapelko, 1972; Hood *et al.*, 1968)
Responses to high frequency of contractions and $[Ca^{2+}]$ increase	Hyperdiastole or similar diastole (Meerson, Kapelko & Shaginova, 1973)	Incomplete diastole (Meerson, Kapelko & Nurmatov, 1971; Meerson & Kapelko, 1972)
Ventricular fibrillation threshold	Increased[10]	Reduced[12]
Expression of Ca-ATPase and Na,K-ATPase genes	?	Reduced[13,14]

[a] References shown in parentheses in TABLES 1–3 are available in the book by F. Z. Meerson.[11]

TABLE 2. Differential Contractile Function of the Trained Heart and of the Heart Subjected to Prominent Hypertrophy Due to Continuous Compensatory Hyperfunction

Index	Trained Heart	Heart in Compensatory Hypertrophy
Content of myosin L-chains	Increased,[15] (Medugorac et al., 1975)	Decreased (Wikman-Coffelt et al., 1975, 1976)
ATPase activity of myofibrils	Increased (Bhan & Scheuer, 1972; Wikman-Coffelt et al., 1975, 1976)	Decreased (Wikman-Coffelt et al., 1975, 1976)
Contraction velocity	Increased,[16] (Meerson, Kapelko et al., 1976)	Decreased (Meerson & Kapelko, 1970; Meerson & Pshennikova, 1965)
Maximum minute volume and external work	Increased (Markovskaya, 1957; Meerson & Chashchina, 1978)	Decreased (Meerson & Larionov, 1975)
Oxygen consumption per unit performance	Decreased. Efficiency of performance increased (Markovskaya, 1957; Hollman, 1959)	Increased (Meerson & Larionov, 1975; Coleman & Gunning, 1970)
Expression of myosin genes	?	Myosin isozymes with reduced ATPase activity are coded[17]

ATPases are localized; these membranes play a decisive role in relaxation, by removing Ca^{2+} from the sarcoplasm and myofibrils, and also reduce the Ca-load on mitochondria. Thus they enable the coupling to phosphorylation, *i.e.*, the ATP resynthesis and the efficiency of oxygen utilization, which have been proved both in animals and in direct studies of trained humans. In these studies Heiss *et al.*[22] showed that the heart of an athlete consumes 1.5 to 2 times less oxygen at equal work. Thus the selective increase of a certain structure causes a huge effect by the parameters of organ capacity and economy, the expenditure of both energy and structures being more economic.

It is interesting that nature uses this way of optimizing functions of the organism not only in ontogenesis, in individual adaptation but also in phylogenesis, in genotypic adaptation. For instance, Weller and Forssman[23] using a method of intravital fixation with peroxidase labelling have calculated the volumes of SR T-system elements, SR longitudinal channels and mitochondria by electronograms. They compared rat with the heart rate of 250 bpm, ordinary mice with the heart rate of 400 to 500 bpm and Japanese "dancing" mice, which have a record heart rate among other mammals, of 700 to 900 bpm. It appeared that in rats the volume of T-system comprised 0.95%, the volume of SR longitudinal elements was 0.23%, and the mitochondrial volume was 29% of the myocardium volume; in ordinary mice the values were 1.2, 0.38, and 30%, respectively; and in Japanese "dancing" mice the same indices were 1.33, 0.53, and 35%, respectively. Therefore, in these species under comparison, the threefold increase in the heart rate was accompanied by the enhancement of T-system volume in 1.5 times, of SR longitudinal channel volume in 2.3 times and of mitochondrial volume by as little as 6%. The most probable explanation of these ratios is that the species with higher heart rate and greater Ca^{2+} influx into cells have correspondingly more potent SR, which is necessary for Ca^{2+} elimination from the cell. When Ca^{2+} is eliminated in a timely

TABLE 3. Differential Energy Supply to the Trained Heart and to the Heart Subjected to Prominent Hypertrophy Due to Continuous Compensatory Hyperfunction

Index	Trained Heart	Heart in Compensatory Hypertrophy
Number of coronary capillaries per unit myocardial mass	Increased (Petren *et al.*, 1937; Tepperman & Pearlman, 1961)	Decreased (Wearn, 1941; Honig *et al.*, 1974)
Oxygen diffusion distance	Decreased[18]	Increased (Honig *et al.*, 1974)
Coronary reserve	Increased[18]	Decreased (Honig *et al.*, 1974; Marchetti *et al.*, 1972)
Mitochondrial surface per unit myocardial volume	Increased[19]	Decreased (Zak & Fishman, 1971; Goldstein *et al.*, 1974)
Activities of respiratory chain enzyme	Slightly increased[20]	Decreased (Wollenberger & Schultze, 1963)
Activities of hexokinase and glycolytic enzymes	Increased (Walpurger & Anger, 1970; Scheuer *et al.*, 1970)	Unchanged[11]

way, mitochondrial potency proves sufficient to provide the increasing contractile function with energy.

On the whole the above-mentioned supports the well-known Baer's law that "ontogenesis repeats phylogenesis" and reminds us again that, in any approach, adaptation is not only a medical but first of all also a general biological problem.

In terms of our presentation it is important to underline that these are just the selective gene expression and the selective growth of structures that provide the most efficient adaptation of the heart and, presumably, of any other organ under normal periodic load, with a slight increase in the organ mass.

The systemic structural trace of adaptation to hypoxia is no less complicated and ramified (see scheme in FIG. 2).

More than 15 years ago it was shown and subsequently confirmed that in the very first days of the exposure to hypoxia the formation of this and other components of the systemic structural "trace" manifests itself as enhanced RNA and

TABLE 4. Structural Ratio in Myocardial Cells in Heart Adaptation[a]

Index[b]	Control	Swimming	p
Mitochondrium volume	0.314 ± 0.011	0.361 ± 0.038	
Number of mitochondria[c]	0.670 ± 0.041	0.872 ± 0.088	<0.05
Surface of mitochondrial external membranes	2.043 ± 0.125	2.616 ± 0.055	<0.01
Surface of longitudinal channels	1.787 ± 0.037	2.636 ± 0.362	<0.05
Golgi apparatus volume	0.00105 ± 0.00016	0.00296 ± 0.0009	<0.005

[a] Each group contained three animals; analysis was performed using 72 electron graphs.
[b] Per tissue unit volume.
[c] Per section unit area.

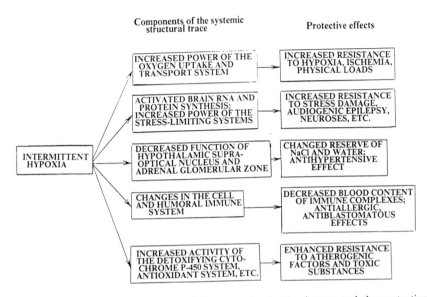

FIGURE 2. The major components of the systemic structural trace and the protective effects of adaptation to intermittent hypoxia.

protein synthesis in the lungs, heart, coronary vessels,[1,4] bone marrow,[24] and the sympathetic neurons innervating the heart.[25]

This activation results in increased growth of cellular structures responsible for the uptake and transport of oxygen, namely, increased mass of the lungs, their surface and number of lung alveoli, moderate hypertrophy and increased functional capacity of the heart, increased density of vascular network in the heart, brain and skeletal muscles and increased capacity of the coronary bed, increased mass of red cells and increased hemoglobin content in the blood, and increased myoglobin concentration in the skeletal muscles. At the same time the power of the energy supply system grows at the level of cells in the heart and other organs. This is evident as an increased amount of mitochondria, activated enzymes of the respiratory chain, and enhanced power of the glycolytic system.[a]

This component of the systemic structural "trace" allows the adapted organism to increase the maximal respiratory volume, the coefficient of oxygen utilization, the efficiency of energy generation and energy utilization, the contractile capacity of the heart, the oxygen capacity of the blood, and the tissue capacity to utilize oxygen. Simultaneously adaptation provides a decrease in basal metabolism and economical oxygen utilization by tissues. This results in decreased oxygen consumption by organs, tissues and the whole organism at sea level[1,4] and sufficiently high oxygen consumption at higher altitude.

In this process, organismic resistance to altitude increases (direct protective effect) along with resistance to exercise (cross protective effect) as is shown by the scheme in FIGURE 2. It is seen that the activated synthesis and increased

---

[a] For references see Chapter 3 in the book by F. Z. Meerson.[3]

content of RNA and proteins in the brain cortex and subcortical structures[1] as well as the increased activities of antioxidant enzymes in the brain, liver, and heart are attended by a whole group of cross protective effects. Among these are increased resistance to stress damage[26] and prevention of audiogenic convulsions.[1,27] Apparently the same shifts may play a role in the therapeutic effect of adaptation to intermittent hypoxia in newly diagnosed paranoid schizophrenia[3] and neurasthenia.[26] Furthermore, FIGURE 2 shows that the components of systemic structural trace play a role in antihypertensive,[1] antiarrhythmic[28] and antiatherogenic[3,6] cross protective effects of this adaptation.

With regard to our presentation, selective expression of strictly definite genes plays a crucial role in the formation of the ramified systemic structural trace of adaptation to hypoxic or ischemic hypoxia. The most striking example of selective and successive gene expression occurring during the adaptive formation of the systemic structural trace is the increased growth of coronary blood vessels in the adaptation of the heart to ischemia. Experiments carried out by W. Schaper and co-workers[29] have shown that many genes may be activated in adaptation to hypoxia, for example, genes coding blood vessel growth factors TGF-b, b-ECGF, bFGF or HBFG-1 (heparin-binding growth factor-1, which was recently discovered by W. Schaper in cardiac ischemia), especially as the increase in coronary vascularization and in blood flow are well known in adaptation to hypoxia.

Adaptation to hypoxia is one more example of adaptation in which the principle of successive and selective gene activation is realized during the formation of the systemic structural trace. This occurs in particular by an increased expression of erythropoietin in kidneys.[30] Erythropoietin, in its turn, induces an increase in red cell mass by stimulating the formation and differentiation of erythroid precursor cells in bone marrow. This increases the blood oxygen capacity and as a result limits tissue hypoxia.

The Role of Stress-Limiting Systems and the Phenomenon of Adaptive Stabilization of Structures (PhASS) in the Protective Effects of Adaptation

The cross protective effects of adaptation appeared even more pronounced in adaptation to brief immobilization stress. Besides protection against prolonged and intense stress exposure,[10] such adaptation provided a considerable increase in resistance to sublethal hypoxia,[31] arrhythmogenic and necrotic damage to the heart,[10,26] chemical damage to the stomach,[32] effects of chemical mutagens,[33] and other factors. It recently appeared that adaptation to stress increases the resistance to damage not only of the whole organism but also of isolated organs and, first of all, of the heart.[34]

It is presently known that such a broad spectrum of cross protective effects is based on at least two phenomena. The first phenomenon is the activation of so-called stress-limiting systems, which restrict the excitation of stress-realizing systems and block the effect of stress hormones at the level of target organs.[26] The second phenomenon is a direct increase in resistance of cell structures at the expense of the activated ancient mechanism expression of special genes and the accumulation of stress proteins with a molecular weight of 70–72 kDa in cells.[3,34]

The broad range of cross protective effects of adaptation to stress along with the well-known ability of stress reaction to transform the protective to the damaging effect warrants the consideration of the major factors characteristic of this adaptation. It was shown that adaptation to repeated stress exposure, on the one hand, increases several times the activity of tyrosine hydroxylase and the content of catecholamines in cerebral neurons,[35,36] and, on the other hand, reduces the elevation of plasma catecholamines in stressful exposures.[37] Likewise, the release of corticosterone from the adrenal gland into blood induced by the first stress exposure is quite considerable, while that in response to the fifth exposure is substantially decreased. Furthermore, the release of this hormone into blood in response to administration of a standard dose of ACTH is much higher in animals adapted to stress than in nonadapted ones.[38] Thus there is no exhaustion of the stress-realizing sympathoadrenal system in correct adaptation to stress. On the contrary, its potency is increased, though the stress reaction to the usual stress factor is clearly reduced.

In analyzing this paradoxical phenomenon, we have put forward a concept of so-called stress-limiting systems of the organism.[26] The essence of this hypothesis is that the organism possesses regulatory and modulatory systems, which are coupled with the stress-realizing hypothalamo-hypophysial-adrenal and sympathetic systems, are activated in any stress action, and limit the intensity and duration of stress reaction. The central stress-limiting systems include the GABAergic system, the system of benzodiazepine receptors, the opioidergic, serotonergic, dopaminergic and other brain systems. Local stress-limiting systems, which operate mainly at the level of target organs, include the systems of prostaglandins, antioxidants, adenosine, etc. Multiple stress enhances the functional capacities of the stress-limiting systems. They begin to limit more efficiently the duration and the intensity of excitation of the nerve center which determine the stress reaction, and to block, more completely the action of stress hormones at the level of target organs. As a result of these adaptive changes the organism resistance to the damaging action of stressful situations and to other environmental factors increases.

This hypothesis of stress-limiting systems is supported by numerous facts, considered in detail in a separate review.[26] The principal facts are as follows:

1. In the process of evolution, cells of the nervous system and executive organs have formed a reliable coupling between activation of the stress-realizing system on the one hand and synthesis of metabolites of central and local stress-limiting systems on the other hand. We will present here only two schemes reflecting the above-mentioned coupling; (i) the schematic mechanism via which the stress-realizing system activates the GABAergic stress-limiting system in the brain (see FIG. 3) and (ii) the schematic mechanism via which stress can activate adenosine synthesis and the adenosinergic protective effect (see FIG. 4). Similar mechanisms have been studied for many stress-limiting systems.

2. In the process of adaptation to repeated restraint or emotional painful stress, there occurs activation of synthesis and accumulation of metabolites or mediators of the above-listed stress-limiting systems: opioid peptides, serotonin, GABA, dopamine, antioxidants, prostaglandins, etc.

3. Pharmacologic factors acting like the metabolites of stress-limiting systems, for example, agonists of benzodiazepine receptors or synthetic analogues of leu-enkephalin, antioxidants, etc., protect against stress damage like adaptation to stress.

It can be expected that the inherited or acquired increase in efficiency of stress-limiting systems plays a role in the prevention of stress-induced diseases, whereas the inherited or acquired decrease in the efficiency of these systems would promote development of such diseases. At the same time it is obvious that many protective

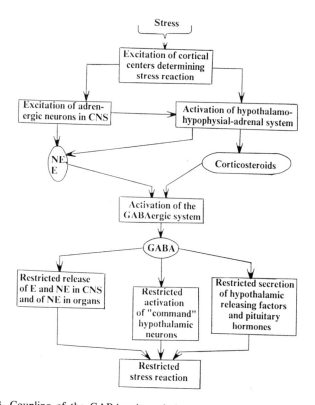

FIGURE 3. Coupling of the GABAergic and the stress-realizing systems, and GABA-mediated restriction of the stress reaction. For explanation see text.

effects of adaptation against direct injuries, especially induced by chemical and thermal factors, sublethal hypoxia, and necrotizing (heart) ischemia, are hardly attributable exclusively to the regulatory defense, *i.e.*, by the action of metabolites of stress-limiting systems. This brings up an idea that the repeated action of mediators of the stress-limiting system can induce expression of definite genes in cell nuclei to form correspondent proteins, which provide direct protection of cellular structures immediately at the cell level.

To test this hypothesis we initially elucidated whether the cardioprotective effect of adaptation persists in the performing heart isolated by Langendorff. It appeared that, in such conditions, *i.e.*, beyond the influence of neuroendocrine factors, the heart of the adapted animal is strikingly more resistant to ischemia and subsequent reoxygenation, toxic concentrations of catecholamines or Ca^{2+}, hot (42°C) perfusion solution.[26,34] Under the action of either factor, the heart of a control animal developed a contracture and ventricular extrasystoles and released CPK from myocardial cells through the damaged sarcolemma into the perfusate. In the heart of the adapted animal, these phenomena were 3–6 times less pronounced than in the control and sometimes were even absent. When the isolated papillary muscle was exposed to a hyposodium solution, the contracture in the

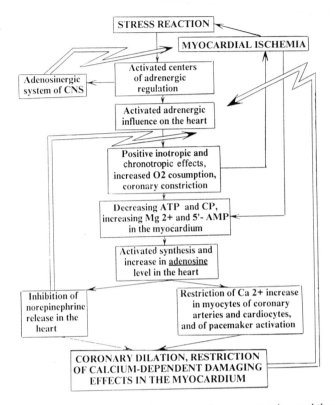

FIGURE 4. Coupling of the adenosinergic system to the stress reaction, and the cardioprotective effect of adenosine. For explanations see text.

control was evident as the sixfold increased rest tension and it was attended by a considerable decrease in the rest potential (RP). In adaptation, this contracture was slight, and the RP decrease was halved. Hyposodium solution is known to induce a massive Ca^{2+} influx in the cell. This is precisely the cause of the contractural effect. The decrease in this effect, as the decrease in all above-listed disorders of the function of isolated heart, can very probably depend on the increased activity of the SR Ca^{2+} pump and on its increased resistance to autolysis.[26] Inactivation of mitochondrial respiration and phosphorylation in the myocardium of adapted animals also occurred slower than in mitochondria from control animals.[26]

On the whole the data evidence a stabilization of cytoplasmic structures, SR, mitochondria, and sarcolemma, in adaptation to stress.

The question of the effect of such an adaptation on the resistance of cardiomyocyte nuclei has been explored in special experiments,[39] in which the DNA content was measured in a suspension of isolated nuclei using a cytofluometric method. Single-strand DNA, which is known to activate nuclear proteases, was added to the suspension. Histograms obtained in these experiments (FIG. 5) demonstrate the effect of adaptation on the magnitude of fluorescence peak of myocardial nuclei with normal DNA content. After the addition of single-strand DNA, a dramatic decrease in the fluorescence peak was observed to indicate the nuclei destruction in control animals. In adaptation this phenomenon was 5.5 times less pronounced. When the single-strand DNA concentration was increased, this protective effect of adaptation remained. Thus the PhASS occurs not only in cytoplasmic structures but also at the level of the DNA genetic matrix.

Evaluating possible molecular mechanisms of PhASS, one could have suggested that it is in part the adaptive activation of local stress-limiting systems, such as the antioxidant, prostaglandin and adenosinergic ones. However, against this suggestion is an important fact established in our laboratory in studying adaptation to intermittent hypoxia. This adaptation induced a potent activation of the prostaglandin, antioxidant and adenosinergic systems. It exerted a strong antiischemic effect at the level of heart. However, in this adaptation, the PhASS was much weaker than in adaptation to stress, and the protection at the level of cell nuclei, which we discussed just now, was totally absent. This suggests that the PhASS is based on some more ancient and, correspondingly, more efficient cellular mechanism, which possesses a very broad range of protective effects.

Indeed, further studies carried out by the method of two-dimensional gel electrophoresis have shown that the cytoplasm and nuclei of myocardial cells accumulate heat shock proteins (HSP 70) in the course of adaptation to repeated restraint stress. The phenomenon of HSP 70 accumulation was characterized by at least three features.[34,40]

1. The maximal HSP 70 accumulation was observed after 8 days following the onset of adaptation. This coincided with all above-mentioned manifestations

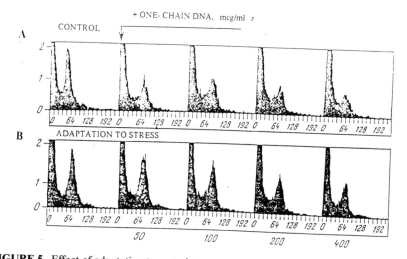

FIGURE 5. Effect of adaptation to restraint stress on the resistance of nuclear DNA from myocardial cells to damaging action of one-chain exogenous DNA. **(A)** Histograms of the nuclear DNA distribution in control. **(B)** The same after adaptation to restraint stress. Histograms: *ordinates*: number of nuclei, thousands; *abscissas*: fluorescence intensity of DNA-bound dye in relative units; to the *left of the arrow*: distribution histograms of nuclear suspension in control and at adaptation without addition of one-chain DNA; to the *right of the arrow*: histograms after the addition of one-chain DNA in concentration of 50, 100, 200, and 400 mg/ml (as indicated in the lower part of the figure).

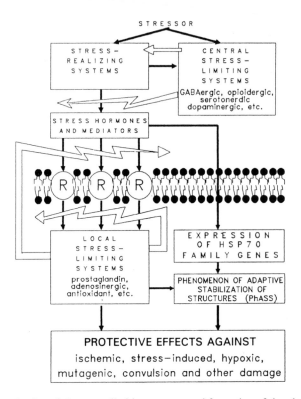

FIGURE 6. Activation of the stress-limiting systems and formation of the phenomenon of adaptive stabilization of structures in adaptation to stress.

of the PhASS. By the 30th day after the onset of the experiment, HSP 70 disappeared or decreased to a minimum; the same happened with the PhASS manifestations.

2. In gradual adaptation to intermittent hypoxia, cytoplasmic HSP 70 were slightly detectable whereas nuclear HSP 70 were completely absent. The PhASS was insignificantly pronounced at the level of the whole heart and was absent at the level of the SR and nuclei.

3. The HSP 70 accumulation induced by adaptation to stress was of a generalized nature: these proteins accumulated in the heart, liver and brain. Consistent with this, the PhASS was generalized as well. For instance, in sublethal hypoxia (6% O_2 in inspired air), the death rate was 6.5 times lower in animals adapted to stress than in control while in animals adapted to hypoxia itself the death rate was only two times lower.[31]

Taken together these facts led to the idea that HSP 70 may play an important role in the PhASS formation.

FIGURE 6 presents a schematized hypothesis of the coordination of stress-limiting systems and PhASS. Intracellular regulatory mechanisms activating the HSP expression are discussed in detail in our recent book.[40]

The mechanisms, via which the protective effect of HSP 70 can occur in the cell are as follows:

1. Fatty acid binding and restriction of damage to membranes and membrane proteins.
2. Enhancement of potency of cell antioxidant systems and restriction of free radical damage to DNA.
3. Disaggregation of damaged preribosomes, contractile and other proteins.
4. Binding to calmodulin and restriction of toxic effects of Ca^{2+} excess.

Further investigations of PhASS have shown that this phenomenon exerts significant antihypoxic[26,34] and antimutagenic[33] effects. It was also shown that PhASS could be obtained using a mild transcranial electric stimulation (applicable in physiotherapy) instead of immobilization of animals. Therefore, the matter is a biological phenomenon that is promising for medicine.

CONCLUSION

Therapy and prophylaxis by adaptation to a broad range of factors have been empirically used for several thousand years. However, many principal scientific notions about this field are comparatively young. They include the ratio of phenotype and genotype in the architecture of structural traces of various adaptations; studying and prediction of positive and negative cross effects of these adaptations; combinations of factors beneficial or, on the contrary, hazardous for the organism; the ratio of adaptive and pharmacologic methods of therapy; adaptational therapy and prophylaxis of those diseases; drug therapy, which leaves something to be desired; and, finally, genetic provision of adaptation, its structural cost and dose. All these problems appeared comparatively recently, and they are unresolved in many respects. They are worthy of the attention of researchers engaged in basic investigations and of physicians in general practice. These problems comprise a perspective of adaptive medicine.

REFERENCES

1. MEERSON, F. Z. 1984. Adaptation, Stress and Prophylaxis. Springer-Verlag. Berlin.
2. MEERSON, F. Z. & V. V. DIDENKO. 1992. Role of the cellular oncogenes in the development of cardiac adaptation to the increased load and ischemia (in Russian). Kardiologiya 32(2): 82–90.
3. MEERSON, F. Z. 1994. Essentials of Adaptive Medicine: Protective Effects of Adaptation. Hypoxia Medical LTD. Moscow, Geneva.
4. MEERSON, F. Z. 1973. Common Mechanism of Adaptation and Prophylaxis (in Russian). Meditzina. Moscow.
5. SALGANIK, R. I., N. M. MANANKOVA & L. A. SEMENOVA. 1977. Hypocholesterolemic effect of induction of liver microsomal enzymes in rats (in Russian). Voprosy med. khimii 4: 468–473.
6. KIENS, B., H. LITHELL & B. VOSSBY. 1984. Further increase in high density lipoproteins in trained males after endurance training. Eur. J. Appl. Physiol. 52: 426–430.
7. KUKKONEN, K., R. RAURAMAA, E. VONTILAINEN & E. LANSIMIES. 1982. Physical training of middle-aged men with borderline hypertension. Ann. Clin. Res. 14(Suppl. 34): 139–145.
8. SULLIVAN, L. 1982. Obesity, diabetes mellitus and physical activity—metabolic responses to physical training in adipose and muscle tissues. Ann. Clin. Res. 14(Suppl. 34): 51–62.

9. LECLERC, L. & A. FREMINET. 1982. Effect de l'entrainement physique sur la reponse metabolique a l'hypoxie du coeur isole de rat. J. Physiol. (Paris) **77:** 905–910.

10. MEERSON, F. Z. & M. G. PSHENNIKOVA. 1988. Adaptation to stressful situations and physical loads (in Russian). Meditzina. Moscow.

11. MEERSON, F. Z. 1983. The failing heart: adaptation and deadaptation. A. M. Katz, Ed. Raven Press. New York.

12. VASILENKO, V. KH., S. B. FELDMAN & N. K. KHITROV. 1989. Myocardiodystrophy (in Russian). Meditzina. Moscow.

13. DELA BASTIE, D., D. LEVITSKY, L. RAPOPORT, J-J. MERCADIER, F. MAROTTE, C. WISNEWSKY, V. BROVKOVICH & K. SCHWARTZ. 1989. Sarcoplasmatic reticulum Ca ATPase in pressure overload in the rat heart function and gene expression. J. Mol. Cell. Cardiol. **21**(Suppl. III): S.2 (Abst. 5).

14. CHARLEMAGNE, D., J. ORLOWSKI, P. OLIVERO & L. LANE. 1989. Expression of Na/K ATPase p and c subunit mRNAs in hypertrophied rat heart. J. Mol. Cell. Cardiol. **21**(Suppl. III): S.4 (Abst. 10).

15. RESINK, T., W. GEVERS, T. D. NOAKES & L. H. OPIE. 1981. Increased cardiac myosin ATPase activity as a biochemical adaptation to running training: enhanced response to catecholamines and a role for myosin phosphorilation. J. Mol. Cell. Cardiol. **13:** 679–694.

16. MEERSON, F. Z. & A. I. SAULYA. 1984. Prevention of disturbances of the heart contractile function in stress by preliminary adaptation of animals to physical load (in Russian). Kardiologiya. **24**(6): 19–23.

17. YAZAKI, Y. & I. KOMURO. 1989. Molecular analysis of cardiac hypertrophy due to overload. J. Mol. Cell. Cardiol. **21**(Suppl. III): S29.

18. WYATT, H. L. & J. MITCHEL. 1978. Influences of physical conditioning and deconditioning on coronary vasculature of dogs. J. Appl. Physiol. **45:** 619–625.

19. PENPARGKUL, S., A. SCHWARTZ & J. SCHEUER. 1976. Effect of physical conditioning on rat heart mitochondria. Circulation **54**(Suppl. 2): 114.

20. SEGEL, L. & D. T. MASON. 1978. Effects of exercise and conditioning on rat heart glycogen synthesis. J. Appl. Physiol. **44:** 183–189.

21. GUSKI, H., F. Z. MEERSON & G. WASSILEV. 1981. Comparative study of ultrastructure and function of rat heart hypertrophied by exercise or hypoxia. Exp. Pathol. **20:** 108–120.

22. HEISS, H. W., J. BARMEYER & K. WINK. 1975. Durchblutung und Substratumsatz des gesunden menschlichen Herzens in Abhangigkeit vom Trainingszustand. Verh. Dtsch. Ges. Kreislaufforsch. **41:** 247–252.

23. WELLER, K. & W. G. FORSSMANN. 1972. Ultrastructure of the T-system in the hearts of animals with extremely high heart rates. *In* Colloque Europeen sur les Surcharges Cardiaques. P. Y. Hatt, Ed. 59–61. INSERM. Paris.

24. BLAGOVESTOVA, N. P., E. V. LOGINOVA & E. E. SIMONOV. 1968. Duration of the bone marrow response to hypoxic acclimation (in Russian). Probl. Kosm. Biol. **8:** 198–201.

25. PSHENNIKOVA, M. G. 1973. Protein synthesis in neurons and glial cells in stellate ganglia of rats in adaptation to the action of high altitude hypoxia (in Russian). Fiziol. Zhurnal SSSR **59**(3): 421–428.

26. MEERSON, F. Z. 1991. Adaptive Protection of the Heart: Protecting against Stress and Ischemic Damage. CRC Press. Boca Raton.

27. MEERSON, F. Z., V. G. PINELIS, V. B. KOSHELEV, L. YU. GOLUBEVA, T. V. RYASINA, E. N. ARSENJEVA, A. L. KRUSHINSKY & T. P. STOROZHEVYKH. 1993. Adaptation to intermittent hypoxia restricts subdural hemorrhages in rats in audiogenic epileptiform convulsions (in Russian). Byull. Eksper. Biol. i Med. **116**(12): 572–573.

28. MEERSON, F. Z., E. E. USTINOVA & E. H. ORLOVA. 1987. Prevention and elimination of heart arrhythmias by adaptation to intermittent high altitude hypoxia. Clin. Cardiol. **12:** 783–787.

29. SHARMA, H. S., M. WUNSCH, R. J. SCHOTT, R. KANDOLF & W. SCHAPER. 1991. Angiogenic growth factors possibly involved in coronary collateral growth. J. Mol. Cell. Cardiol. **32**(Suppl. 5): 19.

30. SCHOLZ, H., H. J. SCHUREK, K. U. ECKARDT & C. BAUER. 1990. Role of erythropoietin in adaptation to hypoxia. Experientia **46:** 1197–1201.
31. MEERSON, F. Z., V. POZHAROV & T. MINYAILENKO. 1994. Superresistance against hypoxia after preliminary adaptation to repeated stress. J. Appl. Physiol. **76:** 1856–1861.
32. WALLACE, J. & M. COHEN. 1984. Gastric mucosal protection with chronic mild restraint: role of endogenous prostaglandins. Am. J. Physiol. **247:** G127–G132.
33. MEERSON, F. Z., K. V. KULAKOVA & V. A. SALTYKOVA. 1993. Byull. Eksper. Biol. i Med. The antimutagenic effect of adaptation to stress. **116**(9): 292–294.
34. MEERSON, F. Z., I. YU. MALYSHEV & A. V. ZAMOTRINSKY. 1992. Phenomenon of the adaptive stabilization of structures and protection of the heart. Can. J. Cardiol. **8**(9): 965–974.
35. ZIGMOND, M. J. & E. M. STICKER. 1985. Adaptive properties of monoaminergic neurons. *In* Handbook of Neurochemistry. Vol. **9:** 87–102. Plenum Press. New York.
36. KVETNANSKY, R., V. WEISE & I. J. KOPIN. 1970. Elevation of adrenal tyrosine hydroxilase and phenylethanolamine-N-methyltransferase by repeated immobilization of rats. Endocrinology **87:** 744–749.
37. PSHENNIKOVA, M. G., B. A. KUZNETZOVA, M. V. SHIMKOVICH, V. I. VOVK & YU. N. KOPYLOV. 1991. Adaptation to stress exposures and adaptation to altitude hypoxia activate the prostaglandin system and attenuate adrenergic response in acute stress. *In* Proceedings of the 1st Congress of the International Society for Pathophysiology. 256 (abst.).
38. MIKULAJ, L., R. KVETNANSKY & K. MURGAS. 1974. Changes in adrenal response during intermittent and repeated stress. Rev. Czech. Med. **20**(3): 162–169.
39. MEERSON, F. Z., I. YU. MALYSHEV, E. YU. VARFOLOMEEVA, D. B. VARFOLOMEEV & A. N. NOSKIN. 1991. Adaptation of the organism to stress exposures increases the resistance of cardiomyocyte nuclei to the damaging effect of one-chain exogenous DNA (in Russian). Byull. Eksper. Biol. i Med. **114**(5): 460–462.
40. MEERSON, F. Z. & I. YU. MALYSHEV. 1993. Phenomenon of adaptive stabilization of structures and protection of the heart (in Russian). Nauka. Moscow.

Pharmacologic Myocardial Preconditioning with Monophosphoryl Lipid A (MLA) Reduces Infarct Size and Stunning in Dogs and Rabbits

GARY T. ELLIOTT[a]

Ribi ImmunoChem Research, Inc.
553 Old Corvallis Road
Hamilton, Montana 59840

INTRODUCTION

A very interesting phenomenon first reported by Murry, Jennings and Reimer in 1986 illustrates what appears to be an endogenous protective mechanism which enhances the ability of myocardium to withstand injury from prolonged ischemia.[1] Specifically, Murray *et al.* and then others reported that transient ischemic events, which are in and of themselves sufficiently brief to avoid irreversibly damaging myocardium, are capable of initiating unidentified biochemical events which limit infarct size and the occurrence of reperfusion arrhythmias following prolonged myocardial ischemia.[1–4] This phenomenon termed ischemic preconditioning has been observed in rats, dogs, rabbits, swine and presumably humans.[1–8]

Protection was initially reported to develop within minutes of transient ischemia followed by reperfusion and to subsequently last for approximately one to two hours. Yellon *et al.* have described a second window of preconditioning (SWOP) which reappears within 24 hours of the transient ischemic event and which may be prolonged in duration.[9]

Considerable effort has been expended to identify the biochemical and physiologic events associated with ischemic preconditioning. Depending on the species under investigation, adenosine, norepinephrine and bradykinin have been implicated as agonists which through stimulation of G protein-coupled receptors leads to activation of phospholipids and kinases, including PKC specifically, and elaboration of nitric oxide.[10–16]

Many investigations suggest that priming or opening of ATP-sensitive potassium (K_{ATP}) channels is a late event in the signal transduction pathway induced by ischemic preconditioning.[14,17–21]

The fact that the ATP-sensitive potassium channel appears to be a phosphorylation substrate and that phosphorylation of K_{ATP} channel modulates ion flux[22] suggests that activation of kinases by ischemic preconditioning may be involved in the ultimate priming of K_{ATP} channel.

Various approaches to pharmacologically mimic ischemic preconditioning have met with some success at least in preclinical settings. Adenosine, A_1-specific

[a] Address correspondence to: Gary T. Elliott, Pharm.D., Ph.D., Division of Pharmaceutical Development, Ribi ImmunoChem Research, Inc., 553 Old Corvallis Road, Hamilton, MT 59840. Tel.: (406) 363-6214; Fax: (406) 363-6129.

adenosine receptor agonists, potassium (K_{ATP}) channel openers, acetylcholine, PMA and L-arginine have all been reported to be protective in models of myocardial ischemia/reperfusion.[23-30]

A report published by Berg *et al.* in 1990 suggested that the ubiquitous gram negative microbial toxin endotoxin protected mice from pulmonary fibrosis and lethality of hyperbaric oxygen exposure.[31] Brown *et al.* at about the same time described endotoxin as cardioprotective in a rat heart Langendorff model of global ischemia/reperfusion.[32] Protection was associated with induction of myocardial catalase.[33] These three reports suggested that endotoxin treatment might induce antioxidant defenses capable of protecting various organs from oxidative free radical damage associated with ischemia/reperfusion injury.

The search for a derivative of endotoxin with reduced "toxic" activity which still enjoyed some of the desirable effects of the parent molecule such as immunostimulatory activity appears to have borne fruit in the characterization of monophosphoryl lipid A (MLA).[34-36] Differing structurally from the minimal toxic pharmacophore of endotoxin, namely, lipid A (FIG. 1), by the removal of a phosphoester from the reducing sugar of the disaccharide and additionally the saponification of a long chain beta-hydroxy ester from the three position hydroxyl group of the reducing glucosamine,[37,38] MLA has been under development as a novel vaccine adjuvant and prophylactic treatment for septic shock.[39]

For approximately four years an effort has been underway to determine the potential utility of MLA as a cardioprotective agent to ameliorate ischemia/reperfusion injury. Preclinical results generated in various species indicate that MLA reduces contractile dysfunction and limits infarct size following regional or global cardiac ischemia followed by reperfusion. Intravenously administered to healthy humans, MLA appeared safe at dose levels up to at least 20 μg/kg.[39] Presently MLA is being evaluated in dose escalation studies in patients scheduled for coronary artery bypass engraftment surgery.

Infarct Size Is Limited by Single Dose Pretreatment with MLA in Dogs and Rabbits

Intravenous pretreatment with MLA formulated as a triethylamine buffered aqueous solution when administered as a single dose between 30 and 100 μg/kg reduced infarct size 40 to 60 percent (FIG. 2).[40,41] Infarct size following 1 hour ischemia and 4–5 hours reperfusion was reduced across a range of collateral myocardial blood flow with the drug having no effect on collateral flow, area at risk, contractility, heart rate or peripheral vascular tone at periischemic time points. Infarct size was reduced using a 24- but not a 1-hour pretreatment with MLA. Significantly reduced neutrophil infiltration, as measured by myeloperoxidase activity, was noted in viable myocardium in postischemic regions of the heart (FIG. 3). Interestingly, myocardial catalase was not significantly induced by microgram per kilogram cardioprotective doses of MLA.

Recent canine studies utilizing a 10% ethanol, 40% propylene glycol, water for injection formulation of MLA indicates that doses of 10 μg/kg or higher significantly reduce infarct size in the dog (FIG. 4).[42]

In an intact model of regional myocardial ischemia (30 minutes) and reperfusion (3 hours) in the rabbit, MLA pretreatment reduced infarct size 70 percent at doses of 35 μg/kg (FIG. 5).[44-46] Protection was observed when treatment was administered 12 or 24 hours prior to ischemia. Cardioprotection was not associated with induction of heat shock protein-70 at the time of ischemia. When isolated

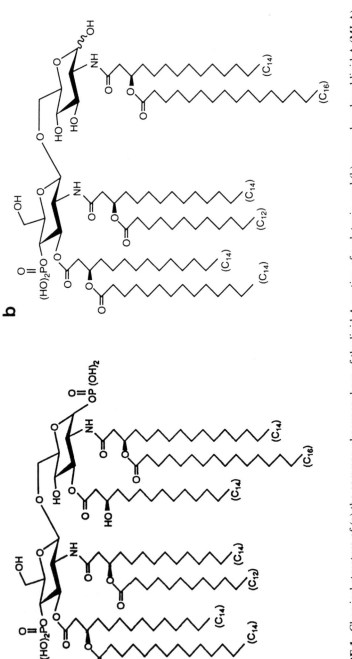

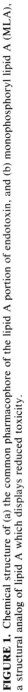

FIGURE 1. Chemical structure of (a) the common pharmacophore of the lipid A portion of endotoxin, and (b) monophosphoryl lipid A (MLA), a structural analog of lipid A which displays reduced toxicity.

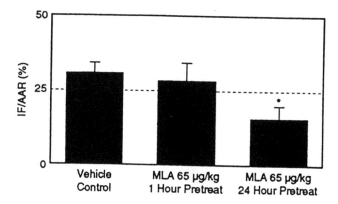

FIGURE 2. Infarct size expressed as a per cent of the area at risk (means ± SEM). Effect of timing of MLA administration relative to time of ischemia upon cardioprotective effect. *p <0.05.

rabbit hearts from pretreated animals were rendered ischemic and reperfused, cardioprotection as evaluated by infarct size reduction and functional recovery was not apparent.[45,46] It was suggested by the investigators that protection elicited by MLA *in situ* may require drug effect on some blood borne element such as inflammatory cell subsets or humoral factor or upon autonomic tone to the heart, features which are not present in a buffer-perfused isolated heart model.

Myocardial Contractile Dysfunction following Ischemia/Reperfusion in Dogs Is Improved with MLA Pretreatment

Transient, intermittent ischemia (6 sequential periods of 5 minutes ischemia and 10 minutes reperfusion) normally results in a pronounced, reversible regional

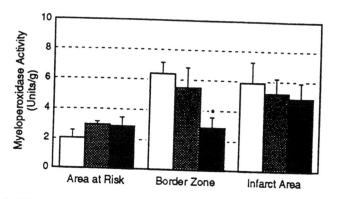

FIGURE 3. MLA treatment related effect on myeloperoxidase (MPO) activity in overall myocardium at risk, viable at risk tissue adjacent to necrotic regions (border region) and infarcted regions. A significant reduction in MPO activity (*p <0.05) was observed in border region of hearts from the 24-hour pretreatment group (■) in comparison with a one-hour pretreatment group (▨) or a vehicle control group (□).

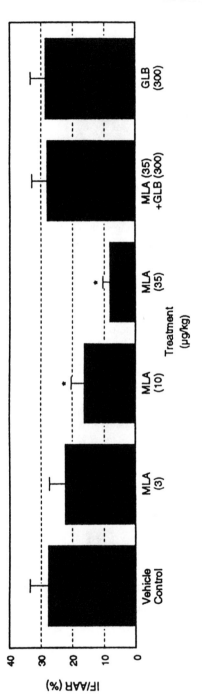
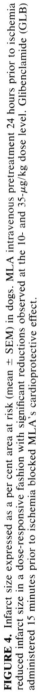

FIGURE 4. Infarct size expressed as a per cent area at risk (mean ± SEM) in dogs. MLA intravenous pretreatment 24 hours prior to ischemia reduced infarct size in a dose-responsive fashion with significant reductions observed at the 10- and 35-μg/kg dose level. Glibenclamide (GLB) administered 15 minutes prior to ischemia blocked MLA's cardioprotective effect.

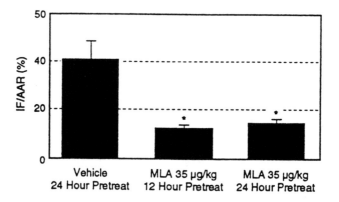

FIGURE 5. Infarct size expressed as a per cent area at risk (mean ± SEM) in rabbits. MLA administered intravenously 12 or 24 hours prior to ischemia at a dose of 35 μg/kg reduced infarct size (*p <0.05) compared to vehicle-treated control animals.

contractile dysfunction in postischemic myocardium. Pretreatment with MLA (35 μg/kg) 24 but not 1 hour prior to ischemia significantly improved contractility during both intermittent and prolonged reperfusion periods with 50% return of baseline function observed in MLA-treated animals versus 20% contractile recovery in control animals (FIG. 6).[47]

Global ventricular function in a canine model of normothermic cardiopulmonary bypass also showed improvement with MLA pretreatment.[48] Left ventricular performance (stroke work ÷ end diastolic length in dyn/cm^2 × 10^3) was improved in treated animals at 30 and 60 minutes postbypass (TABLE 1).

MLA Pretreatment May Pharmacologically Mimic Ischemic Preconditioning

It is generally appreciated that a downregulation of myocyte metabolism is associated with ischemic preconditioning (IP) leading to preservation of ATP and creatine phosphate pools during ischemia.[49,50]

In a rabbit model of cardiogenic shock associated with prolonged (90 minute) regional ischemia and reperfusion (6 hours), MLA-pretreated animals in addition

TABLE 1. Left Ventricular Performance (Load-Independent) in Dogs Subjected to 30 Minutes Normothermic Cardiopulmonary Bypass^a

	Preischemia	Reperfusion	
		30 Min	60 Min
Vehicle control	80.21 ± 5.3	41.35 ± 7.8^b	53.21 ± 5.8^b
MLA (35 μg/kg)	78.70 ± 8.1	54.47 ± 2.3^b	74.38 ± 3.9^c

^{a} Ventricular performance (stroke work/end dyastolic length in dyn/cm^2 × 10^3), mean ± SEM.
^{b} p <0.05 vs preischemia.
^{c} p <0.05 vs control.

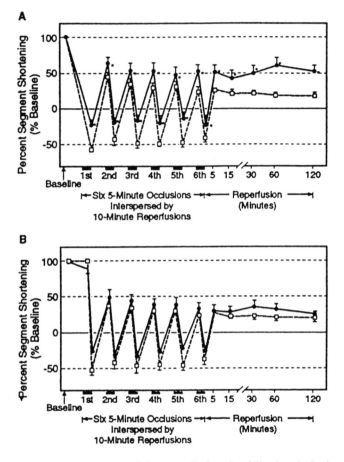

FIGURE 6. Regional canine myocardial contractile function following six 5-minute cycles of ischemia interspersed with 10-minute reperfusions, followed by 2 hours of continuous reperfusion. Contractile function in postischemic regions as assessed by per cent segment shortening was improved both during cyclical ischemia/reperfusion and during subsequent prolonged reperfusion when MLA pretreatment (●) was administered 24 hours **(A)** but *not* 1 hour **(B)** prior to ischemia in comparison with control animals (○).

to displaying significantly improved left ventricular developed pressure, rate-pressure product, dp/dt and mean arterial pressure during reperfusion (TABLE 2), experienced preservation of ATP and ADP pools at the end of ischemia (TABLE 3).[51,52] Reduced accumulation of adenosine catabolites and induction of adenosine kinase was also observed.

In a side-by-side comparison of ischemic preconditioning and MLA pretreatment, Przyklenk *et al.* recently reported preservation of 5'nucleotidase in both IP and MLA treatment groups (TABLE 4). Ischemic preconditioning using 5 cycles of 5 minutes ischemia, interspaced with 5-minute reperfusion cycles, preceded 1 hour ischemia by 15 minutes after the last preconditioning cycle. MLA pretreatment (35 μg/kg) preceded 1 hour ischemia by 24 hours.

It has been well established that IP cardioprotection can be pharmacologically blocked with K_{ATP} channel antagonists such as glibenclamide.[14,18,19] In the dog, MLA's ability to reduce infarct size can likewise be inhibited by glibenclamide (FIG. 4).[42]

Measurement of epicardial monophasic action potential (Mono AP) suggested that the duration of Mono AP significantly shortened in MLA-pretreated dogs during the first 5 minutes of ischemia in comparison with controls. This shortening of Mono AP by MLA could be blocked by glibenclamide and is similar to the electrophysiologic effect of K_{ATP} channel openers.[19]

The kinetics of cardioprotection achieved with MLA, unapparent immediately following dosing yet developing by 12 to 24 hours following drug administration, is temporally similar to that of the second window of preconditioning (SWOP). It has been suggested that SWOP may be associated with induction of HSP-70.[9] HSP-70 overexpressor mice are resistant to the development of ischemia/reperfusion injury,[14] and heat stress preconditions myocardium.[18] If similarities exist

TABLE 2. Hemodynamic Variables at Baseline and Indicated Times during Ischemia and Reperfusion[a]

Hemodynamic Variables	Non-Isch Vehicle Sham	Vehicle Control	35 μg/kg MLA 24-Hr Pretreatment	35 μg/kg MLA 0.5 Hr Postischemia
LVDP (mm Hg)				
Baseline	79 ± 3	89 ± 2	88 ± 4	86 ± 3
Isch 90 min[b]	74 ± 4	71 ± 2	74 ± 2	69 ± 3
Rep 180 min	78 ± 4	68 ± 3	83 ± 3[c]	62 ± 3
Rep 240 min	75 ± 4	64 ± 4	80 ± 5[c]	63 ± 4
Rep 300 min	76 ± 4	68 ± 4	74 ± 4	58 ± 4
Rep 360 min	74 ± 4[c]	58 ± 2	79 ± 3[c]	54 ± 4
LV + dP/dt (mm Hg/s)				
Baseline	2440 ± 132	2628 ± 118	2644 ± 141	2632 ± 143
Isch 90 min[b]	2468 ± 118	2187 ± 95	2232 ± 175	2032 ± 120
Rep 180 min	2338 ± 146	1922 ± 150	2456 ± 157	1592 ± 144
Rep 240 min	2300 ± 219	1733 ± 186	2328 ± 234	1584 ± 156
Rep 300 min	2188 ± 217	1623 ± 139	2036 ± 211	1592 ± 175
Rep 360 min	2070 ± 120[c]	1373 ± 96	2176 ± 172[c]	1208 ± 109
LV − dP/dt (mm Hg/s)				
Baseline	1862 ± 91	2190 ± 120	2104 ± 121	2112 ± 91
Isch 90 min[b]	1992 ± 157	1680 ± 96	1720 ± 101	1680 ± 127
Rep 180 min	2024 ± 95	1692 ± 129	2084 ± 118	1448 ± 129
Rep 240 min	2048 ± 201	1538 ± 199	1992 ± 168	1376 ± 120
Rep 300 min	1928 ± 150[c]	1353 ± 173	1712 ± 149	1272 ± 120
Rep 360 min	1804 ± 90[c]	1230 ± 101	1816 ± 114[c]	1128 ± 99
MAP (mm Hg)				
Baseline	70 ± 3	78 ± 2	73 ± 2	71 ± 3
Isch 90 min[b]	63 ± 3	61 ± 2	61 ± 2	55 ± 3
Rep 180 min	70 ± 4[c]	55 ± 3	70 ± 3[c]	48 ± 3
Rep 240 min	63 ± 5	51 ± 5	70 ± 5[c]	49 ± 4
Rep 300 min	63 ± 4[c]	47 ± 5	63 ± 4[c]	44 ± 4
Rep 360 min	62 ± 3[c]	44 ± 3	67 ± 5[c]	40 ± 3

[a] Values are mean ± SEM. Isch, ischemia; Rep, reperfusion; LVDP, left ventricular developed pressure; MAP, mean arterial pressure.

[b] Sham animals underwent additional 90 minutes of nonischemic baseline evaluation.

[c] $p < 0.05$ vs vehicle control.

TABLE 3. Effect of MLA on Adenine Nucleotide and Metabolite Pools at the End of Myocardial Ischemia (90 Min)[a]

Adenine Nucleotides + Metabolites (nmol/gm Wet Tissue Weight)	Nonrisk		Postischemic	
	Vehicle Control	MLA	Vehicle Control	MLA
ATP	2455.4 ± 182.2	2678.2 ± 117.1	788.0 ± 106.6	1215.3 ± 121.9[b]
ADP	1838.1 ± 92.4	1985.1 ± 70.1	958.7 ± 94.0	1248.8 ± 96.4[b]
AMP	1461.0 ± 146.4	1591.9 ± 96.7	1392.9 ± 217.0	1365.3 ± 110.1
Adenosine	8.2 ± 1.3	6.9 ± 1.2	26.2 ± 2.2	23.1 ± 2.1
Inosine	43.7 ± 6.1	30.4 ± 2.4	352.7 ± 60.1	199.1 ± 38.5[b]
Hypoxanthine	321.2 ± 50.3	254.5 ± 16.5	490.1 ± 41.7	345.3 ± 38.6[b]
Xanthine	38.5 ± 4.7	36.8 ± 3.3	46.5 ± 5.1	34.0 ± 5.6
Uric acid	9.8 ± 1.8	6.8 ± 0.9	52.3 ± 9.3	28.3 ± 5.1[b]
Purine nucleoside ratio: $\frac{[ATP] + [ADP] + [AMP]}{[ADO] + [INO] + [HYP] + [XAN] + [UA]}$	16.72 ± 0.75	19.52 ± 1.00	3.76 ± 1.84	9.40 ± 1.76[b]
Group size	n = 9	n = 10	n = 9	n = 11

[a] Values are mean ± SEM.
[b] $p < 0.05$ vs respective control data.

TABLE 4. Myocardial Ectosolic 5'Nucleotidase (5'NT, nmol/mg Protein/Min) Activity in Dogs

Treatment	Ischemic Endocardial Blood Flow	Infarct Size	Ectosolic 5'NT	
			LAD	Cx
Vehicle control	0.07 ± 0.02	$20 \pm 5\%$	5.6 ± 1.1	8.5 ± 1.7
Ischemic preconditioning	0.06 ± 0.03	$6 \pm 3\%^a$	10.5 ± 2.1^b	12.6 ± 2.1^b
MLA (35 μg/kg)	0.06 ± 0.02	$9 \pm 3\%^a$	7.8 ± 1.3^a	11.1 ± 1.9^a

[a] $p < 0.05$ vs control.
[b] $p < 0.01$ vs control.
[c] $p < 0.05$ vs Cx bed.

between the mechanisms of SWOP and MLA pretreatment, they must reside in mechanisms other than HSP-70 induction. The role of K_{ATP} channel opening in SWOP is as yet unknown, although investigations with MLA suggest that experiments designed to address this question should be undertaken.

DISCUSSION OF FUTURE RESEARCH DIRECTIONS

The issue of whether MLA directly modulates K_{ATP} channel needs to be clarified using patch clamp techniques. If we fail to establish a direct effect of MLA on the ion channel, the possibility that a humoral factor elaborated in response to MLA administration is capable of modulating K_{ATP} channels should be evaluated. Humoral factors known to be induced by endotoxin which subsequently can lead to K_{ATP} modulation include bradykinin and adrenomedullin.[11,14,15,56–61] The possibility of direct induction of inducible nitric oxide synthase by MLA also needs to be evaluated as a possible mechanism of K_{ATP} activation.[62]

As K_{ATP} channel may be a kinase phosphorylation substrate, and appreciating the fact that some of the biological effects of endotoxin appear to require PTK or PKC kinase activation,[63] the ability of MLA to prime K_{ATP} channel through kinase activation should be evaluated.

Monophosphoryl lipid A represents a novel means of preconditioning myocardium to withstand ischemia/reperfusion injury. Safety in humans established at MLA dose levels up to at least 20 μg/kg (higher doses not evaluated) when combined with cardioprotection being realized at dose levels of 5 to 10 μg/kg in various preclinical models suggests an opportunity may exist to effectively precondition human myocardium at well tolerated doses in anticipation of planned ischemic events such as cardiopulmonary bypass surgery.

SUMMARY

As the mechanism of ischemic preconditioning unfolds, various strategies for inducing pharmacologic preconditioning become apparent. Adenosine receptor agonists, K_{ATP} channel activators, and endothelial-neutrophil adhesion antagonists have enjoyed cardioprotective activity against ischemia/reperfusion injury in at least some preclinical models. Monophosphoryl lipid A (MLA), a structural derivative of the pharmacophore of endotoxin, enjoys an improved therapeutic index in relation to the parent biological product. MLA has found clinical application as a vaccine adjuvant and protects from sepsis and septic shock in the preclinical setting. In animal models of myocardial ischemia/reperfusion injury, pretreatment 12–24 hours prior to ischemia with a single IV bolus injection of MLA limits infarct size 50 to 75 percent in standard canine and rabbit models at doses of 10–35 μg/kg. Regional myocardial stunning following multiple 5-minute ischemic episodes as assessed by segment shortening is reduced in dogs pretreated 24 but not 1 hour prior to ischemia. Global cardiac function, as evaluated by pressure-volume constructs generated in dogs being weaned from cardiopulmonary bypass, recovers more quickly in animals pretreated with MLA. Cardiac protection in various models is associated with preservation of ATP during ischemia, induction of 5′ nucleotidase and enhancement of calcium reuptake by SR during reperfusion. Limitation of infarct size by MLA in dogs and rabbits can be reversed by the administration of glibenclamide just prior to ischemia, suggesting a role for K_{ATP} channel opening during the first minutes of sustained ischemia. A clinical formulation of MLA (MPL®-C) is currently undergoing clinical investigation in the Phase II setting in coronary artery bypass surgical patients. MLA may represent a novel means of inducing pharmacologic preconditioning, with potential for clinical application as a pretreatment before planned myocardial ischemia.

REFERENCES

1. MURRY, C. E., R. B. JENNINGS & K. A. REIMER. 1986. Preconditioning with ischemia: a delay of lethal cell injury in ischemic myocardium. Circulation 74: 1124–1136.
2. LI, G. C., J. A. VASQUEZ, K. P. GALLAGHER & B. R. LUCCHESI. 1990. Myocardial protection with preconditioning . Circulation 82: 609–619.
3. OVIZE, M., R. A. KLONER, S. L. HALE & K. PRZYKLENK. 1992. Coronary cyclic flow variations "preconditions" ischemic myocardium. Circulation 85: 779–789.
4. PARRATT, J. R. 1994. Protection of the heart by ischemic-preconditioning: mechanisms and possibilities for pharmacologic exploitation. TIPS 15: 19–25.
5. YTREHUS, K., Y. LIU & J. M. DOWNEY. 1994. Preconditioning protects ischemic rabbit heart by protein kinase C activation. Am. J. Physiol. 266 (Heart Circ. Physiol. 35): H1145–H1152.
6. SCHOTT, R. J., S. ROHMANN, E. R. BROWN & W. SCHAPER. 1990. Ischemic preconditioning reduces infarct size in swine myocardium. Circ. Res. 66: 1133–1142.
7. DEUTOSCH, E., M. BERGER, W. G. KUSS MAUL, J. W. HIRSHFELD, H. C. HEIRMANN & W. K. LOSKEY. 1990. Adaption to ischemia during percutaneous transluminal coronary antioplasty: clinical hemodynamic and metabolic features. Circulation 82: 2044–2051.
8. LUI, Y. & J. M. DOWNEY. 1992. Ischemic preconditioning protects against infarction in rat heart. Am. J. Physiol. 263: H1107–H1112.
9. MARBER, M. S., D. S. LATCHMAN, J. M. WALKER & D. M. YELLON. 1993. Cardiac stress protein elevation 24 hours after brief ischemia or heat stress is associated with resistance to myocardial infarction. Circulation 88: 1264–1272.
10. LIU, G. S., J. THORTON, D. M. VAN WINKLE, A. W. H. STANLEY, R. A. OLSSON & J. M. DOWNEY. 1991. Protection against infarction afforded by preconditioning is mediated by A_1 adenosine receptors in rabbit heart. Circulation 84: 350–356.
11. THORNTON, J. D., C. S. THORNTON & J. M. DOWNEY. 1993. Effect of adenosine receptor blockage: preventing protective preconditioning depends on time of initiation. Am. J. Physiol. 265: H504–H505.

12. YTEHUS, K., Y. LIU & J. M. DOWNEY. 1994. Preconditioning protects ischemic rabbit heart by protein kinase C activation. Am. J. Physiol. **266:** H1145–H1152.
13. SPLECHLY-DICK, M. E., M. M. MOCANU & D. M. YELLON. 1994. Protein kinase C: its role in ischemic preconditioning in the rat. Circ. Res. **75:** 586–590.
14. YAO, Z. & G. J. GROSS. 1993. Role of nitric oxide, muscarinic receptors, and the ATP-sensitive K$^+$ channel in mediating the effects of acetylcholine to mimic preconditioning in dogs. Circ. Res. **73:** 1193–1201.
15. WALL, T. M., R. SHEEHY & J. C. HARTMAN. 1994. Role of bradykinin in myocardial preconditioning. J. Pharmacol. Exp. Ther. **270:** 681–689.
16. GATO, M., Y. LUI, X-M. YANG, J. L. ARDELL, M. V. COHEN & J. M. DOWNEY. 1995. Role of bradykinin in protection of ischemic preconditioning in rabbit hearts. Circ. Res. **77:** 611–621.
17. GROSS, G. J. & J. A. AUCHAMPACH. 1992. Blockade of ATP-sensitive potassium channel prevents myocardial preconditioning in dogs. Circ. Res. **70:** 223–233.
18. YAO, Z. & G. J. GROSS. 1994. The ATP-dependent potassium channel: an endogenous cardioprotective mechanism. J. Cardiovasc. Pharmacol. **24**(Suppl. 4): S28–S34.
19. ROHMANN, S., H. WEYGANDT, P. SCHELLING, L. KIE SOLI, P. D. VERDOUW & I. LUES. 1994. Involvement of ATP-sensitive potassium channels in preconditioning protection. Basic Res. Cardiol. **89:** 563–576.
20. KIRSCH, G. E., J. CODINA, L. BEINBAWMER & A. M. BROWN. 1990. Coupling of ATP-sensitive K$^+$ channels to A$_1$ receptors by G proteins in rat ventricular myocytes. Am. J. Physiol. **259** (Heart Circ. Physiol. **28**): H820–H826.
21. WALL, T. M., A. L. FARRELL & J. C. HARTMAN. 1995. The temporal relationship between bradykinin and K$_{ATP}$ channels in the mechanism of cardioprotective ischemic preconditioning. Circ. Suppl. **92:** I-252.
22. NICHOLS, C. G. & W. J. LEDERER. 1991. Adenosine triphosphate-sensitive potassium channels in the cardiovascular system. Am. J. Physiol. (Heart Circ. Physiol. **30**) **26:** H1675–H1686.
23. THORTON, J. D., G. S. LIU, R. A. OLSSON & J. M. DOWNEY. 1992. Intravenous pretreatment with A$_1$-selective adenosine analogs protects the heart against infarction. Circulation **85:** 659–665.
24. GROSS, G., G. PIEPER, N. L. FARBER, D. WARLTIER & H. HARDMAN. 1989. Effects of nicorandil on coronary circulation and myocardial ischemia. Am. J. Cardiol. **63:** 11J.
25. GROVER, G. L., P. G. SLEPH & S. DZWONCZYK. 1992. Role of myocardial ATP-sensitive potassium channels in mediating preconditioning in the dog heart and their possible interaction with adenosine A$_1$ receptors. Circulation **86:** 1310–1316.
26. GROVER, G. J., S. DZWONCZYK, C. S. PARHAM & P. G. SLEPH. 1990. The protective effects of cromakalim and pinacidil on reperfusion function and infarct size in isolated perfused rat hearts and anesthetized dogs. Cardiovasc. Drug Ther. **4:** 465–474.
27. YAO, Z. & G. J. GROSS. 1994. Effects of the K$_{ATP}$ channel opener bimakalim on coronary blood flow, monophasic action potential duration and infarct size in dogs. Circulation **89:** 1769–1775.
28. LIN, Y., K. YTREHUS & J. M. DOWNEY. 1994. Evidence that translocation of protein kinase C is a key event during ischemic preconditioning of rabbit myocardium. J. Mol. Cell. Cardiol. **26:** 661–668.
29. ARMSTRONG, S. & C. E. GANOTE. 1994. Preconditioning of isolated rabbit cardiomyocytes: effects of glycolytic blockade, phorbol esters, and ischemia. Cardiovasc. Res. **28:** 1700–1706.
30. NAKANISHI, K., J. VINTEN-JOHANSEN, D. J. LEFER et al. 1992. Intracoronary L-arginine during reperfusion improves endothelial function and reduces infarct size. Am. J. Physiol. **263** (Heart Circ. Physiol. **32**): H1650–H1658.
31. BERG, J. T., R. C. ALLISON & A. E. TAYLOR. 1990. Endotoxin extends survival of adult mice in hyperoxia. Proc. Soc. Exp. Biol. Med. **193:** 167–170.
32. BROWN, J. M., M. A. GROSSO, L. S. TERADA et al. 1989. Endotoxin pretreatment increases endogenous myocardial catalase activity and decreases ischemia-reperfusion injury of isolated rat hearts. Proc. Natl. Acad. Sci. USA **86:** 2516–2520.

33. BENSARD, D. D., J. M. BROWN, B. O. ANDERSON et al. 1990. Induction of endogenous tissue antioxidant enzyme activity attenuates myocardial reperfusion injury. J. Surg. Res. **48:** 001–006.
34. TAKAYAMA, K., E. RIBI & J. L. CANTRELL. 1981. Isolation of a non-toxic lipid A fraction containing tumor regression activity. Cancer Res. **41:** 2654–2657.
35. TAKAYAMA, K., N. QURESHI, E. RIBI & J. L. CANTRELL. 1984. Separation and characterization of toxic and nontoxic forms of lipid A's. Rev. Infect. Dis. **6:** 439–443.
36. RIBI, E. 1984. Beneficial modification of the endotoxin molecule. J. Biol. Response Modif. **3:** 1–9.
37. QURESHI, N., K. TAKAYAMA & E. RIBI. 1982. Purification and structural determination of nontoxic lipid A obtained from lipopolysaccharide of *Salmonella typhimurium*. J. Biol. Chem. **257:** 11808–11815.
38. MYERS, K. R., A. T. TRUCHOT, J. WARD, Y. HUDSON & J. T. ULRICH. 1990. A critical determinant of lipid A endotoxic activity. *In* Cellular and Molecular Aspects of Endotoxin Reactions. A. Nowotny, J. J. Spitzer & E. J. Ziegler, Eds. 145–156. Elsevier Science Publishers B.V. (Biomedical Division).
39. ASTIZ, M. E., E. C. RACKOW, J. G. STILL et al. 1995. Pretreatment of normal humans with monophosphoryl lipid A induces tolerance to endotoxin: a prospective, double-blind, randomized, controlled trial. Crit. Care Med. **23:** 9–17.
40. YAO, Z., J. A. AUCHAMPACH, G. M. PIEPER & G. GROSS. 1993. Cardioprotective effects of monophosphoryl lipid A, a novel endotoxin analogue, in the dog. Cardiovasc. Res. **27:** 832–838.
41. YAO, Z., J. L. RASMUSSEN, J. L. HIRT, D. A. MEI, G. M. PIEPER & G. J. GROSS. 1993. Effects of monophosphoryl lipid A on myocardial ischemia/reperfusion injury in dogs. J. Cardiovasc. Pharmacol. **22:** 653–663.
42. MEI, D. A., G. T. ELLIOTT & G. J. GROSS. 1995. ATP-sensitive K$^+$ channels mediate the cardioprotective effect of monophosphoryl lipid A. Circulation 92(Suppl. I): I-388.
43. KUKREJA, R. C., K. YOSHIDA, J. B. SHIPLEY et al. 1995. Pharmacologic 'preconditioning' with monophosphoryl lipid A in the rabbit heart is not mediated by the synthesis of a 70-kilodalton heat shock protein. J. Mol. Cell. Cardiol. **27:** A164.
44. YOSHIDA, K-I., M. M. MAAIEH, J. B. SHIPLEY et al. 1996. Monophosphoryl lipid A induces pharmacologic "preconditioning" in rabbit hearts without concomitant expression of 70-kilodalton heat shock protein. Mol. Cell. Biochem. **156:** 1–8.
45. BAXTER, G. F., R. W. GOODWIN, M. J. WRIGHT, M. KERAC, R. J. HEADS & D. M. YELLON. 1996. Myocardial protection after monophosphoryl lipid A: studies of delayed antiischemic properties in the rabbit heart. Br. J. Pharmacol. **117:** 1685–1692.
46. BAXTER, G. F., R. W. GOODWIN, M. J. WRIGHT, M. KERAC & D. M. YELLON. Delayed myocardial protection following monophosphoryl lipid A treatment in the rabbit is not associated with elevation of 70-kDa stress protein. Circulation. In press.
47. YAO, Z., G. T. ELLIOTT & G. J. GROSS. 1995. Monophosphoryl lipid A (MLA) preserves myocardial contractile function following multiple, brief periods of coronary occlusion in dogs. Pharmacology **51:** 152–159.
48. ABD-ELFATTAH, A. S., J-H. GUO, N. R. EL-SIGABY & G. T. ELLIOTT. 1995. Intravenous administration of monophosphoryl lipid A (MLA) 24 hours before aortic cross-clamping attenuates myocardial stunning in dogs. J. Mol. Cell. Cardiol. **27:** A49.
49. KIDA, M., H. FUJIWARA, M. ISHIDA et al. 1991. Ischemic preconditioning preserves creatine phosphate and intracellular pH. Circ. Res. **84:** 2595–2603.
50. MURRY, C. E., V. J. RICHARD, K. A. REIMER & R. B. JENNINGS. 1990. Ischemic preconditioning slows energy metabolism and delays ultrastructural damage during a sustained ischemic episode. Circ. Res. **66:** 913–931.
51. ZHAO, L., C. C. KIRSCH, S. R. HAGEN & G. T. ELLIOTT. 1996. Preservation of global cardiac function in the rabbit following protracted ischemia/reperfusion using monophosphoryl lipid A (MLA). J. Mol. Cell. Cardiol. **28:** 197–208.
52. ELLIOTT, G. T., C. C. KIRSCH & L. ZHAO. 1995. Monophosphoryl lipid A (MLA) in a rabbit model of prolonged regional ischemia and reperfusion induces functional and biochemical cardioprotection. J. Mol. Cell. Cardiol. **27:** A19.
53. PRZYKLENK, K., L. ZHAO, R. A. KLONER & G. T. ELLIOTT. 1995. Monophosphoryl

lipid A (MLA) is a "preconditioning-mimetic" in the canine model. Circulation **92**(Suppl. I): I-388.

54. MARBER, M. S., R. MESTRIL, D. M. YELLON & W. H. DILLMAN. 1994. A heat shock protein 70 transgene results in myocardial protection. Circulation **90:** I-536.

55. QIAN, Y-Z., M. C. KONTOS, Y. GU & R. C. KUKREJA. 1994. Quercetin blocks ischemic tolerance in heat stressed rat hearts. Circulation **90:** I-536.

56. WHALLEY, E. T., J. A. SOLOMON, D. M. MODAFFERI, K. A. BONHAM & J. C. CHERONIS. 1992. CP-0127, a novel potent bradykinin antagonist, increases survival in rat and rabbit models of endotoxin shock. AAS 38/III. *In* Recent Progress on Kinins. 413–442. Birkhauser Verlag. Basel.

57. TRABER, D. L., H. REDL, G. SCHLAG *et al.* 1988. Cardiopulmonary responses to continuous administration of endotoxin. Am. J. Physiol. (Heart Circ. Physiol.) **254:** H833–H839.

58. BERG, J. T., R. C. ALLISON & A. E. TAYLOR. 1990. Endotoxin extends survival of adult mice in hyperoxia. Proc. Soc. Exp. Biol. Med. **193:** 167–170.

59. KITAMURA, K., K. KANGAWA, M. KAWAMOTO *et al.* 1993. Adrenomedullin: a novel hypotensive peptide isolated from human pheochromocytoma. Biochem. Biophys. Res. Commun. **192:** 553–560.

60. SUGO, S., N. MINAMINO, H. SHAJI *et al.* 1995. Interleukin-1, tumor necrosis factor and lipopolysaccharide additively stimulate production of adrenomedullin in vascular smooth muscle cells. Biochem. Biophys. Res. Commun. **207:** 25–32.

61. PIGOTT, J., T. GARNER, B. BOONE, J. K. CHANG, A. HYMAN & H. LIPPTON. 1994. Adrenomedullin (ADM): an endogenous coronary (COR) vasodilator peptide. Circulation **90**(Pt. 2): I-257.

62. SHINDO, T., U. IKEDA, F. OHKAWA *et al.* 1994. Nitric oxide synthesis in rat cardiac myocytes and fibroblasts. Life Sci. **55:** 1101–1108.

63. GENG, Y., B. ZHANG & M. LOTZ. 1993. Protein tyrosine kinase activation is required for lipopolysaccharide induction of cytokines in human blood monocytes. J. Immunol. **151:** 6692–6700.

Prevention of Post-Pump Myocardial Dysfunction by Glutathione[a]

KAILASH PRASAD,[b] WING P. CHAN, JAWAHAR KALRA,[c]
AND BAIKUNTH BHARADWAJ[d]

Departments of Physiology and [c]Pathology
College of Medicine
University of Saskatchewan
and
Royal University Hospital
Saskatoon, Saskatchewan, Canada
and
[d]Division of Cardiothoracic Surgery
Foothills Hospital
Calgary, Alberta, Canada

INTRODUCTION

Cardiac dysfunction following cardiopulmonary bypass has been reported by numerous investigators in patients[1-4] and in experimental animals.[5-7] There are various sources for an increase in the levels of oxygen free radicals (OFRs) including polymorphonuclear leukocytes (PMNLs),[4] xanthine-xanthine oxidase system,[8] autooxidation of catecholamines.[9] There is an increase in the activated complements (C_{3a}, C_{5a}) during cardiopulmonary bypass,[10,11] which are known to activate PMNLs.[12] Ischemia, which is present during cardiopulmonary bypass, is known to increase levels of xanthine and xanthine oxidase.[13] Levels of catecholamines are increased during cardiopulmonary bypass. Activation of PMNLs would produce OFRs and hypochlorous acid (HOCl).[14,15] Highly reactive OFRs act on unsaturated fatty acids of cell lipid membrane to produce lipid peroxides, malondialdehyde (MDA) that change membrane fluidity and permeability with loss of cell integrity.[16,17] It is also known that OFRs and HOCl depress cardiac function and contractility.[18-20]

We hypothesize that post-pump cardiac dysfunction may be due to elevation of OFRs and HOCl as a result of increased production. Decrease in myocardial contractility may be due to a decrease in the Ca^{++}-uptake and binding by cardiac sarcoplasmic reticulum (SR). Therefore, we investigated the effects of cold crystalloid cardioplegia on the cardiac function and contractility, OFR producing activity of PMNLs (PMNL-CL), blood MDA, coronary sinus plasma creatine kinase (CK) and MB isoenzyme of CK (MBCK), and Ca^{++} binding and uptake by cardiac SR

[a] This work was supported by a grant from the Heart and Stroke Foundation of Saskatchewan.

[b] Address for correspondence: K. Prasad, M.D., Ph.D., FRCP(C), FACC, FICA, FACA, Department of Physiology, College of Medicine, University of Saskatchewan, 107 Wiggins Road, Saskatoon, SK, S7N 5E5 Canada. Tel.: (306) 966-6539; Fax: (306) 966-8718.

in dogs after 2 hours of reperfusion following $1\frac{1}{2}$ hours of ischemic cardiac arrest. We also investigated the effects of glutathione (scavengers of OFRs) and quencher of HOCl on the above-mentioned parameters during and after cardiopulmonary bypass.

METHODS

Healthy mongrel dogs of either sex weighing between 25 and 35 kg were anesthetized with pentobarbital sodium (35 mg/kg intravenously). The trachea was intubated with a closed cuff endotracheal tube, and the lungs were ventilated with a mixture of room air and oxygen using a respiratory pump with a volume of 20 ml/kg and a respiratory rate of 20 breaths/min.

Hemodynamic measurements were made by the previously described method.[19,21] Mean aortic pressure, mean right atrial pressure, left ventricular pressures and rate of rise of left ventricular pressure ($+$dp/dt), and heart rate were recorded. Cardiac index (CI) and left ventricular work index (LVWI) were calculated from the hemodynamic parameters by the previously described method.[19,21] Left ventricular end diastolic pressure (LVEDP), CI and LVWI were used to assess cardiac function. Left ventricular contractility was measured by using the following formula: (dp/dt)(IIP/HR)/CPIP where IIP is the integrated isolemumic pressure measured by using the method described by Yang *et al.*[22] CPIP is common peak isovolumic pressure. This parameter is the true index of myocardial contractility because it is not affected by preload, afterload and heart rate.

The method used for extracorporeal circulation was as described previously.[5-7] In short, the dogs under anesthesia were placed on total cardiopulmonary bypass using an oxygenator gassed with 95% O_2 and 5% CO_2. The extracorporeal circuit consisted of a disposable pediatric Bentley-5-bubble oxygenator and heat exchanger. The system was primed with solution described earlier.[5-7] After initiation of complete cardiopulmonary bypass with left ventricle decompressed, the systemic temperature was lowered to 22°C to 24°C. The ascending aorta was then clamped and cold (4°C) crystalloid cardioplegic solution (200 ml) of the composition described earlier[5-7] was injected in the aortic root. Reinjections of 100 ml of solution were repeated every 20 min for 90 min of the ischemic cardiac arrest period. After $1\frac{1}{2}$ hrs, the cross clamp was removed to restore perfusion and rewarming started. Defibrillation was started when the cardiac muscle temperature was close to 34°C. After $\frac{1}{2}$ hr of reperfusion and warming, cardiopulmonary bypass was discontinued. Hemodynamic stability was achieved through transfusion of left over blood and perfusion fluid. Hemodynamic measurements were made $1\frac{1}{2}$ hrs after discontinuation of bypass.

The dogs were divided into three groups: Group I, 6 dogs (sham bypass); the dogs were put on cardiopulmonary bypass for 2 hrs followed by off bypass for $1\frac{1}{2}$ hrs. The temperature during $1\frac{1}{2}$ hrs of bypass was 22°C to 24°C. The remaining period of $\frac{1}{2}$ hr during bypass was for rewarming to 34°C. Group II, 8 dogs (cold crystalloid cardioplegia); the dogs in this group underwent 90 min ischemic cardiac arrest followed by 30 min for rewarming and $1\frac{1}{2}$ hrs of reperfusion after discontinuation of bypass. Group III, 6 dogs (cold crystalloid cardioplegia with glutathione); all the procedures similar to Group II but these dogs received glutathione 74 mg/kg twice during the procedure. The first dose was given I.V. before initiation of bypass, and the second dose was added 5 min before declamping of aorta in the bubble oxygenator. Hemodynamic measurements were made before opening the chest (pre-op), after opening the chest but before starting on bypass (pre-pump) and 90 min off bypass. Initial blood samples were taken before opening the chest (S_0) from the peripheral veins for measurement of various biochemical parameters [chemiluminescent activity of PMNLs, malondialdehyde (MDA), creatine kinase (CK) and MB-isoenzyme of CK (MBCK)]. The subsequent blood samples were taken from the coronary sinus before clamping the aorta (S_1), 5 min after declamping of aorta (S_2), 5 min off pump (S_3), 30 min off pump (S_4), 60 min off pump (S_5) and 90 min off pump (S_6) for measurement of various biochemical parameters. Oxygen free radical-producing activity of PMNLs was measured as chemiluminescent activity of PMNLs (PMNL-CL) by the previously described method.[19] The results are expressed as superoxide dismutase-inhibitable OFRs (mv.min/10^6 PMNLs). Blood MDA was estimated by the previously described method.[19] Serum CK and MBCK were measured by the methods using creatine kinase reagent test kit.[23] Creatine kinase-isoenzymes were separated by using the column chromatography method of Mercer.[24] Ca^{++}-binding and uptake by cardiac SR were measured by the method of Narayanan.[25]

Statistical analysis for the comparison between the two groups was made using nonparametric statistical Mann-Whitney Rank Sum Test. Analysis of variance and covariance with repeated measures were used for comparison within groups at various times.

RESULTS

The pre-operative and pre-pump hemodynamic values were similar in all the groups, and the post-pump hemodynamic values have been expressed as a percent of pre-operative values. The results for LVEDP, CI and LVWI in the three groups are summarized in FIGURE 1. There was an increase in LVEDP and a decrease in the CI and LVWI in Group I at 90 minutes post-pump as compared to pre-operative values. These changes in Group II were similar to those in Group I. The values for LVEDP were lower and those for CI and LVWI were higher in Group III as compared to Group II.

The changes in the index of myocardial contractility in the three groups are summarized in FIGURE 2. The index of myocardial contractility decreased in Group I and Group II. The values for Group II were lower than those of Group I. The index of contractility was higher in Group III as compared to Groups I and II.

Calcium uptake by cardiac SR from the three groups are summarized in FIGURE 3. Calcium uptake decreased in the cold crystalloid group. It was significantly higher in the cold crystalloid plus glutathione group as compared to the cold crystalloid group. The values for Ca^{++} uptake were similar in the sham and cold crystalloid with glutathione groups. The Ca^{++}-binding by SR decreased in the cold crystalloid group (FIG. 4). It was higher in the cold crystalloid plus glutathione group as compared to that in the cold crystalloid groups but was similar to Group I.

The changes in PMNL-CL for the three groups are summarized in FIGURE 5. The PMNL-CL activity increased in Group I and Group II and there were no differences in the activity between Group I and Group II. The activity in Group III was lower than that in Groups I and II.

Blood MDA increased in all the groups starting 5 min after declamping the aorta (S_2) (FIG. 6). It increased progressively in Group II but remained stationary in Groups I and III thereafter. The values for MDA levels in Groups I and III were similar but lower than in Group II.

The changes in the plasma CK and MBCK are summarized in FIGURES 7 and 8. The post-pump plasma CK activity increased in all the three groups, the increase being greater in Group II than in Groups I and III, where the increases were

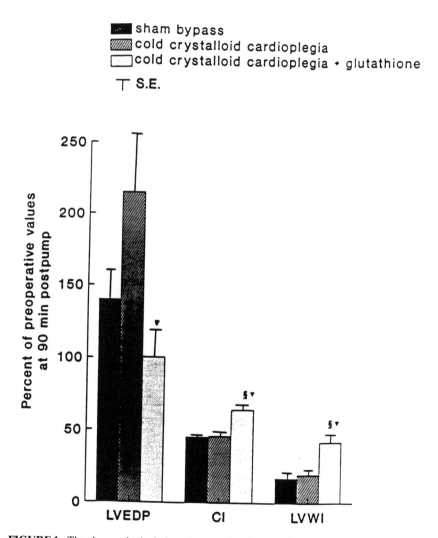

FIGURE 1. The changes in the index of myocardial function in the three groups. The results are presented as percent of the pre-operative values and expressed as mean ± SE. LVEDP, left ventricular end-diastolic pressure; CI, cardiac index; LVWI, left ventricular work index. §p <0.05, sham bypass vs cold crystalloid cardioplegia with or without glutathione. ▼p <0.05, cold crystalloid cardioplegia vs cold crystalloid cardioplegia with glutathione.

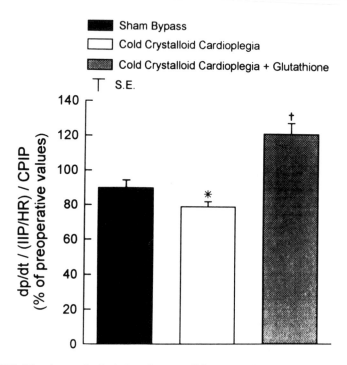

FIGURE 2. The changes in the index of myocardial contractility in the three experimental groups. The results are expressed as mean ± SE. $*p < 0.05$, sham bypass vs cold crystalloid cardioplegia with or without glutathione. $\dagger p < 0.05$, cold crystalloid cardioplegia vs cold crystalloid cardioplegia with glutathione.

similar. There was a progressive and moderate increase in the plasma MBCK 5 min after declamping of the aorta in Group I. The increases in plasma MBCK in Group II were greater than those in Group I. The values for plasma MBCK were significantly lower in Group III than in Groups I and II.

DISCUSSION

There were decreases in CI, LVWI and dp/dt/(IIP/HR)/CPIP and increases in LVEDP in the sham bypass group. The decreases in cardiac function and contractility were further enhanced in Group II (the cold crystalloid cardioplegic group). In the present study, glutathione, an antioxidant and quencher of HOCl, prevented the decline in cardiac function and contractility observed in the cold crystalloid cardioplegic group.

Decreases in cardiac function and contractility were reported previously in sham bypass[4-7] and bypass with cold crystalloid cardioplegia.[4-7] The decreases in cardiac function and contractility in the bypass group may largely be due to the complement-induced PMNL activation and subsequent release of OFRs and

HOCl. Cardiopulmonary bypass with pump oxygenator is associated with activation of complement C_3, C_4 and C_5.[10,11] The results of the present study show that PMNL-CL activity in Group I was increased. Further decreases in cardiac function and contractility in Group II could possibly be due to a further increase in the levels of OFRs through various mechanisms including xanthine-xanthine oxidase, auto-oxidation of catecholamines and arachidonic acid metabolism. Ischemia (ischemic cardiac arrest) increases levels of xanthine and xanthine oxidase activity,[13,26] which in the presence of tissue oxygen (reperfusion following cardiac arrest) would produce OFRs.[8] Elevated systemic levels of arachidonic acid metabolites (prostacyclin and thromboxane A_2) have been reported during cardiopulmonary bypass.[27] OFRs are produced during prostaglandin synthesis.[28] OFRs depress cardiac function and contractility.[18–20] The decrease in contractility could be due

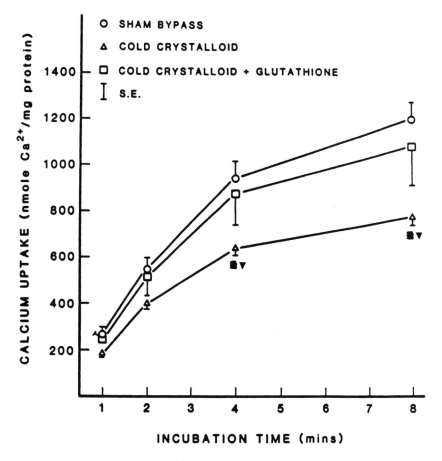

FIGURE 3. The time course of Ca^{++} uptake by cardiac sarcoplasmic reticulum in the three experimental groups. The results are expressed as mean ± SE. ■p <0.05, sham bypass vs cold crystalloid with or without glutathione. ▼p <0.05, cold crystalloid vs cold crystalloid with glutathione.

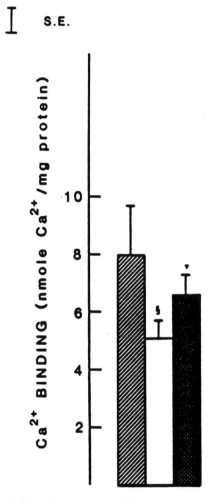

FIGURE 4. Ca^{++}-binding by cardiac SR in the three experimental groups. The results are expressed as mean ± SE. §p <0.05, sham bypass vs cold crystalloid with or without glutathione. ▼p <0.05, crystalloid cardioplegia vs crystalloid cardioplegia with glutathione.

to the depressant effect of OFRs on the contractile apparatus including sarco-lemmal Na^+-K^+ ATPase,[29] Ca^{++} pump,[30] and sarcoplasmic reticular ATPase.[31,32] OFRs could also damage the cell through lipid peroxidation of membrane and hence reduce the contractility. In the present study we observed a decrease in the Ca^{++}-binding and uptake by cardiac SR. This could explain the decrease in the cardiac contractility.

The protective effect of glutathione (Group III) against cold crystalloid car-dioplegic cardiac arrest was associated with a decrease in the oxygen producing

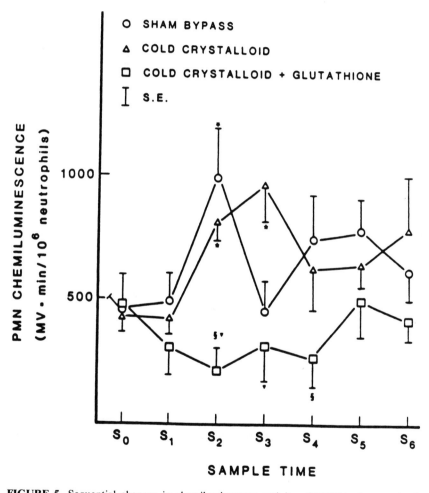

FIGURE 5. Sequential changes in chemiluminescent activity of PMN leukocytes in the three groups. The results are expressed as mean ± SE. S_0, pre-operative; S_1, pre-pump; S_2, 5 min off clamp; S_3, 5 min off pump; S_4, 30 min off pump; S_5, 60 min off pump; S_6, 90 min off pump. *p <0.05, comparison of the values at various times with respect to S_0 in the respective groups. §p <0.05, sham bypass vs cold crystalloid with or without glutathione. ▼p <0.05, cold crystalloid vs cold crystalloid with glutathione.

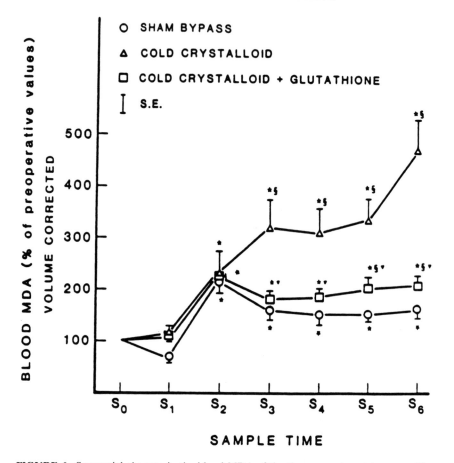

FIGURE 6. Sequential changes in the blood MDA of the three experimental groups. The results are expressed as mean ± SE. The notations for time period are the same as in FIG. 5. *p <0.05, comparison of values at various times with respect to S_0 time in the respective groups. §p <0.05, sham bypass vs cold crystalloid with or without glutathione. ▼p <0.05, cold crystalloid vs cold crystalloid with glutathione.

activity of PMNLs, blood MDA, plasma CK and MBCK, which suggests that glutathione decreased levels of OFR through a decrease in OFR produced by PMNLs. Glutathione is important in protecting cells from oxidant injury.[33] H_2O_2 (oxygen radicals) is broken down by glutathione peroxidase, which requires glutathione as a substrate yielding oxidized glutathione which is re-reduced by the action of glutathione reductase.[34] It quenches triplet carbonyls formed during lipid peroxidation,[35] and acts as a competitive substrate for oxidizing agents, particularly HOCl.[36]

The increase in the PMNL-CL suggests an increased ability of PMNLs to produce OFRs. Increased PMNL-CL activity has also been observed in patients undergoing aortocoronary bypass surgery using cardiopulmonary bypass.[4] As discussed before, the increased PMNL-CL could be due to sensitization of PMNLs by activated complements (C_{3a}, C_{5a}). Increase in blood MDA could be due to increased lipid peroxidation as a result of increased levels of OFRs. It is important to emphasize that the increase in blood MDA is not because of its release from the heart alone but also because of its release from other organs affected by

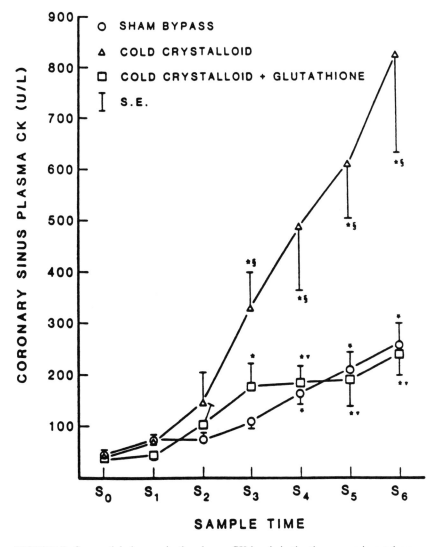

FIGURE 7. Sequential changes in the plasma CK levels in the three experimental groups. The results are expressed as mean ± SE. The notations for time period are the same as in FIG. 5. *p <0.05, comparison of the values at various times with respect to zero time (S_0) in the respective groups. §p <0.05, sham bypass vs cold crystalloid with or without glutathione. ▼p <0.05, cold crystalloid vs cold crystalloid with glutathione.

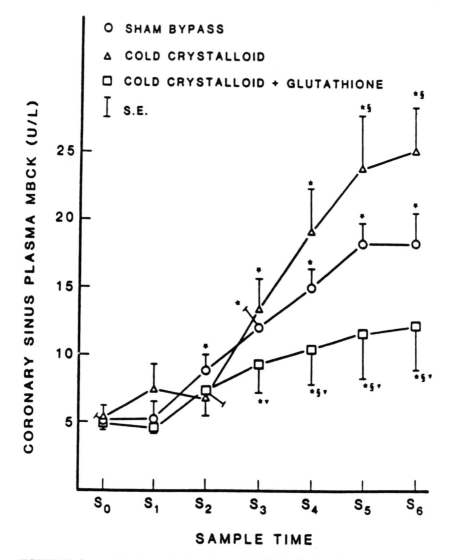

FIGURE 8. Sequential changes in the plasma MBCK levels in the three experimental groups. The results are expressed as mean ± SE. The notations for time period are the same as in FIG. 5. *$p < 0.05$, comparison of value at various times with respect to zero time (S_0) in the respective groups. §$p < 0.05$, sham bypass vs cold crystalloid with or without glutathione. ▼$p < 0.05$, cold crystalloid vs cold crystalloid with glutathione.

cardiopulmonary bypass. Increase in blood MDA has also been reported in patients undergoing cardiopulmonary bypass.[4] The decrease in blood MDA in the glutathione-treated group could be due to the decrease in the levels of OFRs because of its antioxidant activity.

A marked increase in CK and MBCK in Group II as compared to Groups I and III suggests significant damage of cardiac tissue. Increases in plasma CK and MBCK have also been reported during and following cardiopulmonary bypass.[5-7] Prevention of a rise in plasma CK and MBCK by glutathione suggests a protective effect of glutathione against cardioplegic cardiac arrest and cardiopulmonary bypass-induced cellular damage. This protective effect of glutathione is probably due to its antioxidant activity and quenching of HOCl.

The present studies show that the decrease in cardiac function and contractility with the cold crystalloid cardioplegia group was associated with a decrease in Ca^{++} uptake and binding by cardiac SR. Also, recovery in cardiac function and contractility with glutathione was associated with a recovery of Ca^{++} uptake and binding by SR towards control values. OFRs have been reported to depress Ca^{++}-binding and uptake by cardiac SR *in vitro*.[31-32] OFRs are known to depress sarcolemmal Ca^{++} ATPase and the sarcolemmal Ca^{++} pump.[29-31] A decrease in the amount of Ca^{++} being accumulated in cardiac SR would result in a decrease in Ca^{++} being released for muscle contraction. The recovery of Ca^{++}-binding and uptake with glutathione could be due to a decrease in the levels of OFRs.

In summary, the results indicate that a post-pump decrease in cardiac function and contractility was associated with an increase in the OFR-producing activity of PMNLs, blood MDA, and plasma CK and MBCK, and a decrease in Ca^{++}-binding and uptake by cardiac SR. Prevention of post-pump cardiac dysfunction by glutathione was associated with a decrease in the OFR-producing activity of PMNLs, blood MDA, plasma CK and MBCK and an increase in Ca^{++}-binding and uptake by cardiac SR to control levels. In conclusion, these results suggest that post-pump depression of cardiac function and contractility could be due to depression of Ca^{++}-binding and uptake by cardiac sarcoplasmic reticulum as a result of increased levels of oxygen radicals and hypochlorous acid, and that glutathione, a scavenger of oxygen radicals and quencher of hypochlorous acid, may be effective in preventing the post-pump cardiac dysfunction and contractility.

REFERENCES

1. BRODY, W. R., B. A. REITZ, M. J. ANDREWS, W. C. ROBERTS & L. L. MICHAELIS. 1975. Long-term morphologic and hemodynamic evaluation of the left ventricle after cardiopulmonary bypass. J. Thorac. Cardiovasc. Surg. **70:** 1073–1087.
2. BUCKBERG, G. D., G. N. OLINGER, D. G. MULDER & J. V. MALONEY, JR. 1975. Depressed postoperative cardiac performance. Prevention by adequate myocardial protection during cardiopulmonary bypass. J. Thorac. Cardiovasc. Surg. **70:** 974–988.
3. KIRKLIN, J. W. & R. A. THEYE. 1963. Cardiac performance after intracardiac surgery. Circulation **28:** 1061–1070.
4. PRASAD, K., J. KALRA, B. BHARADWAJ & A. K. CHAUDHARY. 1992. Increased oxygen free radical activity in patients on cardio-pulmonary bypass undergoing aorto-coronary bypass surgery. Am. Heart J. **123:** 37–45.
5. PRASAD, K. & B. BHARADWAJ. 1987. Effect of crystalloid cardioplegia and verapamil on cardiac function and cellular biochemistry during hypothermic cardiac arrest. Can. J. Cardiol. **3:** 293–299.
6. PRASAD, K. & B. BHARADWAJ. 1987. Influence of diltiazem on cardiac function at organ and molecular level during hypothermic cardiac arrest. Can. J. Cardiol. **3:** 351–356.
7. CARD, R. T., K. PRASAD, B. BHARADWAJ, L. A. P. HNATUK & M. A. MACFADYEN. 1988. High 2,3-DPG blood cardioplegia and myocardial preservation during cardiopulmonary bypass. Angiology **39:** 123–131.
8. McCORD, J. M. 1985. Oxygen derived free radicals in post-ischemic tissue injury. N. Engl. J. Med. **312:** 159–163.

9. GRAHAM, D. G., S. M. TIFFANY, W. R. BELL & W. F. GUTKENCHT. 1978. Autoxidation versus covalent binding of quinones as the mechanism of toxicity of dopamine, 6-hydroxydopamine, and related compounds towards C1300 neuroblastoma cells *in vitro*. Mol. Pharmacol. **14:** 644–653.

10. CHENOWETH, D. E., S. W. COOPER, T. E. HUGLI, R. W. STEWARD, E. H. BLACKSTONE & J. W. KIRKLIN. 1981. Complement activation during cardiopulmonary bypass. Evidence for generation of C3a and C5a anaphylatoxins. N. Engl. J. Med. **304:** 497–503.

11. CHIU, R. C. J. & R. SAMSON. 1984. Complement (C3, C4) consumption in cardiopulmonary bypass, cardioplegia and protamine administration. Ann. Thorac. Surg. **37:** 229–232.

12. WEBSTER, R. O, S. R. HONG, R. B. JOHNSTON, JR. & P. M. HENSON. 1980. Biological effects of the human complement fragments C5a and C5a des Arg on neutrophil function. Immunopharmacology **2:** 201–219.

13. CHAMBERS, D. E., D. A. PARKS, G. PATTERSON, R. ROY, J. M. McCORD, S. YOSHIDA, L. F. PARMLEY & J. M. DOWNEY. 1985. Xanthine oxidase as a source of free radical damage in myocardial ischemia. J. Mol. Cell. Cardiol. **17:** 145–152.

14. BABIOR, B. M. 1984. The respiratory burst of phagocytes. J. Clin. Invest. **73:** 599–601.

15. FANTONE, J. C. & P. A. WARD. 1982. Role of oxygen-derived free radicals and metabolites in leukocyte-dependent inflammatory reactions. Am. J. Pathol. **107:** 397–417.

16. FREEMAN, B. A. & J. D. CRAPO. 1982. Biology of disease. Free radicals and tissue injury. Lab. Invest. **47:** 412–426.

17. MEERSON, F. Z., V. E. KAGON, Y. P. KOZLOV, L. M. BELKINA & Y. V. ARKKHIPENKO. 1982. The role of lipid peroxidation in pathogenesis of ischemic damage and antioxidant protection of the heart. Basic Res. Cardiol. **77:** 465–485.

18. PRASAD, K., J. KALRA, W. P. CHAN & A. K. CHAUDHARY. 1989. Effect of oxygen free radicals on cardiovascular functions at organ and cellular level. Am. Heart J. **117:** 1196–1202.

19. PRASAD, K., J. KALRA, A. K. CHAUDHARY & D. DEBNATH. 1990. Polymorphonuclear leukocyte activation and cardiac function at organ and cellular level. Am. Heart J. **119:** 538–550.

20. PRASAD, K., J. KALRA & L. BHARADWAJ. 1993. Cardiac depressant effects of oxygen free radicals. Angiology **44:** 257–270.

21. PRASAD, K., P. LEE & J. KALRA. 1991. Influence of endothelin on cardiovascular function, oxygen free radicals and blood chemistry. Am. Heart J. **121:** 178–187.

22. YANG, S. S., L. G. BENTIVOGLIO, V. MARNHAE & H. GOLDBERG. 1972. From Cardiac Catheterization Data to Hemodynamic Parameters. 172. F. A. Davies Company. Philadelphia.

23. KAPOOR, R., J. KALRA & K. PRASAD. 1992. Beneficial effects of methionine on myocardial hemodynamic and cellular function in hemorrhagic shock. Angiology **43:** 294–305.

24. MERCER, D. W. 1974. Separation of tissue and serum creatine kinase isoenzymes by ion exchange column chromatography. Clin. Chem. **20:** 36–40.

25. NARAYANAN, N. 1983. Effects of adrenalectomy and *in vivo* administration of dexamethasone on ATP-dependent calcium accumulation by sarcoplasmic reticulum from rat heart. J. Mol. Cell. Cardiol. **15:** 7–15.

26. JENNING, R. B. & K. A. REIMER. 1982. Lethal myocardial ischemia injury. Am. J. Pathol. **102:** 241–255.

27. TEOH, K. H., S. E. FREMES, R. D. WERSEL, G. T. CHRISTAKIS, S. J. TEASDALE, M. M. MADONILS, J. IVANOV, A. V. MEE & P. Y. WONG. 1987. Cardiac release of prostacyclin and thromboxane A_2 during coronary revascularization. J. Thorac. Cardiovasc. Surg. **93:** 120–126.

28. PANGANAMALA, R. V., H. M. SHARMA, J. C. HEIKKILA, J. C. GEER & D. G. CORNWELL. 1976. Role of hydroxyl radical scavengers, dimethyl sulfoxide, alcohol and methanol in the inhibition of prostaglandin biosynthesis. Prostaglandins **11:** 599–607.

29. KANEKO, M., P. K. SINGAL & N. S. DHALLA. 1990. Alterations in heart sarcolemmal Ca^{++}-ATPase and Ca^{++}-binding activities due to oxygen free radicals. Basic Res. Cardiol. **85:** 45–54.

30. KANEKO, M., V. ELIMBAN & N. S. DHALLA. 1989. Mechanism for depression of heart sarcolemmal Ca^{++} pump by oxygen free radicals. Am. J. Physiol. **257:** H804–H811.
31. KRAMER, J. H., I. T. MAK & W. B. WEGLICKI. 1984. Differential sensitivity of canine cardiac sarcolemmal and microsomal enzyme inhibition by free radical-induced lipid peroxidation. Circ. Res. **55:** 120–124.
32. OKABE, E., K. KUSE, T. SEKISHITA, N. SUYAMA, K. TANAKA & H. ITO. 1991. The effect of raynodine on oxygen free radical-induced dysfunction of cardiac sarcoplasmic reticulum. J. Pharmacol. Exp. Ther. **256:** 868–875.
33. HARLAN, J. M., J. D. LEVINE, K. S. CALLAHAN & B. R. SCHWARTZ. 1984. Glutathione redox cycle protects cultured endothelial cells against lysis by extracellularly generated hydrogen peroxide. J. Clin. Invest. **73:** 706–713.
34. THOMPSON, J. A. & M. L. HESS. 1986. The oxygen free radical system: a fundamental mechanism in the production of myocardial necrosis. Prog. Cardiovasc. Dis. **18:** 449–462.
35. ENCINAS, M. V., E. A. LISSI & A. F. OLEA. 1985. Quenching of triplet benzophenone by vitamin E and C and by sulphur-containing amino-acids and peptides. Photochem. Photobiol. **42:** 347–352.
36. WINTERBOURN, C. 1985. Comparative reactivities of various biological compounds with myeloperoxidase-hydrogen peroxide-chloride, and similarity of the oxidant to hypochlorite. Biochim. Biophys. Acta **840:** 204–210.

Increased Myocardial Tolerance to Ischemia-Reperfusion Injury by Feeding Pigs with Coenzyme Q_{10}

TETSUYA YOSHIDA,[a] GAUTAM MAULIK,
DEBASIS BAGCHI, SITA K. DASH,
RICHARD M. ENGELMAN, AND DIPAK K. DAS

University of Connecticut School of Medicine
Farmington, Connecticut

Creighton University
Omaha, Nebraska

U.A.S. Laboratories
Minnetonka, Minnesota

INTRODUCTION

Several recent studies indicate that Coenzyme Q_{10} (CoQ_{10}), a lipid soluble benzoquinone, may act as potent antioxidant in biological systems and can inhibit the process of lipid peroxidation.[1] Since ischemia and reperfusion are associated with the development of oxidative stress and lipid peroxidation, and antioxidants have been shown to be beneficial for ischemic myocardium,[2] we hypothesized that stimulation of CoQ_{10} may protect hearts from ischemia-reperfusion injury. To test this hypothesis, a group of adult pigs were fed a CoQ_{10}-supplemented diet for four weeks, while another group of pigs were fed regular diets for the same period of time. Previous studies demonstrated that exogenous CoQ_{10} is nonspecifically incorporated into various subcellular fractions including mitochondria and sarcoplasmic reticulum.[3] The results of our study demonstrated an increased amount of CoQ_{10} in mitochondria in the CoQ_{10}-fed pigs in concert with reduced formation of malonaldehyde, a presumptive marker for lipid peroxidation, and improved postischemic ventricular recovery.

MATERIALS AND METHODS

Experimental Protocol

Yorkshire pigs of either sex, weighing 20–25 kg, were fed coenzyme Q_{10} (2 mg/kg) (U.A.S. Laboratories, Minnetonka, MN) for 3 weeks. Age-matched pigs were used for control study. At the end of 3 weeks, the animals were tranquilized with ketamine (Ketaject, 20 mg/kg) and anesthetized with an intravenous injection

[a] Corresponding author: Dr. Tetsuya Yoshida, Cardiovascular Division, Dept. of Surgery, University of Connecticut School of Medicine, 263 Farmington Ave., Farmington, CT 06030-1110.

of sodium pentobarbital (Nembutal, 10 mg/kg). Each animal was supported by controlled respiration with room air by a Harvard respirator and the chest was opened through a median sternotomy as described elsewhere.[4] The azygos vein was ligated. After heparinization with sodium heparin (300 units/kg), cardiopulmonary bypass with a membrane oxygenator (Bentley Univox-IC, Baxter Healthcare Corp., Irvine, CA) primed with 800 ml plasmalyte solution was begun. Arterial inflow was via the ascending aorta, and venous drainage was via a cannula placed in the right ventricle. Another cannula was placed in the left atrium. The heart was isolated from the systemic circulation and maintained in a perfused, oxygenated state by cross clamping the cannulated ascending aorta as described previously.[4] The systemic perfusion was then discontinued. After the systemic circulation was drained into the oxygenator, both the superior and inferior vena cavae were ligated. The heart was perfused at a constant pressure of 75 mmHg with normothermic (37°C) blood.

Left Ventricular Global and Regional Functions

LV pressure measurements were performed with a Millar Mikro-Tip catheter transducer (Millar Instruments, Inc., Houston, TX), which was placed inserted into the left ventricle through an apical stab wound.[4] The maximum and minimum of the first derivative of LV pressure (LV dp/dt max and LV dp/dt$_{min}$) and LV developed pressure (LVDP) were also measured. Sonometric dimension crystals (6 mm diameter) made of 3 MHz piezoelectric crystals (Triton Technologies Inc., San Diego, CA) were placed at the endocardial surface across the anteroposterior minor axis, the septal-free wall minor axis, and the base-apex major axis of the left ventricle as described previously.[4] Functional data were obtained by adding 60 ml of saline to raise the LVEDP and then withdrawing to create pressure-volume loops.

Baseline measurements were taken after stabilization at normothermic perfusion, consisting of left ventricular (LV) developed pressure, LV dp/dt$_{max}$, LV dp/dt$_{min}$, coronary blood flow (CBF) and malonaldehyde (MDA) formation. The left anterior descending (LAD) coronary artery was then occluded distal to the first diagonal branch for 10 min. After 10 min of LAD occlusion, the aortic perfusion was stopped, and 200 ml of cold (4°C) blood cardioplegia was infused into the aortic root to arrest the heart. Blood cardioplegia reinfusion was made every 15 min during 60 min of cardioplegic arrest. The LAD snare was removed just before the second injection of cardioplegia. The myocardial temperature was monitored by inserting a thermometer into ventricular septum and maintained with cold saline between 6 and 10°C during cardioplegia. Normothermic reperfusion was performed for 60 min following cardioplegic arrest. In each study, the heart was paced both pre- and postischemically at 120 beats/min by ventricular pacing. Hemodynamic and metabolic measurements were taken after 15 min and 60 min of reperfusion. At the end of each experiment, LV biopsies were taken for biochemical determination.

Estimation of Malonaldehyde

Malonaldehyde was assayed as described previously to estimate lipid peroxidation.[5] In short, weighed heart biopsies were homogenized in 2 ml of 20% trichloroacetic acid and 5.3 mM sodium bisulfite, kept on ice for 10 min, and centrifuged at 3,000 g for 10 min. The supernatants were then collected, derivatized with 2,4-

dinitrophenylhydrazine (DNPH), and extracted with pentane. Aliquots of 25 μl in acetonitrile were injected onto a Beckman Ultrasphere C_{18} (3 μm) column. The products were eluted isocratically with a mobile phase containing acetonitrile-water-acetic acid (40 : 60 : 0.1, v/v/v) and measured at three different wavelengths (307, 325 and 356 nm) using a Waters M-490 multichannel ultraviolet (UV) detector.

Estimation of Myocardial CoQ_{10}

For CoQ_{10} assay, the left ventricular biopsies were quickly frozen at liquid N_2. The frozen tissues were stored at $-70°C$ for subsequent determination of CoQ_{10}. The tissue was homogenized and treated with 2% $FeCl_3$ to convert the reduced form of ubiquinone into the oxidized form which was extracted with n-hexane. The solvent was evaporated at 30°C under N_2. The residue was dissolved in isopropylalcohol and analyzed by HPLC.[6] CoQ_{10} was eluted with methanol/ethanol (1 : 1, v/v) by passing through a C_{18} column. UV absorbance of the elute was monitored at 275 nm.

RESULTS AND DISCUSSION

Feeding CoQ_{10} to the pigs increased the myocardial content of CoQ_{10} (TABLE 1). The results of our study clearly demonstrate the beneficial effects of CoQ_{10} in myocardial protection during ischemia and reperfusion. As shown in TABLE 2, left ventricular developed pressure (LVDP) dropped significantly after ischemia in both groups. However, in the CoQ_{10} group LVDP was significantly higher during the postischemic reperfusion period. The maximum first derivative of LVDP (LV_{max} dp/dt) followed a similar pattern. The left ventricular end-diastolic pressure (LVEDP) was lower in the treated group prior to ischemia. LVEDP increased in both groups during the postischemic reperfusion, but the values were lower in the treated group as compared to the control group. CoQ_{10} did not affect the heart rate.

There is much evidence that reactive oxygen species play a role in the pathophysiology of ischemic reperfusion injury.[7] The presence of the hydroxyl radical (OH·) has been confirmed in the reperfused myocardium.[7] Membrane lipids are potential targets for free radical attack, and this causes lipid peroxidation. The extent of lipid peroxidation was lower in the CoQ_{10}-fed hearts as evidenced by the reduced amount of MDA formation (FIG. 1). CoQ_{10} was previously shown to block the lipid peroxidation process.[1] It is generally believed that CoQ_{10} exhibits its protective effect either by preventing the formation of lipid free radicals or by directly scavenging them. The results of our study support this notion and further suggest that CoQ_{10} reduces myocardial ischemia-reperfusion injury by reducing the oxidative stress.

TABLE 1. Myocardial Content of Coenzyme Q_{10}

	Baseline	Ischemia	Reperfusion
$-$Coenzyme Q_{10}	21.5 ± 0.7	19.2 ± 0.9	18.7 ± 0.8
$+$Coenzyme Q_{10}	24.0 ± 0.5*	23.1 ± 0.7*	22.9 ± 0.4*

* p <0.05 compared to coenzyme Q_{10}.

TABLE 2. Effect of Coenzyme Q_{10} on Postischemic Ventricular Recovery

		Baseline	Reperfusion			
			15 min	30 min	45 min	60 min
LVDP	Control	198.0 ± 35.2	67.5 ± 18.9	91.0 ± 19.95	80.8 ± 15.7	83.3 ± 13.2
(mmHg)	Treatment	211.8 ± 31.2	105 ± 17.7	108.0 ± 9.6	102.2 ± 9.4	109.7 ± 7.1
LVEDP	Control	24.7 ± 3.8	27.8 ± 6.7	24.2 ± 3.8	20.7 ± 0.8	21.3 ± 2
(mmHg)	Treatment	13.4 ± 1.8	185. ± 2.7	18.8 ± 2.7	16.8 ± 2.7	16.7 ± 3.3
LV_{max} dp/dt	Control	2887 ± 943	487 ± 2.7	601 ± 67	572 ± 157	630 ± 136
(mmHg/sec)	Treatment	4993 ± 884	1248 ± 425	916 ± 135	859 ± 148	823 ± 136
LV_{min} dp/dt	Control	-1793 ± 746	-360 ± 159	-473 ± 116	-403 ± 105	-434 ± 95
(mmHg/sec)	Treatment	-2986 ± 442	-820 ± 316	-682 ± 193	-700 ± 177	-711 ± 170

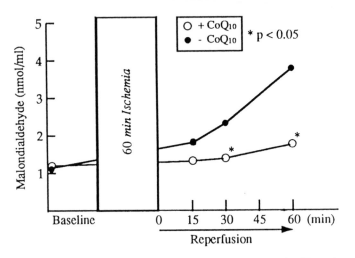

FIGURE 1. Amount of malonaldehyde produced in the perfusate obtained from the coronary effluent at baseline and during postischemic reperfusion. Perfusates were withdrawn at the indicated time points, and malonaldehyde was assayed by HPLC after having been derivatized with DNPH as described in Methods. *p <0.05 compared to nontreated group.

REFERENCES

1. FREI, B., M. C. KIM & B. N. AMES. 1990. Uniquinol-10 is an effective lipid-soluble antioxidant at physiological concentrations. Proc. Natl. Acad. Sci. USA **87:** 4879–4883.
2. DAS, D. K. & N. MAULIK. 1994. Evaluation of antioxidant effectiveness in ischemia reperfusion tissue injury methods. Methods Enzymol. **233:** 601–610.
3. NAKAMURA, T., H. SAMMA, M. HIMENO & K. KATO. 1980. Transfer of exogenous coenzyme Q to the inner membrane of heart mitochondria in rats. *In* Biomedical and Clinical Aspects of Coenzyme Q. K. Volkers, Y. Yamamura & Y. Ito, Eds. Vol. 2: 3–14. Elsevier. North Holland.
4. ENGELMAN, D. T., M. WATANABE, N. MAULIK, G. A. CORDIS, R. M. ENGELMAN, J. A. ROUSOU, J. E. FLACK, D. W. DEATON & D. K. DAS. 1995. L-arginine reduces endothelial inflammation and myocardial stunning during ischemia/reperfusion. Ann. Thorac. Surg. **60:** 1275–1281.
5. CORDIS, G. A., N. MAULIK, D. BAGCHI, R. M. ENGELMAN & D. K. DAS. 1993. Estimation of the extent of lipid peroxidation in the ischemic and reperfused heart by monitoring lipid metabolic products with the aid of high-performance liquid chromatography. **632:** 97–103.
6. HORISHIMA, O., Y. YAMANO, H. TAKAHIRA, T. NAITO, S. ISHIKAWA, E. ARAKI & G. KATUI. 1985. Rapid method for determination of ubiquinone in biological materials by high-performance liquid chromatography. Vitamin **59:** 457–463.
7. TOSAKI, A., D. BAGCHI, D. HELLEGOUARCH, T. PALI, G. A. CORDIS & D. K. DAS. 1993. Comparisons of ESR and HPLC methods for the detection of hydroxyl radicals in ischemic/reperfused hearts. A relationship between the genesis of oxygen-free radicals and reperfusion-induced arrhythmias. Biochem. Pharmacol. **45:** 961–969.

Changes in Atrial Natriuretic Factor (ANF) and Ca^{++} ATPase mRNA Transcriptional Activity Are Markers of Myocardial Integrity during Continuous Warm Blood Cardioplegia (CWBCP) in Rats

E. S. REMSEY, M. A. BAIG,[a] J. G. KRAL,[b]
K. D. EGHBALI, M. VARGA, R. B. WAIT, AND
M. A. Q. SIDDIQUI[a]

*Department of Surgery
and [a]Department of Anatomy and Cell Biology
State University of New York Health Science Center
at Brooklyn
Box 40
450 Clarkson Avenue
Brooklyn, New York 11203*

INTRODUCTION

Normothermic blood cardioplegia is often termed "aerobic" or nonischemic cardioprotection.[1] However, significant elevations in lactate production have been demonstrated during CWBCP, implying ischemia.[2] Hypoxia causes increases in atrial natriuretic factor (ANF) levels.[3] It has been proposed that ANF exerts a cytoprotective effect by cyclic guanosine 3'-5' monophosphate (c-GMP) activating c-GMP-dependent protein kinase. Protein kinase acts by a conformational change of the L-type Ca^{++} channel, which is inhibited and consequently decreases intracellular calcium.[5] Administration of ANF has been shown to prevent ischemia and reperfusion injury.[4] During cardiac overload,[6] heart failure[7] and ischemic cardiomyopathy,[8] there is upregulation of ANF mRNA transcriptional activity, and it is inversely related to L-type Ca^{++} ATPase mRNA transcription.[9] We hypothesized that CWBCP causes transient ischemia, which results in changes in ANF and Ca^{++} ATPase gene expression. These changes, in turn, influence myocardial metabolism and cardiac performance, since some reports suggest that ANF has direct hemodynamic effects.[6-10]

METHODS

Transcriptional activity of ANF and Ca^{++} ATPase was analyzed quantitatively in atrial and ventricular myocardium by RT-PCR[11-12] on 5 μg of total RNA. Peak

---

[b] Corresponding author.

left ventricular pressure (LVP), ($\pm$) dP/dt, LV end diastolic pressure (LVEDP), heart rate (HR) and coronary flow (CF) were measured in blood perfused rat hearts (n = 10) in Langendorff mode before and after one hour of CWBCP. In % of prearrest values this model achieves means ($\pm$ SEM) of 97.5 $\pm$ 2.7% of LVP, 98.9 $\pm$ 5.35% of ($\pm$) dP/dt, 105.0 $\pm$ 2.3% of HR and 117 $\pm$ 2.8% of CF after one hour of continuous warm blood cardioplegia and 30 minutes of reperfusion. There was 100% spontaneous defibrillation without arrhythmia. Performance parameters and myocardial tissue were analyzed at baseline (BL), and subsequently after 30 minutes of equilibration (EQ), after EQ plus 60 minutes of CWBCP and after EQ + CWBCP plus 30 minutes of reperfusion (R). Lactate in the inflow (IF) and outflow (OF) perfusate was measured spectrophotometrically at 540 nm with a diagnostic kit from Sigma Co. Lactate production in mg/ml = (IF-OF)/CF. Beating hearts perfused by modified Krebs-Henseleit buffer were used as temporal controls (sham) at 90 minutes (n = 6) for CWBCP and 120 minutes (n = 6) for reperfusion.

RESULTS

From BL to EQ both atrial and ventricular myocardial ANF and Ca^{++} ATPase gene expression (TABLE 1) were downregulated (p <0.05). During CWBCP there was a significant upregulation of ANF mRNA transcriptional activity in the atrium and ventricle compared to EQ. Ca^{++} ATPase mRNA, on the other hand, was only upregulated in the ventricle during CWBCP compared to EQ (p <0.05), (TABLE 2). During reperfusion ANF gene expression both in atrial and ventricular myocardium reverted to the same level as during EQ; however, atrial and ventricular Ca^{++} ATPase levels were significantly reduced below EQ compared to CWBCP (p <0.01). Gene expression data of ANF and Ca^{++} ATPase in both atrium and ventricle during CWBCP were higher than in the 90-minute beating heart controls (p <0.05). After reperfusion there was a significant downregulation in atrial and ventricular Ca^{++} ATPase compared to the 120-minute controls (p <0.01), and there was no difference in ANF mRNA transcription. During reperfusion atrial ANF mRNA transcriptional activity was inversely related to dP/dt (r = 0.83; p <0.05) and inversely related to heart rate (r = 0.89; p <0.001). Lactate production during the CWBCP after 30 minutes was 0.08 $\pm$ 0.02 mg/ml and after 60 minutes was 0.11 $\pm$ 0.03 mg/ml (n.s.).

TABLE 1. Transcriptional Activity[a] of Atrial Natriuretic Factor mRNA

	Experimental Group				Sham Group	
	Baseline n = 10	Equilibration n = 10	CWBCP[b] n = 10	Reperfusion n = 10	90 min n = 6	120 min n = 6
Atrium	2685 $\pm$ 31	1527 $\pm$ 60[c]	2107 $\pm$ 67[d]	1739 $\pm$ 69[e]	1560 $\pm$ 43[f]	1509 $\pm$ 54
Ventricle	1935 $\pm$ 72	1204 $\pm$ 58[c]	1962 $\pm$ 65[d]	1501 $\pm$ 78[e]	1477 $\pm$ 55[f]	1357 $\pm$ 96

[a] Transcriptional activity results expressed in DPM counts (means $\pm$ SEM).
[b] CWBCP: continuous warm blood cardioplegia.
[c] p <0.05 vs baseline.
[d] p <0.05 vs equilibration.
[e] p <0.05 vs CWBCP.
[f] p <0.05 vs CWBCP at 90 min.

TABLE 2. Transcriptional Activity[a] of Ca^{++} ATPase mRNA

	Experimental Group				Sham Group	
	Baseline n = 10	Equilibration n = 10	CWBCP[b] n = 10	Reperfusion n = 10	90 min n = 6	120 min n = 6
Atrium	2039 ± 52	1358 ± 69[c]	1519 ± 67	675 ± 38[e]	1287 ± 40[f]	1180 ± 159[g]
Ventricle	2151 ± 72	1408 ± 48[c]	1949 ± 77[d]	720 ± 38[e]	1379 ± 61[f]	1343 ± 145[g]

[a] Transcriptional activity results expressed in DPM counts (means ± SEM).
[b] CWBCP: continuous warm blood cardioplegia.
[c] $p < 0.05$ vs baseline.
[d] $p < 0.05$ vs equilibration.
[e] $p < 0.01$ vs CWBCP.
[f] $p < 0.05$ vs CWBCP at 90 min.
[g] $p < 0.05$ reperfusion vs sham at 120 min.

DISCUSSION

Upregulation of ANF and Ca^{++} ATPase gene expression during CWBCP implies the existence of mild transient ischemia, which is not reflected in lactate levels. This finding may indicate that changes in ANF and Ca^{++} ATPase mRNA transcription are more sensitive markers of ischemia than lactate. The time courses of the recovery of ANF and Ca^{++} ATPase gene expression are different, which may be due to an interactive underlying mechanism for the regulation of their expression in the ischemic myocardium.[8,9] This finding supports earlier data showing an inverse relationship between ANF mRNA and Ca^{++} ATPase mRNA transcription in acute heart failure[6] and ischemic cardiomyopathy.[7] Cardiac performance as dP/dt and heart rate was reflected in atrial ANF gene expression. Based on earlier reports it is possible that the concomitant changes in (atrial) ANF and sarcoplasmic Ca^{++} ATPase in concert may play compensatory roles in ischemic and also in acute and severely failing myocardium.[8–9]

We conclude that significant upregulation of ANF and Ca^{++} ATPase mRNA transcriptional activity during continuous warm blood cardioplegia suggests that there is a mild ischemia during CWBCP. The inverse relationship between atrial ANF mRNA transcription and heart performance parameters implies that ANF may be involved in maintaining myocardial integrity during warm cardioprotection. Potentially it may help to prevent reperfusion injury of the heart as has been shown in other tissue.[4]

REFERENCES

1. LICHTENSTEIN, S. V., A. A. KASSAM, E. D. DALATI, R. J. CUSIMANO, A. PANOS & A. S. SLUTSKY. 1989. Warm heart surgery. J. Thorac. Cardiovasc. Surg. **101:** 269–274.
2. YAU, T. M., J. S. IKONOMIDIS, R. D. WEISEL, D. A. MICKLE, N. HAYASHIDA, J. IVANOV, S. CARSON, M. K. MOHABEER & L. C. TUMIATI. 1993. Which techniques of cardioplegia prevent ischemia? Ann. Thorac. Surg. **56:** 1020–1028.
3. BAERTSCHI, J. A., C. HAUSMANINGER, R. S. WALSH, R. M. MENTZER, D. A. WYATT & R. A. PENCE. 1986. Hypoxia-induced release of atrial natriuretic factor (ANF) from the isolated rat and rabbit heart. Biochem. Biophys. Res. Commun. **140:** 427–433.
4. BILZER, M., R. WITTHAUS, G. PAUMGARTNER & A. L. GERDES. 1994. Prevention of

ischemia/reperfusion injury in the rat liver by atrial natriuretic peptide. Gastroenterology **106:** 143–151.

5. TOHSE, N., H. NAKAYA, Y. TAKEDA & M. KANNO. 1995. Cyclic GMP-mediated inhibition of L-type Ca^{++}-channel activity by human natriuretic peptide in rabbit heart cells. Br. J. Pharmacol. **114:** 1076–1082.

6. DREXLER, H., J. HANZE, M. FINCK, W. LU, H. JUST & R. E. LANG. 1988. Atrial natriuretic peptide in a rat model of cardiac failure. Circulation **79:** 620–633.

7. WANGLER, R. D., B. A. BREHAUS, H. O. OTERO, D. A. HASTINGS & M. D. HOLZMAN. 1985. Coronary vasoconstrictor effects of atriopeptin II. Science **230:** 558–561.

8. TAKAHASHI, T., P. D. ALLEN & S. IZUMO. 1992. Expression of A-, B-, and C-type natriuretic peptide genes in failing and developing human ventricle. Circ. Res. **71:** 9–17.

9. ARAI, M., H. MATSUI & M. PERIASAMY. 1993. Sarcoplasmic reticulum gene expression in cardiac hypertrophy and heart failure. (Review). Circ. Res. **74:** 555–564.

10. FERRARI, R. & G. AGNOLETTI. 1989. Atrial natriuretic peptide: its mechanism of release from the atrium. Int. J. Cardiol. **24:** 137–149.

11. CHOMCZYNSKI, P. & N. SACCHI. 1987. Single-step method for RNA isolation by acid guanidium thiocyanate-phenol-chloroform extraction. Anal. Biochem. **162:** 156–159.

12. SAIKI, R. K., D. H. GELFAND, S. STOFFEL, S. J. SHARF, R. F. HIGUCHI, G. T. HORN, K. B. MULLIS & H. A. EHRLICH. 1988. Primer directed enzymatic amplification of DNA with a thermostable DNA polymerase. Science **239:** 487–491.

An Approach to a Definition of the Limits of Adaptive Reorganization of Capillary Endothelium in Ischemic Myocardium Based on Ultrastructural Analysis

A. M. VOLKOV, G. M. KAZANSKAYA,
A. M. KARAS'KOV, AND A. V. SHUNKIN

Laboratory of Electron Microscopy
Research Institute of Circulation Pathology
Novosibirsk, Russia

Endothelial cells (EC) with different opaque densities of cytoplasm and different package densities of organelles are occasionally seen in the same capillary under the electron microscope.[1] The question is, what may be the relative proportions of morphological variants in these myocardial ECs under normal and pathological conditions? It is also unclear what changes in these proportions may be adaptive in providing tolerance of ischemic myocardial damage by endothelial monolayer.

With the use of electron microscopy, the ECs of myocardial capillaries were analyzed in models of ischemia in dogs: (1) occlusion of coronary arteries for 150 min under normothermia, 3 dogs; (2) total ischemia of the myocardium for 30 min under normothermia, 6 dogs; (3) total ischemia of the myocardium for 60 min under hypothermic protection (22–24°C), 6 dogs. Tissue samples were obtained at the end of the ischemic period in all the models and additionally during resumption of cardiac activity in models (2) and (3). Dogs sacrificed under anesthesia served as controls.

Thus, the control endothelium mainly consists of cells, which we designated as having moderately dense cytoplasm, or cells of the main type. Their morphological characteristics generally conformed to those amply described for normal capillary endothelium.[2–4] In addition, ECs conventionally called light or dark occasionally were seen in the capillaries of the left ventricle. The optical density of light ECs is lower than that of cells of the main type. Organelles occur less frequently, the numbers of cytogranules and plasmolemmal vesicles are reduced. In spite of this, all the structures are quite uniformly distributed within the cell. In dark ECs, the optical density of cytoplasm is higher than that of cells of the main type. A distinguishing feature is the great amount of plasmolemmal vesicles lying freely in the cytoplasm or attached to the luminal-abluminal surfaces of the cell.

Stereological analysis confirmed the differences between the three morphological variants of the ECs. The number of freely lying vesicles per unit area of cell is significantly greater in the dark (29.4 ± 1.8 vesicle/μm^2) than light cells (12.9 ± 1.0 vesicle/μm^2) or cells of the main type (16.4 ± 1.3 vesicle/μm^2).

Single ECs with sharply changed ultrastructure occur in the control capillaries and their presence in normal endothelium reflects natural death of endotheliocytes which have passed through their cell cycle. The control percentages of the five

TABLE 1. Relative Proportions of Five Morphological Variants of Capillary Endothelial Cells in Regional and Total Models of Myocardial Ischemia

Experiment	Cell Differentiation According to Density of Cytoplasm (% of Total)				
	Moderate Density (Main Cell Type)	Light	Dark	Swollen	Necrotized
1. Control	68	15	15	1	1
2. Regional ischemia for 150-min coronary artery occlusion					
End of occlusion	22	18	36	7	17
3. Total ischemia for 30-min under normothermia					
End of occlusion	33	25	32	7	3
Reperfusion	24	21	31	8	16
4. Total ischemia for 60 min under deep (22–24°C) hypothermia					
End of occlusion	41	15	38	3	3
Reperfusion and rewarming (to 35–36°C)	49	11	35	4	1

morphological variants are as follows: 68% for main type cells, 15% for light, 15% for dark, 1% for swollen and 1% for necrotized ECs.

Analysis of capillary endothelium of the left ventricle by the end of 150 min occlusion of the coronary artery and of 30 min of total myocardial ischemia demonstrated a sharp decrease in the number of cells of the main type. In contrast, the proportion of swollen and necrotized ECs is increased (TABLE 1).

In all the morphological variants of ECs, organelles show characteristic changes. Cytoplasm and nuclei start to swell in the light cells and swelling continues increasing in the already swollen cells. In contrast, nuclei become denser in cells of the main type and dark ones. Many clumps of inactive chromatin accumulate in their karyoplasm. All the variants showed swollen mitochondria. The dystrophic changes developed in all the variants were similar. However, changes were less conspicuous in main type cells than in light and dark.

In model 2, after removal of occlusion of the major vessels, the number of main type cells further decreased compared to the occlusion period (TABLE 1). Dystrophic changes became more marked in all the morphological variants of ECs. Plasmolemma lost its integrity in many cells which were subjected to lysis.

In model 3, the relative proportions of the five variants also changes. In this model, the number of cells of the main type remained much higher than in the two other models (TABLE 1). In all the morphological variants, the degree to which the organelles were damaged was moderate. Of all the morphological variants, cells of the main type were most tolerant to hypothermic heart occlusion. Some showed only mild ultrastructural changes even after long ischemia. The general architectonics of such cells was preserved, their plasmolemma was distinct, and there were many free and attached plasmolemmal vesicles in cytoplasm.

After removal of total ischemia and restoration of cardiac activity, the proportion of main type cells increased (TABLE 1). Dark and light ECs showed only some evidence of normalization of ultrastructure at this step. In contrast, many cells of the main type showed distinct evidence of regeneration. Granularity of euchromatin in nuclei appeared quite uniformly distributed throughout karyoplasm, although there were small condensations of chromatin. Thick walled vesicles branched off from Golgi cisternae, frequently from their ends (FIG. 1). A branching network of channels of rough endoplasmic reticulum was encountered

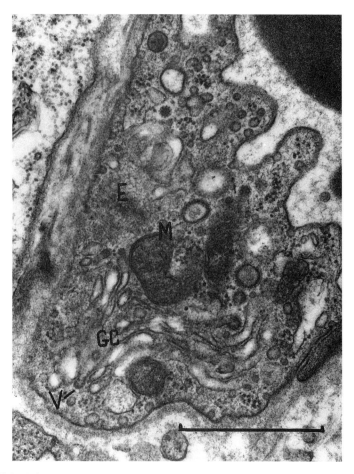

FIGURE 1. A fragment of left ventricle capillary endothelium (E) after removal of 60 min total ischemia under deep hypothermia, restoration of cardiac activity and rewarming of dogs to an oesophagal temperature of 35–36°C. The Golgi complex (GC) appears as a pile of semicircular cisternae, vacuoles and vesicles. Thick-walled vesicles (V) branch off from cisternae, frequently from their ends. Small vesicles are either smooth or bristled at their surfaces. Many free ribosomes are prominent in the cytoplasm. The matrix is of normal density in mitochondria (M) showing distinct outer and inner membranes (39,000×).

in cells of the main type. Their membranes were tightly covered by ribosomes. There were also many free ribosomes in cytoplasm.

Our broad approach to ultrastructural analysis demonstrated that the ECs of the main type are the most tolerant to ischemia because of the dynamic equilibrium established between the development of organelles involved in transport and synthesis. Hyperfunction of the organelles involved in transport in dark cells and the initial underdevelopment of all organelles in light cells restrict their tolerance of ischemia-reperfusion.

This present ultrastructural analysis of capillaries in models of ischemia differing in duration and extent of myocardial damage allowed us to define the limits of reorganization of endothelium which are compatible with life after ischemic challenge. As demonstrated by the experiment with hypothermic cardiac arrest, it is of vital importance that not less than a third of main type cells be involved in adaptive reorganization during ischemia. Deviations from this third may cause a breakdown in the structural and functional adaptation of capillary endothelium and make necrotic processes prominent.

REFERENCES

1. CHERNYKH, A. M., P. N. ALEKSANDROV & O. B. ALEKSEEV. 1975. Microcirculation. A. M. Chernykh, Ed. Medicine. Moscow.
2. RHODIN, J. A. G. 1968. J. Ultrastruct. Res. **25:** 452–500.
3. SHERF, L., Y. BEN-SHAUL & Y. LIEBERMAN. 1977. Am. J. Cardiol. **39:** 599–608.
4. HORMIA, M. & I. VIRTANEN. 1988. Med. Biol. **64:** 247–266.

Implication of DNA Damage during Reperfusion of Ischemic Myocardium

GERALD A. CORDIS,[a] DEBASIS BAGCHI,
WALTER RIEDEL, SIDNEY J. STOHS, AND
DIPAK K. DAS

University of Connecticut School of Medicine
Farmington, Connecticut

Creighton University School of Pharmacy
Omaha, Nebraska

Max-Planck Institut
Bad Nauheim, Germany

INTRODUCTION

Numerous studies indicate that reperfusion of ischemic myocardium is associated with generation of reactive oxygen species that attack membrane lipids causing lipid peroxidation.[1] Although DNA is also a potential target for free radicals, little evidence exists to indicate the role of ischemia/reperfusion in DNA damage. The most common method used to assess the DNA damage is the estimation of DNA strand break.[2] Based on the fact that hydroxyl radical (OH•) has been detected in the ischemic reperfused heart[3] and that deoxyguanosine is a preferential target for OH• in hepatic DNA,[4] we examined the possible presence of DNA-OH• conjugate, 8-hydroxydeoxyguanosine (8-OHDG), in the ischemic reperfused myocardium.

MATERIALS AND METHODS

Isolated Rat Heart Preparation

Isolated perfused rat hearts were prepared and perfused by Langendorff mode as described previously.[5] Hearts were equilibrated for 10 min by perfusing with oxygenated normothermic Krebs-Henseleit buffer (KHB). Hearts were then divided into two groups. The first group of hearts were subjected to 30 min of ischemia followed by 30 min of reperfusion, while the second group of hearts were perfused with OH• generating system (100 μM xanthine, 8 mU/ml xanthine oxidase, 100 μM FeCl$_3$ and 100 μM EDTA). Experiments were terminated at different time points, rapidly frozen in liquid N$_2$, and stored at $-70°C$ for subsequent DNA isolation.

[a] Correspondence: University of Connecticut School of Medicine, 263 Farmington Ave., Farmington, CT 06030-1110.

Isolation of DNA

Rat hearts (1 gm) were homogenized in 10 ml solution containing 1% SDS and 1 mM EDTA using a Polytron homogenizer, and the homogenates incubated at 38°C for 30 min with proteinase K (500 mg/ml).[6] 0.5 ml of 1 M Tris-HCl buffer, pH 7.4, was added to the homogenate, and the resulting solution was extracted with 1 volume of phenol: Sevag (1 : 1 v/v) and Sevag.

The phases were separated by centrifugation, and the aqueous phases collected and pooled. DNA was precipitated with 0.1 vol of 5 M NaCl and 1 vol of ethanol at −20°C. After centrifugation and a 70% ethanol rinse, the DNA was dissolved in 2 ml of 1.5 mM NaCl, 150 μM Na-citrate, 1 mM EDTA. The solution was incubated for 30 min at 38°C with RNase T_1 (50 units/ml) and RNase A (100 μg/ml). The DNA solutions were extracted with Sevag and precipitated with NaCl and ethanol.[6]

DNA Hydrolysis

The DNA pellets were dissolved in 0.5 ml of 20 mM sodium acetate, pH 4.8, and incubated for 30 min at 37°C with 63 mg of nuclease P_1. 50 μl of 1 M Tris-HCl, pH 7.4, was added, and the nucleotides incubated for 60 min at 37°C with 6.3 units of *E. coli* alkaline phosphatase.[4]

HPLC of Bases

A 25 μl of the filtered aliquot of the hydrolyzed DNA was injected onto a C_{18} Beckman Ultrasphere column (3 μm particle size, 7.5 cm × 4.6 mm) equipped with a Waters HPLC chromatograph containing Millenium software and the 996 photodiode array detector. The sample was run isocratically for 10 min using a mobile phase containing 4% acetonitrile and 0.1% acetic acid. The DNA-OH• conjugate, 8-OHDG, was detected at a retention time of 3.8 min using a wavelength of 297 nm. Purity of 8-OHDG was determined by the UV scan of the authentic standard with comparison to the rat heart 8-OHDG.

RESULTS AND DISCUSSION

Damage of DNA by oxygen free radicals results in the production of a large number of lesions, which can be grouped into strand breaks and base modification

TABLE 1. Production of 8-OHDG in the Ischemic Reperfused Heart[a]

Experimental Condition	8-OHDG Formed (pmol/mg DNA)
Baseline	1008 ± 98
30 min ischemia	1079 ± 103
30 min ischemia + 10 min reperfusion	857 ± 87
30 min ischemia + 20 min reperfusion	1547 ± 121*
30 min ischemia + 30 min reperfusion	1500 ± 118*

[a] Results are means ± SE of six samples per group; * p <0.05 compared to baseline.

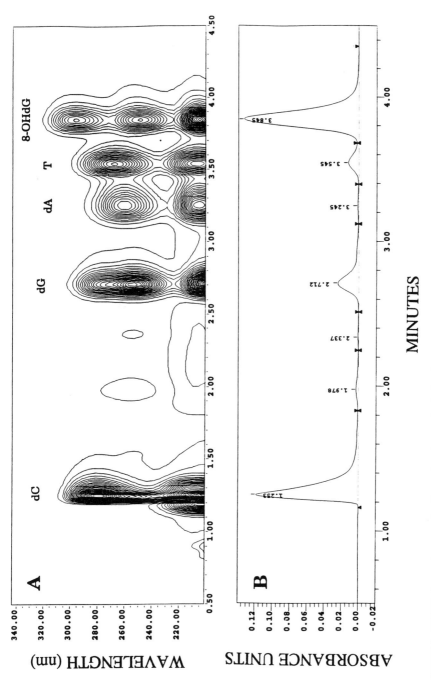

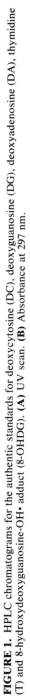

FIGURE 1. HPLC chromatograms for the authentic standards for deoxycytosine (DC), deoxyguanosine (DG), deoxyadenosine (DA), thymidine (T) and 8-hydroxydeoxyguanosine-OH· adduct (8-OHDG). (A) UV scan. (B) Absorbance at 297 nm.

TABLE 2. Production of 8-OHDG in Heart during Perfusion with OH•
Generating System[a]

Time of Perfusion with OH• Generating System	8-OHDG Formed (pmol/mg DNA)
Baseline	1008 ± 98
10 min	2109 ± 193*
20 min	2367 ± 208*
30 min	2076 ± 187*

[a] Results are means ± SE of six samples per group; * $p < 0.05$ compared to baseline.

products. At least three modified bases, 8-hydroxyguanine, 5-hydroxymethyl-uracil, and thymine glycol, are formed when OH• attacks a DNA molecule.[7] In this study we clearly detected the formation of 8-OHDG in the heart. As shown in FIGURE 1, HPLC chromatograms of the authentic standards for deoxycytosine (DC), deoxyguanosine (DG), deoxyadenosine (DA), thymidine (T) and 8-hydroxydeoxyguanosine-OH• adduct (8-OHDG) showed retention times of 1.3 min, 2.7 min, 3.2 min, 3.5 min and 3.8 min, respectively. 8-OHDG was detected in the normal heart (TABLE 1). The amount of 8-OHDG increased significantly after 20 min of reperfusion following 30 min of ischemia and maintained up to 30 min of reperfusion. As shown in TABLE 2, the amount of 8-OHDG increased by 2-fold after 10 min of perfusing the hearts with OH• generating system. This increased 8-OHDG level was also maintained up to 30 min of perfusion with OH• generating system.

The results of this study provided evidence for the first time that the reperfusion of ischemic myocardium results in the DNA modification producing 8-OHDG. The formation of 8-OHDG can serve as a sensitive marker for the development of oxidative stress associated with ischemia and reperfusion.

REFERENCES

1. DAS, D. K. & N. MAULIK. 1994. Evaluation of antioxidant effectiveness in ischemia reperfusion tissue injury methods. Methods Enzymol. **233:** 601–610.
2. BRAWN, K. & I. FRIDOVICH. 1981. DNA strand scission by enzymatically generated oxygen radicals. Arch. Biochem. Biophys. **206:** 414–419.
3. TOSAKI, A., D. BAGCHI, D. HELLEGOUARCH, T. PALI, G. A. CORDIS & D. K. DAS. 1993. Comparisons of ESR and HPLC methods for the detection of hydroxyl radicals in ischemic/reperfused hearts. A relationship between the genesis of oxygen-free radicals and reperfusion-induced arrhythmias. Biochem. Pharmacol. **45:** 961–969.
4. AGARWAL, S. & H. H. DRAPER. 1992. Isolation of a malonaldehyde-deoxyguanosine adduct from rat liver DNA. Free Radical Biol. Med. **13:** 695–699.
5. MAULIK, N., D. K. DAS, M. GOGINENI, G. A. CORDIS, N. AVROVA & N. DENISOVA. 1993. Reduction of myocardial ischemic reperfusion injury by sialylated glycosphingo-lipids, gangliosides. J. Cardiovasc. Pharmacol. **22:** 74–81.
6. GUPTA, R. C. 1984. Nonrandom binding of the carcinogen N-hydroxy-2-acetylamino-fluorene to repetitive sequences of rat liver DNA *in vitro*. Proc. Natl. Acad. Sci. USA **81:** 6943–6947.
7. FLOYD, R. A. & J. E. SCHNEIDER. 1990. Hydroxy free radical damage to DNA. *In* Membrane Lipid Oxidation. Vol. 1. C. Vigo-Pelfrey, Ed. CRC Press. Boca Raton, FL.

Oxidative Damage to Myocardial Proteins and DNA during Ischemia and Reperfusion

GAUTAM MAULIK,[a] GERALD A. CORDIS, AND
DIPAK K. DAS

University of Connecticut School of Medicine
Farmington, Connecticut

INTRODUCTION

Oxygen-derived free radicals play a significant role in the pathophysiology of ischemia reperfusion injury.[1] The generation of oxygen free radicals has been demonstrated directly using ESR and HPLC techniques,[2] and indirectly by the formation of lipid peroxidation products.[3] Although proteins and DNA are well-known targets of free radical attack, little attention has been paid to the injury of protein and DNA molecules of ischemic reperfused hearts. This study was undertaken to examine the role of protein and DNA in myocardial ischemia/reperfusion injury.

MATERIALS AND METHODS

Sprague-Dawley male rats of 250–300 gm body weight were anesthetized with intraperitoneal pentobarbitol. After intravenous administration of heparin, hearts were rapidly excised and mounted on a nonrecirculating Langendorff perfusion apparatus.[4] Retrograde perfusion was established at a pressure of 100 cm water with oxygenated normothermic Krebs-Henseleit bicarbonate (KHB) buffer previously equilibrated with 95% O_2/5% CO_2, pH 7.4 at 37°C. Hearts were subjected to 30 min of ischemia followed by 10, 20, and 30 min of reperfusion. In a separate set of experiments, hearts were perfused with hydroxyl radical (OH•)-generating system (100 μM xanthine, 8 mU/ml xanthine oxidase, 100 μM $FeCl_3$, and 100 μM EDTA)[4] for 10, 20 and 30 min. At the end of the experiments, all hearts were frozen in liquid N_2 and stored at -70°C. Carbonyl content was estimated both in the soluble protein fraction (198,000 g) and in the SR fraction, while DNA unwinding was performed in nuclear fraction.

Preparation of Sarcoplasmic Reticulum (SR)

The hearts were excised, minced and homogenized using a Polytron homogenizer with 3 volumes of 10 mM/liter imidazole buffer, pH 7.0. The homogenate

---

[a] Correspondence: University of Connecticut School of Medicine, 263 Farmington Ave., Farmington, CT 06030-1110.

was then centrifuged at 4,080 g for 20 min, filtered through cheese cloth and centrifuged at 51,000 g for 60 min as described previously.[5] The resultant pellet was then suspended in 1 M/liter KCl and 10 mM/liter imidazole buffer, pH 7.0, and centrifuged at 198,000 g for 60 min. The final pellet, designated as SR, was then resuspended in 5 volumes of 30% sucrose and 20 mM/liter imidazole buffer, pH 7.0.

Preparation of Extracts

Protein oxidation was measured in the 100,000 g supernatant soluble protein as described.[6] Frozen hearts were homogenized in buffer (pH 7.4) containing 137 mM NaCl, 4.6 mM KCl, 1.1 mM KH_2PO_4, 0.6 mM $MgSO_4$, 10 mM Hepes, protease inhibitors (leupeptin, 0.5 μg/ml, pepstatin, 0.7 μg/ml, aprotinin, 0.5 μg/ml, PMSF, 40 μg/ml), and 1.1 mM EDTA and centrifuged at 100,000 g for 5 min.

Carbonyl Assay

The protein concentration of the soluble protein fraction and SR preparation were determined by the Pierce BCA method. The protein carbonyl content was estimated spectrophotometrically using 2,4-dinitrophenylhydrazine methods.[7] The protein hydrazone derivatives were sequentially extracted with 10% (w/v) trichloroacetic acid, treated with ethanol/ethylacetate (1 : 1 v/v), and reextracted with 10% trichloroacetic acid. The resulting precipitate was dissolved in 6 M guanidine hydrochloride, and the difference spectrum of the sample treated with DNPH in HCl was determined versus the sample treated with HCl alone. Results are expressed as nmoles of DNPH incorporated per mg protein calculated from the extinction coefficient of 22 $mM^{-1}cm^{-1}$.

Fluorescence Analysis of DNA Unwinding

For this, hearts were homogenized in 3 volumes of 0.25 M sucrose-3 mM $MgCl_2$.[8] The homogenate was centrifuged at 800 g for 10 min and filtered. The crude nuclear pellet was washed and further purified by centrifugation through 2.2 M sucrose-1 mM $MgCl_2$ at 75,000 g for 60 min. The nuclei were washed once in homogenization medium followed by four times in saline. Nuclei were suspended in PBS buffer. The FADU method[9] uses the fluorescence data from test samples (P) as well as from reference samples (T and B). The first set (B) shows the lowest level of fluorescence. 0.5 ml of the samples are lysed by addition of 0.5 ml of 0.1 N NaOH, sonicated, incubated at 20°C for the whole unwinding period (30 min) and subsequently neutralized by addition of 0.5 ml of 0.1 N HCl and resonicated.

The second reference set (T) is used for estimating total fluorescence. 0.5 ml of nuclear extract are lysed by the addition of 0.5 ml of 0.1 N NaOH comixed with 0.5 ml of 0.1 N HCl, incubated at 20°C for 30 min and sonicated afterward.

The third reference set (P) is used to estimate the unwinding rate of damaged DNA. The nuclear extract is exposed to alkaline conditions, which bring about partial unwinding of the DNA. The difference (P-B) provides an estimate of the amount of DNA that remains double stranded, thus indicating the amount of the induced DNA damage. 0.5 ml of the extract are lysed by gentle addition of 0.5 ml of 0.1 N NaOH without mixing, followed by incubation at 20°C for 30 min. The tubes are shielded from light and vibrations to avoid artificially induced strand breaks. After DNA unwinding, the P samples are neutralized by the addition of 0.5 ml of 0.1 N HCl (pH 7.1–7.6) and sonicated.

All samples (B, T, and P) then receive 0.5 ml of fluorochrome-containing buffer (1.25 μM bisbenzamide in 0.15 M phosphate buffer, pH 7.6). After mixing, relative fluorescence intensities are read from a spectrofluorometer operating at 355 nm (excitation) and 450 nm (emission). The percentage of fraction of double-stranded DNA (F) is calculated according to F = (P-B)/(T-B) × 100 where T, P, and B are fluorescence intensities of the T, P, and B samples, respectively.

RESULTS AND DISCUSSION

Numerous evidence supports the notion of the generation of oxygen free radicals and development of oxidative stress during the reperfusion of ischemic myocardium.[1] The generation of free radicals has been confirmed directly using ESR and HPLC techniques,[2] and indirectly by measuring the extent of lipid peroxidation.[3] Peroxidation of lipid occurs when oxygen free radicals directly interact with the polyunsaturated fatty acids of the membrane lipids. However, in addition to membrane lipids, proteins and DNA molecules are also potential targets of free radical attack. Recent studies of Pacifici and Davies have suggested the protein degradation as an indicator for oxidative stress.[10] Oxidative modification of proteins generates a variety of products including carbonyl compounds, which have been detected in tissues when exposed to oxidative stress.[11] In this study, we found that while ischemia does not cause the generation of carbonyl compounds, reperfusion of ischemic myocardium leads to the production of carbonyl contents (FIG. 1A). Carbonyl contents of whole heart as well as SR fraction were increased progressively as the function of the time of reperfusion. In order to confirm that the production of the carbonyl content was due to the free radicals, we perfused the hearts with the OH•-generating system. As shown in FIGURE 2A, carbonyl content of the whole heart and SR increased as the time of perfusion (with OH•) progressed.

In order to examine the role of DNA modification in ischemic reperfusion injury, we performed fluorometric analysis of DNA unwinding. As shown in FIGURE 1C, relative percent of double-stranded DNA was decreased continuously with the reperfusion time. A significantly lower amount of double-stranded DNA was found after 30 min of reperfusion as compared to baseline controls. Again, perfusing the hearts with the OH•-generating system resulted in the reduction of double-stranded DNA, as shown in FIGURE 2C. It was shown previously that oxyradicals could cause DNA strand breaks in the target cells.[12] Oxygen free radicals, specifically OH•, have been shown to cause extensive damage to DNA resulting in the DNA strand breaks.[13] The fact that reperfusion of ischemic myocardium is associated with the generation of OH• radicals[2] and that OH• caused DNA strand breaks in our study, suggests that OH• produced in the ischemic reperfused myocardium is instrumental for the DNA damage observed in our study.

In summary, we have demonstrated that reperfusion of ischemic myocardium caused the increase in carbonyl contents of heart in concert with causing damage to DNA molecules. It is our belief that elucidation of the mechanism of DNA and protein injury in the ischemic reperfused heart will contribute significantly to myocardial preservation during ischemia.

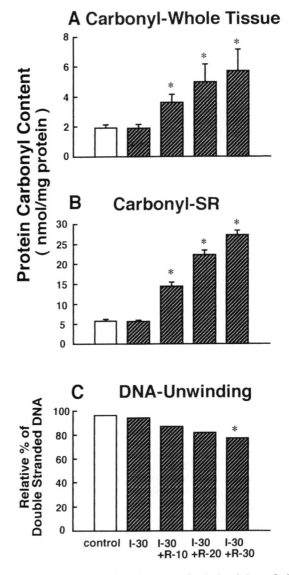

FIGURE 1. (A) Changes in protein carbonyl content after ischemia/reperfusion (I/R) injury in rat heart. Soluble protein fractions were prepared from hearts of rats subjected to various conditions of ischemia and reperfusion. Results (nmol/mg protein) are expressed as means ± SD for n = 6 for each group. *p <0.001 compared to control. **(B)** Changes in protein carbonyl content of SR preparation from hearts subjected to various conditions of ischemia and reperfusion. Results (nmol/mg protein) are expressed as means ± SD for n = 6 for each group. *p <0.001 compared to control. **(C)** Changes in relative percentage of double-stranded DNA remaining in nuclear DNA of rat hearts subjected to various conditions of ischemia and reperfusion. Results are expressed as means ± SD. *p <0.001 compared to control.

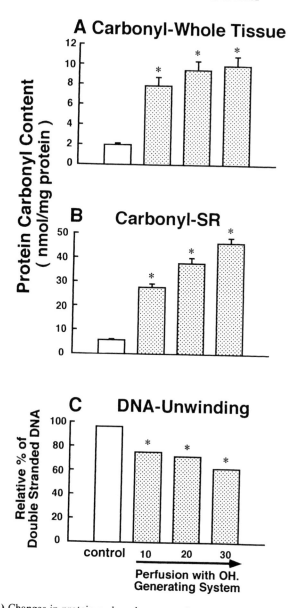

FIGURE 2. (A) Changes in protein carbonyl content of soluble protein fractions prepared from rat hearts that had been perfused with the OH•-generating system for the indicated time periods. Results (nmol/mg protein) are expressed as means ± SD for n = 6 for each group. *p <0.001 compared to control. **(B)** Changes in protein carbonyl content of SR preparation prepared from rat hearts that had been perfused with the OH•-generating system for the indicated time periods. Results (nmol/mg protein) are expressed as means ± SD for n = 6 for each group. *p <0.001 compared to control. **(C)** Changes in relative percentage of double-stranded DNA remaining in nuclear DNA of rat hearts that had been perfused with the OH•-generating system for the indicated time periods. Results are expressed as means ± SD. *p <0.001 compared to control.

REFERENCES

1. DAS, D. K. & R. M. ENGELMAN. 1990. Mechanism of free radical generation in ischemic and reperfused myocardium. *In* Oxygen Radicals: Systemic Events and Disease Processes. D. K. Das & W. B. Essman, Eds. 97–128. Krager. Basel.
2. TOSAKI, A., D. BAGCHI, D. HELLEGOUARCH, T. PALI, G. A. CORDIS & D. K. DAS. 1993. Comparisons of ESR and HPLC methods for the detection of hydroxyl radicals in ischemic/reperfused hearts. A relationship between the genesis of oxygen-free radicals and reperfusion-induced arrhythmias. Biochem. Pharmacol. **45:** 961–969.
3. CORDIS, G. A., N. MAULIK & D. K. DAS. 1995. Detection of oxidative stress in heart by estimating the dinitrophenylhydrazine derivative of malonaldehyde. J. Mol. Cell. Cardiol. **27:** 1645–1653.
4. BAGCHI, D., D. K. DAS, R. M. ENGELMAN, M. R. PRASAD & R. SUBRAMANIAN. 1990. Polymorphonuclear leucocytes as potential source of free radicals in the ischemic-reperfused myocardium. Eur. Heart J. **11:** 800–813.
5. HESS, M. L., M. F. WARNER, A. D. ROBBINS, S. CRUTE & L. J. GREENFIELD. 1981. Characterization of the excitation-contraction coupling system of the hypothermic myocardium following ischemia and reperfusion. Cardiovasc. Res. **15:** 390–397.
6. OLIVER, C. N., P. E. STARKE-REED, E. R. STADTMEN, G. J. LIU, J. M. CARNEY & R. A. FLOYD. 1990. Oxidative damage to brain proteins, loss of glutamine synthetase activity, and production of free radicals during ischemia/reperfusion-induced injury to gerbil brain. Proc. Natl. Acad. Sci. USA **87:** 5144–5147.
7. LEVINE, R. L., D. GARLAND, C. N. OLIVER, A. AMICI, I. CLIMENT, A. LENZ, B. AHN, S. SHALTIEL & E. R. STADTMAN. 1990. Determination of carbonyl content in oxidatively modified proteins. Methods Enzymol. **186:** 464–478.
8. CESARONE, C. F., C. BOLOGNESI & L. SANTI. 1979. Improved microfluorometric DNA determination in biological material using 33258 Hoechst. Anal. Biochem. **100:** 188–197.
9. BAUMSTARK-KHAN, CHRISTA. 1994. Alkaline elution versus fluorescence analysis of DNA unwinding. Methods Enzymol. **234:** 88–102.
10. PACIFICI, R. E. & K. J. A. DAVIES. 1990. Protein degradation as an index of oxidative stress. Methods Enzymol. **186:** 485–502.
11. STADTMAN, E. R. 1990. Metal ion-catalyzed oxidation of proteins: biochemical mechanism and biological consequences. Free Radical Biol. Med. **9:** 315–325.
12. BIRNBOIM, H. C. 1982. DNA strand breakage in human leukocytes exposed to a tumor promoter, phorbol myristate acetate. Science **215:** 1247–1249.
13. TULLIUS, T. D. 1987. Chemical "snapshots" of DNA: using the hydroxyl radical to study the structure of DNA and DNA-protein complexes. Trends Biochem. Sci. **12:** 297–300.

Severe Isolated Aortic Stenosis with Advanced Left Ventricular Dysfunction

Results of Aortic Valve Replacement

U. F. TESLER[a] B. TOMASCO,[a] R. FLORILLI,[b]
AND R. LUPINO[a]

Divisions of [a]Cardiovascular Surgery and [b]Cardiology
Ospedale San Carlo
Potenza, Italy

INTRODUCTION

Untreated severe aortic stenosis (AS) with advanced left ventricular (LV) dysfunction carries a grave prognosis. With the onset of severe symptoms (angina at rest, pulmonary edema, syncope, paroxysmal nocturnal dyspnea, congestive heart failure) the average life expectancy is reported between one and three years.[1,2]

Advanced LV dysfunction and severe clinical symptomatology have been identified as significant risk factors for operative mortality in patients (pts) undergoing aortic valve replacement (AVR),[3,4] while reports on the reversal of the LV dysfunction are contradictory.[3,4] In order to investigate early and late surgical results and the potential recovery of LV function in such clinical setting, we undertook a retrospective analysis of a group of consecutive pts who underwent AVR for isolated AS an advanced LV dysfunction, arbitrarily defined as a left ventricular ejection fraction (EF) lower than 40%.

CLINICAL MATERIAL AND METHODS

Fifty-seven pts, aged 26–78 years (mean 58.8 years), with severe isolated AS and markedly reduced EF, underwent AVR between July 1982 and December 1994. There were 44 men and 13 women. This cohort represents the 5.6% of pts who underwent isolated AVR and the 8.3% of pts operated for pure or prevalent AS at our institution. All pts were symptomatic: eleven were in Class IV, thirty-five in Class III and eleven in Class II of the NYHA Functional Classification; twenty had angina pectoris, thirteen had syncopal episodes, twenty-five had congestive heart failure and fifteen had experienced one or more episodes of acute pulmonary edema. Many had a combination of symptoms. Mean EF was 32% (range 15–40%); mean aortic valve area index was 0.28 cm^2/m^2. No pt was denied surgery. AVR was performed under standard cardiopulmonary bypass with moderate systemic hypothermia with intermittent cold oxygenated cristalloid or blood cardioplegia. Mechanical valves were generally employed in pts below the age of 70 years and biological valves in pts over 70 years of age. Six pts had concomitant coronary artery disease and underwent coronary artery by-pass at the time of aortic valve replacement. Three pts had aortic root enlargement, one had a septal myomectomy and one a reduction aortoplasty.

RESULTS

There were 6 hospital deaths with a mortality of 11% without statistical correlation to age, severity of symptoms or degree of LV dysfunction. The follow-up time ranged from six months to 12 years. There were six late deaths, five of which were cardiac-related. All surviving pts underwent systematic cardiological follow-up, including serial echocardiographic studies, in the hospital out-patient clinic. Overall survival at ten years was 74%. Most pts showed a remarkable improvement both in their clinical status and in reversal of the ventricular dysfunction, both without statistical correlation with the severity of preoperative symptoms or degree of LV dysfunction: most pts are now in Functional Class I of the NYHA classification, while the mean left ventricular ejection fraction has increased from 32% to 58%.

CONCLUSIONS

The relatively low hospital mortality, the encouraging long-term survival, the marked improvement in the clinical picture and in the ventricular function in this group of severely disabled pts lead us to conclude that pts with severe aortic stenosis should be submitted to aortic valve replacement, even in the presence of gravely impaired left ventricular function.

REFERENCES

1. ROSE, J. JR. & E. BRAUNWALD. 1968. Aortic stenosis. Circulation 38(Suppl. V): 61–67.
2. FRANK, S., A. JOHNSON & J. ROSS. JR. 1973. Natural history of valvular aortic stenosis. Br. Heart J. 35: 41–46.
3. MORRIS, J. J., H. V. SCHAFF, C. J. MULLANY, A. RASTOGI, C. G. A. MCGREGOR, R. C. DALY, R. L. FRYE & T. A. ORSZULAK. 1993. Determinants of survival and recovery of left ventricular function after aortic valve replacement. Ann. Thorac. Surg. 56: 22–30.

Postnatal Developmental Profiles of Antioxidant Enzymes in Heart[a]

NILANJANA MAULIK,[b] JOHN E. BAKER,
RICHARD M. ENGELMAN, AND DIPAK K. DAS

University of Connecticut School of Medicine
Farmington, Connecticut

Medical College of Wisconsin
Milwaukee, Wisconsin

Baystate Medical Center
Springfield, Massachusetts

INTRODUCTION

Reactive oxygen species are implicated in a variety of myocardial parthophysio-logical conditions including ischemic heart disease, heart attack, atherosclerosis, and hypertrophy.[1-4] The fact that oxygen free radicals are also implicated in the aging process, and that neonatal hearts are more susceptible to cellular injury compared to adult hearts, prompted many investigators to examine the antioxidant reserve of the neonates. For example, earlier studies demonstrated that in porcine myocardium, major antioxidant enzymes—SOD, catalase, GSH peroxidase, GSH reductase—all increase up to 8–10 days after birth.[5,6] SOD activity was found to be higher in 3-month-old rat heart compared to that for 18-month-old heart.[7] GSH level of adult (12-month) rat heart was lower compared to young (3-month) rat heart.[8] Increasing evidence thus suggests a link between the occurrence of cardio-vascular diseases and the aging process with the development of oxidative stress.[9]

In this study, we measured the major antioxidant enzymes and the GSH content of rabbit heart in five different age groups between newborn and 49 day old. The results of our study not only show definitive developmental profiles of antioxidant enzymes in heart, but also demonstrate a difference in enzyme activities between left and right ventricles.

MATERIALS AND METHODS

Neonatal Heart Preparation

Time date pregnant New Zealand white rabbits were purchased at the Univer-sity of Wisconsin, Milwaukee (JEB). Neonates (day 0, 7, 14, 35, and 49) were

[a] This study was supported in part by NIH Grants HL 34360 and HL 22559 and by a Grant-In-Aid from the American Heart Association.

[b] Correspondence: University of Connecticut School of Medicine, 263 Farmington Ave., Farmington, CT 06030-1110.

delivered by caesarean section and sacrificed immediately. Hearts were immediately excised, the left and right ventricles were separated and cut out, and immediately frozen at liquid N_2 temperature. The biopsies were then packed in dry ice and shipped to the cardiovascular laboratory (NM, DKD), where the enzyme assays were performed.

Processing of Biopsies

The tissue (LV and RV) homogenate was prepared by homogenizing weighed amounts of ventricular biopsies in a measured volume of ice-cold Tris-sucrose buffer [0.25 mol/L sucrose, 10 mmol/L Tris-HCl, pH 7.5, 1 mmol/L EDTA, pH 7.5, 0.5 mmol/L DTT and 0.1 mmol/L phenyl methyl sulfoxide (PMSF)]. After centrifugation at 3,000 g for 10 min, the resultant supernatant was centrifuged at 10,000 g for 20 min to obtain a mitochondrial pellet, which was further purified by repeated centrifugation and used as a source for Mn-SOD. This supernatant was recentrifuged at 105,000 g for 1 hr, and the supernatant fluid thus obtained was used as a source for the assay of cytosolic antioxidant enzymes, GSH peroxidase, GSH reductase, catalase, Cu/Zn-SOD and G-6-P dehydrogenase. Protein content was estimated by using a BCA protein assay reagent kit (Pierce, Rockford, IL).

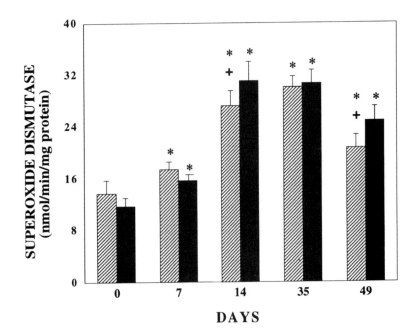

FIGURE 1. Activities of SOD at birth, and at 7, 14, 35 and 49 days of age. ▨ LV, ■ RV. *p <0.05 compared to newborn; +p <0.05 compared to RV.

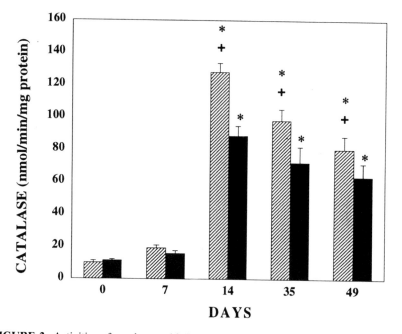

FIGURE 2. Activities of catalase at birth, and at 7, 14, 35 and 49 days of age. ▨ LV,
■ RV. *$p < 0.05$ compared to newborn; +$p < 0.05$ compared to RV.

Enzyme Assays

Superoxide dismutase activity was assayed by its inhibitory action on the superoxide dependent reduction of ferricytochrome by xanthine-xanthine oxidase.[10] The final concentrations in the assay medium (total volume 1 ml) were: 100 μM cytochrome C, 100 μM hypoxanthine, 10 mM Tris/HCl, and 50–80 μg of enzyme protein. The reaction was initiated by addition of 8 mU xanthine oxidase. Total SOD was calculated by adding mitochondrial and cytosolic SOD contents. Catalase was estimated by measuring the decreases in the absorbance of H_2O_2 at 240 nm.[11] Final concentrations in the assay medium (total volume 1 ml) were: 35 mM phosphate buffer, pH 7.2, 0.02% Triton X-100, and 30–50 μg enzyme protein. The reaction was started by the addition of 30 μl of 1% H_2O_2 and monitored by the decrease in absorbance of H_2O_2 at 240 nm. Glutathione peroxidase was estimated by measuring the decrease in absorbance of NADPH at 340 nm.[12] The final concentrations in the assay medium (total volume 1 ml) were: 62 mM Tris/HCl, pH 7.6, 0.2 mM NADPH, 0.1 mM EDTA, 0.5 mM GSH, and 1 U/ml GSSG reductase. The reaction was initiated by adding 100 μl 2 mM cumene hydroperoxide. Glutathione reductase activity was estimated by measuring the decrease in absorbance of NADPH at 340 nm.[13] The final concentrations in the assay buffer (1 ml total volume) were: 90 mM Tris/HCl, pH 7.8, 0.8 mM EDTA, and 0.2 mM NADPH, and the decrease in OD was followed at 340 nm for 10 minutes. The protein-free supernatant was used to measure the amount of GSH in the sample.[14]

The reaction mixture contained (3 ml total volume) 1 M Tris/HCl buffer, pH 8.0, 5-5'-dithiobis-(2-nitrobenzoic acid) (DTNB) (0.8 mg/ml) and the absorbance was read at 412 nm.

RESULTS

The activities of antioxidant enzymes in heart were increased significantly after birth. For example, SOD activity was enhanced by 27% in LV and 34% in RV after 7 days, and 98% in LV and 165% in RV after 14 days of birth (FIG. 1). This level was maintained up to 35 days, and then dropped by 31% in LV and 19% in RV after 49 days. The activities of SOD were 51% and 112% higher in LV and RV, respectively, after 49 days as compared to those after birth. Catalase activity was very low after birth (FIG. 2). The activities were increased by 90% in LV and 39% RV after 7 days; and 1170% in LV and 683% in RV after 14 days. After 35 days the enzyme activity waş lowered by 23% in LV and 18% in RV, this level was maintained up to 49 days. GSH peroxidase activity was enhanced by 33% in LV and 44% in RV after 7 days; and 172% in LV and 105% in RV after 14 days of birth (FIG. 3). The activities were then dropped, and after 35 days they became 43% lower in LV and 61% lower in RV. These levels, which were similar to those after birth, were

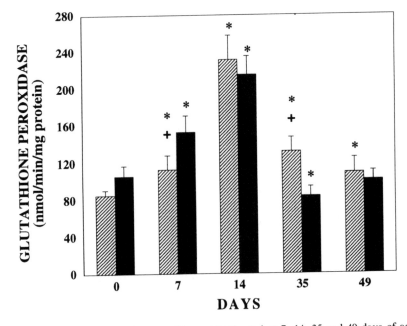

FIGURE 3. Activities of GSH peroxidase at birth, and at 7, 14, 35 and 49 days of age. ▨ LV, ■ RV. *$p < 0.05$ compared to newborn; +$p < 0.05$ compared to RV.

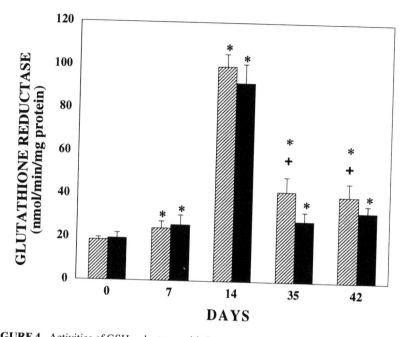

FIGURE 4. Activities of GSH reductase at birth, and at 7, 14, 35 and 49 days of age. ▨ LV, ■ RV. $*p < 0.05$ compared to newborn; $+p < 0.05$ compared to RV.

maintained up to 49 days. GSH reductase activity was enhanced by 30% in LV and 33% in RV after 7 days, and then further enhanced by 430% in LV and 369% in RV after 14 days (FIG. 4). The activities were then dropped substantially by 58% in LV and 69% in RV after 35 days. The activities were maintained up to 49 days. G-6-P dehydrogenase activity was enhanced by 70% in LV but remained unaltered in RV after 7 days; and then increased by 335% in LV and 237% in RV after 14 days (FIG. 5). These activities were dropped by 74% in LV and 65% in RV after 35 days and then leveled off.

We also measured the glutathione content of the LV and RV. As shown in FIGURE 6, GSH content was increased by 27% in LV and 70% in RV after 7 days, and 95% in LV and 119% in RV after 14 days. The amount of GSH level was then dropped appreciably by 76% in LV and 78% in RV after 35 days. The amount of GSH in LV was maintained up to 49 days, but further dropped by 90% in RV. When the antioxidant levels were compared between LV and RV, significant differences were also noticed. For example, catalase activity was 45% higher in LV compared to that in RV after 14 days of birth (FIG. 2). GSH peroxidase and GSH reductase levels were also 50% and 57% higher, respectively, in LV compared to those in RV after 35 days of birth (FIGS. 3 and 4). The G-6-P dehydrogenase level was 123% and 82% higher in LV as compared to RV after 7 days and 14 days, respectively (FIG. 5). The activities did not vary between LV and RV in the case of SOD and GSH.

DISCUSSION

Our results indicate that activities of the myocardial antioxidant enzymes increase progressively and steadily until the neonates attain the age of 14 days, and then begin to decline. For example, SOD which dismutates O_2^- into H_2O_2, becomes double in 14 days in LV, and triple in RV, maintains these levels up to 35 days, and then declines significantly after 49 days. The H_2O_2 formed by the dismutation reaction is removed by catalase. The activity of catalase increases significantly within a week, is enhanced 7-fold in LV and 8-fold in RV after 14 days, and maintains the level in LV but drops by 30% in RV after 49 days. A number of studies have confirmed the biologic importance of SOD and catalase in the prevention of oxygen free radical cytotoxicity. When the presence of SOD and catalase in a tissue is not adequate to prevent the free radicals, the generated toxic radicals attack the unsaturated lipids in the cell causing lipid peroxidation. These toxic lipid peroxides are converted into hydroxy fatty acids which are then metabolized by the β-oxidation pathway (FIG. 7). The enzyme which is responsible for this conversion is GSH peroxidase. Activity of this enzyme in newborn rabbits is about 20% higher in RV compared to LV, and increases 1.5 times in both LV and RV in 7 days and 3 times in LV and 2 times in RV in 14 days, then drops slightly in LV but significantly to approximately 50% in RV.

Since GSH is essential for the normal function of myocardial cells, it must be regenerated to ensure proper repair and proliferation of myocardial cells. The

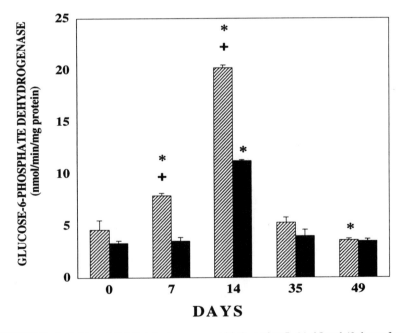

FIGURE 5. Activities of G-6-P dehydrogenase at birth, and at 7, 14, 35 and 49 days of age. ▨ LV, ■ RV. *p <0.05 compared to newborn; +p <0.05 compared to RV.

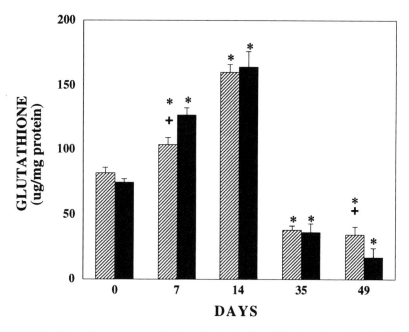

FIGURE 6. Glutathione content at birth, and at 7, 14, 35 and 49 days of age. ▨ LV, ■ RV.
*p <0.05 compared to newborn; ^+p <0.05 compared to RV.

reducing equivalents used by GSH peroxidase are regenerated by GSH reductase, which transfers the reducing equivalents from reduced nicotinamide adenine dinucleotide phosphate (NADPH) to produce intracellular supplies of reduced GSH. Our results indicate a slight increase in these enzyme activities from newborn to 7 days after birth, which are then enhanced 5-fold in both LV and RV in 14 days, dropped 50% in LV 70% in RV after 35 days, and maintained at these levels up to 49 days.

When the supply becomes low, NADPH can be regenerated through the action of pentose phosphate shunt enzyme, G-6-P dehydrogenase, which is abundantly present in myocardial tissue. It appears from our results that this enzyme also undergoes significant developmental changes. For example, it increased 1.8-fold in LV after 7 days of birth while no change was noticed in RV during that period; was enhanced 4-fold in LV and 3-fold in RV in 14 days, maintained this level in LV, but dropped appreciably to 30% of this level in RV after 49 days. The presence of a relatively lower level of this enzyme in 49-day-old rabbit hearts also suggests that these hearts may be less susceptible to peroxidative injury, since not only is lipid peroxidation in biologic tissue not only checked by G-6-P dehydrogenase activity on lipid peroxides, but also lipid peroxidase may actually be prevented by this enzyme as a result of direct scavenging of highly toxic OH• radicals.[15] In addition to providing the necessary supply of NADPH, G-6-P dehydrogenase may be a critical ingredient for the biosynthesis of adenine nucleotides and fatty acids essential for the repair of free radical-induced damaged myocardium.[16] However, although we did not measure malic enzyme and 6-phosphogluconate dehydrogenase activities in heart, it may be equally interesting to know the developmental

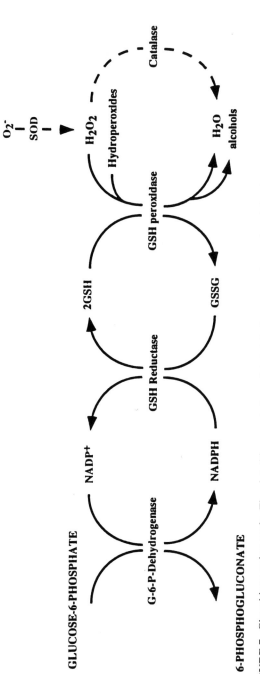

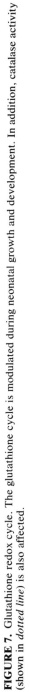

FIGURE 7. Glutathione redox cycle. The glutathione cycle is modulated during neonatal growth and development. In addition, catalase activity (shown in *dotted line*) is also affected.

profiles of these two enzyme activities since they are also able to regenerate necessary NADPH when the supply becomes low.[16]

GSH is the most abundant nonprotein thiol in heart and serves as an important intracellular antioxidant. The aging process is known to be associated with a decrease in GSH level in heart.[17] In another study, the GSH level of both LV and RV of rat was found to decrease as a function of age.[8] In contrast, Slivka *et al.*[18] did not find any difference in glutathione content during aging. Rikans and Moore[19] also did not find a difference in GSH level in rat heart between 6 and 26 months of age. In our study GSH increased nearly 2-fold from 0 to 14 days after birth, and then dropped significantly to below baseline level after 35 days. This level was maintained up to 49 days. Thus, it appears that the GSH level increases only during the early neonatal growth and development, and then decreases. This reduced level is maintained during the adult age.

The findings of this study are also clinically relevant. Recent studies demonstrated that adults are more susceptible to the ischemic injury than neonates.[20] Numerous reports exist in the literature to indicate that ischemia/reperfusion is associated with the development of oxidative stress and generation of oxygen free radicals.[1] The decreased susceptibility of neonatal heart to ischemia/reperfusion injury may be explained by the presence of increased levels of antioxidant enzymes in these hearts.

In summary, the results of this study indicate that glutathione redox cycle (shown in Fig. 7) of heart undergoes significant alterations after birth. Although a large number of data are available regarding the fate of glutathione and antioxidant enzymes during adult and old ages, only a limited number of reports are available in the literature regarding the regulation of these antioxidants during early neonatal life. Our results demonstrate that major antioxidant enzymes as well as glutathione content are enhanced after birth, reaching the maximal level between the age of 14 and 21 days, and then drop gradually and progressively to baseline or below baseline levels, which are maintained during further growth and development. It is tempting to speculate that after coming out of the womb, where a relatively hypoxic milieu is maintained, newborns are likely to be subjected to oxidative stress. Such oxidative stress may be instrumental for the stimulation of glutathione and the enzymes of the glutathione redox cycle, because oxidative stress has been found to stimulate the antioxidants/antioxidant enzymes.[21] Such increased antioxidants may be necessary for the survival of newborn hearts because of the exposure of the newborn hearts to increased amounts of potentially harmful toxic oxygen metabolites such as superoxide anions and hydroxyl radicals.

REFERENCES

1. Das, D. K. & R. M. Engelman. 1990. Mechanism of free radical generation during reperfusion of ischemic myocardium. *In* Oxygen Radicals: Systemic Events and Disease Processes. D. K. Das & W. B. Essman, Eds. 97–121. Karger. Basel.
2. Tosaki, A., D. Bagchi, T. Pali, G. A. Cordis & D. K. Das. 1993. Comparisons of ESR and HPLC methods for the detection of OH• radicals in ischemic/reperfused hearts. Biochem. Pharmacol. **45:** 961–969.
3. Prasad, K. & J. Kalra. 1993. Oxygen free radicals and hypercholesterolemic atherosclerosis: effect of vitamin E. Am. Heart J. **125:** 958–973.
4. Bolli, R., M. O. Jeroudi, B. S. Patel, O. I. Aruoma, B. Halliwell, E. K. Lai & P. B. McCay. 1989. Marked reduction of free radical generation and contractile dysfunction by antioxidant therapy begun at the time of reperfusion. Circ. Res. **65:** 607–622.

5. DAS, D. K., D. FLANSAAS, R. M. ENGELMAN, J. A. ROUSOU, R. H. BREYER, R. JONES, S. LEMESHOW & H. OTANI. 1987. Age-related development profiles of the antioxidative defense system and the peroxidative status of the pig heart. Biol. Neonate **51:** 156–169.
6. DAS, D. K., R. M. ENGELMAN, D. FLANSAAS, H. OTANI, J. ROUSOU & R. H. BREYER. 1987. Developmental profiles of protective mechanisms of heart against peroxidative injury. Basic Res. Cardiol. **82:** 36–50.
7. SOHAL, R. S., L. A. ARNOLD & B. H. SOHAL. 1990. Age-related changes in antioxidant enzymes and prooxidant generation in tissues of the rat with special reference to parameters in two insect species. Free Radical Biol. Med. **10:** 495–500.
8. VEGA, J. A., C. CAVALLOTTI, W. L. COLLIER, D. V. GIUSEPPE, I. ROSSODIVITA & F. AMENTA. 1992. Changes in glutathione content and localization in rat heart as a function of age. Mech. Ageing Dev. **64:** 37–48.
9. HARMAN, D. 1982. The free radical theory of aging. *In* Free Radicals in Biology. Vol. 6. W. A. Pryor, Ed. 255–275. Academic Press. New York.
10. CRAPO, J. D., J. M. McCORD & I. FRIDOVICH. 1978. Preparation and assay of super-oxide dismutase. Methods Enzymol. **53:** 382–393.
11. BEERS, R. F., JR. & I. W. SIZER. 1952. A spectrophotometric method for measuring and breakdown of hydrogen peroxide by catalase. J. Biol. Chem. **195:** 133–140.
12. PAGLIA, D. E. & W. N. VALENTINE. 1967. Studies on the quantitative and qualitative characterization of erythrocyte glutathione peroxidase. J. Lab. Clin. Med. **70:** 158–169.
13. PINTO, R. E. & W. BARTLEY. 1969. The effect of age and sex on glutathione reductase and glutathione peroxidase activities and on aerobic glutathione oxidation in rat liver homogenates. Biochem. J. **112:** 109–115.
14. STEVENSON, T. D., B. L. McDONALD & S. ROSTON. 1960. Colorimetric method for determination of erythrocyte glutathione. J. Lab. Clin. Med. **56:** 157–160.
15. McCAY, P. B., D. D. GIBSON, K. L. FONG & K. R. HORNBROOK. 1976. Effect of glutathione peroxidase activity on lipid peroxidation in biological membranes. Biochim. Biophys. Acta **431:** 459–468.
16. TIERNEY, D. F., L. AYERS, S. HERZOG & J. YANG. 1973. Pentose pathway and produc-tion of reduced nicotinamide adenine dinucleotide phosphate. Am. Rev. Respir. Dis. **108:** 1348–1351.
17. HAZELTON, G. A. & C. A. LANG. 1980. Glutathione contents of tissues in the aging mouse. Biochem. J. **188:** 25–30.
18. SLIVKA, A., C. MYTILINEOU & G. COHEN. 1987. Histochemical evaluation of gluta-thione in brain. Brain Res. **409:** 275–284.
19. RIKANS, L. E. & D. R. MOORE. 1988. Effect of aging on aqueous-phase antioxidants in tissues of male Fischer rats. Biochim. Biophys. Acta **966:** 269–275.
20. NAKANASHI, T., H. H. YOUND, T. SHIMIZU, D. NISHIOKA & J. M. JARMAKANI. 1984. The relationship between myocardial enzyme release and Ca^{2+} uptake during hypoxia and reoxygenation in the newborn and adult heart. J. Mol. Cell. Cardiol. **16:** 519–532.
21. MAULIK, N., R. M. ENGELMAN, Z. WEI, D. LU, J. A. ROUSOU & D. K. DAS. 1993. Interleukin-1α preconditioning reduces myocardial ischemia reperfusion injury. Circulation **88:** 387–394.

Age-Related Changes in Lipid Peroxidation and Antioxidant Defense in Fischer 344 Rats[a]

MANASHI BAGCHI,[b] DEBASIS BAGCHI,
ERIC B. PATTERSON, LIN TANG, AND SIDNEY J. STOHS

Creighton University Health Sciences Center
Department of Biomedical Sciences
Omaha, Nebraska 68178

INTRODUCTION

In recent years, the free radical theory of aging has generated much interest. The cascade of events which occurs during aging is not known. Aging is the progressive accumulation of changes with time that are responsible for the ever increasing likelihood of disease and death.[1] A current hypothesis of aging postulates that deleterious reactions initiated by partially reduced oxygen species are an underlying factor in the causation of the aging process in multicellular organisms. Free radicals such as superoxide anions, hydrogen peroxide (H_2O_2) and hydroxyl radicals promote cellular damage by reacting with lipids, proteins and nucleotides.[2] These radicals have been implicated in the pathogenesis of many diseases, and may play a vital role in the process of aging.[3] Numerous pathways have been attributed to the action of these partially-reduced oxyradicals. The dominant and landmark theory of aging contends that senescent changes are a consequence of the accumulated action of oxygen free radicals.[3]

Oxidative stress is believed to be associated with the aging process, and changes in antioxidant defenses may also be involved. In the present study, age-related alterations in superoxide dismutase (SOD) and catalase (CAT) activities, glutathione (GSH) content, and lipid peroxidation (LP) were measured in the heart and liver of Fischer 344 rats at ages 4, 16, 22 and 29 months. To determine if the age-related changes in the activities of SOD and catalase were due to the changes in transcription, the levels of the mRNA species coding for these enzymes were determined by RNA/cDNA hybridization.

EXPERIMENTAL PROCEDURES

Male specific-pathogen-free Fischer 344 rats (4, 16, 22 and 29 months) were obtained from National Institute of Aging, Indianapolis, IN. The animals were killed by decapitation, and the liver and hearts were removed. All tissues

[a] This work was supported in part by a grant from California Age Research Institute.
[b] Corresponding author.

were immediately frozen in liquid nitrogen and stored at −80°C until used. Heart and liver homogenates were prepared by homogenizing the organs in Tris KCl buffer (pH 7.4) containing 150 mM KCl, 1 mM EDTA, 1 mM dithiothreitol (DTT) and 10% glycerol with a Potter Elvehjem homogenizer.[4] Protein concentrations were determined by the standard method of Lowry,[5] using bovine serum albumin as the standard. Membrane lipid peroxidation was determined colorimetrically according to the method of Buege and Aust,[6] using malondialdehyde as the standard, with a molar extinction coefficient of 1.52×10^5 at 535 nm. Catalase activity was assayed spectrophotometrically at 480 nm according to the method of Ohia et al.[7] by following the disappearance of added 6 mM H_2O_2 and 0.01 $NKMnO_4$. Superoxide dismutase (SOD) activity and glutathione (GSH) content were determined colorimetrically using Bioxy Tech SOD-525 and GSH-400 kits (Cedex, France), respectively. Protein kinase C (PKC) was measured by the nonradioactive method described by Yano.[8]

Hearts were homogenized in guanidinium thiocyanate, and RNA was isolated by cesium chloride density gradient as described by Chirgwin et al.[9] Northern blot analysis of RNA isolated from different aged hearts of Fischer 344 rats was performed according to Sambrook et al.[10] RNA/cDNA hybridization was performed according to the procedure of Thomas.[11]

RESULTS AND DISCUSSION

The results clearly show a marked increase in free radical production in aged animals, as evidenced by enhanced lipid peroxidation in the heart and liver. Increases in lipid peroxidation of 2.4- to 3.5-fold occurred in heart and liver homogenates, respectively, in 29-month-old rats as compared to 4-month-old rats (TABLE 1).

The glutathione (GSH) contents in the heart and liver decreased by 15% to 77% in 29-month-old rats as compared to 4-month-old rats (TABLE 1). Catalase activity decreased 42% and 63% in heart homogenate, and hepatic microsomes of 29-month-old rats, respectively, as compared to 4-month-old rats (TABLE 1). The age-related decrease in catalase activity may facilitate membrane damage due to the accumulation of H_2O_2. The SOD activity decreased by approximately 19% in hepatic microsomes in 29-month-old rats as compared to 4-month-old rats (TABLE 1), but not in the heart. PKC activity in heart and liver homogenates isolated from 16-month-old and 22-month-old Fischer 344 rats was also measured (data not shown). PKC activity was approximately 2.0-fold higher in old animals as compared to 4-month-old rats.

The results support a scenario in which the age-related increases in the production of reactive oxygen species and lipid peroxidation, the decreases in catalase activity and glutathione (GSH) content and the inability to induce superoxide dismutase (SOD) contribute to the observed increase in tissue damage with increased age. In a related preliminary study catalase and SOD RNA levels in homogenized hearts from Fischer 344 rats at different ages were assessed. The reduced specific activity observed for catalase does not appear to be due to a reduction in steady state RNA levels for catalase as detected by Northern dot blot analysis. Furthermore, the specific total RNA for SOD appeared to be in greater abundance in younger rats. Additional studies will be required to elucidate the mechanisms associated with the production of reactive oxygen species with aging, and to determine whether transcriptional or translational events are involved in the changes in catalase and SOD protein activities with aging.

TABLE 1. The Effect of Age on Lipid Peroxidation, Catalase Activity, Glutathione Content, and Superoxide Dismutase (SOD) Activity in Heart and Liver of Fischer 344 Rats[a]

Age (Months)	Lipid Peroxidation (nmol/mg Protein)		Catalase Activity (Units/mg Protein/min)		Glutathione Content (μmol/gm Tissue)		Superoxide Dismutase Activity (Units/mg Protein)	
	Heart Homogenate	Liver Microsomes	Heart Homogenate	Liver Microsomes	Heart Homogenate	Liver Microsomes	Heart Homogenate	Liver Microsomes
4	3.6 ± 0.2^a	3.2 ± 0.4^a	4.5 ± 0.3^a	8.7 ± 0.5^a	4.5 ± 0.6^a	10.2 ± 1.1^a	7.4 ± 0.8^a	10.8 ± 1.7^a
16	6.4 ± 0.5^b	7.1 ± 0.2^b	3.7 ± 0.3^b	5.1 ± 0.3^b	$3.9 \pm 0.5^{a,b}$	8.3 ± 0.9^b	7.5 ± 0.9^a	$9.2 \pm 1.1^{a,b}$
22	8.3 ± 0.8^c	9.5 ± 0.8^c	2.6 ± 0.5^c	4.0 ± 0.4^c	$3.7 \pm 0.4^{a,b}$	6.9 ± 0.8^c	7.3 ± 0.6^a	8.5 ± 1.4^b
29	9.4 ± 0.7^c	11.2 ± 0.6^d	2.1 ± 0.5^c	3.3 ± 0.5^c	3.2 ± 0.4^b	5.4 ± 0.6^c	7.2 ± 0.9^a	7.7 ± 1.2^b

[a] Lipid peroxidation is expressed as the content of thiobarbituric acid reactive substances (TBARS) per mg of protein. Malondialdehyde was used as the standard. Catalase activity was performed using 6 mM H_2O_2 as the substrate. Reactions were continued for 3 min and stopped using 6N H_2SO_4. Spectrophotometric measurements were made at 480 nm. Total glutathione content was determined colorimetrically using a Bioxy Tech S.A. GSH-400 kit, Cedex, France at 400 nm. Superoxide dismutase activity was determined colorimetrically using a Bioxy Tech SOD-525 kit at 525 nm. Each value is the mean $\pm$ SD of 4 to 6 animals. Values with nonidentical superscripts are significantly different ($p < 0.05$).

REFERENCES

1. UPTON, A. C. 1977. Pathobiology. *In* The Biology of Aging. C. E. Finch & L. Hayflick, Eds. 513–535. New York.
2. BANDY, B. & A. J. DAVISON. 1990. Free Radical. Biol. Med. **8:** 523.
3. HARMAN, D. (1986). J. Gerontol. **23:** 476–482.
4. OHIA, S. E., M. BAGCHI & S. J. STOHS. 1994. Res. Commun. Mol. Pathol. Pharmacol. **85:** 21–31.
5. BAGCHI, M. & S. J. STOHS. 1993. Free Radical. Biol. Med. **14:** 11–18.
6. LOWRY, O. H., N. J. ROSEBROUGH, A. L. FARR & R. J. RANDALL. 1951. J. Biol. Chem. **193:** 265–275.
7. BUEGE, J. A. & S. A. AUST. 1978. Methods Enzymol. **105:** 305–310.
8. YANO, T. 1991. Biochem. Biophys. Res. Commun. **175:** 1144–1148.
9. CHIRGWIN, J. J., A. E. PRZYBYLA, R. J. MACDONALD & W. J. RUTTER. 1979. Biochemistry **18:** 5294–5299.
10. SAMBROOK, J., E. F. FRITSCH & T. MANIATIS. 1989. Molecular Cloning: a Laboratory Manual. 779–782. Cold Spring Harbor Press. Cold Spring Harbor, NY.
11. THOMAS, P. S. 1980. Proc. Natl. Acad. Sci. USA **77:** 5201–5205.

Intracellular Signal Transduction in T Cells in Takayasu's Arteritis

B. K. SHARMA,[a] S. JAIN, AND N. K. GANGULY[b]

Departments of Internal Medicine and [b]Experimental Medicine
Postgraduate Institute of Medical Education and Research
Chandigarh-160012, India

INTRODUCTION

Takayasu's arteritis (TA) is a chronic inflammatory disease characterized by involvement of the aorta and its major branches and occasionally the pulmonary and coronary arteries. Several immunological changes occurring in TA suggest an autoimmune mechanism in its pathogenesis.[1-3] To study the cellular and biochemical mechanisms involved in T cell activation after an antigenic challenge, we studied the proliferative response of T cells to various antigens and mitogens in this disease. We estimated the activity of protein kinase C (PKC), intracellular calcium and inositol-1,4,5-triphosphate (IP3) levels to delineate the signal transduction cascade in the activated T cells and studied the role of cAMP, cGMP and cytokines IL-2 and IL-4 in the disease process.

MATERIALS AND METHODS

The study group comprised 20 patients of angiographically proven TA and 10 age and sex matched controls. 20 ml peripheral blood was collected at the time of first examination and subjected to analysis. Peripheral blood mononuclear cells were separated from the heparinized blood by density centrifugation and T cells were enriched by nylon wool column. These T cells reacted with anti-CD3 monoclonal antibody and their viability was checked by trypan blue exclusion test. Earlier, we described the methods to estimate protein kinase C and intracellular calcium.[1] For IP3 estimation, cells in 24-well culture trays were incubated with different stimulants like phytohemagglutinin and the reaction was terminated by addition of 20% ice-cold perchloric acid. The proteins were removed by centrifugation at 2000 g for 20 min at 4°C. The supernatant was titrated to pH 7.5 with cold 1ON KOH. Amprep minicolumns SAX; 100 mg code RPN 1908 (Amersham) were prepared and the cell suspension extracted with perchloric acid was applied to the sample column and eluted with 5 ml water. 5 ml of 0.17 M $KHCO_3$ eluted IP3. Eluant was collected in scintillation vials and radioactivity incorporated was measured. cAMP assay was done using cAMP (^3H) assay system (Amersham). Similarly, cGMP assay was done using Amersham kit containing (8-^3H) guanosine 3',5'-cyclic monophosphate. IL-2/IL-4 were measured by their effect on prolifera-

[a] Address for correspondence: Prof. B. K. Sharma, M.D., FAMS., Professor and Head, Dept. of Internal Medicine, and Director, Postgraduate Institute of Medical Education and Research, Chandigarh-160012, India.

TABLE 1. cGMP Levels in TA Patients (pmol/million cells)

Group	Basal	PHA
TA	0.606 ± 0.36	1.714 ± 0.260*
Controls	0.54 ± 0.034	1.40 ± 0.094

* $p < 0.01$.

tion of IL-2- and IL-4-dependent cell line HT2. Anti-IL-4 and anti-IL-2 monoclonal antibodies were used for differential blocking.

RESULTS

Total T cells in TA patients (65.8 ± 7.6%) were significantly higher ($p < 0.01$) as compared to controls (58.4 ± 3.32%), while total B cells in TA patients were not significantly different from controls. CD^{4+} inducer/helper cells were higher in patients with TA (43.5 ± 2.6%) than controls (30.83 ± 1.5%) ($p < 0.01$). CD^{8+} suppressor/cytotoxic cell percentage (34.4 ± 5.8%) was also higher than controls (30.3 ± 1.25%) ($p < 0.01$). CD^4/CD^{8+} ratio in TA was increased (1.28 ± 0.18) compared with controls (1.01 ± 0.04). A higher T cell proliferative response was seen in TA patients (13.22 ± 0.56 × 10^3 cpm) after stimulation with phorbol-myristate acetate (PMA) as compared to controls (7.5 ± 0.66) ($p < 0.01$). The basal level of PKC (1.074 ± 0.233 mmol/mg protein/min) and intracellular calcium (177.07 ± 12.56 nmol/L) in TA were higher than that of controls (0.57 ± 0.12) ($p < 0.01$) and (112.83 ± 10.6) ($p < 0.001$), respectively. There was a further rise in intracellular calcium on stimulation. PHA-stimulated T cells in TA cases showed significantly high counts indicating high IP3 levels in the cells of these patients (14.51 ± 3.48 × 10^3 cpm) ($p < 0.01$) as compared to controls. [cAMP in T cells of TA (1.12 ± 0.169 pmol/million cells) was lower than controls (1.544 ± 0.02 pmol/million cells) ($p < 0.05$).] cGMP levels in unstimulated T cells and stimulated cells with PHA are shown in TABLE 1.

IL-2 levels in TA cases were significantly raised in response to PHA (20.90 ± 1.90 U/ml) as compared to controls (12.54 ± 0.58) ($p < 0.001$), while IL-4 levels were not significantly different in the two groups (TABLE 2).

DISCUSSION

Our findings suggest that TA may be a consequence of an immunological dysregulation. In earlier studies, an elevated CD^{4+} subset of T lymphocytes,

TABLE 2. Cytokine IL-2/IL-4 Levels in 24-hr T Lymphocyte Culture in TA Patients (Stimulation with PHA*)

Group	IL-2 Levels U/ml	IL-4 Levels U/ml
TA	20.90 ± 1.908**	4.59 ± 0.46
Controls	12.54 ± 0.58	4.90 ± 0.66

* Phytohemagglutinin.
** $p < 0.001$.

increased serum levels of immunoglobulin IgG and a reduction in serum complement (C3 and C4) have been documented.[1] However, the molecular mechanisms underlying the abnormal immunological dysfunction at the level of signal transduction pathway is not known.

In the present study, we showed an increase in total T cells, CD^{4+} subset of T cells and an increased CD^{4+}/CD^{8+} cell ratio in patients with TA, suggesting that cell-mediated immunity is involved in this disease. These findings are in agreement with a previous study of Sagar *et al.*[3] However, Scott *et al.*[4] have shown a predominant infiltration of CD^{8+} cells in the arterial wall of the patients of TA.[5] Recently, Seko *et al.*[5] have shown that the infiltrating cells in the aortic tissue consists of killer cells, especially $\gamma\delta$T lymphocytes, and release a cytolytic factor, perforin. A high basal PKC and intracellular calcium in circulating lymphocytes suggest that these cells are presensitized and activated. On stimulation, a high level of intracellular calcium and IP3 and low levels of cAMP favor an activation of PKC-calcium pathway in TA. IL-2 production was enhanced in TA indicating TH1 response sensitive to PKC predominates in the disease state and could be important in the pathogenesis of the disease. However, the exact inciting stimulus or the antigen for this phenomenon remains unknown.

REFERENCES

1. DHAR, J., N. K. GANGULY, S. KUMAR & B. K. SHARMA. 1995. Role of calcium and protein kinase C in activation of T cells in Takayasu's arteritis. Jpn. Heart J. **36:** 341–348.
2. GUPTA, S. 1981. Surgical and immunological aspects of Takayasu disease. Ann. R. Coll. Surg. Engl. **63**(5): 325–332.
3. SAGAR, S., N. K. GANGULY, M. KOICHA & B. K. SHARMA. 1992. Immunopathogenesis of Takayasu's arteritis. Heart Vessels 7(Suppl.): 85–90.
4. SCOTT, D. G., M. SALMON, D. L. SCOTT *et al.* 1986. Takayasu's arteritis—a pathogenetic role for cytotoxic T lymphocytes. Clin. Rheumatol. **5**(4): 517–522.
5. SEKO, Y., S. MINOTA, A. KAWASAKI *et al.* 1994. Perforin secreting killer cell infiltration and expression of a 65-kd heat shock protein in aortic tissue of patients with Takayasu's arteritis. J. Clin. Invest. **93:** 750–758.

Why Is the Hamster Heart Resistant to Calcium Paradox?[a]

M. RAY[b,c] AND S. C. MAITRA[d]

cDivision of Physiology
dElectron Microscopy Unit
Central Drug Research Institute (CDRI)
Lucknow 226 001 (U.P.), India

INTRODUCTION

During perfusion of the isolated mammalian heart, a brief withdrawal of calcium from the perfusion medium followed by its restitution results in a rapid severe injury to myocytes, the calcium paradox (CP). However, the hamster heart does not exhibit the pathophysiological changes of the CP under the usual conditions.[1]

METHODS

Adult male golden hamster and albino Sprague-Dawley rats from the CDRI animal house were used. Hearts were perfused retrogradely. The composition of HEPES-Tyrode (HT) was (in mM) NaCl 137, KCl 5.4, $CaCl_2$ 1.8, $MgCl_2$ 1.0, glucose 11.2 and HEPES 3.0. Normal salt solution (NS) composition (in mM) NaCl 142.92, Na_2HPO_4 2.05, KCl 4.05, KH_2PO_4 0.15, CaCl 1.8, glucose 5. Calcium chloride was omitted in the calcium-free buffer (CF). The experimental protocol was 30 minutes of calcium equilibration, 15 min (CF) followed by 30 min of normal buffer. For ultrastructure study papillary muscle was processed after calcium repletion as previously reported.[2]

RESULTS

Rat heart went into a state of contracture, whereas hamster heart did not in HT perfusing medium (FIG. 1). When NS with 3 mM KCl was used in place of HT during CF, the hamster heart went into a state of contracture. Addition of NaH_2PO_4 (10 mM) to the Ca-free (CF) HT resulted in 65 ± 7% recovery following reperfusion with HT. In another set of experiments, CF perfusion with low KCl-HT, there was time-dependent inhibition of force of contraction, at 5 min, there was 25 ± 5% contraction, and at 15 min irreversible contracture was observed.

---

[a] CDRI Communication No.
[b] Corresponding author.

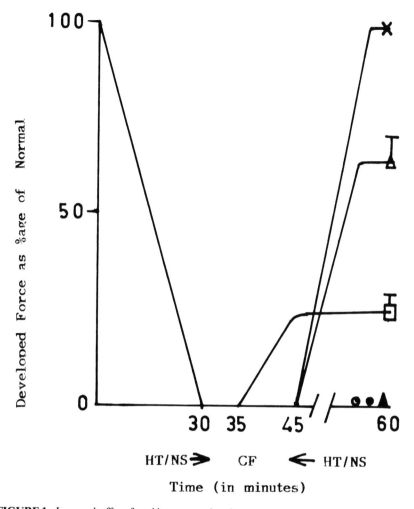

FIGURE 1. Langendorff perfused hamster and rat heart subjected to calcium repletion after calcium-free perfusion. Values are SEM from five experiments. ×——× Hamster in HT; ⊙——⊙ rat in HT; ●——● hamster in NS hypokalemic; △——△ hamster in HT with phosphate; □——□ hamster in HT hypokalemic (5 min); ▲——▲ hamster in HT hypokalemic (15 min).

Papillary muscle of hamster heart treated with low KCl-NS showed two distinct populations of cells. Some myocytes were hypercontracted with detached sarcolemma and ejected mitochondria (FIG. 2D); often juxtaposed were cells with relaxed myofibrils and mitochondria with well organized cristae (FIG. 2C). Heart from rat subjected to CP showed a prominent contraction band (FIG. 2A), whereas hamster hearts maintained their contacts at the intercalated disks. The sarcolemma was intact with relaxed myofilaments (FIG. 2B).

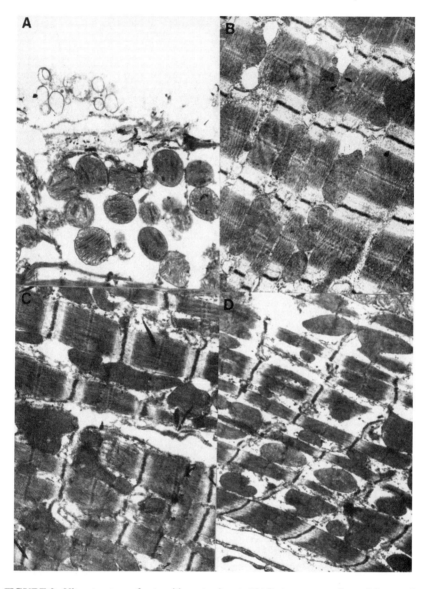

FIGURE 2. Ultrastructure of rat and hamster heart. **(A)** Rat myocytes after calcium repletion in HT. **(B)** Hamster myocytes after Ca repletion in HT. **(C)** and **(D)** Hamster myocytes
subjected to NS after hypokalemic calcium-free perfusion. Magnification for all electron
micrographs: × 15600.

DISCUSSION

Results obtained in the present investigation indicate that the hamster heart can be provoked into a state of contracture with two interventions: one with low KCl containing NS and the other when HT with low KCl is used; both interventions were during the CF state. Both procedures resulted in loss of contractility and damaged myocytes, although the damage caused by the second intervention was time dependent. Addition of 10 mM phosphate results in an increase in ^{45}Ca (calcium-45) uptake. Phosphate provides a donor that exchanges for matrix hydroxide ions on the phosphate hydroxide antiporter.[3] The entry of H_3PO_4 is followed by loss of a proton to the alkaline matrix; the excess anion provides the milieu for accumulation of calcium as the phosphate salt.

K concentration during zero-calcium does not have a measurable effect on calcium efflux. If K concentration determines the calcium movement, it would seem necessary to look for shifts within the several compartments for calcium rather than for changes in total contents.[4] The reason for the critical importance of the $[K^+]$ during CF perfusion on the effects of subsequent restoration of Ca^{2+} to the perfusate is still not clear. Some still unidentified change in the muscle induced by low external $[K^+]$ may be involved.

It is reported that there is a decrease in the intramembrane particles of bilayer during the CF state.[5] Hypokalemic HT-perfused heart showed partial resistance to CP, which is time dependent. It is possible that in the hamster, calcium bonded to the cell surface plays a major role. There is no difference between normal and myopathic hamster heart as seen in the kinetics of Ca exchange or the role of $[Ca^{2+}]$ in the excitation-contraction coupling process.[6]

REFERENCES

1. RAY, M. & R. ROY. 1992. J. Mol. Cell. Cardiol. **24**(Suppl. 1): P-02-11.
2. TRIPATHI, O., M. MEHROTRA, V. K. VAJPAI, A. BHATNAGAR, C. SINGH, A. C. SHIPSTON & B. N. DHAWAN. 1988. Biomed. Biochim. Acta **17**: 901–914.
3. LANGER, G. A. & L. M. NUDD. 1980. Am. J. Physiol. **237**: H239–H246.
4. LEE, Y. C. P. & M. B. VISSCHER. 1970. Am. J. Physiol. **219**: 1937–1941.
5. FRANK, J. S., T. L. RICH, S. BEYDLER & M. KREMAN. 1982. Circ. Res. **51**: 117–130.
6. MA, T. & L. BAILEY. 1979. Cardiovasc. Res. **13**: 487–498.

Effects of Cromakalim and Glibenclamide in Ischemic and Reperfused Hearts

ARPAD TOSAKI,[a] RICHARD M. ENGELMAN,
AND DIPAK K. DAS

The University of Connecticut Health Center
School of Medicine
Farmington, Connecticut 06030-1110

INTRODUCTION

To date, adenosine triphosphate sensitive (K_{ATP}) channel openers have been extensively studied in hearts obtained from healthy animals, but, to our knowledge, such a study has not yet been carried out in diseased hearts. K_{ATP} channel blockers (*e.g.*, glibenclamide) could reduce the intracellular K^+ loss via the K_{ATP} channels during or after an ischemic episode leading to a reduced incidence of arrhythmias. The application of K_{ATP} channel opener (*e.g.*, cromakalim) could increase the incidence of arrhythmias by the acceleration of K^+ efflux in ischemic/reperfused diabetic hearts. Our previous studies show[1-3] that K_{ATP} channel blockers protected the nondiabetic myocardium against ischemia/reperfusion-induced damage, and K_{ATP} channel openers aggravated postischemic cardiac function. The main objective of the present investigation is to use isolated working diabetic rat hearts to study the effects of cromakalim and glibenclamide on the incidence of reperfusion-induced arrhythmias.

METHODS

Male Sprague-Dawley rats were used for all studies. Diabetes was induced by an intraperitoneal injection of streptozotocin (65 mg/kg) dissolved in 0.1 M citrate buffer. Nondiabetic age-matched control animals were injected with an equivalent volume of the vehicle. Rats were anesthetized with an intraperitoneal injection of pentobarbital (60 mg/kg body weight) and then given intravenous heparin (500 IU/kg). After thoracotomy, the heart was excised, the aorta was cannulated, and the heart was perfused according to the Langendorff method followed by working mode as previously described by Tosaki and Hellegouarch.[3] After a 10-min aerobic perfusion of the heart, the left atrial inflow and aortic outflow lines were clamped at a point close to their origin. Reperfusion was initiated by unclamping the atrial

[a] Correspondence: Arpad Tosaki, University of Connecticut Health Center, School of Medicine, Farmington, CT 06030-1110. Tel.: (860)-679-2727; Fax: (860)-679-2451.

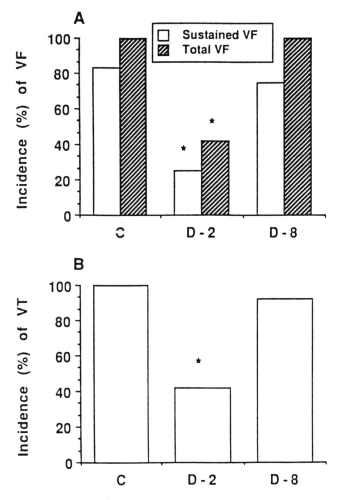

FIGURE 1. Rats (n = 12 in each group) were subjected to 0 (age-matched control), 2 (D-2), or 8 (D-8) weeks of diabetes before the induction of 30 min ischemia followed by 30 min of reperfusion in isolated hearts. The incidence of reperfusion-induced VF **(A)** during reperfusion is shown as sustained VF (*open columns*) and total (sustained plus nonsustained) VF (*hatched columns*). **(B)** The incidence of reperfusion-induced VT during reperfusion. Comparisons were made to the nondiabetic age-matched control group. *$p < 0.05$.

inflow and aortic outflow lines. The electrocardiograms were analyzed to determine the incidence of ventricular fibrillation (VF) and ventricular tachycardia (VT) and whether VF was nonsustained or sustained. Hearts (n = 12 in each group) were obtained from three populations of rats: (i) age-matched nondiabetic control rats and diabetic rats that had been injected with streptozotocin (65 mg/kg, i.p.) two (ii) and eight (iii) weeks prior to the isolation of hearts and the induction of

30 min ischemia followed by 30 min of reperfusion. The duration of diabetes, the concentrations of K_{ATP} channel opener and blocker were chosen according to our previous studies.[1-4] A change of $p < 0.05$ was considered significant.

RESULTS

The results demonstrate (FIG. 1A) that in rats subjected to 2 weeks of diabetes, paradoxically, the incidence of reperfusion-induced sustained and total VF was

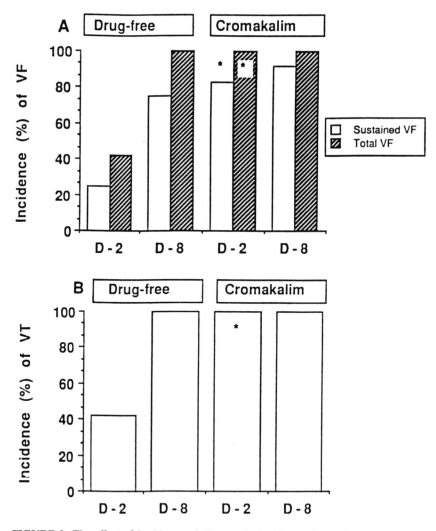

FIGURE 2. The effect of 3 μM cromakalim on the incidence of reperfusion-induced VF **(A)** and VT **(B)** in hearts obtained from 2- (D-2) and 8-week (D-8) diabetic rats. n = 12 in each group; comparisons were made to the drug-free age-matched diabetic groups. *$p < 0.05$.

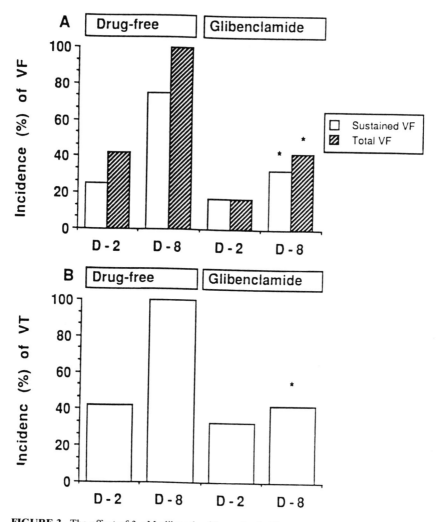

FIGURE 3. The effect of 3 μM glibenclamide on the incidence of reperfusion-induced VF **(A)** and VT **(B)** in hearts obtained from 2- (D-2) and 8-week (D-8) diabetic rats. n = 12 in each group; comparisons were made to the drug-free age-matched diabetic groups. *p <0.05.

reduced from their nondiabetic control values of 83% and 100% to 25% (p <0.05) and 42% (p <0.05), respectively. With progressive diabetes (after 8 weeks) this initial protection was abolished. The incidence of VT showed the same pattern (FIG. 1B). Hearts obtained from 2-week diabetic rats treated with 3 μM of croma-kalim before the induction of ischemia and reperfusion, had an increase in the incidence of reperfusion arrhythmias. Thus, the incidence of sustained and total VF was significantly increased from their 2-week diabetic drug-free values (FIG. 2A). The incidence of VT followed the same pattern (FIG. 2B). FIGURE 3 shows the effects of glibenclamide on the incidence of reperfusion-induced arrhythmias in diabetic hearts. In the 8-week diabetic group, 3 μM of glibenclamide significantly reduced the incidence of reperfusion-induced sustained and total VF from their drug-free diabetic values of 75% and 100% to 33% (p <0.05) and 42% (p <0.05), respectively (FIG. 3A). The same reduction in the incidence of reperfusion-induced VT was observed (FIG. 3B).

DISCUSSION

Although the effects of diabetes[5] and K_{ATP} channel blockers[6] on cardiac performance have been investigated in ischemic and reperfused diabetic hearts, no data have yet been published, to our knowledge, regarding the effects of K_{ATP} channel openers in diseased (myopathic or hypertrophic) hearts. The cardiac effect of K_{ATP} channel openers has been extensively studied in nondiabetic "healthy" hearts[7] rather than diabetic subjects. The results of our study show that streptozotocin-induced diabetes results in a reduced, then later an increased susceptibility to reperfusion-induced arrhythmias in the rat heart. Cromakalim, a K_{ATP} channel opener, significantly increased the incidence of reperfusion-induced arrhythmias in the two-week diabetics, whereas glibenclamide, a K_{ATP} channel blocker, reduced the incidence of such arrhythmias after 8 weeks of diabetes. We have shown that in the incidence of VF in the presence of an acute ischemic/reperfused event, cromakalim increases the potential for the development of VF in postischemic diabetic hearts. Clinical evaluation of ATP-sensitive K^+ channel openers in patients with essential hypertension suggests therapeutic efficacy with an incidence of dose-related side effects of edema formation, palpitation and ventricular tachycardia.[8–9] Our data show that the use of K_{ATP} channel openers as anti-ischemic agents may be of particular concern in that population of postinfarction diabetic patients who are known to be at high risk of sudden coronary death.

REFERENCES

1. TOSAKI, A., P. SZERDAHELYI & D. K. DAS. 1992. Reperfusion-induced arrhythmias and myocardial ion shifts: pharmacologic interaction between pinacidil and cicletanine in isolated rat hearts. Basic Res. Cardiol. **87:** 366–384.
2. TOSAKI, A., P. SZERDAHELYI, R. M. ENGELMAN & D. K. DAS. 1993. Potassium channel openers and blockers: do they possess proarrhythmic or antiarrhythmic activity in ischemic and reperfused rat hearts? J. Pharmacol. Exp. Ther. **267:** 1355–1362.
3. TOSAKI, A. & A. HELLEGOUARCH. 1994. Adenosine triphosphate-sensitive potassium channel blocking agent ameliorates, but the opening agent aggravates, ischemia/reperfusion-induced injury: heart function studies in nonfibrillating isolated hearts. J. Am. Coll. Cardiol. **23:** 487–496.
4. TOSAKI, A., D. T. ENGELMAN, R. M. ENGELMAN & D. K. DAS. 1996. The evolution of diabetic cardiomyopathic response to ischemia/reperfusion and preconditioning in isolated working rat heart. Cardiovasc. Res. **31:** 526–536.
5. BEATCH, G. N. & J. H. MCNEILL. 1988. Ventricular arrhythmias following coronary artery occlusion in the streptozotocin diabetic rat. Can. J. Physiol. Pharmacol. **66:** 312–317.
6. SCHAFFER, S. W., B. A. WARNER & G. L. WILSON. 1993. Effects of chronic glipizide treatment on the NIDD heart. Horm. Metab. Res. **25:** 348–352.
7. CHI, L., S. C. BLACK, P. I. KUO, S. O. FAGBEMI & B. R. LUCCHESI. 1993. Actions of pinacidil at a reduced potassium concentration: a direct cardiac action possibly involving the ATP-dependent potassium channel. J. Cardiovasc. Pharmacol. **21:** 179–190.

8. AHNFELT-RONNE, I. 1988. Pinacidil: history, basic pharmacology, and therapeutic implications. J. Cardiovasc. Pharmacol. **12**(Suppl. 2): S1–S4.
9. GOLDBERG, M. R., C. S. SUSHAK, F. W. ROCKHOLD & W. L. THOMPSON. 1988. Vasodilator monotherapy in the treatment of hypertension: comparative efficacy and safety of
pinacidil, a potassium channel opener, and prazosin. Clin. Pharmacol. Ther. **44**: 78–92.

Myocardial Angiotensin II (Ang II) Receptors in Diabetic Rats

JAGDISH C. KHATTER,[a,b,c,d] PARISA SADRI,[c]
MEI ZHANG,[b,d] AND ROBERT J. HOESCHEN[b,d]

[b]Department of Medicine (Cardiology)
[c]Department of Pharmacology & Therapeutics
University of Manitoba
[d]Health Sciences Centre and St. Boniface General Hospital
Winnipeg, Manitoba, Canada R3E 0Z3

INTRODUCTION

It is now well recognized that the renin-angiotensin system is not only an endocrine but also an autocrine or paracrine system, since all its components are found to be generated at the tissue level.[1] Various components of the renin-angiotensin system and Ang II receptors have been identified in cardiac tissue.[2-4] mRNAs for renin[5] and angiotensinogen[5,6] have also been identified in rat heart. Recent evidence also emphasized that the tissue angiotensin-forming system appears to play a more important role than previously thought. Ang II stimulates protein synthesis and cell growth in cultured chick heart cells.[7] Both chronotropic and positive inotropic effects of Ang II have been demonstrated in various animal species.[8-12] High affinity and low capacity membrane Ang II receptor sites have also been identified in various mammalian species[10-12,13] including rat heart.[4] Moreover, a role of Ang II in pathological conditions is suggested by the beneficial effects conferred by treatment with angiotensin-converting enzyme (ACE) inhibitors.[14]

In the streptozotocin (STZ)-induced diabetic rat, a model of type I diabetes, abnormalities of cardiac function may be seen as early as seven days after the induction of diabetes.[15] There is evidence suggesting a downregulation of the plasma renin-angiotensin system in STZ- or alloxan-induced diabetes rats.[16,17] Plasma renin activity and the threshold pressor dose of Ang II are significantly decreased in the diabetic rats, which correlate inversely with the severity of diabetes.[18] In addition, ACE inhibitors appear to provide a protective effect against glomerular and microvascular complications of the diabetic state.[19] Ang II has been implicated in the regulation of cellular growth[20,21] and cardiocyte hypertrophy.[22] In this study, we used diabetic rats, induced by a single injection of 60 mg/kg STZ, to characterize myocardial Ang II receptors. In addition, the effects of treatment with insulin and/or an ACE inhibitor captopril on Ang II receptor characteristics were investigated.

[a] Address all correspondence: Dr. J. C. Khatter, GF328-700 William Avenue, Winnipeg, Manitoba, Canada R3E 0Z3.

MATERIALS AND METHODS

Male Sprague-Dawley rats, weighing between 175 and 200 g, were used for the present study. The proposed investigations were carried out 6 weeks after the induction of diabetes.

Induction of Diabetes

Rats were made diabetic by a single intravenous injection of STZ. Streptozotocin solution was prepared in 0.1 M citrate buffer (pH 4.5) and used within 30–45 min of preparation. Animals were divided into two groups; one group was injected with 60 mg/kg STZ via the tail vein and the other group was injected with equal volume of citrate buffer. After the injection, both groups of animals were maintained on normal rat chow diet and water. Plasma glucose levels of the animals were measured randomly between 36 and 48 hours of injection (using glucose kit 510 purchased from Sigma) of streptozotocin. More than 95% of the animals were found diabetic within this period.

Membrane Preparation

The method employed in the preparation of the sarcolemmal membrane vesicles was essentially the same as described by us earlier.[23] Briefly, after 6 weeks of induction of diabetes, rats were decapitated and the hearts quickly removed and chilled on ice. Blood was flushed out of the hearts with saline, the atria and connective tissue were trimmed, and the ventricles were weighed. Approximately 6 g of ventricular tissue was used for each preparation. The ventricles were minced in a small volume of ice-cold buffer (600 mM sucrose in 10 mM imidazole, pH 7.0). Then the minced tissue was homogenized three times in the above buffer (4 vol/g tissue) using polytron PT20 with 15 sec cooling intervals. The homogenate was centrifuged at 10,000 g (4°) for 20 min in a Beckman J2-21 centrifuge (rotor JA20). The supernatant was then diluted 5-fold with 160 mM NaCl, 20 mM 3-(*N*-morpholino) propanesulfonic acid (MOPS), (NaCl/MOPS), pH 7.4, and centrifuged at 96,000 g for 60 min in a Beckman L3-40. The pellet was suspended in 2 mL NaCl/MOPS and layered over 15 mL of 30% sucrose solution containing 0.3 M NaCl, 50 mM sodium pyrophosphate and 0.1 M Tris-HCl, pH 8.3, and centrifuged at 95,000 g for 75 min. The white band at the sample-sucrose interface was pipetted out, diluted with 5 vol of NaCl/MOPS, and centrifuged at 100,000 g for 30 min. The pellet was resuspended in either NaCl/MOPS (for Na^+-loaded vesicles) or KCl/MOPS (for K^+-loaded vesicles) to a protein concentration of 1 mg/mL. The protein concentration in the final suspensions was determined by the method of Lowry *et al.*[24] using bovine serum albumin as standard specific ^{125}I-[sar', Ile^8]-Ang II binding.

Portions of the sarcolemmal fraction isolated by the above described procedures were used for the investigation of the binding properties of Ang II. At 2, 3, 6 and 12 weeks after the induction of diabetes, 50–100 μg of isolated membrane protein was incubated in the medium containing 10 mM sodium phosphate (pH 7.4), 145 mM sodium chloride, 5 mM $MgCl_2$ and 1 mM EDTA at 37°C. After 5 min of preincubation, the reaction was started by the addition of 100 pM ^{125}I-[sar', Ile^8]-Ang II (specific activity 400–500 mci/mmol) and incubated for 30 min. Nonspecific binding was determined by incubation with 5 μM nonlabelled Ang II in the medium and subtracted from total ^{125}I-[sar', Ile^8]-Ang II binding. At the end of the incubation period, ice-cold buffer was added to the incubation tubes and filtered immediately through GF/C millipore glass fiber filters using a constant vacuum suction system. The filters are washed with 10 mM ice-cold phosphate buffer (pH 7.4), dried and added to aquasol scintillation fluid and counted. The data were analyzed by using Scatchard plot.

Myocardial Ang II Receptor Characterization in Diabetic Rat

Radiolabelled ^{125}I-[sar', Ile^8]-Ang II binding to the isolated myocardial sarco-lemmal membranes were studied 2, 3, 6, and 12 weeks after the induction of diabetes. In each case a parallel study was carried out in controlled nondiabetic rats injected with citrate buffer. In one set of experiments, a group of rats, after they were confirmed diabetic, were made euglycemic with 6 u/day insulin for 6 weeks. ^{125}I-[sar', Ile^8]-Ang II binding was then studied and compared with 6 week diabetic rats and a parallel 6 week control group. In a second set of experiments, a group of diabetic rats were given 12 mg/day captopril in water for 6 weeks and the binding compared with 6 week diabetic and parallel control rats. In a third set of experiments, the treatment included both 6 u/day insulin and 12 mg/day captopril in water for 6 weeks after the injection with STZ. The data obtained were analyzed by Student t test and linear regression analysis.

RESULTS

Specific ^{125}I-[sar', Ile^8]-Ang II binding in isolated sarcolemmal membranes was saturable and demonstrated a single class of receptor sites. The equilibrium binding was achieved within 25–30 minutes. A time course of specific Ang II receptor binding, determined in the presence of 100 pM ^{125}I-[sar', Ile^8]-Ang II at 37°C and pH 7.4, is shown in FIGURE 1. The values at different time periods represent mean ± SE of 3–4 experiments.

TABLE 1 shows ^{125}I-[sar', Ile^8]-Ang II binding, analyzed by Scatchard plot, after 2–12 weeks of induction of diabetes. The specific binding of ^{125}I-[sar', Ile^8]-Ang II increased significantly from 32 ± 5 f moles/mg prot. to 47 ± 6 after 2 weeks and to 98 ± 5 f moles/mg prot. after 6 weeks of induction of diabetes. The specific binding obtained at 12 weeks was not significantly different from that obtained after 6 weeks of diabetes. The affinity of the receptor sites for Ang II, as indicated by negative reciprocal of the slope of the plot, was quantitatively unchanged even after 6–12 weeks of diabetes. As can be seen in TABLE 1, the dissociation constant (Kd) remained unchanged throughout the diabetic period studies.

Treatment with Insulin and Captopril

FIGURE 2 shows specific ^{125}I-[sar', Ile^8]-Ang II binding with isolated mem-branes after 6 weeks of diabetes without any treatment with insulin (6 u/day) or captopril. After 6 weeks of diabetes, the myocardial Ang II receptor density increased from 32 ± 5 f moles to 98 ± 6 f moles/mg protein. Treatment with

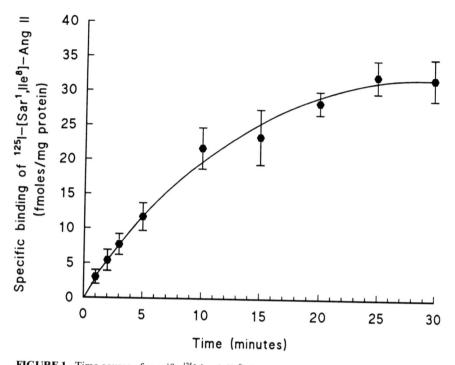

FIGURE 1. Time course of specific ^{125}I-[sar′, Ile^8]-Ang II binding with isolated sarcolemmal membranes from rat heart. Each value is a mean ± SE of 4–5 experiments.

insulin for 6 weeks limited increase in the receptor density to 58 f moles/mg protein, whereas treatment with captopril (12 mg/day) for 6 weeks limited the increase to only 50 f moles/mg prot. A combined treatment with 6 u/day insulin and 12 mg/day captopril resulted in complete prevention of any increase in the myocardial receptor density of Ang II.

TABLE 1. Changes in Myocardial Ang II Receptor Density (βmax) and Their Affinity (Kd) for Ang II with the Severity of Diabetes^a

No. of Weeks Diabetic	βmax f moles/mg prot.	Kd ($\times$ 10^{-9} M)	Correlation Coefficient
Control (non-diabetes)	32 ± 5	2.13 ± 0.1	0.901
2.0	47 ± 6*	2.10 ± 0.09	0.897
3.0	78 ± 9*	2.15 ± 0.12	0.884
6.0	98 ± 5*	2.16 ± 0.13	0.917
12.0	102 ± 11*	2.10 ± 0.10	0.906

^{a} The values represent the means ± SE of 3–4 experiments in each case.
* Indicates statistical significance (p <0.05).

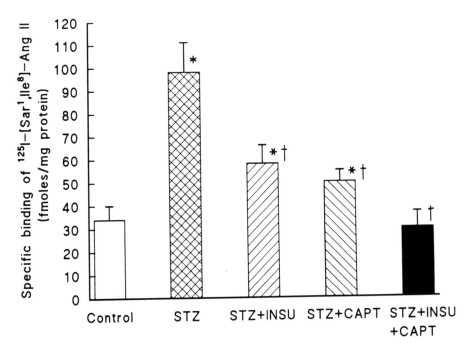

FIGURE 2. Effects of insulin ▨ and captopril ▧ treatment, individually and in combination ■, on ^{125}I-[sar', Ile^8]-Ang II binding in STZ-induced ▩ diabetic rat. The values represent mean ± SE of 4–5 experiments. * represents significant difference ($p < 0.05$) from nondiabetic controls □. + represents significant difference ($p < 0.05$) from diabetic control ▩.

DISCUSSION

The results of this study clearly demonstrate that myocardial Ang II receptors are increased within 2 weeks and continue to increase until after 6 weeks of the induction of diabetes. No significant increases in the density of the receptor sites were observed between 6–12 weeks of diabetes. Furthermore, the affinity of the receptor sites for Ang II remained unchanged throughout the diabetic period studied. Increase in the myocardial Ang II receptor density may reflect increased myocardial renin-angiotensin system activity due to primary myocardial metabolic disturbances associated with diabetes.[25,26] Treatment with insulin, in doses sufficient to maintain euglycemia, substantially reduced the cardiac disturbances[26] and the increase in Ang II receptor density. An increased expression of AT1 Ang II subtype receptor in cardiac tissue was recently reported[27] in STZ-induced diabetic rat heart. Normal levels of renin mRNA in the kidney and decreased level of angiotensinogen mRNA in the liver were earlier reported in STZ-induced diabetic rats, whereas other studies found increased levels of renin mRNA in the kidney of rats with genetically induced diabetes.[30] These observations clearly indicate a propensity for tissue-specific changes in the local renin-angiotensin system in diabetes.

Sechi *et al.*[27] (1992) reported that plasma renin concentration does not change in STZ-induced diabetic rats. Chronic infusion of Ang II in doses sufficient to suppress plasma renin concentration also did not alter renin or angiotensinogen mRNA levels in either control or diabetic rats suggesting that the expression of these genes in the heart is not under the influence of circulating angiotensin II.[27] That the alterations in the myocardial Ang II receptor density, observed by us, are more likely to reflect abnormal Ang II generation in the cardiac tissue is supported by the fact that chronic treatment with captopril, an ACE inhibitor, significantly lowered the increase in the receptor density of Ang II in this study. Chronic treatment with captopril, combined with insulin treatment, completely blocked any increase in the Ang II receptor density. These data confirmed that the abnormal renin-angiotensin system occurs in cardiac tissue with cronic diabetes. We further conclude that treatment with insulin alone may not be sufficient to prevent the cardiac disturbances in diabetes.

REFERENCES

1. DZAU, V. J. 1988. Circulating versus local renin-angiotensin system in cardiovascular homeostasis. Circulation 77(Suppl.): I4–I13.
2. RE, R. 1987. The myocardial intracellular renin-angiotensin system. Am. J. Cardiol. 59: A56–A58.
3. FABRIS, B., B. JACKSON, R. CUBELA, F. A. O. MENDELSOHN & C. I. JOHNSTON. 1989. Angiotensin converting enzyme in rat heart: studies of its inhibition *in vitro* and *in vivo*. Clin. Exp. Pharmacol. Physiol. 16: 309–313.
4. SECHI, L. A., C. A. GRIFFIN, E. F. GRANDY, J. E. KALINYAK & M. SCHAMBELAIN. 1992. Characterization of Ang II receptor subtypes in rat heart. Circ. Res. 71: 1482–1489.
5. DZAU, V. J., K. E. ELLISOIN, T. BRODY, J. INGELFINGER & R. PRATT. 1977. A comparative study of the distribution of renin and angiotensinogen mRNA in rat and mouse tissue. Endocrinology 120: 2334–2338.
6. KUNAPULI, S. P. & A. KUMAR. 1987. Molecular cloning of human angiotensinogen cDNA and evidence for presence of its mRNA in the rat heart. Circ. Res. 60: 786–790.
7. BAKER, K. M. & J. F. ACETO. 1990. Angiotensin II stimulation of protein synthesis and cell growth in chick heart cells. Am. J. Physiol. 259: H610–H618.
8. FREER, R. J., A. J. PAPPANO, M. J. PEACH, K. T. BING, M. J. MCLEAN, S. VOGEL & N. SPERELAKIS. 1976. Mechanism for the positive inotropic effect of angiotensin II on isolated cardiac muscle. Circ. Res. 39: 178–183.
9. KOBAYASHI, M., Y. FURUKAWA & S. CHIBA. 1978. Positive chronotropic and inotropic effect of angiotensin II in the dog heart. Eur. J. Pharmacol. 50: 17–25.
10. HIRAKATA, H., F. M. FOUAD & F. M. BUMPS. 1990. Enhanced positive inotropic response to Ang I in isolated cardiomyopathic hamster heart in the presence of captopril. Circ. Res. 66: 891–899.
11. DEMPSEY, P. J., Z. T. McCALLUM, K. M. KENT & T. COOPER. 1971. Direct myocardial effects of angiotensin II. A. J. Physiol. 220: 477–481.
12. HEYNDRICKX, G. R., D. H. BOETTCHER & S. F. VATNER. 1976. Effects of angiotensin vasopressin and methoxamine on cardiac function and blood flow distribution in conscious dogs. A. J. Physiol. 231: 1579–1587.
13. BAKER, K. M. & H. A. SINGER. 1988. Identification and characterization of guinea pig Ang II ventricular and atrial receptors: coupling to inositol phosphate production. Circ. Res. 62: 896–904.
14. PFEFFER, J. M., M. A. PFEFFER, C. STEINBURG & P. FINN. 1985. Survival after an experimental myocardial infarction: beneficial effects of long term therapy with captopril. Circulation 72: 406–412.
15. LITWIN, S. E., T. E. RAYA, P. G. ANDERSON, S. DAUGHERTY & S. GOLDMAN. 1990.

Abnormal cardiac function in the streptozotocin-diabetic rat: changes in active and passive properties of the left ventricle. J. Clin. Invest. **86:** 481–488.

16. CHRISTLIEB, A. R. 1974. Renin-angiotensinogen and norepinephrine in alloxan diabetes. Diabetes **23:** 962–970.

17. CHRISTLIEB, A., R. LON & R. UNDERWOOD. 1979. Renin-angiotensin-aldosterone system, electrolyte homeostasis and blood pressure in alloxan diabetes. Am. J. Med. Sci. **277:** 295–303.

18. CASSIS, L. A. 1992. Down regulation of the renin-angiotensin system in STZ-diabetic rats. Am. J. Physiol. **262:** E105–E109.

19. ANDERSON, S. H., D. G. RENNKE, D. GARCIA & B. BRENNER. 1989. Short and long term effect on antihypertensive therapy in the diabetic rat. Kidney Int. **36:** 526–536.

20. ACETO, J. F. & K. M. BAKER. 1990. Ang II receptor-mediated stimulation of protein synthesis in chick heart cells. Am. J. Physiol. **258:** H806–H813.

21. BEINLICK, C. J., G. J. WHITE, K. M. BAKER & H. E. MORGAN. 1991. Angiotensin II and left ventricular growth in new born pig heart. J. Mol. Cell. Cardiol. **23:** 1031–1038.

22. SHELLING, P., H. FISCHER & D. GANTEN. 1991. Angiotensin and cell growth: a link to cardiovascular hypertrophy. J. Hypertens. **9:** 3–15.

23. KHATTER, J. C., M. AGBANYO, S. NAVARATNAM & R. J. HOESCHEN. 1989. Mechanism of developmental increase in the sensitivity to ouabain. Dev. Pharmacol. Ther. **12:** 128–136.

24. LOWRY, O. H., M. J. ROSEBROUGH, A. L. FARR & R. J. RANDALL. 1951. Protein measurement with the folin phenol reagent. J. Biol. Chem. **193:** 265–275.

25. KHATTER, J. C. & M. AGBANYO. 1990. Mechanisms of increased digitalis tolerance in ST-induced diabetic rat myocardium. Biochem. Pharmacol. **40**(12): 2707–2711.

26. NAVARATNAM, S. & J. C. KHATTER. 1989. Influence of the diabetic state on digitalis-induced cardiac arrhythmias in rat. Arch. Int. Pharmacodyn. Ther. **301:** 151–164.

27. SECHI, L. A., A. G. CHANDI & M. SCHAMBERLAIN. 1994. The cardiac renin-angiotensin system in STZ-induced diabetes. Diabetes **43:** 1180–1184.

28. KALINYAK, J. C., L. A. SECHI, C. A. GRIFFIN, B. R. DON, T. TAVANGAR, G. B. KRAEMER, A. R. HOFFMAN & M. SCHAMBERLAIN. 1993. The renin-angiotensin system in streptozotocin-induced diabetes mellitus in the rat. J. Am. Soc. Nephrol. **4:** 1337–1345.

29. CORREA-ROTTER, R., T. H. HOSTETTERS & M. E. ROSENBERG. 1992. Renin and angio-tensinogen expression in experimental diabetes mellitus. Kidney Int. **41:** 796–804.

30. ANDERSON, S., B. BOUYOUNES, L. E. CLAREY & J. R. INGELFINGER. 1990. Internal renin-angiotensin system (RAS) in experimental diabetes (abstract). J. Am. Soc. Nephrol. **1:** A621.

Dietary and Physiological Studies Involving Magnesium Homeostasis in the Heart[a]

BRENDA I. HUSTLER, JAIPAUL SINGH,[b]
JOHN J. WARING, AND FRANK C. HOWARTH

Cell Communication Group
Department of Applied Biology
University of Central Lancashire
Preston, Lancashire PR1 2HE, England

INTRODUCTION

Molecular evolution in mammals has resulted in the development of over 300 magnesium (Mg^{2+})-dependent enzymes.[1,2] Hence Mg^{2+} regulates many cellular processes and has an integral role in muscle contraction and synthesis of proteins, lipids, carbohydrates, nucleic acids and nucleotides. It has been suggested that Mg^{2+} deficiency or reduced dietary Mg^{2+} intake may play an important role in the etiology of many diseases including many of those involving the cardiovascular system, such as hypertension, cardiac arrhythmias, atherosclerosis and ischemic heart disease.[3,4] Magnesium deficiency is common in patients who have suffered acute myocardial infarction, and studies have shown that intravenous infusion of Mg^{2+} in the acute phase of a myocardial infarction significantly reduces arrhythmias and mortality.[5,6] It is therefore of some interest to understand the mechanisms of Mg^{2+} homeostasis in the heart. Hence, the effects of (a) elevated extracellular Mg^{2+} concentration ($[Mg^{2+}]_o$) on amplitude of contraction and (b) catecholamines, forskolin (10^{-5} M), elevated extracellular (181.5 mM) Na^+ concentration ($[Na^+]_o$), and sucrose (72.6 mM) on Mg^{2+} efflux, were investigated in isolated Langendorff hearts taken from 3-month-old rats fed on standard CRM rat feed. Weanling rats aged 4 weeks were maintained on dietary regimes that were either deficient in Mg^{2+} or contained excess Mg^{2+}. Magnesium and calcium (Ca^{2+}) status were determined in hearts, plasma and other organs from these rats.

METHODS

Perfusion of Isolated Hearts

Adult Sprague-Dawley rats of either sex and weighing 250–300 g were killed by a blow to the head and cervical dislocation. The hearts were rapidly excised and cannulated via the aorta using Langendorff's technique and perfused (5 ml

[a] This work was supported by the British Heart Foundation.
[b] Address for correspondence: Professor Jaipaul Singh, Cell Communication Group, Department of Applied Biology, University of Central Lancashire, Preston PR1 2HE, Lancashire, England. Tel.: +44(0)-1772-893515/893500; Fax: +44(0)-1772-892929.

min^{-1}) with Krebs-Henseleit (KH) solution at 37°C containing (mM) NaCl, 118; KCl, 4.8; $CaCl_2$, 1.25; $NaHCO_3$, 27.2; KH_2PO_4, 1.0; $MgSO_4$, 1.2 and glucose, 11.1. The hearts were electrically paced (3–6 Hz frequency, 20 V, 1 msec pulse width) and amplitude of contraction was measured by an isometric transducer attached to the apex of the heart by a silk suture. These experiments have been described in detail elsewhere.[7]

Effects of Catecholamines, Forskolin, Elevated $[Na^+]_o$ and Sucrose on Mg^{2+} Fluxes

Briefly, hearts were perfused with KH containing 1.2 mM Mg^{2+} for a stabilization period and then perfused with Mg^{2+}-free KH solution (control) for the remainder of the experimental period. After 20 min Mg^{2+}-free KH perfusion, the heart was stimulated with either isoprenaline (10^{-7} M) for 3 min, forskolin (10^{-5} M), elevated NaCl (181.5 mM) or sucrose (72.6 mM) for 10 min. Effluent samples were collected every 30 sec and analyzed for Mg^{2+} content using a Pye Unicam SP9 atomic absorption spectrophotometer (AAS) (Model 2280). The absorbance of the unknown samples was read at 285 nm, and Mg^{2+} concentrations were measured against a standard calibration curve. All values were expressed in ng (100 mg tissue)$^{-1}$.

Effects of Dietary Mg^{2+} on Mg^{2+} and Ca^{2+} Status in the Heart and Plasma

The effects of dietary Mg^{2+} intake, very low (39 mg kg^{-1}), low (88 mg kg^{-1}), high (681 mg kg^{-1}) and normal (control, 516 mg kg^{-1}) on Mg^{2+} and Ca^{2+} status in weanling rat hearts, plasma and other organs was investigated. Weanling Lister rats aged 4 weeks at the start of the experiment were maintained on one of the four dietary regimes for a period of 28 days. Food intake and weight gain were recorded regularly throughout the experiment and the behavior and condition of the rats was noted. At the end of the dietary period the rats were killed and bled and the blood centrifuged immediately to obtain plasma. The hearts and other organs were removed, weighed and acid digested and analyzed by AAS for Mg^{2+} and Ca^{2+} content using wavelengths of 285 nm and 435.5 nm, respectively.

Statistical Analysis

Data were expressed as mean ± standard error of the mean (SEM) (n = 3 to 8) and were compared by Mann-Whitney non-parametric test, analysis of variance test and Student t test (Minitab statistical software). Values with $p < 0.05$ were accepted as significant.

RESULTS AND DISCUSSION

Physiological Studies

FIGURE 1 shows the total net Mg^{2+} efflux over a 10-min sampling period employing different stimulatory parameters. Isoprenaline and forskolin evoked

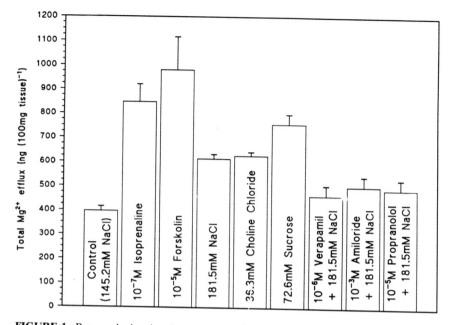

FIGURE 1. Bar graph showing the net total Mg^{2+} efflux from hearts perfused for 10 min with Mg^{2+}-free KH solution containing control $[Na^+]_o$ (145.2 mM), isoprenaline (10^{-7} M), forskolin (10^{-5} M), elevated $[Na^+]_o$ (181.5 mM by addition of 36.3 mM NaCl), choline chloride (36.3 mM), sucrose (72.6 mM) and elevated $[Na^+]_o$ (181.5 mM) in the presence of verapamil (10^{-6} M), amiloride (10^{-3} M) and propranolol (10^{-5} M). Data are mean $\pm$ SEM (n = 3–8).

large and highly significant increases in Mg^{2+} efflux. Propranolol (10^{-5} M), a beta-adrenergic antagonist, inhibited Mg^{2+} efflux in response to isoprenaline.[7] Verapamil (10^{-6} M), a calcium antagonist, and propranolol (10^{-5} M) inhibited Mg^{2+} efflux under control conditions and in response to elevated $[Na^+]_o$. A 25% increase (36.3 mM) in $[Na^+]_o$, as NaCl, evoked a significant increase in Mg^{2+} efflux, which was not associated with LDH release. Sucrose (72.6 mM) and choline chloride (36.3 mM) evoked similar significant increases in Mg^{2+} efflux. The effect of elevated $[Na^+]_o$ was attenuated by 10^{-3} M amiloride. There was a concomitant increase in force of contraction of the heart during stimulation. The results indicate that Mg^{2+} efflux is not due to cell damage in the heart, but may be associated with a cyclic AMP mechanism, with an Na^+/Mg^{2+} counterport mechanism or with osmotic shock.

Dietary Studies

Rats maintained on the very low and low Mg^{2+} diet (VLM and LM rats) consumed 20% less food than those on the normal (control) and high Mg^{2+} diets (CM and HM rats), but their weight gain was 50–53% less than that of the latter two groups. This reduction is attributed to changes in insulin-like growth factor and growth hormone accompanying Mg^{2+} deficiency.[8] The VLM

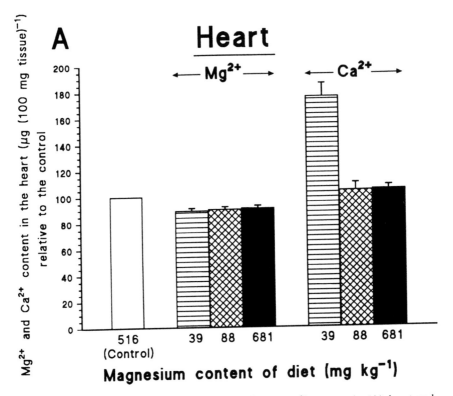

FIGURE 2. Bar graphs showing the relative Mg^{2+} and Ca^{2+} content in **(A)** heart and **(B)** plasma of rats fed a very low (39 mg kg^{-1}), low (88 mg kg^{-1}) and high (681 mg kg^{-1}) Mg^{2+} diet expressed as a percentage of the content (mg (100 mg tissue^{-1})) of the normal (control, 516 mg kg^{-1}) Mg^{2+} diet. Each point is mean ± SEM (n = 10).

and LM rats became increasingly nervous and hyperexcitable as the dietary period progressed and there was slight fur loss and reddening of exposed skin areas in these rats. FIGURE 2 shows changes in Mg^{2+} and Ca^{2+} contents in the heart (A) and plasma (B) relative to the control. Heart Mg^{2+} in VLM and LM rats was relatively well conserved at 89% and 90%, respectively, of the CM rats (FIG. 2A) but there was a significant reduction in plasma Mg^{2+} to approximately 34% in both groups (FIG. 2B). There was a degree of hypercalcemia in the hearts of VLM rats with Ca^{2+} content being 176% of the control (FIG. 2A). Heart Ca^{2+} levels in LM rats were relatively unchanged at 105% of the control. Heart and plasma Mg^{2+} and Ca^{2+} status in HM rats was similar to that in CM rats (FIG. 2). Analysis of other organs in VLM and LM rats showed that the greatest loss of both Mg^{2+} and Ca^{2+} was from bone. In general these results suggest that there is a high degree of buffering of Mg^{2+} content in the heart. Nevertheless, within a relatively short time (28 days) on a low Mg^{2+} diet, significant changes in Mg^{2+} content do occur, which may be sufficient to affect organ function and may predispose the tissue to degenerative changes.[3]

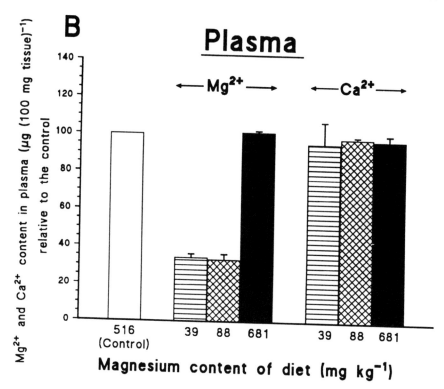

FIGURE 2. (*Continued*)

Overall, these results indicate that hypomagnesemia is associated with decreased levels of Mg^{2+} and increased levels of Ca^{2+} in the heart and that Mg^{2+} fluxes in the heart may occur by several mechanisms.

REFERENCES

1. FLATMAN, P. W. 1991. Mechanisms of magnesium transport. Annu. Rev. Physiol. **53:** 259–271.
2. WACKER, W. E. C. 1968. The biochemistry of magnesium. Ann. N. Y. Acad. Sci. **162:** 717–726.
3. ALTURA, B. M. & B. T. ALTURA. 1995. Magnesium in cardiovascular biology. Sci. Am. Sci. Med. **2**(3): 28–37.
4. MURPHY, E., C. C. FREUDENRICH & M. LIEBERMAN. 1991. Cellular magnesium and Na/Mg exchange in heart cells. Annu. Rev. Physiol. **53:** 273–287.
5. ABBOTT, L. G. & R. K. RUDE. 1993. Clinical manifestation of magnesium deficiency. Miner. Electrolyte Metab. **19:** 314–322.
6. WOODS, K. L. & S. FLETCHER. 1994. Long-term outcome after intravenous magnesium sulphate in suspected acute myocardial infarction: the second Leicester Intravenous Magnesium Intervention Trial (LIMIT-2). The Lancet **343:** 816–819.

7. HOWARTH, F. C., J. J. WARING, B. I. HUSTLER & J. SINGH. 1994. Effects of extracellular magnesium and beta adrenergic stimulation on contractile force and magnesium mobilization in the isolated rat heart. Magnesium Res. **7**(3/4): 187–197.
8. CHARLTON, J. A. & D. G. ARMSTRONG. 1989. The effect of varying the sodium or potassium intake, or both, on magnesium status in the rat. Br. J. Nutr. **62:** 399–406.

Stress Relief Protein Modulation by Calnexin

T. VINAYAGAMOORTHY[a] AND A. R. J. RAJAKUMAR[b]

[a]Department of Dermatology
University of Alberta
Alberta, Edmonton, Canada
and
[b]Department of Medicine
Royal University Hospital
Saskatoon, Saskatchewan, Canada

INTRODUCTION

Cardiovascular disease is the number two cause of death in North America. Within it, the incidence of myocardial infarction is significant. This is due to a prolonged ischemic condition of the heart where myocardial cells are subjected to hypoxia leading to intracellular stress and death. In the recent past researchers have been studying the cellular response to stress. This had led to the study of a new group of genes/proteins called "stress relief genes/proteins."

This includes various intracellular antioxidants such as glutathione, alpha loco-phenol, ascorbic acid, betacarotene and antioxidant enzymes such as superoxide dismutase (SOD) catalase, and glutathione peroxidase.[1] Further expression of these genes could form the first line of defense, buffering and nullifying the intra-cellular effects of the oxidative stress elements such as oxygen free radicals, and preventing them from causing damage to more vital intracellular molecules such as DNA-strand break, protein-degradation and lipid peroxidation. Among the various stress response genes identified, heat shock protein (HSP) is the most common in prokaryotic as well as eukaryotic cells including heart myocardial cells.[2,3] HSP is a class of housekeeping proteins varying in molecular size ranging from 15 KDa to 110 KDa, expressed at low level in normal cells, but elevated under cellular stress. In the recent past it was shown that the HSP 70 is induced in heart muscle by ischemia/reperfusion, oxidative stress, hypoxia/reoxygenation and hyperthermia.[1,4] Among this family of proteins, HSP 70 has been reported to be elevated following ischemia in heart myocardial cells.[5]

In studying melanoma/melanogenesis-associated protein, we isolated and identified an endoplasmic reticulum (ER) membrane protein calnexin.[6] Further studies have shown that calnexin is a "chaperone" protein targeting cellular proteins to their respective sites.[7] Therefore, we hypothesize that calnexin may be involved in sorting and directing stress relief protein HSP 70 to the respective target site. In this report we present the data based on computer analysis and the possible mechanism for calnexin to be involved in the processing of HSP.

MATERIALS AND METHOD

The nucleotide sequence of human calnexin and HSP 70 cDNA were analyzed, using the Gene Runner program (Hasting Software, NY). Analysis by this software

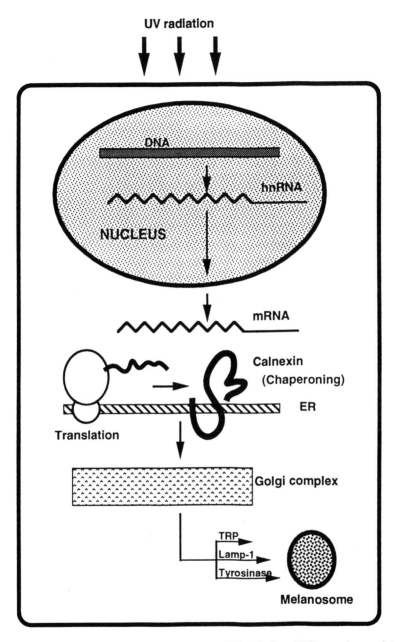

FIGURE 1. Cellular response by melanocytes to UV radiation. TRP: tyrosinase-related proteins; Lamp: lysozomal-associated membrane proteins; ER: endoplasmic reticulum.

TABLE 1. Potential Functional Motifs of Heat Shock Protein 70

Sites Pattern[a]	Functional Motifs
1. X-G-(RK)(RK)	amidation site
2. (RK) (2)-X-(ST)	cAMP & cGMP protein kinase phosphorylation site
3. S-G-X-G	glycosaminoglycan attachment site
4. (IV)D-L-G-T-T-X-S	heat shock 70 protein family signature
5. D-(LF)-G(3)-T-F-D	heat shock protein family signature
6. (RK)-X(2)((DE)-X-(3)-Y	tyrosinase kinase phosphorylation site
7. N-P-(ST)-P	N-glycosylation site
8. (ST)-X-(RK)	protein kinase C phosphorylation site
9. G-(EDRKHPFYW)-X(2)(STAGCN)-(P)	N-myristolylation site
10. ST-X(2)-(DE)	caesin kinase II phosphorylation site

[a] X = variable amino acids.

program identifies conserved amino acid sequences with 10% homology to already known functional sequences (motifs) in other reported proteins in data bank.

RESULTS AND DISCUSSION

Cellular organelles such as unit membranes and macrobiomolecules such as DNA are potential targets for damage by oxygen free radicals. The potential damage by these free radicals is prevented by vitamin C, vitamin E, and carotene.

Recently, another family of stress relief proteins was reported particularly in myocardial cells. Recent studies[8] postulated that "the stress protein HSP 70 is able to alter the resistance of the heart to subsequent ischemic and nonischemic injury." Further, studies[9] show that "HSP 70 mRNA is expressed under anaerobic conditions in rat hearts, and the cessation of anaerobic metabolism in severe ischemic hearts is associated with shut down of HSP 70 mRNA expression."

In our earlier studies we reported the correlation of cellular stress and the response.[10] Radiation by UV B induces formation of oxygen free radicals in the cells. It has been documented that formation of melanin is the cellular protective response to radiation stress by UV B. Melanin scavenges the free radicals as well as it absorbs UV radiation. After repeated UV B exposure there was increased expression of proteins involved in the melanogenesis cascade (tyrosinase, Lamp-1 and TRP-1) as well as melanin, the end product to relieve the intracellular stress created by UV B radiation (FIG. 1). These melanogenesis-associated proteins are localized in the subcellular organelle, melanosome, where melanin is produced. Therefore, formation of these proteins in the ER necessitates a mechanism by which these proteins could be directed to the target sites. We simultaneously isolated and identifed an ER-based Ca^{++} phosphoprotein, calnexin. Thus calnexin became the potential candidate for chaperoning these proteins from the ER including posttranslational modification, sorting and posting to target sites in the cell.[11]

The computer analysis of the heat shock protein cDNA by gene analysis (Gene Runner, Hasting Software Inc., New York) reveals the protein motifs specifying the HSP 70 family signature (IV)DLGTTXS and D(LF)G(S)TFD (TABLE 1). In addition it shows an N-glycosylation site. It also carries potential phosphorylation sites (tyrosinase kinase phosphorylation, caesin kinase II phosphorylation, protein kinase C phosphorylation and cAMP-, cGMP-dependent protein kinase phos-

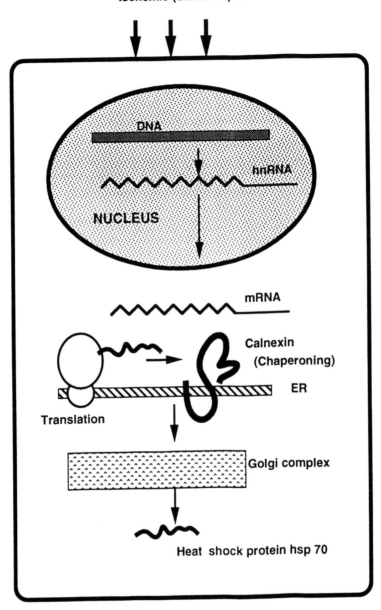

FIGURE 2. Cellular response by myocardial cells to oxidative stress. ER: endoplasmic reticulum; hsp: heat shock protein.

phorylation sites. This not only exhibits possible interaction with other proteins through phosphorylation, but also signals for sorting and posting as well.

Based on the above information we postulate that like the stress response proteins in melanogenesis, stress relief protein HSP 70 in myocardial cells may also be modulated by the same resident "chaperon" protein calnexin at the endoplasmic reticulum (Fig. 2)!

SUMMARY

Oxygen free radical (OFR)-mediated oxidative stress in myocardial cells following ischemia could damage unit membrane and macromolecules such as nucleic acids (DNA). It is being reported that under this condition these cells produce antioxidants and heat shock proteins (HSP 70). It is implied that this family of proteins could function as a "molecular chaperon" in the cell and hence has to be transported to various target sites. This proces is comparable to the induction of oxygen free radicals in melanocytes and its response, melanin production following UV light exposure stress. Lamp-1, trp-1 and tyrosinase are melanosomal-associated stress relief proteins which are involved in the production of melanin in the subcellular organelle, melanosomes. UV exposure studies as well as gene transfection studies and antisense hybridization in human melanoma cells clearly indicated an increase and marked coordinated interaction of all these stress relief proteins in melanogenesis. These proteins are synthesized in the endoplasmic reticulum and have to undergo posttranslation modification, sorting and posting to their respective target sites. We simultaneously identified and characterized an ER resident protein, calnexin. It became the potential candidate for "chaperoning" these proteins following translation. Based on the computer analysis of HSP 70 cDNA, we postulate that similar to stress response proteins in melanogenesis, stress relief proteins in myocardial cells may also be modulated by the same ER resident protein, calnexin.

REFERENCES

1. DAS, D. K., N. MAULIK & I. I. MORARA. 1995. Gene expression in acute myocardial stress. Induction by hypoxia, ischemia, reperfusion, hypothermia and oxidative stress. J. Mol. Cardiol. **27:** 181–193.
2. LINQUIST, S. & E. A. CRAIG. 1988. The heat shock proteins. Annu. Rev. Genetics **22:** 631–677.
3. YELLON, D. M. & D. S. LATCHAMAN. 1992b. Stress proteins and myocardial protection. J. Mol. Cardiol. **24:** 113–124.
4. HEADS, R. J., D. S. LATCHAMAN & D. M. YELLON. 1995. Differential stress protein mRNA expression during early ischaemic preconditioning in the rabbit heart and its relationship to adenosine receptor function. J. Mol. Cell. Cardiol. **27:** 2133–2148.
5. LEUNG, K. C. T., Y. M. RAJENDRAN, C. MONIFRIES, C. HALL & L. LIM. 1990. The human heat shock protein family. Biochem. J. **267:** 12–132.
6. DAKOUR, J., T. VINAYAGAMOORTHY, H. CHEN, D. LOU, W. DIXON & K. JIMBOW. 1993. Cloning and identification of a Ca^{++} binding p90 phosphoprotein (calnexin-like) on melanosomes on normal and malignant human melanocytes. Exp. Cell Res. **209:** 288–300.
7. WADAL, D., P. H. RINDRESS, CAMERON, WEI-JIAOU, J. J. DOHERTY, D. LOUVARD, A. W. BELL, D. DIGHARD, D. Y. THOMAS & J. J. M. BERGERON. 1991. SSRx and associated calnexin, one major calcium binding protein of the endoplasmic reticulum membrane. J. Biol. Chem. **266:** 19599–19610.

8. YELLON, D. M. & M. S. MARBER. 1994. Hsp 70 in myocardial ischemia. Experimentia **50**(11–12): 1075–1084.
9. MYREMEL, T., J. D. McCULLY, L. MALIKIN, B. KRUKENKAMPL & S. LEVITSKY. 1994. Heat shock protein 70 mRNA is induced by anerobic metabolism in rat hearts. Circulation **90**(5p.2): 11299–11305.
10. JIMBOW, K., H. HARA, T. VINAYAGAMOORTHY, D. LUO, J. DAKOUR, K. YAMADA & W. DIXON. 1994. Molecular control of melanogenesis in malignant melanoma: functional assessment of tyrosinase and Lamp gene families by UV exposure and gene co-transfection, and cloning of a cDNA encoding calnexin, a possible melanogenesis "chaperon." J. Dermatol. **21**(11), 894–906.
11. VINAYAGAMOORTHY, T., J. DAKOUR, W. DIXON & K. JIMBOW. 1993. cDNA based functional domains of a calnexin-like melanosomal protein, p90. Melanoma Res. **3:** 263–269.

Ischemic Preconditioning Involves Phospholipase D[a]

OVIDIU C. TRIFAN,[b] LAURENTIU M. POPESCU,[c]
ARPAD TOSAKI,[b] GERALD CORDIS,[b] AND
DIPAK K. DAS[b]

[b]Surgical Research Center
Department of Surgery
University of Connecticut Health Center
Farmington, Connecticut 06030
and
[c]Department of Cell Biology and Histology
"Carol Davila" University of Medicine and Pharmacy
P.O. Box 35-10
Bucharest, Romania

INTRODUCTION

Brief episodes of myocardial ischemia followed by reperfusion have been shown to render the heart more resistant to prolonged ischemia. This phenomenon is termed preconditioning, but the biochemical pathways are not yet fully known. Several mechanisms are currently hypothesized, including induction of the expression of shock-induced genes, stimulation of different receptors (adenosine A_1, α_1-adrenergic), and slowing of the energy metabolism during ischemia.[1,2] Recent studies have shown that protein kinase C (PKC) activity might play a role in preconditioning effects.[3] PKC is physiologically stimulated by diacylglycerol (DAG). Increased levels of DAG could be a consequence of enhanced myocardial phospholipase C (PLC) and/or phospholipase D (PLD) activity. The pharmacologic preconditioning could involve PLC activation, but little is known about the role of the PLD signaling pathway in the ischemic heart. Thus, in the present study we attempted to ascertain the role of PLD in preconditioning by using inhibitory anti-PLD antibodies.

MATERIALS AND METHODS

Preparation of Inhibitory Anti-PLD Antibodies

Anti-PLD polyclonal antibodies were obtained in rabbits immunized with PLD (from *Streptomyces chromofuscus*) from Sigma Chemical Co., according to the method described by Moraru *et al.*[4] Rat hearts perfused with anti-PLD antibodies have shown a decrease in PLD transphosphatidylation activity quantified using n-[1-^{14}C]butanol. Rabbit IgG (for control) was purchased from Sigma Chemical Co.

[a] This study was partially supported by National Heart, Lung and Blood Institute Grants HL22559 and HL33889. Dr. Ovidiu C. Trifan was supported by National Institutes of Health Grant HL33026.

Isolated Working Rat Heart

Hearts from male Sprague-Dawley rats (300–350 g) sacrificed after anesthesia with 200 mg/kg intraperitoneal sodium pentobarbital were perfused with Krebs-Henseleit (KH) buffer as previously described.[1] After equilibration, the hearts (six in each group) were subjected to different perfusion protocols (see Results). Global normothermic ischemia and normoxic reperfusion were used in all protocols. At the end of perfusion, the ventricles were excised at the atrioventricular junction, frozen in liquid nitrogen and stored at −80°C for further use.

Indices of Myocardial Function and Rhythm Disturbances

The incidence of ventricular fibrillation (VF) and ventricular tachycardia (VT) were determined as previously described.[3] Before and after antibody perfusion, after preconditioning, and after ischemia and reperfusion, the heart rate (HR), coronary flow (CF) and aortic flow (AF) were measured. Left ventricular developed pressure (LVDP) and its first derivative (LVdp/dt$_{max}$) were also recorded.

RESULTS AND DISCUSSION

In this study, our initial goal was to establish the concentration of perfused antibody which would inhibit PLD activity without significant changes in the heart function. Perfusing the hearts for 30 min with 50 μg/ml anti-PLD antibody (in KH buffer) inhibits myocardial PLD activity (quantified using n-[1-^{14}C]butanol; data not shown) without any changes in the functional parameters of the heart (TABLE 1). The preconditioned (PC) group was perfused for 30 min with 50 μg/ml of normal rabbit IgG, followed by four cycles of preconditioning (each consisting of 5 min ischemia and 10 min reperfusion), and by 30 min ischemia and 30 min reperfusion. Compared to the control group (no-PC, 30 min ischemia, 30 min reperfusion), preconditioning significantly decreases the incidence of VT and VF

TABLE 1. Effect of Anti-PLD Antibody on Isolated Rat Heart

Group	HR	CF	AF	LVDP	LVdp/dt$_{max}$
Control baseline	319 ± 5.8	26.5 ± 1.4	51.0 ± 1.5	17.9 ± 0.4	785 ± 30
Control 30 min	312 ± 4.8	26.7 ± 1.1	50.2 ± 1.0	17.9 ± 0.4	787 ± 30
anti-PLD 100 baseline	323 ± 6.0	27.5 ± 1.3	50.8 ± 1.0	17.8 ± 0.3	812 ± 27
anti-PLD 100 30 min	280 ± 6.8	27.2 ± 0.7	38.7 ± 1.9	15.8 ± 0.4	700 ± 34
anti-PLD 50 baseline	321 ± 7.9	27.8 ± 1.2	52.0 ± 1.8	17.9 ± 0.3	783 ± 26
anti-PLD 50 30 min	319 ± 7.4	27.8 ± 0.8	51.0 ± 1.2	17.7 ± 0.3	783 ± 27

[a] Baseline, before perfusion with anti-PLD antibody or rabbit IgG; 30 min, recorded after 30 min of perfusion with anti-PLD antibody/rabbit IgG. Control, perfusion with rabbit IgG; anti-PLD 100, perfusion with 100 μg/ml anti-PLD antibody; anti-PLD 50, perfusion with 50 μg/ml anti-PLD antibody. HR, heart rate (beats/min); CF, coronary flow (ml/min); AF, aortic flow (ml/min); LVDP, left ventricular developed pressure (kPa); LVdp/dt$_{max}$, first derivative of LVDP (kPa/s).

TABLE 2. Values Measured before Ischemia and after 30 Min Ischemia and 30 Min Reperfusion[a]

Group	HR	CF	AF	LVDP	LVdp/dt$_{max}$	VF	VT
Before ischemia							
Control	323 ± 6.5	27.5 ± 1.1	50.7 ± 2.0	17.7 ± 0.4	806 ± 43	0%	0%
PC	310 ± 6.0	28.2 ± 1.0	50.2 ± 1.8	17.8 ± 0.3	777 ± 29	0%	0%
anti-PLD	322 ± 7.0	26.0 ± 1.1	49.0 ± 2.4	17.6 ± 0.4	793 ± 24	0%	0%
After 30 min ischemia and 30 min reperfusion							
Control	295 ± 9	16.7 ± 1.3	10.8 ± 1.0	11.3 ± 0.5	469 ± 17	100%	100%
PC	288 ± 8	16.5 ± 1.1	11.2 ± 1.0	10.7 ± 0.5	454 ± 21	42%	50%
anti-PLD	288 ± 6	15.7 ± 1.2	4.3 ± 1.1	4.9 ± 0.8	333 ± 29	100%	100%

[a] n = 6 in each group. Values are mean ± SEM. Control, no preconditioning, 30 min ischemia and 30 min reperfusion; PC, 30 min perfusion with rabbit IgG, preconditioning (four cycles), 30 min ischemia and 30 min reperfusion; anti-PLD, 30 min perfusion with rabbit anti-PLD antibody, preconditioning, 30 min ischemia and 30 min reperfusion. HR, heart rate (beats/min); CF, coronary flow (ml/min); AF, aortic flow (ml/min); LVDP, left ventricular developed pressure (kPa); LVdp/dt$_{max}$, first derivative of LVDP (kPa/s).

(from 100% to 50% and 42%, respectively; TABLE 2). Perfusion with 50 μg/ml of inhibitory anti-PLD antibodies for 30 min before preconditionign (anti-PLD group) raised the incidence of VF and VT back to 100% (TABLE 2). We previously reported that the decrease in the incidence of VF and VT induced by PC could be an expression of different beneficial cellular effects of preconditioning (*i.e.*, prevention of ionic shifts caused by ischemia/reperfusion, reduced generation of free radicals),[1,2] the triggering mechanisms of which are unknown. Reversing the effect of preconditioning on VF and VT by PLD inhibition strongly suggests that the PLD signaling pathway might play a role in ischemic preconditioning. Physiologically, activation of PLD results in membrane phospholipid hydrolysis, mainly phosphatidylcholine (PC), generating phosphatidic acid (PA) and choline. PA can be hydrolyzed by PA phosphatase into DAG. DAG is produced directly by PLC activity, and can in turn be phosphorylated by DAG kinase to form PA. However, a previous report showed that the PA-DAG interconversion during ischemia occurs mainly from PA to DAG and not in the reverse direction.[5] Therefore, the ultimate effect of increased PLD activity could be an increase in DAG levels resulting in stimulation of PKC. Other recent studies suggest that PKC activity may be an important factor in triggering the preconditioning effect[3] and that PLD activity may be beneficial to restoring myocardial contractility after an ischemic injury.[5] A likely explanation of our results would thus be that one of the intracellular mechanisms of preconditioning is enhanced PLD activity with increased production of PA leading to increased DAG levels and PKC stimulation.

REFERENCES

1. TOSAKI, A., G. A. CORDIS, P. SZERDAHELYI, M. M. ENGELMAN & D. K. DAS. 1994. Effects of preconditioning on reperfusion arrhythmias, myocardial functions, formation of free radicals, and ion shifts in isolated ischemic/reperfused rat hearts. J. Cardiovasc. Pharmacol. 23(3): 365.

2. TOSAKI, A., N. S. BEHJET, D. T. ENGELMAN, M. M. ENGELMAN & D. K. DAS. 1995. Alpha-1 adrenergic receptor agonist-induced preconditioning in isolated working rat hearts. J. Pharmacol. Exp. Ther. **273**(2): 689.

3. BUGGE, E. & K. YTREHNUS. 1995. Ischaemic preconditioning is protein kinase C dependent but not through stimulation of alpha adrenergic or adenosine receptors in the isolated rat heart. Cardiovasc. Res. **29**(3): 401.

4. MORARU, I. I., L. M. POPESCU, C. VIDULESCU & C. TZIGARET. 1987. Antibodies against phospholipase C inhibit smooth muscle contraction induced by acetylcholine and histamine. Eur. J. Pharmacol. **138**: 427.

5. MORARU, I. I., L. M. POPESCU, N. MAULIK, X. LIU & D. K. DAS. 1992. Phospholipase D signaling in ischemic heart. Biochim. Biophys. Acta **1139**: 148.

Nitric Oxide Is Involved in Active Preconditioning in Isolated Working Rat Hearts[a]

P. FERDINANDY,[b] Z. SZILVÁSSY,[c] N. BALOGH,[d]
C. CSONKA, T. CSONT, THE LATE M. KOLTAI,[e]
AND L. DUX

[c]Department of Biochemistry 1st Department of Medicine
Szent-Györgyi University
Szeged, H-6701 Hungary

[d]Department of Biophysics
Biology Research Center
Szeged, Hungary

[e]IPSEN-Beaufour
Paris, France

INTRODUCTION

There are considerable controversies in the literature about the mechanism of ischemic preconditioning (PC). The discrepancies are generally attributed to species differences.[1] However, we recently reported that the mechanism of PC induced by ventricular overdrive pacing (VOP) resulting in high oxygen demand is different from the mechanism of PC induced by no-flow ischemia leading to low oxygen supply in rat hearts.[2] Therefore, PC may be classified as active PC induced by high oxygen demand, and passive PC induced by low oxygen supply.[2] The involvement of nitric oxide (NO) in the mechanism of PC is controversial.[3,4] The objective of the present study was to investigate the involvement of NO in the mechanism of active PC induced by VOP.

METHODS

Hearts were isolated from male Wistar rats (300–350 g) anesthetized with diethyl-ether, and perfused in a working mode.[5] Hearts (n = 8 in each group) were then subjected to an active PC protocol, *i.e.*, 3 intermittent periods of VOP (600 beats/min) of 5-min duration with 5-min interpacing periods, or time-matched non-PC protocol, followed by 10 min of coronary artery occlusion (test ischemia), respectively, as described.[2] PC and non-PC protocols were repeated in the pres-

[a] This work was supported by grants from OTKA F6396, MHB 709/94, Hungarian Space Research Office, Budapest, Hungary and from IPSEN-Beaufour, Paris, France.
[b] Address for correspondence: Peter Ferdinandy, MD, Dept. of Biochemistry, Albert Szent-Györgyi University Medical School, P.O. Box 415, H-6701 Szeged, Hungary. Tel.: +36 62 455096; Fax: +36 62 455097; e-mail: PETER@BIOCHEM.SZOTE.U-SZEGED.HU.

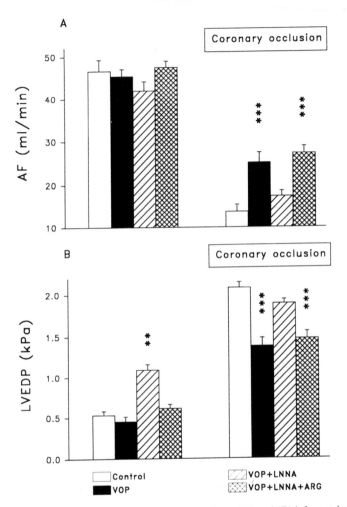

FIGURE 1. Effects of preconditioning on **(A)** aortic flow (AF) and **(B)** left ventricular end-diastolic pressure (LVEDP) measured after the 3rd period of ventricular overdrive pacing (VOP) and at the 10th min of the subsequent coronary artery occlusion (test ischemia). Control: non-preconditioned group; LNNA: 1 mg/L N^G-nitro-L-arginine; ARG: 200 mg/L L-arginine.**p < 0.01 and ***p < 0.001 show significant difference compared to the non-preconditioned control group.

ence of 1 mg/L N^G-nitro-L-arginine (LNNA), 200 mg/L L-arginine (Arg), and their combination. The dose of 1 mg/L LNNA was selected, since it did not affect coronary flow (CF) or ischemic myocardial function during non-PC protocol. However, it considerably decreased myocardial NO content assessed by electron spin resonance (ESR) spectroscopy. Aortic flow (AF), CF, and left ventricular end-diastolic pressure (LVEDP) were recorded as described.[2] Data expressed as means ± SE were statistically analyzed by ANOVA. All groups were then com-

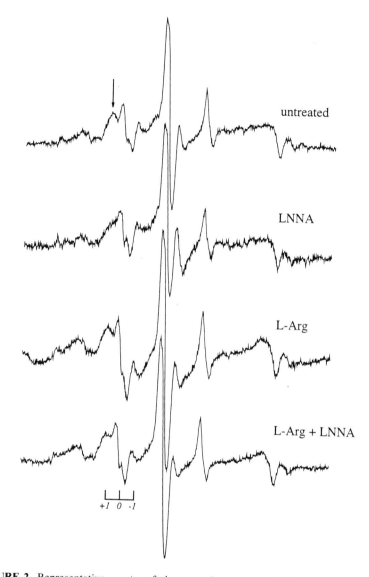

FIGURE 2. Representative spectra of electron spin resonance (ESR) signal of the nitric oxide-Fe^{2+}-diethyl-dithiocarbamate complex in left ventricular tissue. LNNA: 1 mg/kg N^G-nitro-L-arginine; L-Arg: 200 mg/kg L-arginine. ESR conditions: 10 mW microwave power, 2.85 G modulation, 9.2 GHz microwave frequency, and 100 kHz modulation frequency. *Arrow* shows g = 2.047. +1 0 −1 show hyperfine coupling of nitroxyl triplet.

pared to the non-PC control group by a t test with Bonferroni correction for multiple comparisons. To test if 1 mg/kg LNNA decreases NO content of the hearts and 200 mg/kg Arg inhibits the effect of LNNA, in separate experiments the spin-trap diethyl-dithio-carbamate (DETC, 200 mg/kg) and 50 mg/kg $FeSO_4$ were administered intravenously. After isolation of hearts, tissue samples of the left ventricles were assayed for ESR spectra of the $NO-Fe^{2+}$-DETC complex[6] recorded with a Bruker ECS106 (Rheinstetten, Germany) spectrometer operating at X band with 100 kHz modulation frequency at temperature of 160 K, using 10 mW microwave power. Scans were traced with 2.85 G modulation amplitude, 340 G sweep width, and 3356 G central field.

RESULTS

In the non-PC group, test ischemia markedly decreased cardiac performance. Preceding periods of VOP significantly improved ischemic cardiac function (FIG. 1). LNNA (1 mg/L) inhibited the effect of VOP-induced PC. The combination of 1 mg/L LNNA with 200 mg/L Arg did not significantly affect VOP-induced protection. LNNA and/or Arg did not significantly alter myocardial function before and during test ischemia when non-PC protocol was applied (data not shown). However, after the 3rd period of VOP during PC protocol, LNNA decreased cardiac performance. In tissue samples of hearts treated with LNNA, the specific ESR spectra of the $NO-Fe^{2+}$-DETC complex were eliminated. However, the complex reappeared when combined treatment of LNNA and 200 mg/L Arg was applied (FIG. 2).

DISCUSSION

The present results show that LNNA eliminates the ESR spectra of NO in the myocardium, and inhibits the cardioprotective effect of active PC elicited by VOP in the rat. If Arg is combined with LNNA, VOP-induced protection and ESR spectra of NO reappear. These findings strongly suggest that an intact NO metabolism is required to elicit active PC in the rat. In agreement, we previously showed that elevation of myocardial cGMP content was associated with active PC in rabbits.[7,8] Similarly to the present results, Vegh et al.[3] observed that the anti-arrhythmic effect of PC induced by coronary occlusion was abolished by administration of N^G-nitro-L-arginine methyl ester in anesthetized dogs. However, Lu et al.[4] could not confirm these results in anesthetized rats. Nevertheless, in the latter studies, no attempts were made to detect the changes of NO content of the myocardium when NO synthesis was pharmacologically modulated. We conclude that the present study provides strong evidence that a NO-mediated mechanism is involved in active PC.

REFERENCES

1. WALKER, D. M. & D. M. YELLON. 1992. Ischaemic preconditioning: from mechanism to exploitation. Cardiovasc. Res. **26:** 734–739.
2. FERDINANDY, P., Z. SZILVASSY, M. KOLTAI & L. DUX. 1995. Ventricular overdrive pacing-induced preconditioning and no-flow ischemia-induced preconditioning in isolated working rat hearts. J. Cardiovasc. Pharmacol. **25:** 97–104.

3. VEGH, A., L. SZEKERES & J. R. PARRATT. 1992. Preconditioning of the ischemic myocardium; involvement of the L-arginine nitric oxide pathway. Br. J. Pharmacol. **107:** 648–652.

4. LU, H. R., P. REMEYSEN & F. DE CLERCK. 1995. Does the antiarrhythmic effect of ischemic preconditioning in rats involve the L-arginine nitric oxide pathway? J. Cardiovasc. Pharmacol. **25:** 524–530.

5. FERDINANDY, P., D. K. DAS & A. TOSAKI. 1993. Pacing-induced ventricular fibrillation leading to oxygen free radical production in aerobically perfused rat hearts. J. Mol. Cell. Cardiol. **25:** 683–692.

6. TOMINAGA, T., S. SATO, T. OHNISHI & S. T. OHNISHI. 1993. Potentiation of nitric oxide formation following bilateral carotid occlusion and focal cerebral ischemia in the rat: *in vivo* detection of the nitric oxide radical by electron paramagnetic resonance spin trapping. Brain Res. **614:** 342–346.

7. SZILVASSY, Z., P. FERDINANDY, I. JAKAB, J. LONOVICS & M. KOLTAI. 1994. Ventricular overdrive pacing-induced anti-ischemic effect: a conscious rabbit model of preconditioning. Am. J. Physiol. **266:** H2033–H2044.

8. SZILVASSY, Z., P. FERDINANDY, P. BOR, I. JAKAB, J. SZILVASSY, I. NAGY, J. LONOVICS & M. KOLTAI. 1994. Loss of preconditioning in rabbits with vascular tolerance to nitroglycerin. Br. J. Pharmacol. **112:** 999–1001.

The Use of Glucose and Insulin during Hypothermic and Normothermic CABG[a]

VIVEK RAO, GIDEON COHEN, RICHARD D. WEISEL,[b]
FRANK MERANTE, JOHN S. IKONOMIDIS,
JOAN IVANOV, SUSAN M. CARSON,
DONALD A. G. MICKLE, AND GEORGE T. CHRISTAKIS

*Centre for Cardiovascular Research
and
Division of Cardiovascular Surgery
The University of Toronto
Toronto, Ontario M5G 2C4, Canada*

INTRODUCTION

Isolated coronary bypass surgery is now associated with low rates of morbidity and mortality.[1] However, certain groups of patients such as those who present for surgery with unstable angina, poor preoperative left ventricular function or a recent myocardial infarction still face an increased risk for perioperative morbidity. We previously showed that the proportion of these high risk patients presenting for coronary bypass surgery is increasing with time.[2] Therefore, improved methods of perioperative myocardial protection are required to reduce the risks of surgery for these patients.

Glucose and insulin (GI) solutions have been used in a wide variety of clinical settings for patients with coronary artery disease.[3-12] The use of GI in coronary bypass surgery has traditionally been associated with hypothermic, intermittent, crystalloid cardioplegia. Kuntschen *et al.*[13] have demonstrated that glucose metabolism is inhibited during hypothermia. We previously showed a delay in recovery of myocardial metabolism following hypothermic cardioplegic arrest.[14] Insulin-enhanced cardioplegia may provide benefit when given with near continuous, normothermic, blood cardioplegia. Insulin may allow for a more rapid transition from anaerobic to aerobic metabolism following cardioplegic arrest and may therefore provide a form of metabolic resuscitation for high risk patients presenting for coronary artery bypass graft (CABG) with episodes of preoperative ischemia.

[a] Supported by the Heart and Stroke Foundation of Ontario (Grant B2267) and the Medical Research Council of Canada (Grant MT 9829). VR is a Research Fellow of the Heart and Stroke Foundation of Canada. GC is a Surgical Scientist from the Department of Surgery, University of Toronto. RDW is a career investigator of the Heart and Stroke Foundation of Canada. JSI is a Research Fellow of the Heart and Stroke Foundation of Canada. GTC is a Research Scholar of the Heart and Stroke Foundation of Canada.

[b] Address for correspondence: Richard D. Weisel, MD, Division of Cardiovascular Surgery, EN 14-215, The Toronto Hospital, 200 Elizabeth Street, Toronto, Ontario M5G 2C4, Canada.

This study examines the effect of normothermic cardioplegia on glucose metabolism in patients undergoing isolated CABG. In addition, we examined the metabolic and hemodynamic effects of insulin-enhanced cardioplegia.

METHODS

Thirty-eight patients undergoing isolated coronary bypass surgery agreed to participate in this study following appropriate institutional ethics committee approval. Hypothermic (10°C) cardioplegia was employed in 8 patients, normothermic (37°C) cardioplegia in 6 patients and tepid (29°C) cardioplegia in 24 patients. Patients who received tepid cardioplegia were randomized to receive either standard 4 : 1 cardioplegia (n = 11) or insulin-enhanced (10 IU/L Humulin R) cardioplegia (n = 13). Cardioplegic delivery was interrupted when necessary to permit completion of the distal anastamosis. Arterial and coronary sinus blood samples were obtained for analysis of myocardial oxygen, glucose and lactate extraction as well as acid production. Hemodynamic measurements were made intraoperatively and postoperatively at 1, 2, 4, 8 and 24 hours following aortic crossclamp (XCL) removal.

RESULTS

There were no significant differences in clinical outcomes between groups. There was one patient who developed low cardiac output syndrome in the insulin group. This patient had severe chronic obstructive lung disease and suffered a bronchospastic respiratory arrest in the intensive care unit. There were no

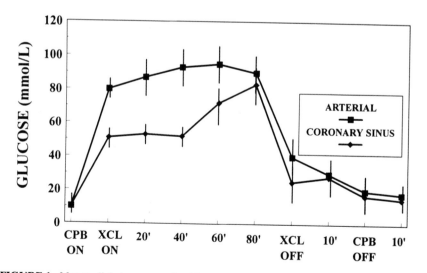

FIGURE 1. Myocardial glucose uptake. Note that coronary sinus blood glucose levels rise 60 minutes following aortic crossclamping.

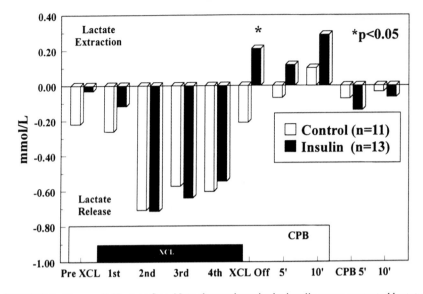

FIGURE 2. Myocardial lactate flux. Note that patients in the insulin group extracted lactate at the time of crossclamp release compared to persistent lactate release in the control group.

perioperative myocardial infarctions or deaths. The perioperative arterial and coronary sinus blood glucose levels are depicted in FIGURE 1. Administration of cardioplegia immediately raised arterial glucose levels. Myocardial glucose extraction diminished after 60 minutes of XCL. Insulin treatment lowered blood glucose levels at each sample interval during the XCL period. Myocardial lactate release persisted throughout the SCL period and early reperfusion. Patients who received insulin cardioplegia displayed an earlier recovery of aerobic metabolism as evidenced by lactate extraction during early reperfusion. (FIG. 2) Patients who received insulin had higher cardiac outputs at two hours following XCL release than the control group (6.1 vs 4.3 L/min, $p < 0.05$).

DISCUSSION

Glucose and insulin containing solutions were first employed in an attempt to reduce ischemic injury during acute myocardial infarction.[3] Unfortunately, a large randomized trial funded by the British Medical Research Council failed to show a beneficial effect of GI in this patient population.[15] Majid et al.[4] subsequently showed a small but statistically significant benefit of GI in patients treated for congestive heart failure. However, the development of alternate myocardial protective agents defused the early enthusiasm surrounding GI therapy, despite the lack of a large prospective trial in patients undergoing cardiac surgery.

More recently, insulin was shown to have positive inotropic action in a canine model,[16] and thus insulin-containing solutions have been employed to treat patients suffering from left ventricular dysfunction following coronary bypass surgery.[7,8,10,11]

We previously showed that hypothermia delays the recovery of normal aerobic metabolism following cardioplegic arrest.[14] In a study employing cold blood (4°C) cardioplegia, glucose uptake during the crossclamp period was negligible.[17] In this study, glucose extraction was significant during the initial crossclamp period. We previously showed that tepid cardioplegia permits myocardial metabolism while reducing ischemic lactate production seen with normothermia. In addition, tepid cardioplegia prevented the depression in postoperative left ventricular function seen with hypothermic cardioplegia.[18] However, even tepid cardioplegia resulted in lactate release at the time of crossclamp removal. In this study, we found that insulin-enhanced cardioplegia resulted in net lactate extraction immediately following the removal of the aortic crossclamp. This improved transition to aerobic metabolism led to improved cardiac outputs for as long as 24 hours following crossclamp removal. Thus, insulin-enhanced cardioplegia may be beneficial to patients undergoing coronary bypass surgery. The results of this clinical study support the need for a large prospective, randomized clinical trial employing insulin-enhanced cardioplegia.

Abnormal Lymphocyte Surface Antigen Expression in Peripheral Blood of a Kuwaiti Population

F. F. MAHMOUD,[a,d] S. A. AL-HARBI,[b] M. McCABE,[a]
D. D. HAINES,[c] J. A. BURLESON,[c] AND D. L. KREUTZER[c]

[a]Faculty of Health Science and Nursing
Kuwait University
Suliebikhat, Kuwait

[b]Kuwait University Faculty of Medicine
Safat, Kuwait

[c]University of Connecticut School of Medicine
Farmington, Connecticut 06030-3105

Human leukocyte cell surface antigens defined by antibody group specificities according to the CD (cluster of differentiation) system can undergo altered expression during active or impending disease states and after exposure to toxic chemicals.[1,2] Because significant amounts of environmental toxins were released following the Gulf War in 1991, alterations in immune status and thus CD expression may occur in individuals suffering from health problems arising as a result of exposure to these substances. Thus we examined the expression of a battery of CD marker proteins, plus kappa and lambda immunoglobulins on peripheral blood mononuclear cells (PBMC) from 13 subjects exposed to pollutants released during or after the conflict and in 7 subjects absent from Kuwait for at least 2 years prior to this study. Our analysis demonstrates significant increases in the percentage of peripheral blood lymphocytes expressing CD10, CD14, CD33 and CD34 for individuals exposed to pollutants compared to unexposed persons. These initial findings may be useful in predicting the risk of future public health burdens in Kuwait and surrounding countries.

Alterations in the normal profile of CD proteins, expressed on the surface of peripheral blood leukocytes are often associated with immune dysfunction[1,2] and may provide an indicator of immune and disease status. Previous studies provided evidence that many environmental toxins can alter CD expression in animals[3] and humans.[4] For example, multiple immune derangements occurring as a result of chemical exposure include altered cell-mediated immunity[5] and hormone production.[6,7] A relationship between exposure to chemicals and increased risk of cancers has also been demonstrated.[1,8] Functional abnormalities in the immune system following toxin exposure include neoplastic disorders such as leukemias, which

[d] Address correspondence to: Fadia F. Mahmoud, PhD, Dept. of Medical Laboratory Sciences, Faculty of Allied Health, Kuwait University, P.O. Box 31470—Suliebikhat, 90805 Suliebikhat, Kuwait.

are seen to be significantly elevated among farmers exposed to agricultural chemicals,[9-11] and among individuals occupationally exposed to petroleum products.[9]

Recently, serious chemical contamination of the human environment occurred as a consequence of the Iraqi occupation of Kuwait. Most of this contamination was due to massive environmental release of crude oil and pyrolytic substances secondary to open burning of the released oil as well as the formation of extensive oil lakes during the spring and summer of 1991. These events resulted in release of benzene and other hydrocarbons into the atmosphere. Additional chemical release occurred due to demolition of abandoned Iraqi ammunition stocks, conducted on a daily basis for a year following the conflict, exposing populations downwind of the demolition sites to vaporized components of the destroyed munitions.

For the present study, we hypothesized that the release of these toxic chemicals may have induced immunological abnormalities in exposed individuals and that alterations in the expression levels for a variety of CD proteins known to be useful in predicting or characterizing various diseases associated with toxin exposure would occur in some of these exposed individuals. For our studies thirteen subjects (11 male and 2 female, mean age 34.6 ± 13.5), present in Kuwait for two years or more following the war, were selected as the exposed group. A control "unexposed" group was selected consisting of 7 individuals (4 male and 3 female, mean age 41.4 ± 11.0) who were absent from Kuwait during the war and returned two years or more after the crisis. All members of both groups were outwardly healthy and showed no obvious signs of disease. Blood samples were provided by local physicians from individuals appearing for routine physical examinations and were contributed to this study on a voluntary basis. Expression levels for fourteen marker phenotypes are reported as percentage of lymphocytes in each sample of peripheral blood, bearing a particular marker on its surface (TABLE 1).

Skewedness within the test groups was compensated for by applying arcsine transformation to each data set, followed by independant t tests, to determine whether exposed subjects differed significantly from unexposed controls in the expression of any particular marker. One-tailed tests of the hypothesis were warranted, in that a marker would never be expected to reflect pathology more for unexposed than for exposed subjects.

Four CD markers showed significant increases in expression (*i.e.*, percentage of peripheral blood lymphocytes bearing a particular marker) in exposed subjects when compared to controls (TABLE 1 and FIG. 1); activated B-cell marker (CD10 ($p < 0.013$), stem cell progenitor marker CD34 ($p < 0.002$) and myeloid markers CD14 ($p < 0.019$) and CD33 ($p < 0.022$) were all elevated. A trend towards elevation in CD4 and HLA-DR expression was also observed (TABLE 1). Antigen density, as determined by mean channel fluorescence was found not to correlate with percentage of cells bearing a particular CD marker (FIG. 1, panels e–i); nor were any significant differences in antigen density detected between the exposed versus unexposed groups for CD10, CD14, CD33 and CD34 (TABLE 1 and FIG. 1). The percentage of cells expressing each of the four elevated markers was found in some cases to positively correlate with expression of one or more of the other markers. However, this was not always the case, and correlations between markers within a group were poor.

Previous studies demonstrated alterations in expression of each of these markers found in association with various diseases. For example, CD10, a 100-kDa transmembrane glycoprotein, is found on 80% of non-T cell acute lymphoblastic leukemia (ALL) tumor cells[12] and in normal individuals is found only on pre-B cells and neutrophils.[13] CD14, a 55-kDa phosphoinositol-linked glycoprotein, is

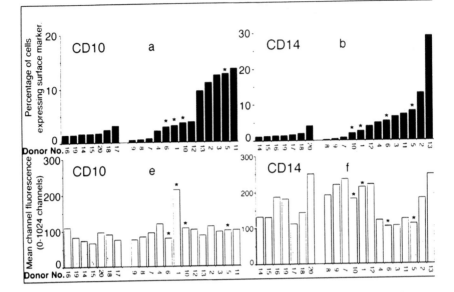

FIGURE 1. Distribution of expression (by percentage of peripheral blood lymphocytes bearing a particular marker) for markers significantly elevated in exposed versus unexposed groups. Expression distributions of leukocyte surface antigens for which percentages of lymphocytes bearing the indicated marker were found to be elevated in peripheral blood of exposed subjects as compared to unexposed control group: CD10 **(a,e)**, CD14 **(b,f)**, CD33 **(c,g)** and CD34 **(d,h)**. Male donors with spouses reporting recent history of recurrent spontaneous abortion (donors 1, 6, 5 and 10) are indicated. Peripheral blood mononuclear cells were prepared from whole, heparinized blood within 3 hours of collection using standard methods.[14] Cells were labeled with fluorophore-conjugated monoclonal antibodies specific for each surface marker evaluated. Antigen density as estimated by mean channel fluorescence was reported in a range of 0–1024 channels. FACS analysis was accomplished with a single laser flow cytometer (EPICS Profile II: Coulter Scientific Inc.). Fluorescent intensity standardization was performed on each day of use. Optical alignment was conducted with 200 μl EPICS Alignment Flourospheres with an emission spectrum ranging from 525–700 nm, with peak excitation wavelength at 488 nm. Lymphocyte subpopulations were identified by position on forward and side scatter plots and gated. Isotype-matched control antibodies were utilized to control for nonspecific fluorescence. Briefly, peripheral blood mononuclear cells from healthy control subjects were labeled with fluorophore-conjugated, nonspecific antibody, chain-matched with the antibody to be used for a particular assay. Background values for antibodies used in assays (*e.g.*, CD34) were based on fluorescence of nonspecific antibodies. Results are reported as percentage cells positive for a particular surface marker or as antigen density estimated by mean channel fluorescence. * Male donors with spouses reporting recent spontaneous abortion.

primarily a mature monocyte marker.[15] It is additionally found on 50–100% of leukemic cells from donors with acute myelomonocytic or acute monocytic leukemia.[16] CD33, a 67-kDa transmembrane glycoprotein is elevated in 85% of acute myelogenous leukemia,[17] and CD34, a 105- to 120-kDa glycophosphoprotein, expressed on most hematopoetic precursor cells[18] is normally seen on only 0.1–0.5% of cells in peripheral blood. Elevated levels of this antigen in peripheral blood may be a predictor of both lymphoid and myeloid leukemias.[19]

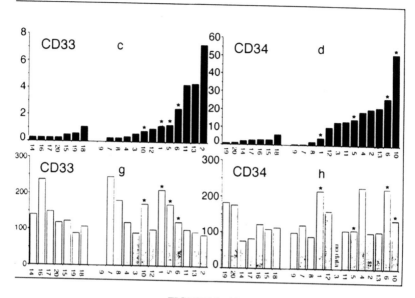

FIGURE 1. (*Continued*)

While the observed immunologic abnormalities may suggest the possibility of an increased future cancer burden in Kuwait, particularly of the reticuloendothelial system, any environmental toxins that have contributed to development of the altered CD protein expression levels need not be restricted to this particular effect. Additional health-related problems may have occurred in response to the same etiological agent or agents that produced the abnormalities described in this report. For example, four out of the 11 males included in the group of 13 exposed subjects reported that their spouses suffer from recurrent spontaneous abortion, as defined by occurrence of 3 or more consecutive abortions (see FIG. 1). Since the percentage risk of premature pregnancy termination varies from 12% for women with no prior history of spontaneous abortion to as high as 45% for women with 2 or more abortions,[20] this observation may be due to chance. Moreover, no female donor in either group claimed to have experienced pregnancy-related disorders. Yet it is anecdotal evidence for possible damage to cells of the male reproductive system and possibly significant in light of a finding that young males exposed to chemical warfare agents during the Iran-Iraq war suffer from defective spermatogenesis three years following exposure.[7]

The scope of this study does not allow firm correlations between any etiological agents present in Kuwait and the observed CD marker expression abnormalities. Nevertheless, the observed cellular responses allow us to suggest an increased susceptibility to certain diseases within the exposed population. These subjects will be longitudinally observed, and future changes in marker expression and/or outward manifestation of diseases will be documented.

Clearly, future in-depth analysis of the various subpopulations, *e.g.*, two color FACS analysis, will be needed before absolute conclusions can be drawn. It is our hope that other investigators will expand on our initial studies so that new

TABLE 1. CD Marker Protein Expression on Peripheral Blood Mononuclear Cells[a]

	Cells Expressing Indicated Marker (%)		
CD Marker	Exposed Group (Mean ± SD)	Unexposed Control Group (Mean ± SD)	p Value
CD3	66.11 ± 2.94	61.64 ± 2.92	0.16(ns)
CD4	43.92 ± 2.43	37.94 ± 2.80	0.075*
CD8	28.22 ± 2.60	26.09 ± 1.67	0.28(ns)
CD10	**5.88 ± 1.41**	**0.96 ± 0.22**	**0.013**
CD14	**6.55 ± 2.13**	**1.91 ± 0.38**	**0.019**
CD20	17.62 ± 2.56	13.69 ± 1.48	0.12(ns)
CD25	19.31 ± 4.97	10.92 ± 1.77	0.16(ns)
CD33	**1.88 ± 0.60**	**0.49 ± 0.11**	**0.022**
CD34	**15.27 ± 3.84**	**2.66 ± 0.060**	**0.002**
CD45	73.85 ± 2.90	75.57 ± 3.86	0.348(ns)
Kappa light chain	13.97 ± 2.34	11.73 ± 0.68	0.27(ns)
Lambda light chain	9.58 ± 1.71	8.11 ± 1.04	0.33(ns)
HLADR	14.93 ± 1.97	11.59 ± 0.67	0.074*

[a] Group averages of percent peripheral blood lymphocytes expressing indicated cell surface antigens. Skewedness for marker expression levels in both the exposed group (n = 13) and the nonexposed control group (n = 7) was reduced using arcsine transformation of values obtained by flow cytometry. Differences in marker expression between these groups were then evaluated using independant t tests. *Boldfaced listing* is given for data sets in which percentage of cells positive for a particular cell surface marker is significantly elevated in exposed relative to unexposed subjects (p <0.05). * Trend towards significant difference in group averages within data set (0.05 <p <0.10). ns, nonsignificant difference in group averages within data set. To eliminate the possibility that elevated levels of CD10 might have arisen from contamination of the lymphocyte gate with neutrophils, flow cytometric printouts were examined to determine whether donors with increased percentage of cells bearing the CD10 antigen also had higher levels of neutrophils than low CD10 expressers. A similar quality control measure was conducted for the CD14 measurements to rule out monocyte contamination of the lymphocyte gate. In neither case was any contamination evident, indicating that marker expression was based on measurement of lymphocytes.

insight into the potential immune alterations which may have occurred as a result of the Gulf War can be developed.

ACKNOWLEDGMENTS

We are grateful to Dr. Barbara Ehrlich of University of Connecticut School of Medicine for her kind assistance in editing this publication, to Yasmine Khan for the assistance in preparation of samples for flow cytometric analysis, to Dr. Robert Vogt of the US Centers for Disease Control and Dr. Howard Shapiro, for their guidance on analysis of our results.

REFERENCES

1. CULLEN, M. R., M. G. CHERNIACK & L. ROSENSTOCK. 1990. N. Engl. J. Med. **332:** 675–683.

2. McConnachie, P. R. & A. C. Zahalsky. 1991. Arch. Environ. Health **46:** 249–253.
3. Vos, J. G. 1977. CRC Crit. Rev. Toxicol. **5:** 67–101.
4. Vojdani, A., M. Ghoneum & N. Brautbar. 1992. Toxicol. Ind. Health **8**(5): 239–254.
5. Vojdani, A. & L. Alfred. 1984. Cancer Res. **44:** 942–945.
6. Azizi, F., M. Amini & P. Arbab. 1993. Exp. Clin. Endocrinol. **101**(5): 303–306.
7. Azizi, F., A. Keshavarz, F. Roshanzamir & M. Nafarabadi. 1995. Med. War **11**(1): 33–34.
8. Whiteside, T., J. Bryant, R. Day & R. B. Heberman. 1990. J. Clin. Lab. Anal. **4:** 104–114.
9. Adamson, R. H. & S. M. Seiber. 1981. Environ. Health Perspect. **39:** 93–103.
10. Milham, S. 1971. Am. J. Epidemiol. **94:** 307–310.
11. McCabe, M. 1984. Med. J. Aust. **141:** 412–414.
12. Ritz, J., L. Nadler, A. Bhan, J. Notix-McConarty, J. Pesando & S. Schlossman. 1981. Blood **48:** 648.
13. Baur, K., R. Duque & T. Shankey. Clinical Flow Cytometry. 444.
14. Coligan, J., A. Kruisbeek, D. Margulies, M. Shevach & W. Strober. 1991. Curr. Protocols Immunol. **1:** 5.3.
15. Bernard, A., L. Bournsell & S. Schlossman. Springer-Verlag. Leukocyte Typing. 108, 407.
16. Griffin, J., R. Mayer, H. Weinstein, D. Rosenthal, F. Coral, R. Beveridge & S. Schlossman. 1983. Blood **62:** 557–563.
17. Griffin, J., D. Lynch, K. Sabbath, P. Larcome & S. Schlossman. 1984. Leuk. Res. **8:** 521.
18. Civin, C., L. Strauss, C. Brovall, M. Fackler, J. Schwartz & J. Shaper. J. Immunol. **133:** 157.
19. Katz, F., R. Tindle, D. Sutherland & M. Greaves. 1985. Leuk. Res. **9:** 1.
20. Gabbe, S., J. Niebyl & J. Simpson. 1991. Obstetrics, Normal & Problem Pregnancies. 2nd Edit. Ch. 21, p. 657.

Hyperoxia Causes Increases in Antioxidant Enzyme Activity in Fetal Type II Pneumocytes

VINEET BHANDARI, NILANJANA MAULIK,[a] AND
MITCHELL KRESCH

Departments of Pediatrics and [a]Surgery
University of Connecticut School of Medicine
Farmington, Connecticut 06030

INTRODUCTION

Exposure to hyperoxia commonly occurs during mechanical ventilation of the sick newborn and is a factor for development of chronic lung disease. Hyperoxic exposure is often accompanied by tissue damage and results in a well-described pathophysiologic response in the lungs of virtually all animals studied.[1,2] The type II alveolar epithelium seems to be resistant to hyperoxia.[3] Neonatal animals of many species are relatively resistant to pulmonary oxygen toxicity when compared to adult animals of the same species,[4] though the same may not be true for the premature fetuses. Antioxidant enzymes such as superoxide dismutase, glutathione reductase, glutathione peroxidase and catalase may protect the cells against oxidant stress. We recently showed increased activities of antioxidant enzymes (AOE) in adult type II pneumocytes exposed to hyperoxia.[5] We hypothesized that fetal type II pneumocytes would show a much decreased response. The goal of the present study was to measure the effects of hyperoxia on the activities of catalase, glutathione reductase (GR), glutathione peroxidase (GPX) and cytosolic superoxide dismutase (SOD) in cultures of 19-day fetal rat type II pneumocytes.

MATERIAL AND METHODS

The type II pneumocytes were obtained from the lungs of 19-day timed Sprague-Dawley rats (Charles River Laboratories, Wellington, MA) and grown to full confluence in pure culture.[6] Control cells were kept in 95% room air/5% CO_2 while the hyperoxia group was exposed to 95% O_2/5% CO_2 for 24 hours. Viability was determined by exclusion of trypan blue. LDH was also assayed to monitor cellular disruption. Measurements of the AOE were done using standard methods.[7]

RESULTS

The results are shown in TABLE 1. Previous data of the adult cells have also been included for comparison. Compared to controls, there is less cell death in fetal type II pneumocytes exposed to hyperoxia. Hyperoxia resulted in increased AOE activity for all enzymes in the adult cells while GPX and SOD increased in

TABLE 1. Effects of Hyperoxia on Cultures of Rat Lung Type II Pneumocytes[a]

	Adult Cells		Fetal Cells	
	Control	Hyperoxia	Control	Hyperoxia
Viability	95%	50%	68%	61%
LDH release	13.2 ± 0.4%	22.3 ± 2.3%*	4.3 ± 0.8%	5.6 ± 1.4%
Catalase	4.7 ± 0.3	15.4 ± 1.4#	8 ± 2	17.7 ± 6
GR	20.6 ± 1.8	68.9 ± 10.8#	27.2 ± 7	40.3 ± 7
GPX	23.9 ± 2.1	71.7 ± 3.7@	21.8 ± 1.9	49.1 ± 9.5*
SOD	5.6 ± 0.6	15 ± 1.8#	2.8 ± 0.3	12 ± 2.7$

[a] Mean ± SEM, n = 3–4; AOE in nmol/min/mg protein, adjusted for cell viability. *$p < 0.05$, #$p < 0.01$, @$p = 0.001$, \$$p < 0.03$ vs respective controls.

the fetal cells. GR and GPX was lower in the hyperoxic fetal type II pneumocytes as compared to the adult cells.

CONCLUSIONS

The fetal type II pneumocytes seem to be resistant to the hyperoxia in this model as compared to the response seen in the adult cells versus their respective controls. Since the AOE activities measured in the fetal cells exposed to hyperoxia were not increased compared to the adult cells, other protective antioxidant factors might account for the better survival of fetal type II pneumocytes in hyperoxia.

REFERENCES

1. WISPE, J. R. & R. J. ROBERTS. 1987. Molecular basis of pulmonary oxygen toxicity. Clin. Perinatol. **14:** 651–666.
2. DENEKE, S. M. & B. L. FANBURG. 1980. Normobaric oxygen toxicity of the lung. N. Engl. J. Med. **303:** 76–86.
3. HOUSSET, B., I. HURBAIN, J. MASILAH, A. LAGHSAL, M. T. CHAUMETTE-DEMAUGRE, H. KARAM & J. PH. DERENNE. 1991. Toxic effects of oxygen on cultured alveolar epithelial cells, lung fibroblasts and alveolar macrophages. Eur. Respir. J. **4:** 1066–1075.
4. FRANK, L., J. R. BUCHER & R. J. ROBERTS. 1978. Oxygen toxicity in neonatal and adult animals of various species. J. Appl. Physiol. **45:** 699–704.
5. BHANDARI, V., N. MAULIK, M. J. KRESCH & D. DAS. 1995. Anti-oxidant enzyme activity increases in adult type II pneumocytes. Am. J. Resp. Crit. Care Med. **151:** A650.
6. KRESCH, M. J., D. W. DYNIA & I. GROSS. 1987. Culture of differentiated and undifferentiated type II cells from fetal rat lung. Biochem. Biophys. Acta **930:** 19–32.
7. LU, D., N. MAULIK, I. I. MORARU, D. L. KREUTZER & D. DAS. 1993. Molecular adaptation of vascular endothelial cells to oxidative stress. Am. J. Physiol. **264**(Cell Physiol 33): C715–C722.

Endotoxemia and Oxidative Stress[a]

UTTARA PATTANAIK AND KAILASH PRASAD[b]

Department of Physiology, College of Medicine
University of Saskatchewan
Saskatoon, Saskatchewan
Canada, S7N 5E5

INTRODUCTION

The pathophysiology of endotoxic shock (ET-shock) is complex. Endotoxin is known to release interleukin-1 (IL-1),[1,2] tumor necrosis factor (TNF)[1] and platelet activating factor (PAF),[3] and to activate complement.[4] IL-1,[5] TNF,[6] activated complement (C_{3a}, C_{5a})[7] and PAF[5] are known to activate polymorphonuclear leukocytes (PMNLs), which on activation leads to increased production of oxygen free radicals (OFRs).[8,9] During ET-shock, OFRs can also be produced by autoxidation of catecholamines,[10] arachidonic acid metabolism[11] and the xanthine-xanthine oxidase system.[12] OFRs are known to depress cardiac function and contractility[9] and cause tissue injury.[13,14] OFRs exert their cytotoxic effects by causing peroxidation of membrane phospholipids, which can change the membrane fluidity and loss of cellular integrity.[13,14] Lipid peroxidation results in the formation of malondialdehyde (MDA). An increase in the level of MDA suggests an increased level of OFRs. We hypothesized that endotoxin-induced cardiac dysfunction and cellular injury is due to increased levels of oxygen free radicals because of increased production and/or decreased destruction. Therefore, we investigated the effects of endotoxin on the OFR-producing activity of PMNL (PMNL-CL), cardiac malondialdehyde (LV-MDA), left ventricular muscle chemiluminescence (LV-CL)—a measure of antioxidant reserve, and cardiac function and contractility in anesthetized dogs.

METHODS

Dogs were anesthetized with sodium pentobarbital (35 mg/Kg, intravenously). The dogs were divided into two groups: Group I, control; Group II, subjected to endotoxic shock by administering endotoxin (5 mg/Kg) intravenously. Hemodynamic measurements and collection of blood samples (for PMNL-CL) were made before and at various times after endotoxin administration. At the end of the protocol, the heart was removed for the measurement of LV-MDA and LV-CL.

Cardiac function was measured by measuring left ventricular work index (LVWI). Cardiac contractility was assessed by using the ratio of dp/dt (rate of left ventricular pressure development) at common peak isovolumetric pressure

[a] This work was supported by a grant from the Heart and Stroke Foundation of Saskatchewan and forms a part of Ms. Pattanaik's thesis for Ph.D degree in Toxicology.

[b] Address for correspondence: K. Prasad, MD, Ph.D, FRCP(C), FACA, FICA, Department of Physiology, College of Medicine, University of Saskatchewan, 107 Wiggins Road, Saskatoon, Sask., Canada, S7N 5E5. Tel.: (306) 966-6539; Fax: (306) 966-8718.

TABLE 1. Changes in Mean Aortic Pressure (mAO), Left Ventricular Work Index (LVWI), dp/dt at CPIP/PAW (Index for Contractility) and Oxygen-Derived Polymorphonuclear Leukocyte Chemiluminescence (PMNL-CL) in Two Groups of Dogs[a]

Parameter	Group	0 Min	15 Min	30 Min	60 Min	90 Min	120 Min	180 Min
mAO (mmHg)	I	132.2 ± 5.7	132.0 ± 6.6	135.9 ± 7.1	129.3 ± 5.0	128.0 ± 7.3	132.6 ± 4.4	136.9 ± 3.7
	II	144.8 ± 5.8	85.7 ± 11.9*†	93.4 ± 9.1*†	79.4 ± 4.5*†	78.8 ± 6.0*†	82.3 ± 9.0*†	88.8 ± 10.7*†
LVWI (Kg · m/min · m²)	I	4.40 ± 0.64	4.55 ± 0.78	4.76 ± 0.80	4.69 ± 0.56	4.25 ± 0.68	3.50 ± 0.56	3.13 ± 0.48
	II	7.90 ± 1.11	2.36 ± 0.62*†	3.02 ± 0.79*	2.28 ± 0.45*†	2.10 ± 0.37*†	2.09 ± 0.45*	2.08 ± 0.53*
dp/dt at CPIP/PAW (sec⁻¹)	I	149.0 ± 25.4	155.2 ± 29.8	143.9 ± 22.8	129.5 ± 28.6	129.2 ± 25.3	140.0 ± 23.6	91.7 ± 15.7*
	II	149.5 ± 16.4	55.1 ± 9.2*†	69.8 ± 14.0*†	82.3 ± 16.3*	79.9 ± 15.0*	96.3 ± 19.2*	98.4 ± 20.3*
PMNL-CL (mv · min/10⁶ PMNL)	I	727.4 ± 167.5	788.5 ± 158.6	782.8 ± 148.1	834.6 ± 154.0	875.2 ± 164.9	867.7 ± 206.5	989.9 ± 293.4
	II	937.1 ± 260.3	3246.8 ± 1416.0*†	1698.3 ± 709.8	2914.85 ± 1552.3	1072.4 ± 294.6	1306.7 ± 410.6	1758.8 ± 883.4

[a] The results are expressed as mean ± SE. CPIP = common peak isovolumetric pressure; PAW = pulmonary arterial wedge pressure.
* $p < 0.05$, comparison of values at various time intervals with respect to preshock (0 min) values in the respective groups.
† $p < 0.05$, control vs ET-shock group.

(CPIP) to pulmonary arterial wedge pressure (PAW). Aortic pressure, cardiac function and contractility were measured by previously described method.[9] Tissue chemiluminescence (LV-CL) was measured by the method of Prasad et al.[15] An increase in LV-CL indicates a decrease in antioxidants and vice-versa. Cardiac MDA was estimated by earlier described method.[16] The method for the measurement of PMNL-CL was as described by Prasad et al.[9]

RESULTS

The changes in the mean aortic pressure (mAO), LVWI, and dp/dt at CPIP/PAW for the two groups are summarized in TABLE 1. The hemodynamic parameters in Group I remained unaltered. Significant decreases in the hemodynamic parameters were observed in Group II. As compared to Group I, the values for mAO in Group II were lower throughout the study. However, the values for LVWI and dp/dt at CPIP/PAW were lower up to 90 min and 30 min, respectively.

The levels of LV-CL and LV-MDA in the two groups are summarized in FIG. 1. There was a significant increase in the levels of LV-CL and LV-MDA in Group II. The changes in PMNL-CL in the two groups are summarized in TABLE 1. It remained unaltered in Group I but increased in Group II being significant at 15 min only.

DISCUSSION AND CONCLUSION

In the present study endotoxin produced depression of cardiac function and contractility, and mAO which were associated with an increased production of

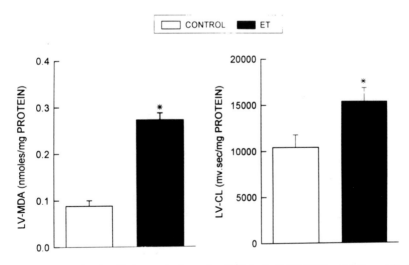

FIGURE 1. The levels of left ventricular malondialdehyde (LV-MDA) and left ventricular chemiluminescence (LV-CL) in the control and ET-shock group. The results are expressed as mean ± SE. *p <0.05, control vs ET-shock.

OFRs by PMNLs. It is known that OFRs and HOCl depress cardiac function and contractility.[9] The increase in the MDA content of the left ventricle suggests lipid peroxidation, which could be due to an increase in levels of OFRs, as suggested by an increase in the production of OFRs by PMNLs. The increase in the levels of OFRs could also be due to a decrease in the antioxidant reserve measured by LV-CL. An increase in production of OFRs and decrease in antioxidants in the cell would lead to lipid peroxidation.

The decrease in the contractility could be due to lipid peroxidation and also due to the effect of OFRs on the contractile apparatus. OFRs are known to depress Ca^{+2}-ATPase.[17] These changes could lead to a decrease in contractility and hence the functions. These results suggest that the endotoxin-induced cardiac depression could be due to increased levels of OFRs because of increased production by PMNLs and decreased destruction because of decreased antioxidant reserve.

In conclusion oxidative stress may be involved in the endotoxin-induced depression of cardiac function and contractility.

REFERENCES

1. WEINBERG, J. R., P. BOYLE, A. MEAGER & A. GUZ. 1992. Lipopolysaccharide, tumour necrosis factor and interleukin-1 interact to cause hypotension. J. Lab. Clin. Med. **120**(2): 205–211.

2. BEDROSIAN, I., R. D. SOFIA, S. M. WOLFF & C. A. DINARELLO. 1991. Taurolidine, an analogue of amino acid taurine, suppresses interleukin-1 and tumour necrosis factor synthesis in human peripheral blood mononuclear cells. Cytokine **3**(6): 568–575.

3. MOZES, T., J. P. HEILIGERS & C. J. TAK. 1991. Platelet activating factor is one of the mediators involved in endotoxic shock in pigs. J. Lipid Mediators **4**(3): 309–325.

4. LUNDSGAARD-HANSEN, P. & B. BLAUHUT. 1992. Markers and mediators in enterogenic infectious-toxic shock. Curr. Stud. Hematol. Blood Transfus. **59**: 163–203.

5. BRAQUET, P., D. HOSFORD, M. BRAQUET, R. BOURGAIN & F. BUSSOLINO. 1989. Role of cytokines and platelet activating factor in microvascular immune injury. Int. Arch. Allergy Appl. Immunol. **88**: 88–100.

6. PAUBERT-BRAQUET, M., M. O. LONGCHAMPT & P. KOLTZ. 1988. Tumour necrosis factor (TNF) primes human neutrophil (PMN) platelet activating factor (PAF) induced superoxide generation. Consequence in promoting PMNL mediated endothelial cell (EC) damages (abstract). Prostaglandin **35**: 803.

7. WEBSTER, R. O., S. R. HONG, R. B. JOHNSTON, JR. & P. M. HENSON. 1980. Biological effects of human complement fragments on C_{5a} and C_{5a} des Arg on neutrophil function. Immunopharmacology **2**: 201–219.

8. BADWAY, J. A. & M. L. KARNOVSKY. 1980. Active oxygen species and the function of phagocytic leukocytes. Annu. Rev. Biochem. **49**: 695–715.

9. PRASAD, K., J. KALRA, A. K. CHAUDHARY & D. DEBNATH. 1990. Effect of polymorphonuclear leukocyte-derived oxygen free radicals and hypochlorous acid on cardiac function and some biochemical parameters. Am. Heart J. **119**: 538–550.

10. GRAHAM, D. G., S. M. TIFFANY, W. R. BELL & W. F. GUTKNECHT. 1978. Autooxidation versus covalent binding of the quinones as the mechanism of toxicity of dopamine, 6-hydroxydopamine and related compounds toward C1300 neuroblastoma cells *in vitro*. Mol. Pharmacol. **14**: 644–653.

11. EGAN, R. W., J. PAXTON & F. A. KHUEHL. 1976. Mechanism of irreversible self deactivation of prostaglandin synthatase. J. Biol. Chem. **251**: 7329–7335.

12. CHAMBERS, D. E., D. A. PARKS, G. PATTERSON, R. ROY, J. M. MCCORD, S. YOSHIDA, L. F. PALMLEY & J. M. DOWNEY. 1985. Xanthine oxidase as a source of free radical damage in myocardial ischemia. J. Mol. Cell. Cardiol. **17**: 145–152.

13. FREEMAN, B. A. & J. D. CRAPO. 1982. Biology of disease. Free radicals and tissue injury. Lab. Invest. **47**: 412–426.

14. MEERSON, F. Z., V. E. KAGON & Y. P. KOZLOV. 1982. The role of lipid peroxidation in the pathogenesis of ischemic damage and antioxidant protection of the heart. Basic Res. Cardiol. **77:** 465–485.
15. PRASAD, K., P. LEE, S. V. MANTHA, J. KALRA, M. PRASAD & J. B. GUPTA. 1992. Detection of ischemia reperfusion cardiac injury by cardiac muscle chemiluminescence. Mol. Cell. Biochem. **115:** 49–58.
16. KAPOOR, R. & K. PRASAD. 1994. Role of oxyradicals in cardiovascular depression and cellular injury in hemorrhagic shock and reinfusion: effect of SOD and catalase. Circ. Shock **43:** 79–94.
17. KRAMER, J. H., I. T. MAX & W. B. WEGLICKI. 1984. Differential sensitivity of the canine cardiac sarcolemma and microsomal enzymes to inhibition by free radical induced lipid peroxidation. Circ. Res. **55:** 120–124.

Myocardial Preservation, Redox Potential Maintenance and Oxidant Injury by Heparin-Coated Carmeda Circuit

PARINAM S. RAO, ROBERT S. PALAZZO,
GREG L. HARLOW, KARL A. BOCCHIERI,
HELENE N. METZ, DAVID W. WILSON,
SRINIVASA K. RAO, AND L. MICHAEL GRAVER

Department of Surgery
Long Island Jewish Medical Center
Long Island Campus of Albert Einstein College of Medicine
New Hyde Park, New York 11042

INTRODUCTION

Carmeda circuit, heparin-coated tubing, improves biocompatibility from blood coagulation and complement activation on CPB.[1] This in turn protects myocardium against oxyradical tissue damage. A study was undertaken to elucidate the mechanism of action of heparin-coated carmeda circuit on oxidants, oxyradicals, redox potential, endothelial, complement, platelet and coagulation cascades in bringing the positive effects of myocardial preservation during CPB.

METHODS

We studied two groups of patients undergoing elective CABG: heparin-coated (H) CPB circuit, n = 20, (Carmeda Bioactive Surface, CBAS) and control (C), n = 20, on standard EC, both with systemic heparinization. We measured apparent redox potentials (E_m) of serum using micro redox electrode Pt/AgCl (MI-800, ME Inc.) and kinetic redox potential (E_0^1) by titrating serum with redox agents of known E_0^1 using a method developed by us. EDRF/NO, PMN elastase, C_3a des arg, GSH and ascorbate were measured by appropriate methods.[2] Serial CK, CK-MB were measured and cumulative CK-MB release (CK-R) and infarct size (IS-g-Eq) were calculated.[3] Data were normalized where necessary.

RESULTS

The data are presented in TABLE 1 and FIGURE 1 (E_m, E_0^1). The data presented here show that carmeda circuit regulates and maintains redox shift in E_m. Measurements of NO showed that it is restored by 72%. The positive effects are also mediated via the protection of GSH, as the concentration of GSH was found to be 78%. This probably resulted in a reduction in the loss of hemoglobin (Hb) by

TABLE 1. Data Obtained from Measurements of Apparent (E_m) and Kinetic (E_0^1) Redox Potential and Other Biochemical Parameters with Carmeda (H) and Controls (C)

	E_m (mV)		E_m^{01} (mV)		NO (μM)		Hb (mg/dL)		C_3a (μg/ml)	
	H	C	H	C	H	C	H	C	H	C
Pre-CPB	−48	−46	2.0	25	.29	.28	13	12	0.9	0.6
CPB	−40*	−22	2.2*	46	.19*	.06	13*	20	1.9	4.4
Post-CPB	−50*	−37	1.5*	32	.21*	.05	13.*	47	3.6*	5.8

* $p < 0.001$.

95%. The reduction in the loss of Hb is much more than the protection given by aprotinin. In addition, it activates C_3a complement by 52%. The CK-MB release (CK-R) is significantly lower in carmeda circuit as compared to controls. The levels dropped to 5.2 from 6.7 IU at 30 min, and to 27.7 from 38.4 IU at 12.5 hours. In addition infarct size (IS-g-Eq) was lower in carmeda circuit (6.6) as compared to controls (9.1).

CONCLUSIONS

The data presented here show that carmeda circuit, heparin-coated tubing, significantly protects against oxidant formation and preserves myocardium as measured by redox potential and endothelial cell damage and as seen by the data on complement, EDRF/NO, reduction in cell damage and blood loss during CPB. Heparin-coated carmeda circuit regulates and maintains redox potential of the plasma. This protection can be monitored by measuring redox potential.

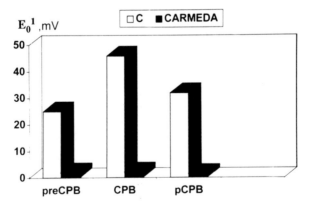

FIGURE 1. Kinetic redox potential of pre-CPB, CPB, and post-CPB (pCPB) of carmeda circuit (Carmeda) are shown in comparison with the controls (C). $p < 0.001$, C vs carmeda: CPB, post-CPB.

REFERENCES

1. BOROWIEC, J. *et al.* 1992. Heparin coated cardiopulmonary bypass circuits: a clinical study. Upsala J. Med. Sci. **97:** 55–66.
2. ZANNIONI, V., M. LYNCH, S. GOLDSTEIN & P. SATO. 1974. A rapid micro method for determination of ascorbic acid in plasma and tissues. Biochem. Med. **11:** 41–44.
3. RAO, P. S., G. S. WEINSTEIN, N. RUJIKARA, J. M. LUBER & D. H. TYRAS. 1990. An HPLC method for *in vivo* quantitation of oxygen free radicals using spin and chemical traps. Chromatographia **30:** 19–23.

Aprotinin Protects against Myocardial and Oxidant Formation and Endothelial Cell Damage during Open Heart Surgery

PARINAM S. RAO, ROBERT S. PALAZZO,
KARL A. BOCCHIERI, GREG L. HARLOW,
HELENE N. METZ, DAVID W. WILSON,
SRINIVASA K. RAO, AND L. MICHAEL GRAVER

Department of Surgery
Long Island Jewish Medical Center
Long Island Campus of Albert Einstein College of Medicine
New Hyde Park, New York 11042

INTRODUCTION

Aprotinin, a specific serine protease and kallikrein-plasmin inhibitor,[1] significantly reduce blood loss during CPB. We present results from data obtained from the experiments designed to elucidate aprotinin's mechanism of action on oxyradicals as studied by redox potential, endothelial, complement, platelet, coagulation cascades and myocardial preservation.

METHODS

We studied 30 patients undergoing elective CABG and divided them into two groups: AP (aprotonin) N (Normal) (n = 10) and C (control) (n = 20). We measured apparent redox potentials (E_m) of serum using micro redox electrode Pt/AgCl (MI-800, ME Inc.) and kinetic redox potential (E_0^1) by titrating serum with redox agents of known E_0^1 by a method developed by us. EDRF/NO, PMN elastase, TXB_2, 6 Keto $PGF_{1\alpha}$, C_3a des arg, GSH and ascorbate were measured by appropriate methods.[2] Serial CK, CK-MB were measured and cumulative CK-MB release (CK-R) and infarct size (IS-g-Eq) were calculated.[3] Data were normalized where necessary.

RESULTS

The data are presented in TABLE 1 and FIGURE 1 (E_m, E_0^1). The data presented here show that aprotinin regulates and maintains redox shift in E_m. Measurements of NO showed that it is restored by 77%. The positive effects are also mediated via the protection of GSH as the concentration of GSH was found to be 78%.

TABLE 1. Data Obtained from Measurements of Apparent (E_m) and Kinetic (E_0^1) Redox Potential and Other Biochemical Parameters with Aprotinin (AP) and Controls (C)

	E_m (mV)		E_m^{01} (mV)		NO (μM)		Hb (mg/μl)		C_3a (μg/ml)	
	AP	C	AP	C	AP	C	AP	C	AP	C
Pre-CPB	−48	−46	+19	+25	0.29	0.28	12.4	12.2	0.8	0.6
CPB	−42*	22	+20*	+46	0.18*	0.06	16.6	20.1	4.2	4.4
Post-CPB	−50*	−37	+15*	+32	0.20*	0.05	28.5*	46.7	4.8*	5.8

* $p < 0.001$.

This probably resulted in a reduction in the loss of hemoglobin by 39%. The CK-MB release (CK-R) is significantly lower in aprotinin-treated patients as compared to controls. The levels dropped to 5 from 6.8 IU at 30 min, and to 26.6 from 37.6 IU at 12.5 hours. In addition, infarct size (IS.-gm-Eq) was lower in aprotinin-treated (6.3) as compared to controls (8.9).

CONCLUSIONS

The data presented here lend support to conclude that aprotinin protects against oxidant formation and endothelial cell damage during CPB and preserves myocardium. Aprotinin regulates and maintains redox potential of the plasma. This protection can be monitored by measuring redox potential.

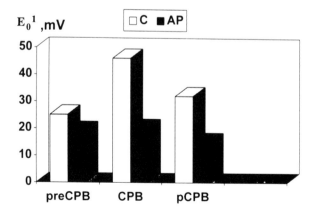

FIGURE 1. Kinetic redox potential of pre-CPB, CPB and post-CPB (pCPB) of aprotinin (AP)-treated and controls (C) are shown. $p < 0.001$, C vs aprotinin: CPB, post-CPB.

REFERENCES

1. ALVEREZ, J. *et al.* 1995. The use of ultra low dose aprotinin to reduce blood loss in cardiac surgery. J. Cardiotho. Vascu. Anasthe. **9**(1): 29–33.
2. ZANNIONI, V., M. LYNCH, S. GOLDSTEIN & P. SATO. 1974. A rapid micro method for determination of ascorbic acid in plasma and tissues. Biochem. Med. **11**: 41–44.
3. RAO, P. S., G. S. WEINSTEIN, N. RUJIKARA, J. M. LUBER & D. H. TYRAS. 1990. An HPLC method for *in vivo* quantitation of oxygen free radicals using spin and chemical traps. Chromatographia **30**: 19–23.

Responses to Acute Myocardial Stress and Prior Drug Therapy on Plasma Levels of Antioxidants and Oxidants and the Proposed Role of Interventions on Molecular Adaptations

RAM B. SINGH,[a] MOHAMMAD A. NIAZ,
SHANTI S. RASTOGI, AND M. ASLAM

Centre of Nutrition and Heart Research Laboratory
Medical Hospital and Reserch Centre
Moradabad, India

INTRODUCTION

Experimental studies by Murry, Reimer and Jennings in 1986 reported that brief periods of transient ischemia can protect the myocardium against subsequent ischemia injury.[1] The mechanism by which such myocardium becomes resistant to ischemia is commonly called preconditioning. This endogenous myocardial protection as described by Downey, may include adenosine receptors having a relatively rapid but short-term effect and a second, slower and more prolonged mechanism involving the synthesis of stress proteins, which enhance the resistance to infarction.[1] However, these changes may be associated with depressed myocardial contractility or stunning and reperfusion arrhythmias with underlying mechanisms of free radical-induced injury and disturbed calcium homeostasis.[1] It is possible that oxidant stress-mediated changes may alter thiol-regulated enzymes, which could lead to their very rapid activation or deactivation. Das and co-workers[2] in 1994 found that intracellular responses due to acute myocardial stress as induction of catalase gene represent myocardial adaptation against stress that is associated with preservation of cells.

In several recent studies,[3-5] lower levels of the antioxidant vitamins A, E and C and carotene, pyridoxine, selenium, zinc, magnesium, potassium and l-carnitine and higher concentrations of copper and iron were described in patients with acute myocardial stress. In victims dying sudden cardiac death, low levels of myocardial magnesium, potassium, menganese, copper and iron and higher concentrations of calcium have been described in the myocardial tissue.[4,6] The exact clinical significance of these responses in the serum or tissue concentrations of antioxidants and oxidants are not known.[4] However, it is possible that these changes in the serum and myocardial tissue concentrations of antioxidants and oxidants can influence molecular adaptation and endogenous myocardial protection. There is evidence that prior drug therapy or treatment of suspected acute myocardial infarction (AMI) with beta blockers and ACE inhibitors can provide protection

[a] Correspondence: Dr. R. B. Singh, MD, Director, Heart Research Laboratory, MHRC, Civil Lines, Moradabad-10, UP, 244001, India. Tel.: (91) 591-317437.

517

against complications and mortality,[7,8] which might influence the myocardial and circulating antioxidant and oxidant levels and calcium homeostasis in these patients. In the present paper, we report the antioxidant vitamin and mineral status in patients with AMI in relation to prior drug therapy.

MATERIALS AND METHODS

Inclusion and exclusion criteria of patients and methods in this study[4] have been reported elsewhere. In brief, of 505 patients admitted in the Medical Hospital, Moradabad with suspicions of AMI within the past 24 hours of the symptoms, those were excluded because of blood urea >40 mg/dl (n = 6), cancer (n = 5), diarrhea or dysentary (n = 14) and death (n = 20). Other patients with acute myocardial stress included proved AMI and possible AMI diagnosed by electrocardiogram and raised cardiac enzymes (n = 387), and unstable angina (n = 19) in this study as reported elsewhere.[16] There were 42 subjects out of 505 subjects who showed no evidence of coronary disease. None of the patients was taking any vitamin or mineral supplement related to our study. History of drug intake was obtained by examination of available record of treatment and drug samples. The duration of drug therapy varied between 3 months to 5 years.

Laboratory data were obtained at entry to the study in all patients. A venous blood sample was obtained immediately after the diagnosis of suspected AMI at admission and analyzed for blood counts, hemoglobin, urea, glucose, cardiac enzyme activity, copper, zinc, iron and vitamin C, lipid peroxides, magnesium, calcium and potassium in all the subjects.[4] Vitamin C was measured within one hour of collection of blood sample.

One-way analysis of variance was used for data analysis. Only p values <0.05 and two-tailed t test were considered statistically significant. Z score test for proportions was used for the comparison of groups.

RESULTS

Of a total of 406 patients, 52 were taking proprandol, 48 captopril, 66 verapamil or nifedipine, and remaining 240 patients were not taking any of these drugs. Previous AMI and angina pectoris were more common in the propranolol group, and known hypertension was more common in the captopril and verapamil groups than in the no drug group. The captopril group also had more patients with previous AMI. Current smokers and exsmokers were also more common in the groups of patients receiving drugs compared to the no drug group. Mean maximum pulse rates were also significantly lower in the drug intake groups than in the no drug group. However, mean peak creatine kinase, left ventricular failure and ventricular ectopics were significantly lower in the propranolol and captopril group compared to the no drug group. The group receiving calcium blockers did not reveal these benefits. The study groups with acute myocardial stress included patients with AMI and possible AMI (387, 95.3%) and unstable angina (group C 19, 4.6%) which were comparable among different drug intake groups and the no drug group. Those subjects with noncardiac chest pain (n = 42) were taken as control. Serum levels of minerals were comparable in the unstable angina and control groups. However, plasma concentrations of vitamin C were significantly lower in unstable angina and lipid peroxides higher compared to the control group. In AMI and possible

TABLE 1. Mineral and Vitamin Levels in Patients with Acute Myocardial Stress and Controls in Relation to Drug Therapy with and without Adjustment for Smoking, Diabetes and Female Sex[a]

	Controls (n = 42)	Propranolol (n = 52)	Captopril (n = 48) (Mean (SD))	Verapamil (n = 66)	No Drug (n = 240)
Serum copper (μg/dl)					
Unadjusted	105(9.8)**	148.4(14.2)*	152.4(13.6)*	162.6(18.0)	170.2(20.6)
Adjusted	108(9.0)**	140.2(10.5)**	155.2(12.0)*	166.0(15.2)	180.4(17.5)
Serum zinc (μg/dl)					
Unadjusted	107(9.8)**	100.2(6.4)*	97.5(7.5)*	85.5(10.2)*	65.6(8.8)
Adjusted	112(11.2)**	110.5(7.8)**	102.2(9.2)*	87.4(11.4)*	70.2(11.4)
Serum iron (μg/dl)					
Unadjusted	122(12.5)**	158.5(20.0)*	166.4(18.2)*	185.4(22.4)	192.6(24.0)
Adjusted	116(11.5)**	152.4(16.1)*	155.4(16.4)*	172.3(20.0)	185.4(21.6)
Vitamin C (μmol/L)					
Unadjusted	24.6(4.3)**	16.8(2.1)**	19.4(3.6)**	9.87(1.7)*	5.44(0.68)
Adjusted	20.0(3.6)**	18.2(2.0)*	22.5(3.8)*	11.6(1.8)	8.3(0.71)
Magnesium (mEq/L)					
Unadjusted	1.72(0.16)*	1.71(0.13)*	1.68(0.16)*	1.68(0.13)*	1.61(0.15)
Adjusted	1.71(0.15)*	1.72(0.13)*	1.69(0.15)*	1.67(0.12)*	1.60(0.15)
Potassium (mEq/L)					
Unadjusted	4.6(0.35)*	4.4(0.42)*	4.7(0.43)*	4.22(0.35)	4.11(0.36)
Adjusted	4.5(0.37)*	4.5(0.43)*	4.7(0.42)*	4.23(0.36)	4.10(0.35)
Calcium (mg/dl)					
Unadjusted	9.2(0.41)*	9.0(0.46)*	9.3(0.45)	9.3(0.51)	9.6(0.53)
Adjusted	9.1(0.42)*	9.0(0.43)*	9.1(0.42)*	9.3(0.50)	9.6(0.52)
Lipid peroxides (pmol/L)					
Unadjusted	1.2(0.21)**	2.46(0.52)*	2.62(0.64)*	3.31(0.70)	3.34(0.82)
Adjusted	1.1(0.11)**	2.41(0.51)*	2.51(0.62)*	3.21(0.68)	3.26(0.76)

[a] p value obtained by comparison of drug intake groups with the no drug group and the no drug group with controls. *$p < 0.05$; **$p < 0.01$.

AMI groups, the changes were more marked; however, in those who received propranolol and captopril, the changes were less marked. Serum levels of copper, iron, lipid peroxides and calcium were significantly higher and serum zinc, vitamin C, magnesium and potassium levels significantly lower in patients with AMI in the no drug group compared to control subjects. (TABLE 1). Prior treatment with propranolol and captopril was associated with only modest increase in copper, iron and lipid peroxides, no increase in calcium and only modest reductions in zinc, vitamin C, magnesium and potassium compared to these changes in the no drug group.

DISCUSSION

This study has demonstrated that the propranolol and captopril groups of patients had only modest increases in serum concentrations of copper, iron, calcium and lipid peroxides and modest reductions in serum concentrations of zinc, magnesium, potassium and vitamin C, which are known to provide beneficial cytoprotective effect in patients with AMI. Copper and iron are oxidants and lipid peroxides are indicators of free radical damage. While propranolol acts by decreasing the release of catecholamines from the adrenals, captopril has a direct antioxidant effect, and it may also prevent the loss of magnesium and potassium from the cells. Inhibition of angiotensin converting enzyme may also cause preservation of antioxidant vitamins and minerals in the circulation. Prior treatment with propranolol and captopril was associated with a lower maximum pulse rate in the first 24 hours, lower mean peak creatine kinase activity and lower incidence of ventricular ectopics compared to the no drug group. The incidence of left ventricular failure was higher in the propranolol group and lower in the captopril group compared to the no drug group.

An increase in iron in association with acute myocardial stress may initiate the induction of the catalase gene, whereas increase in copper migh initiate the superoxide dismutase gene, which may be useful in cell preservation and endogenous myocardial protection. Attenuation of responses in the form of less increase in serum copper and iron in patients with propranolol and captopril therapy in association with lower lipid peroxides indicate that prior treatment with these drugs provides benefit by decreasing the free radical stress and myocardial calcium homeostasis and by increasing cellular levels of vitamin C, zinc, magnesium and potassium, which were less lowered in the propranolol- and captopril-treated patients. It seems that these responses in serum levels of antioxidants are indicators of cell responses which may be associated with enhanced synthesis of stress proteins, & G-protein and gene expression responsible for myocardial protection.[8-10] Intervention trials with these drugs[9] and animal experiments would be necessary to provide further evidence as to whether these drugs can enhance preconditioning or myocardial adaptation.

REFERENCES

1. GAVIN, J. B. & L. MAXWELL. 1995. Advances in myocardial protection: concepts and context. Heart Beat **2:** 3–4.
2. DAS, D. K. 1994. Gene expression in myocardial stress. (Abstract). International Satellite Symposium on Free Radicals in Biology, Chandigarh (India), Sept. 15–17.
3. SINGH, R. B., M. A. NIAZ, J. P. SHARMA, S. S. RASTOGI, S. GHOSH, S. AHMAD, R. KUMAR & M. RAIZADA. 1994. Plasma levels of antioxidant vitamins and oxidative stress in patients with acute myocardial infarction. Acta Cardiol. **49:** 441–452.
4. SINGH, R. B., M. A. NIAZ, S. AHMAD, S. S. RASTOGI, U. SINGH & P. AGARWAL. 1995. Dietary and serum levels of antioxidant minerals in patients with acute myocardial infarction. Trace Elem. Electro. **12:** 148–152.
5. GUPTA, R. 1981. Serum copper in acute myocardial infarction. J. Assoc. Phys. India **29:** 987–990.
6. SPEICH, M., B. BONSQUET & G. NICOLAS. 1980. Concentrations of magnesium, calcium, potassium and sodium in human heart muscle after acute myocardial infarction. Clin. Chem. **26:** 1662–1665.
7. COHEN, L., A. LAOR & R. KITZES. 1984. Serum magnesium in propranolol treated patients with acute myocardial infarction. Magnesium **3:** 138–144.
8. SAVE Investigators. 1992. Effect of captopril on mortality and morbidity in patients with left ventricular dysfunction after myocardial infarction. N. Engl. J. Med. **327:** 669–677.
9. Fourth International Study of Infarct Survival Collaborative Group. 1995. A randomised factorial trial assessing early oral captopril, oral mononitrate, and intravenous magnesium sulphate in 58,050 patients with suspected acute myocardial infarction. Lancet **345:** 669–685.
10. THRONTON, J. C., G. S. LIN & J. M. DOWNEY. 1993. Pretreatment with pertussis toxin blocks protective effects of preconditioning: evidence of a G-protein mechanism. J. Mol. Cell. Cardiol. **25:** 311–320.

Aprotinin Effects Related to Oxidative Stress in Cardiosurgery with Mechanical Cardiorespiratory Support (CMCS)

V. F. BROCHE,[a,c] A. ROMERO SUÀREZ,[b] E. OLEMBE,[a]
G. E. FERNÀNDEZ,[b] E. M. CÉSPEDES,[a] J. C. GARCIA,[a]
E. REYNOSO,[b] P. NÙÑEZ,[b] AND E. PRIETO[a]

[a]Biomedical Research Center "Victoria de Giròn"
Havana, Cuba

[b]Hospital Pediàtrico-Docente "William Soler"
Cardiocentro
Havana City, Cuba

INTRODUCTION

Oxygen reactive species (ORS) are generated during ischemia-reperfusion damage (IRD)[1] due to endogenous mechanisms such as mitochondrial respiratory chain dysfunction and xanthine oxidase (XO) activity.[2]

XO may be converted from its dehydrogenase form (XD) at least by partial proteolitic cleavage.[1,3,4]

During cardiosurgery with mechanical cardiorespiratory support (CMCS) damaged myocardial and systemic tissues release a large amount of proteases whose deleterious effects are recognized upon cells and extracellular matrix.[5]

Physical blood trauma during CMCS leads to leukocyte and arachidonic acid pathway activation; both are sources of ORS, which include protease-mediated steps.[1,6]

A synergism has been suggested among oxidants, phospholipases, proteases and a variety of other agonists derived from activated leukocytes in the pathophysiology of IRD.[6]

Aprotinin, a polivalent protease inhibitor, has been applied lately, achieving an improvement in hemostasis and a better recovery of physiological functions.[5]

In virtue of the accepted relationship between oxidative stress and protease activation,[7] we wondered if aprotinin may exert its protective effects by means of oxidative stress reduction under ischemia-reperfusion conditions.

MATERIALS AND METHODS

A double blind clinical trial was performed with child patients (1–6 years) divided randomly into Group 1 (G-1, nontreated, n = 11) and Group 2 (G-2,

[c] Address for correspondence: Biomedical Research Center "Victoria de Giròn," Divisiòn: Estrés Oxidativo, Calle 146 y Ave. 31, Cubanacàn, Playa, Habana 16, Cuba 11600. Fax: (537) 336257; E-mail: jcarlos@giròn.sld.cu.

treated, n = 8) both submitted to CMCS. Bypass circuit was supplied by DIDECO. A Lactate-Ringer + whole blood cardioplegia was used. Aprotinin was supplied by Bayer (10 000 KIU/ml vials) and perfused before skin opening (30 000 KIU/kg), 30 000 KIU/kg at system feed and 10 000 KIU/kg/hour until the operation was finished.

Blood samples were taken at: T-0: anesthesia induction, T-1: 5 minutes after aortic clamping, T-2: 10 minutes after reperfusion, T-3 and T-4: 24 and 72 hours after the operation. Biochemical indicators include: malonildialdehyde (MDA) (nmoles/ml),[8] phospholipase A_2 (PLA$_2$) activity (U/ml),[9] uric acid (μmoles/1)[10] and activity of catalase (CAT) (KU/1).[11] Low cardiac output and arrythmias were registered, too. An analysis of variance (two way ANOVA) was applied.

RESULTS AND DISCUSSION

MDA levels were significantly lower in G-1 than in G-1 at T-2, T-3 and T-4 as FIGURE 1 shows. PLA$_2$ exhibited a tendency to lower activity in G-2 than in G-1 at T-2, T-3 and T-4, too, without remarkable statistical difference. Uric acid values were significantly higher in G-2 than in G-1 as is shown in FIGURE 2. It showed maximum values after aortic clamping. CAT activity was higher in G-2 than in G-1 at T-2. There was a higher incidence of low cardiac output in G-1 (30%) than in G-2 (10%) during the postoperative period. Incidence of arrythmias was greater in G-1 (60%) than in G-2 (30%).

Overproduction of oxidant species as well as primary reduction of antioxidant reserve generate oxidative stress[2] in child patients who suffer from chronic cardiopathy. During CMCS, neutrophils are activated by mechanical trauma involving an active role of intercellular signaling mediators.[13,14] Free hemoglobin released after erythrocyte disruption can generate ORS by iron catalyzed reactions. Nitric oxide (NO), which plays a role in the regulation of tissular perfusion, can be

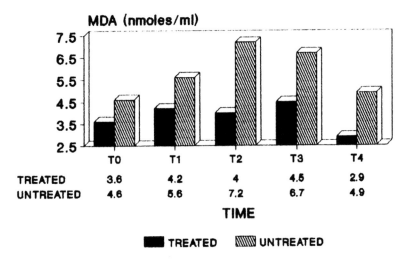

FIGURE 1. MDA levels in treated and untreated groups submitted to CMCS.

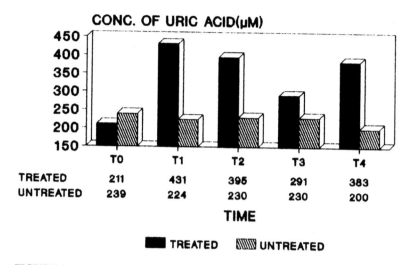

FIGURE 2. Uric acid levels in treated and untreated groups submitted to CMCS.

consumed through Fe^{III} + NO and Fe^{II} + NO cyclic reactions as well as by peroxynitrite formation.[15] MAD levels reflect a systemic oxidative stress and aprotinin may inhibit leukocyte activation and proteolitic conversion of XD to XO. Therefore, the behavior of MDA in G-2 could be explained by this indirect antioxidant effect of the drug.

Extracellular PLA_2 isoform may be inhibited by a reduced formation of lipid peroxides and aprotinin-mediated blockade of kallicrein-quinins cascade. The drug can interact, modulating some of the proteolitic reactions linked to Ca^+ homeostasis, whose intracellular overload can induce PLA_2 activation, too.[18-21]

During ischemia-reperfusion events there is an increase in XO-catalyzed uric acid synthesis, whose direct antioxidant effects are currently well documented. Lower levels of uric acid in G-1 than in G-2 may be due to its consumption by scavenging ORS. Oxidative breakdown of uric acid in humans has been suggested as a defensive mechanism under extreme oxidative stress.[22]

Oxidative inactivation of CAT may be supposed in G-1. Then, in the presence of a large amount of ORS there may be an accelerated consumption of reduced nicotinamide-adenine dinucleotide phosphate (NADPH) by glutathione reductase to supply reduced glutathione to glutathione peroxidase, which reduces its availability for CAT even when the NADPH role for CAT activity is still unclear.

The higher incidence of postoperative low cardiac output and arrythmias in G-1 than in G-2 may be sustained based on the behavior of biochemical indicators of oxidative stress in virtue of its recognized role in myocardial IRD.[1]

Our results suggest that the protective effects of aprotinin are associated with an antioxidant effect. The convenience of using aprotinin to improve preservation of cellular viability in clinical conditions where oxidative stress appears included in its pathophysiology should be taken into consideration.

We consider that the role of endogenous protease inhibitors should be included in basic and clinical research related to cellular adaptation to a broad spectrum of stress conditions.

SUMMARY

There is evidence to support a relationship between oxidative stress and protease release in "ischemia-reperfusion damage." We have proposed that aprotinin may exert an antioxidant effect. A double blind clinical trial was performed with a control (G-1) and treated (G-2) groups, both submitted to CMCS. Blood samples were taken 5 times. Biochemical indicators were measured spectrophotometrically. Aprotinin was supplied by Bayer. Malonildialdehyde levels were greater in G-1 (7.2 ± 3.6 nmoles/ml) than in G-2 (4 ± 1.65) at the time of reperfusion. Phospholipase A_2 exhibited a tendency of higher activity in G-1 than in G-2. Uric acid levels were higher in G-2 (431 ± 274 μmoles/1) than in G-1 (224 ± 188) at 5 minutes after aortic clamping, and catalase activity was greater in G-2 (294 ± 55 KU/1) than in G-1 (118 ± 47) at time of reperfusion. Low cardiac output was 10% in G-2 and 30% in G-1. Arrythmias appeared in 30% of G-2 and in 60% of G-1. These results suggest an antioxidant effect of aprotinin under ischemia-reperfusion conditions.

REFERENCES

1. SIES, H., Ed. 1991. Oxidative Stress: Oxidants and Antioxidants. 2nd edit. Academic Press Inc. San Diego.
2. MARKS, J. 1989. Clinical implications of free radicals. Nanngstorskning **4**: 130–137.
3. FREDERIKS, W. M. & K. S. BOSCH. 1995. Histol. Histopathol. **10**: 111–116.
4. TAN, S., S. GELMAN, J. K. WHEAT & D. A. PARKS. 1995. South. Med. J. **88**: 479–482.
5. SUNAMORI, M., R. INNAMI, J. AMANO, A. SUZUKI & C. E. HARRISON. 1988. J. Thorac. Cardiovasc. Surg. **96**: 314–320.
6. GINSBURG, I., R. MISGAV, A. PINSON, J. VARANI, P. A. WARD & R. KOHEN. 1992. Inflammation **16**(5): 519–538.
7. CARR, F. K. & R. D. GOLDFARB. 1980. Exp. Mol. Pathol. **33**: 36–42.
8. ROCHE, E. & D. ROMERO. 1994. Estrés oxidativo y degradación de proteinas. Med. Clin. (Barc.) **103**: 189–196.
9. OHKAWA, H. 1991. Acta Med. Okayama **44**(2): 103–111.
10. HOTTER, G., O. S. LEÓN, J. ROSELLÓ, M. A. LÓPEZ, P. PUIG, R. HENRIQUEZ, L. FERNÁNDEZ & E. GELPI. 1991. Transplantation **51**(5): 987–990.
11. BARHAM, D. & P. TRINDER. 1972. Analyst **97**: 142–145.
12. GOTH, L. 1991. Clin. Chim. Acta **196**: 143–152.
13. KLEIN, C. L., H. KOHLER, F. BITTINGER, M. OTTO, I. HERMANNS & C. J. KIRKPATRICK. 1995. Pathobiology **63**: 1–8.
14. BUJA, M. & R. J. BICK. 1994. Promega Notes **47**: 6–9.
15. KUBES, P., M. SUZUKI & D. N. GRANGER. 1991. Proc. Natl. Acad. Sci. USA **88**: 4651–4655.
16. ALAYASH, A. I. & R. E. CASHOW. 1995. Mol. Med. Today **4**(3): 122–127.
17. SANFEY, H., M. G. SARR, G. B. BULKLEY & J. L. CAMERON. 1986. Acta Physiol. Scand. **548**: 109–118.
18. VAN DER VUS, G. J., M. VAN BLISEN, T. SONDERKAMP & R. S. RENEMAN. 1990. Hydrolysis of phospholipids and cellular integrity. In Pathophysiology of Severe Ischemic Myocardial Injury. H. M. Piper, Ed. 239–267. Kluwer Academic Publishers. Dordrecht.
19. ENGLEBERGER, W., K. BITTER-SUERMAN & U. HADDING. 1987. Int. J. Immunopharmacol. **9**: 275–282.
20. NAGAOKA, H. & M. KATORI. 1975. Circulation **52**: 325–332.
21. ELLIOT, S. J. & T. N. DOAN. 1993. Biochem. J. **292**(Pt. 2): 385–393.
22. BECKER, B. 1993. Free Radical Biol. Med. **14**: 615–631.

Subject Index

Index of Contributors